MIS Techniques in Orthopedics

MIS Techniques in Orthopedics

Giles R. Scuderi, MD

Attending Orthopedic Surgeon, Department of Orthopedic Surgery, Lenox Hill Hospital, New York; Assistant Clinical Professor of Orthopedics, Albert Einstein College of Medicine, Bronx, New York; Director, Insall Scott Kelly Orthopedics and Sports Medicine, New York

Alfred J. Tria, Jr., MD

Clinical Professor of Orthopedic Surgery, St. Peter's University Hospital, Robert Wood Johnson Medical School, New Brunswick, New Jersey; Institute for Advanced Orthopedic Study, Orthopedic Center of New Jersey, Somerset, New Jersey

Richard A. Berger, MD

Assistant Professor, Special Projects Coordinator, Residency Program, Department of Orthopedic Surgery, Rush-Presbyterian-St. Luke's Medical Center, Chicago, Illinois

Editors

With 315 Illustrations

Springer

Giles R. Scuderi, MD
Attending Orthopedic Surgeon
Department of Orthopedic Surgery
Lenox Hill Hospital
New York, NY
and
Assistant Clinical Professor of Orthopedics
Albert Einstein College of Medicine
Bronx, NY
and
Director
Insall Scott Kelly Orthopedics and Sports Medicine
New York, NY 10128
USA

Alfred J. Tria, Jr., MD
Clinical Professor of Orthopedic Surgery
St. Peter's University Hospital
Robert Wood Johnson Medical School
New Brunswick, NJ
and
Institute for Advanced Orthopedic Study
Orthopedic Center of New Jersey
Somerset, NJ 08873
USA

Richard A. Berger, MD
Assistant Professor
Special Projects Coordinator
Residency Program
Department of Orthopedic Surgery
Rush-Presbyterian-St. Luke's Medical Center
Chicago, IL 60612
USA

Library of Congress Control Number 2005923812

ISBN 10: 0-387-24210-4 Printed on acid-free paper.
ISBN 13: 978-0387-24210-1

Printed in the United States of America. (BS/MVY)

9 8 7 6 5 4 3 2 1 SPIN 10962633

springeronline.com

This book is dedicated to our families,
who allow us to pursue our dreams and careers,
and to our colleagues, with whom we wish to share our ideas.

Preface

Minimally invasive surgery (MIS) is changing the way orthopedic surgery is practiced and is now considered state-of-the-art. There are rapid advances in the surgical techniques with the introduction of navigation and robotics, which assist the surgeon in performing the procedure with limited visualization. This edition of *MIS Techniques in Orthopedics* elaborates on current techniques for the hip and knee, and also introduces the most recent sections on the upper extremity and computer navigation. The contributing authors are experts in the field and share with the reader their experiences and surgical pearls. Keeping pace with new techniques and technologies in orthopedic surgery can be very demanding; our hope is that surgeons will find this text a useful reference as they embark upon minimally invasive surgery.

Giles R. Scuderi, MD
Alfred J. Tria, Jr., MD
Richard A. Berger, MD

Contents

Preface vii
Contributors xiii

Section I The Shoulder and Elbow

Chapter 1 Mini-Incision Bankart Repair for Shoulder Instability 3
Edward W. Lee and Evan L. Flatow

Chapter 2 Mini-Open Rotator Cuff Repair 21
Jason A. Schneider and Frances Cuomo

Chapter 3 Mini-Incision Fixation of Proximal Humeral Four-Part Fractures 32
Jim Hsu and Leesa M. Galatz

Chapter 4 Minimally Invasive Approach for Shoulder Arthroplasty 45
Theodore Blaine, Ilya Voloshin, Kevin Setter, and Louis U. Bigliani

Chapter 5 Mini-Incision Medial Collateral Ligament Reconstruction of the Elbow 71
Steven J. Thornton, Andrew Willis, and David W. Altchek

Chapter 6 Mini-Incision Distal Biceps Tendon Repair 90
Jason A. Schneider and Peter D. McCann

Section II The Hip

Chapter 7 A Technique for the Anterolateral Approach to MIS Total Hip Replacement 103
Richard A. Berger

Chapter 8 The Anterior Approach for Total Hip Replacement: Background and Operative Technique 121
Joel M. Matta

Chapter 9 Posterolateral Minimal Incision for Total Hip Replacement: Technique and Early Results 141
Mark A. Hartzband

Chapter 10 Minimally Invasive Total Hip Arthroplasty Using the Two-Incision Approach 159
Richard A. Berger

Chapter 11 Minimally Invasive Metal-on-Metal Resurfacing Arthroplasty of the Hip 180
Hari P. Bezwada, Phillip S. Ragland, Craig M. Thomas, and Michael A. Mont

Section III The Knee: Unicondylar Knee Arthroplasty

Chapter 12 Minimally Invasive Surgery for Unicondylar Knee Arthroplasty: The Bone-Sparing Technique 193
John A. Repicci and Jodi F. Hartman

Chapter 13 Minimally Invasive Surgery for Unicondylar Knee Arthroplasty: The Intramedullary Technique 214
Richard A. Berger and Alfred J. Tria, Jr.

Chapter 14 Minimally Invasive Surgery for Unicondylar Knee Arthroplasty: The Extramedullary Tensor Technique 230
Paul L. Saenger

Chapter 15 Minimally Invasive Surgery for Unicondylar Knee Arthroplasty: The Extramedullary Technique 257
Giles R. Scuderi

Chapter 16 Minimally Invasive Surgery for Arthroplasty with the UniSpacer 270
Richard H. Hallock

Chapter 17 Minimally Invasive Technique for Insertion of a Unicompartmental Knee Arthroplasty 285
A.J. Price and D.W. Murray

Section IV The Knee: Total Knee Arthroplasty

Chapter 18 Minimal Incision Total Knee Arthroplasty with a Limited Medial Parapatellar Arthrotomy 303
Giles R. Scuderi

Chapter 19 Minimally Invasive Total Knee Replacement with the Quadriceps-Sparing Subvastus Approach . . . 315
Mark W. Pagnano and Giles R. Scuderi

Chapter 20 Mini-Midvastus Total Knee Arthroplasty 324
Steven B. Haas, Andrew P. Lehman, and Mary Ann Manitta

Chapter 21 Minimally Invasive Lateral Approach to Total Knee Arthroplasty 339
Hari P. Bezwada, Michael A. Mont, Peter M. Bonutti, Sandeep K. Chauhan, Phillip S. Ragland, Craig M. Thomas, and Mark Kester

Chapter 22 Minimally Invasive Total Knee Arthroplasty Using the Quadriceps-Sparing Approach 349
Alfred J. Tria, Jr.

Section V Computer Navigation

Chapter 23 Computer-Guided Total Hip Arthroplasty 367
James B. Stiehl

Chapter 24 Computer-Guided Total Knee Arthroscopy 390
Alon Wolf, Branislav Jaramaz, Andrew B. Mor, and Anthony DiGioia III

Index 409

Contributors

David W. Altchek, MD
Associate Professor of Surgery (Orthopedics) at the Weill Medical College of Cornell University; Associate Attending Orthopedic Surgeon, Sports Medicine and Shoulder Service, Hospital for Special Surgery, New York, NY 10021, USA

Richard A. Berger, MD
Assistant Professor, Special Projects Coordinator, Residency Program, Department of Orthopedic Surgery, Rush-Presbyterian-St. Luke's Medical Center, Chicago, IL 60612, USA

Hari P. Bezwada, MD
Fellow, Center for Joint Preservation and Reconstruction, Rubin Institute for Advanced Orthopedics, Sinai Hospital of Baltimore, Baltimore, MD 21215, USA

Louis U. Bigliani, MD
Frank E. Stinchfield Professor and Chairman, Department of Orthopedic Surgery, New York Presbyterian Hospital, Columbia University, New York, NY 10032, USA

Theodore Blaine, MD
Assistant Professor, Department of Orthopedic Surgery, New York Presbyterian Hospital, Columbia University, New York, NY 10032, USA

Peter M. Bonutti, MD
Associate Clinical Professor, Department of Orthopedic Surgery, University of Arkansas, Little Rock; Founder and CEO, Bonutti Clinic, Effington, IL 62401, USA

Sandeep K. Chauhan, MD
Consultant, Department of Orthopaedic Surgery, Sussex Nuffield Hospital, Woodingdean, Brighton, East Sussex, BN2 6DX, UK

Frances Cuomo, MD
Chief, Shoulder and Elbow Service, Beth Israel Medical Center, Insall Scott Kelly Institute for Orthopedics, New York, NY 10128, USA

Anthony DiGioia III, MD
Director, Institute for Computer Assisted Orthopedic Surgery, Western Pennsylvania Hospital, Pittsburgh, PA 15217, USA

Evan L. Flatow, MD
Lasker Professor of Orthopedic Surgery, Chief of Shoulder Surgery, Department of Orthopedic Surgery, Mount Sinai Medical Center, New York, NY 10029, USA

Leesa M. Galatz, MD
Assistant Professor, Shoulder and Elbow Service, Department of Orthopedic Surgery, Washington University School of Medicine/ Barnes-Jewish Hospital, St. Louis, MO 63110, USA

Steven B. Haas, MD, MPH
Associate Chief of the Knee Service, Department of Orthopedic Surgery, Hospital for Special Surgery, New York, NY 10021, USA

Richard H. Hallock, MD, CEO
Orthopedic Institute of Pennsylvania, Camp Hill, PA; Hallock/Fell Research, Hummelstown, PA; Clinical Assistant Professor, Department of Orthopedic Surgery, Penn State University, Camp Hill, PA 17011, USA

Jodi F. Hartman, MS
President, Orthopedic Research and Reporting, Ltd., Gahanna, OH 43230, USA

Mark A. Hartzband, MD
Director, Insall Scott Kelly Institute; Section Chief, Hip Surgery, Beth Israel Medical Center, New York, NY; Director, Total Joint Replacement Service, Department of Orthopedics, Hackensack University Medical Center, Hackensack, NJ; Hartzband Joint Replacement Institute, Paramus, NJ 07652, USA

Jim Hsu, MD
Chief Resident, Shoulder and Elbow Service, Department of Orthopedic Surgery, Washington University School of Medicine/ Barnes-Jewish Hospital, St. Louis, MO 63110, USA

Branislav Jaramaz, PhD
Associate Director and Scientific Director, Institute for Computer Assisted Orthopedic Surgery, Western Pennsylvania Hospital, Pittsburgh, PA 15217, USA

Mark Kester, PhD
Center for Joint Preservation and Reconstruction, Rubin Institute for Advanced Orthopedics, Sinai Hospital of Baltimore, Baltimore, MD 21215, USA

Edward W. Lee, MD
Clinical Shoulder Fellow, Department of Orthopedic Surgery, Mount Sinai Medical Center, New York, NY 10029, USA

Andrew P. Lehman, MD
Fellow, Department of Orthopedic Surgery, Hospital for Special Surgery, New York, NY 10021, USA

Peter D. McCann, MD
Attending Orthopedic Surgeon, Beth Israel Medical Center, Insall Scott Kelly Institute for Orthopedics and Sports Medicine, New York, NY 10128, USA

Mary Ann Manitta, RN
Research Nurse, Department of Orthopedic Surgery, Hospital for Special Surgery, New York, NY 10021, USA

Joel M. Matta, MD
Associate Clinical Professor, USC School of Medicine, Los Angeles, CA 90017, USA

Michael A. Mont, MD
Director, Center for Joint Preservation and Reconstruction, Rubin Institute for Advanced Orthopedics, Sinai Hospital of Baltimore, Baltimore, MD 21215, USA

Andrew B. Mor, PhD
Research Scientist, Institute for Computer Assisted Orthopedic Surgery, Western Pennsylvania Hospital, Pittsburgh, PA 15217, USA

D.W. Murray, MD, FRCS(Orth)
Professor, Department of Orthopaedics, Nuffield Orthopaedic Centre, Headington, Oxford, OX3 7LD, UK

Mark W. Pagnano, MD
Assistant Professor of Orthopedics, Mayo Clinic College of Medicine, Rochester, MN 55905, USA

A.J. Price, DPhil, FRCS(Orth)
Clinical Lecturer, Department of Orthopaedic Surgery, Nuffield Orthopaedic Centre, Headington, Oxford, OX3 7LD, UK

Phillip S. Ragland, MD
Fellow, Center for Joint Preservation and Reconstruction, Rubin Institute for Advanced Orthopedics, Sinai Hospital of Baltimore, Baltimore, MD 21215, USA

John A. Repicci, MD
Joint Reconstruction Orthopedic Center, Buffalo, NY 14226, USA

Paul L. Saenger, MD
Blue Ridge Bone and Joint, Asheville, NC 28801, USA

Jason A. Schneider, MD
Clinical Shoulder Fellow, Beth Israel Medical Center, Insall Scott Kelly Institute for Orthopedics, New York, NY 10128, USA

Giles R. Scuderi, MD
Attending Orthopedic Surgeon, Department of Orthopedic Surgery, Lenox Hill Hospital, New York, NY; Assistant Clinical Professor of Orthopedics, Albert Einstein College of Medicine, Bronx, NY; Director, Insall Scott Kelly Orthopedics and Sports Medicine, New York, NY 10128, USA

Kevin Setter, MD
Fellow, Department of Orthopedic Surgery, New York Presbyterian Hospital, Columbia University, New York, NY 10032, USA

James B. Stiehl, MD
Associate Clinical Professor, Department of Orthopedic Surgery, Medical College of Wisconsin, Milwaukee, WI 53212, USA

Craig M. Thomas, MD
Fellow, Center for Joint Preservation and Reconstruction, Rubin Institute for Advanced Orthopedics, Sinai Hospital of Baltimore, Baltimore, MD 21215, USA

Steven J. Thornton, MD
Attending Surgeon, Sports Medicine and Shoulder Service, Hospital for Special Surgery, New York, NY 10021, USA

Alfred J. Tria, Jr., MD
Clinical Professor of Orthopedic Surgery, St. Peter's University Hospital, Robert Wood Johnson Medical School, New Brunswick, NJ; Institute for Advanced Orthopedic Study, Orthopedic Center of New Jersey, Somerset, NJ 08873, USA

Ilya Voloshin, MD
Fellow, Department of Orthopedic Surgery, New York Presbyterian Hospital, Columbia University, New York, NY 10032, USA

Andrew Willis, MD
Fellow, Department of Orthopedics, Sports Medicine and Shoulder Service, Hospital for Special Surgery, Weill Medical College of Cornell, New York, NY 10021, USA

Alon Wolf, PhD
Research Scientist, Institute for Computer Assisted Orthopedic Surgery, Western Pennsylvania Hospital, Pittsburgh, PA 15217, USA

Section I

The Shoulder and Elbow

1

Mini-Incision Bankart Repair for Shoulder Instability

Edward W. Lee and Evan L. Flatow

The tenuous balance between stability and motion of the glenohumeral joint often results in one of the most common problems encountered by the orthopedic surgeon. Historically, surgical treatment of glenohumeral instability was generally indicated only for recurrent anterior dislocations. The breadth of operative procedures to treat anterior shoulder instability has included staple capsulorraphy,[1] subscapularis transposition,[2] shortening of the subscapularis and anterior capsule,[3] transfer of the coracoid,[4] and osteotomies of the proximal humerus[5] or the glenoid neck.[6] In terms of measuring clinical success based on recurrence of dislocation, these various procedures were very effective. However, restricted external rotation and overhead motion sacrificed stability at the expense of function and led to the recognition of late glenohumeral osteoarthrosis following some of these repairs.[7–11] Furthermore, the traditional limited operative indications failed to account for the growing awareness of subluxations as a source of symptomatic instability.[12–15] Better understanding of glenohumeral joint biomechanics, the role of the capsuloligamentous structures, and their modes of failure has led to an emphasis on restoration of normal anatomic relationships.

Anatomy and Biomechanics

Multiple structures are involved in maintaining stability of the shoulder. The balance between stability and permitting a wide range of motion is provided by the interaction of dynamic and static factors. The static stabilizers include the glenoid, labrum, capsule, glenohumeral ligaments, and the rotator interval. The role of the biceps tendon as a static stabilizer is unclear but is also thought to contribute to glenohumeral joint stability.

The glenoid provides a small, shallow surface to articulate with the humeral head and provides little constraint for the glenohumeral joint. The fibrocartilaginous labrum attaches to the glenoid rim and increases its effective depth and surface area. Isolated labral deficiency has been shown not to allow glenohumeral dislocation without associated injury to the capsule, emphasizing the crucial role of the capsuloligamentous structures in maintaining stability.

The three major glenohumeral ligaments function as *check-reins* toward the extremes of motion while remaining relatively lax in the mid-range to allow normal joint translation. Turkel et al.[16] found that the contributions of these structures were position dependent. The superior glenohumeral ligament, coracohumeral ligament, and the rotator interval (between the leading edge of the supraspinatus and the superior edge of the subscapularis) restrain anterior humeral head translation in 0 degrees of abduction and external rotation. With increasing abduction to 45 degrees, the middle glenohumeral ligament provides the primary anterior restraint. Finally, the inferior glenohumeral ligament (IGHL) tightens and becomes the prime anterior stabilizer at 90 degrees of abduction and 90 degrees of external rotation. Biomechanical study of the IGHL demonstrated tensile failure at the glenoid insertion or in midsubstance. Significant deformation, however, was observed in midsubstance even if the ultimate site of failure occurred at the insertion.[17]

The rotator cuff and scapular stabilizers serve as dynamic restraints in normal shoulder biomechanics. A primary role of the rotator cuff is to resist translational forces on the joint through compression of the humeral head into the glenoid cavity. Scapular winging, an imbalance of the scapular stabilizing musculature, has been implicated in pain and instability of the glenohumeral joint. Operative intervention addressing scapulothoracic dysfunction may lead to elimination of symptoms in select cases.

Clinical Features

Patient History

Critical to the evaluation of glenohumeral instability is a careful history and physical examination. The nature of the injury surrounding the onset of symptoms should be determined and is particularly useful in identifying the type of instability. Position of the arm at the time of injury or circumstances that provoke symptoms often indicates the direction of instability. Reproduction of a patient's symptoms in a position of abduction, external rotation, and extension suggests anterior instability. Flexion, internal rotation, and adduction, in contrast, would more likely point to posterior instability.

In determining the degree and etiology of instability, the history should ascertain whether the initial and any subsequent episodes of instability were elicited by high-energy trauma (such as violent twisting or fall), minimal repeated trauma (such as throwing a ball), or no trauma (such as reaching a high shelf). An initial dislocation resulting from a single traumatic episode frequently produces a Bankart lesion. In contrast, capsular laxity and absence of a Bankart lesion often is found in those patients who suffer an atraumatic dislocation, multijoint laxity, and several shoulder subluxations prior to a frank dislocation. The type of reduction required (i.e., was the shoulder self-reduced or did it require manipulation by another person?) may also provide additional information about the extent of joint laxity.

Acquired instability was described by Neer in which cumulative enlargement of the capsule results from repetitive stress.[18] Overhead athletes develop isolated shoulder laxity from overuse with no evidence of laxity in other joints. These patients may become symptomatic after years of microtrauma or only after a frank dislocation following a single traumatic event. This patient group demonstrates that multiple etiologies may contribute to instability and underscores the need for careful diagnosis and treatment to address coexisting pathologic entities.

Voluntary control of instability must be carefully sought as this may change the ultimate course of treatment. Patients with psychiatric disorders may use a concomitant ability to dislocate the shoulder for secondary gain. While operative intervention in this situation would likely fail, treatment options exist for other forms of voluntary subluxation. Surgery may benefit patients who can subluxate the shoulder by placing the arm in provocative positions. Biofeedback techniques, however, may help those patients who sublux through selective muscular activation.[19]

Detailed record of prior treatment should also be obtained, including the type and duration of immobilization, rehabilitative efforts, and previous surgeries. Knowledge of failed interventions helps guide future treatment in the recurrent dislocator.

Pain as an isolated symptom does not typically reveal much useful information. Anterior shoulder pain may indicate anterior instability as well as other common disorders including subacromial impingement. Similarly, posterior shoulder pain is nonspecific and may represent a range of pathology from instability to cervical spine disorders. Location of the pain in combination with provoking arm positions and activities, however, may aid in making a diagnosis of instability. Altered glenohumeral kinematics in throwers, for example, may result in posterior shoulder pain during late-cocking (internal impingement).[20]

Patients may also report other symptoms consistent with subtle shoulder instability. Rowe and Zarins[21] described a phenomenon termed the *dead-arm syndrome* in which paralyzing pain and loss of control of the extremity occurs with abduction and external rotation of the shoulder. A similar phenomenon may be seen in patients with inferior subluxation when they carry heavy loads in the affected arm.

Finally, determining the patient's functional demands and level of impairment is important prior to formulating a therapeutic plan. The different expectations of a sedentary patient with minimal functional loss versus the high-performance athlete with pain and apprehension may affect the type of prescribed treatment.

Physical Examination

A thorough physical examination is equally essential in making an accurate diagnosis and recommending the appropriate intervention. Both shoulders should be adequately exposed and examined for deformity, range of motion, strength, and laxity. Demonstration of scapular winging may accompany instability, particularly of the posterior-type, and should be considered a potential cause of symptoms. Generalized ligamentous laxity may also contribute to instability and can be elicited with the ability to touch the thumb to the forearm and hyperextend the

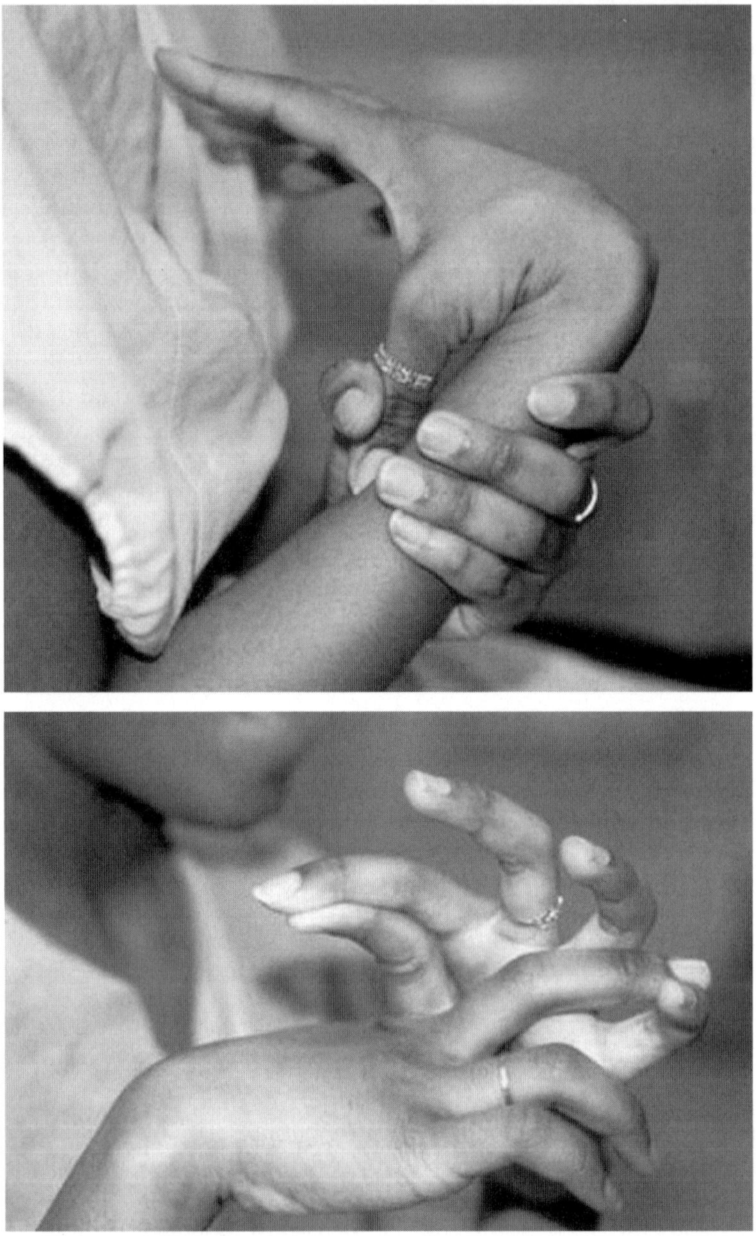

A

B

Figure 1.1. Tests for generalized ligamentous laxity. (A) Thumb-to-Forearm. (B) Index metacarpophalangeal joint hyperextension.

index metacarpophalangeal joint beyond 90 degrees (Figure 1.1). Operative reports and evidence of healed anterior or posterior scars from previous instability repairs will indicate what has been done and may provide a rationale for the patient's current symptoms.

Tenderness to palpation of the acromioclavicular joint should be sought and may represent the source of symptoms in a patient with an asymptomatic loose shoulder. Pain along the glenohumeral joint line can be associated with instability but is a nonspecific finding.

Typically, there is a full range of motion with the exception of guarding at the extremes as the shoulder approaches unstable positions. Clinical suspicion should be raised, however, in the patient older than 40 years of age who is unable to actively abduct the arm after a primary anterior dislocation. It has been shown that a high percentage of these patients will have a concurrent rupture of the rotator cuff with restoration of stability following repair.[22]

Various basic provocative tests can be used to reproduce the patient's symptoms and confirm the diagnosis. In order to minimize the effects of muscle guarding, these maneuvers should be performed first on the unaffected side and then in succession of increasing discomfort. The *sulcus test* evaluates inferior translation of the humeral head with the arm at the side and in abduction[23] (Figure 1.2). Significant findings would include an increased palpable gap between the acromion and humeral head compared to the opposite side as well as translation below the glenoid rim. Incompetence of the rotator interval will not reduce the gap with performance of the test in external rotation.

Laxity can be further evaluated by anterior and posterior drawer or load-and-shift tests.[24] The proximal humerus is shifted in each direction while grasped between the thumb and index fingers. Alternatively, with the patient supine, the scapula is stabilized while the humeral head is axially loaded and translated anteriorly and posteriorly. Translation greater than the opposite shoulder or translation over the glenoid rim indicates

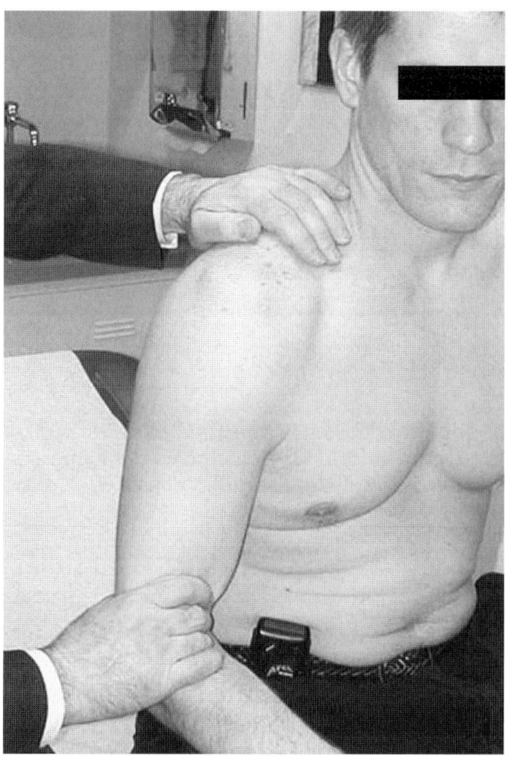

Figure 1.2. Sulcus sign. Downward traction of the arm will create a gap between the acromion and the humeral head.

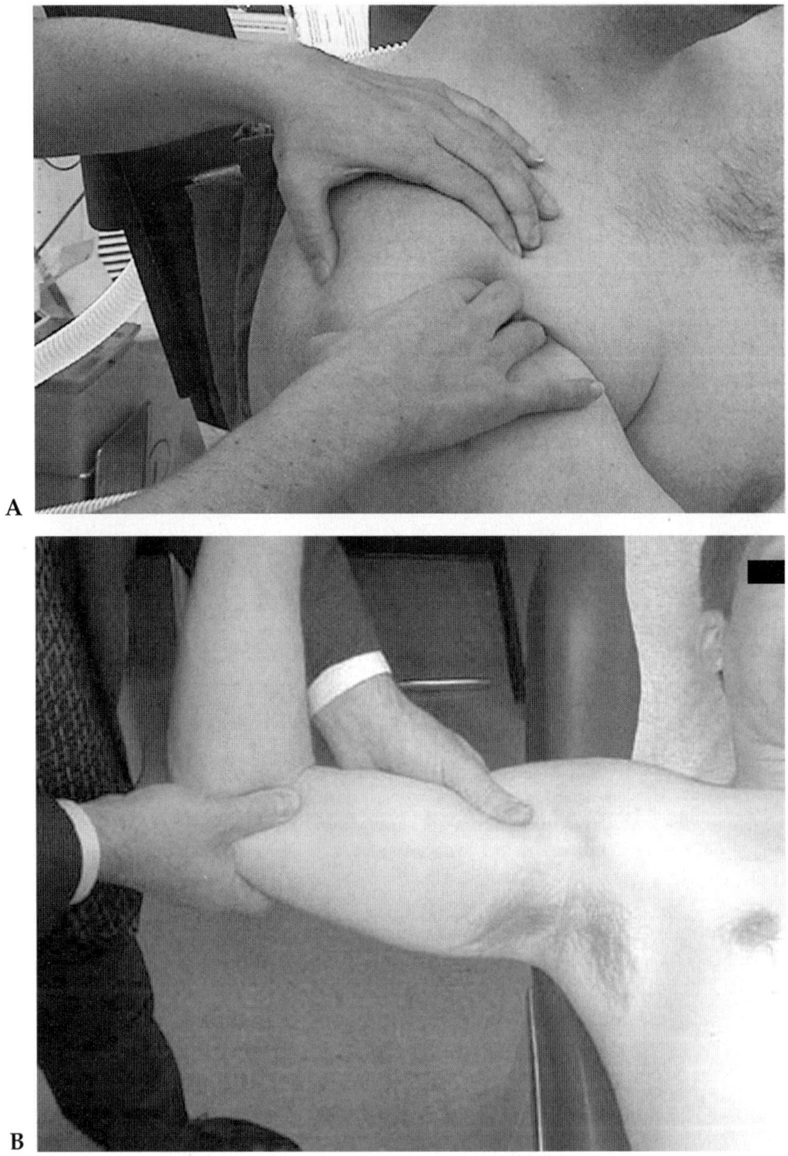

Figure 1.3. (A) Anterior/posterior drawer: translation of the humeral head held between the thumb and index finger and stabilization of the scapula with the other hand. (B) Load-and-shift: simultaneous axial loading and translation of the humeral head.

significant laxity. Only translations which reproduce the patient's symptoms are considered as demonstrating instability (Figure 1.3).

The anterior apprehension test is performed by externally rotating, abducting, and extending the affected shoulder while stabilizing the scapula or providing an anteriorly directed force to the humeral head with the other hand. Significant findings would include a sense of impending subluxation or dislocation, or guarding and resistance to further rotation secondary to apprehension.[25] Pain as an isolated finding is nonspecific and may indicate other pathology such as rotator cuff disease. *Jobe's relocation test* is done in the supine position, usually accompanying the apprehension test. As symptoms are elicited with progressive external rotation, the examiner applies a posteriorly directed force to the humeral head. A positive test is signified by alleviation of symptoms[26] (Figure 1.4).

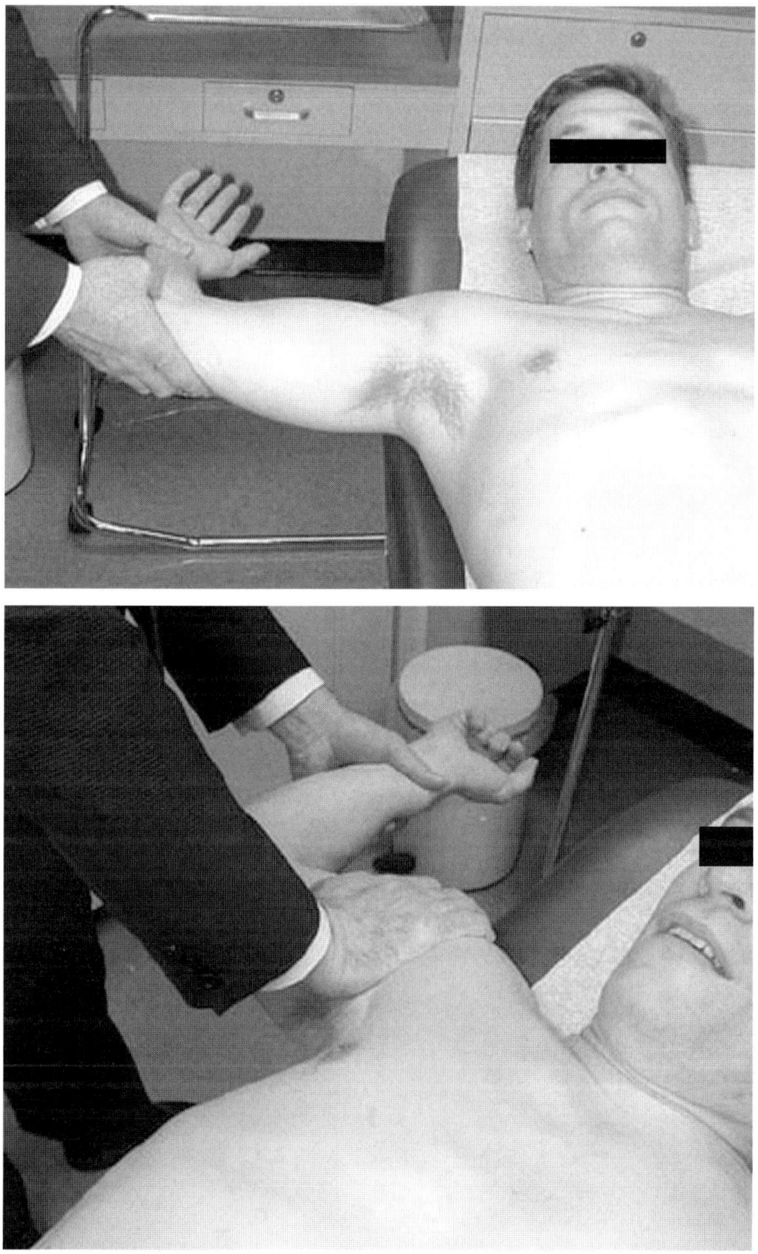

A

B

Figure 1.4. (A) Apprehension test: abduction and external rotation will produce sense of impending subluxation/dislocation with anterior glenohumeral instability. (B) Relocation test: posterior-directed force on the humeral head will alleviate symptoms.

Posterior instability can be elicited with the *posterior stress test*. As one hand stabilizes the scapula, a posteriorly directed axial force is applied to the arm with the shoulder in 90 degrees of flexion, abduction and internal rotation. Unlike the anterior apprehension test, the posterior stress test usually produces pain rather than true apprehension.[27]

Radiographic Features

Though the history and physical examination are the key elements in patient evaluation, a series of radiographic studies may be helpful in confirming the diagnosis and defining associated pathology. Anteroposterior (AP) radiographs in internal and external rotation, a lateral view in the scapular plane (scapular-Y view), and a lateral of the glenohumeral joint (i.e., a standard supine axillary or Velpeau axillary view) should be obtained in the initial evaluation. A Hill-Sachs lesion (posterolateral impression fracture) of the humeral head is best seen on the AP radiograph in internal rotation (Figure 1.5) or on specialized views such as the Stryker Notch.[28] Fractures or erosions of the glenoid rim can be detected on an axillary or apical oblique view (Garth).[29]

Other more specialized imaging studies are not routinely obtained in the initial evaluation of instability but may be useful in a preoperative workup. Computed tomography can assist in further assessment of fractures and glenoid erosions or altered glenoid version as well as detect subtle subluxation of the humeral head.[30,31] MRI and MR arthrography can identify associated pathology of the labrum, glenohumeral ligaments, and the rotator cuff.[32–34] The addition of abduction and external rotation has been shown to increase the sensitivity of MR arthrography in delineating tears of the anterior labrum.[35,36] More

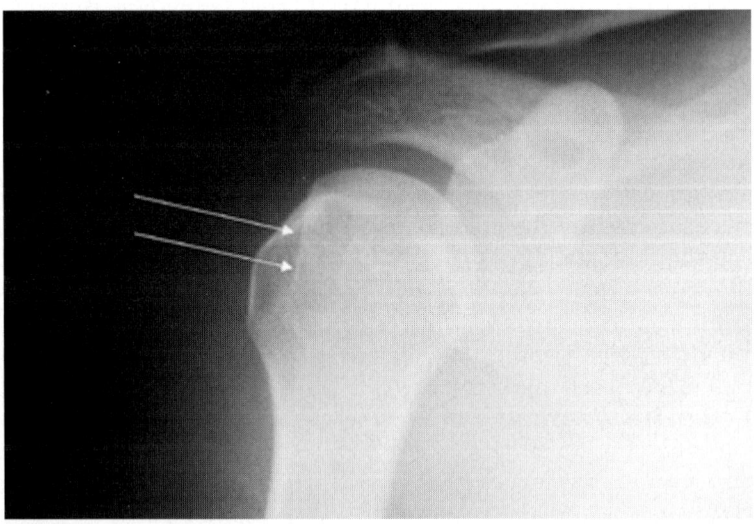

Figure 1.5. Hill-Sachs lesion. An impaction fracture of the posterolateral humeral head associated with an anterior glenohumeral dislocation is depicted by the small white arrows on this internally rotated anteroposterior radiograph.

recent radiographic modalities such as dynamic MR imaging currently have no defined indications but may become a useful adjunct in evaluating glenohumeral instability.[37]

Treatment

Nonoperative Treatment

Although the results vary with age and associated bone and soft-tissue injury, nonoperative treatment consisting of a period of immobilization followed by rehabilitation is typically successful in managing the majority of patients with glenohumeral instability. Early studies of young (less than 20 years old), athletic patients, however, found a recurrence rate as high as 90% after a primary dislocation.[38,39] While subsequent studies have reported lower numbers,[40,41] clearly the risk for subsequent dislocations is higher with earlier onset of instability.

The length and type of immobilization remains a matter of debate. Several published series have advocated immobilization for a few days to several weeks. However, studies by Hovelius[41] and Simonet and Cofield[40] have found no difference in outcome from either the type or length of immobilization. In general, younger patients (less than 30 years of age) sustaining a primary dislocation are preferably immobilized for approximately 3 to 4 weeks. Older patients, who have a smaller risk of recurrent instability but a higher susceptibility to stiffness, may be immobilized for shorter periods.

Rehabilitation efforts are aimed at strengthening the dynamic stabilizers and regaining motion. Progressive resistive exercises of the rotator cuff, deltoid, and scapular stabilizers are recommended. Stress on the static restraints (i.e., capsuloligamentous structures) should be prevented in the immediate postinjury period by avoidance of vigorous stretching and provocative arm positions.

Operative Treatment

Failure of conservative management for glenohumeral instability is an indication for proceeding with operative intervention. Open procedures are currently the gold standard for repair of the disrupted soft-tissue shoulder stabilizers.

Modern techniques emphasize anatomic restoration of the soft-tissue structures. Based on the work of Perthes in 1906,[42] Bankart,[43] in 1923, popularized repair of the capsule to the anterior glenoid without shortening of the overlying subscapularis. After modifications to his original description, reconstruction of the avulsed capsule and labrum to the glenoid lip is commonly referred to today as the *Bankart repair*. Several capsulorraphy procedures have also been described to address capsular laxity and the increase in joint volume. These procedures allow tightening of the anterior capsule in combination with reattachment of a capsulolabral avulsion.

The inferior capsular shift was first introduced by Neer and Foster for multidirectional instability.[44] This procedure can reduce capsular volume through overlap of capsular tissue on the side of greatest instability and reducing tissue redundancy by tensioning the inferior capsule and opposite side. For anterior inferior instability, we prefer to use a modified inferior capsular shift procedure, in essence, a laterally based T capsulorraphy, which allows us to adapt the repair to each individual.[45,46]

The rationale behind this universal approach to instability is predicated on several factors. First, the capsule is shaped like a funnel with a broader circumferential insertion on the humeral side. Implementing a laterally based incision allows the tissue to be shifted a greater distance and reattached to the broader lateral insertion, thus allowing more capsular overlap. Second, following intraoperative assessment of the inferior pouch and capsular redundancy, the inferior shift procedure permits variable degrees of capsular mobilization around the humeral neck to treat different grades of tissue laxity. Third, use of a T capsulorraphy permits independent tensioning of the capsule in the medial-lateral and superior-inferior directions. Medial-lateral tensioning is usually a secondary concern, and if overdone, may result in loss of external rotation. Fourth, a lateral capsular incision affords some protection to the axillary nerve, particularly during an inferior dissection as the nerve traverses under the inferior capsule. Finally, capsular tears/avulsions from the humeral insertion, although rare, are more readily identified and repaired with a laterally based incision.

The patient is placed in a beach-chair position although slightly more recumbent than when performing a rotator cuff repair. We prefer interscalene regional block anesthesia at our institution because of its safety and ability to provide adequate muscle relaxation. Examination under anesthesia should be performed prior to breaching the soft tissues to confirm the predominant components of instability. The key to a mini-open Bankart procedure is the use of a concealed anterior axillary incision starting approximately 3 cm below the tip of the coracoid and extending inferiorly for 7 cm to 8 cm into the axillary recess (Figure 1.6). Local anesthetic is injected into the inferior aspect of the wound where thoracic cross-innervation prevents a complete block in this area. Full-thickness subcutaneous flaps are mobilized until the inferior aspect of the clavicle is palpated. The deltopectoral interval is then developed taking the cephalic vein laterally with the deltoid. If needed, the upper 1 cm to 2 cm of the pectoralis major insertion may be released to gain further exposure. The clavipectoral fascia is then gently incised lateral to the strap muscles, which are gently retracted medially. Osteotomy of the coracoid should not be necessary and may endanger the medial neurovascular structures. A small, medially based wedge of the anterior fascicle of the coracoacromial ligament may be excised to increase visualization of the superior border of the subscapularis muscle, rotator interval, and anterior aspect of the subacromial space.

The upper and lower borders of the subscapularis are identified. The anterior humeral circumflex vessels are carefully isolated and ligated. Preservation of the inferior border of the subscapularis to provide protection to the axillary nerve has been suggested.[47] This may be a reasonable option in true unidirectional instability cases; however, inadequate exposure of the inferior capsule may compromise the

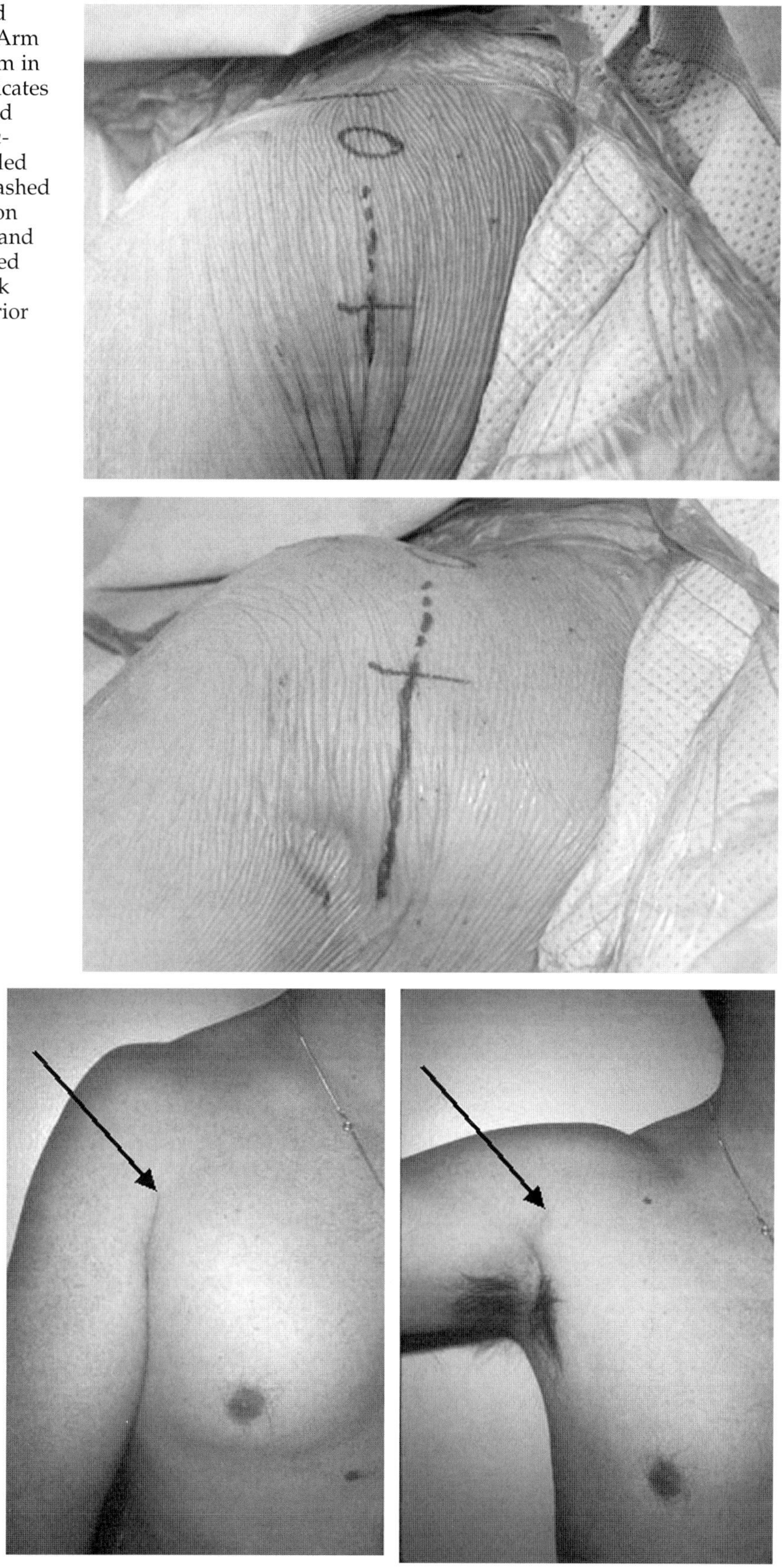

Figure 1.6. Concealed axillary incision. (A) Arm at the side and (B) arm in abduction. Circle indicates coracoid process. Solid line indicates true *concealed* incision; if needed for more exposure, dashed line indicates extension toward coracoid. (C) and (D) demonstrate healed axillary incision. Black arrows indicate superior extent of incision.

ability to correct any coexisting inferior laxity component. Another approach splits the subscapularis longitudinally in line with its fibers making visualization of the glenoid rim more difficult but motion is less restricted postoperatively. This approach may be useful in athletes who throw, in whom any restriction in external rotation postoperatively should be avoided.[48] We prefer to detach the tendon 1 cm to 2 cm from its insertion onto the lesser tuberosity, careful not to stray too medial into the muscle fibers and compromise the subscapularis repair. Blunt elevation of the muscle belly from the capsule medially may permit easier identification of the plane between the two structures.

Examination of the rotator interval is essential during dissection of the capsule and subscapularis. As one of the primary static stabilizers of the glenohumeral joint, the rotator interval can be an important component of recurrent anterior instability. We repair it when it is widened, aware that overly tightening the gap will limit external rotation.

The capsule is then incised laterally leaving a 1-cm cuff of tissue for repair while placing traction sutures in the free edge. Placing the arm in adduction and external rotation maximizes the distance between the incision and axillary nerve which should be palpated and protected throughout the procedure.

The extent of capsular dissection and mobilization depends on the components of instability. Unidirectional anterior instability will only require dissection of the anterior capsule. Bi-directional anterior-inferior instability requires the addition of inferior capsular mobilization to eliminate the enlarged capsule. In these cases, the shoulder is gradually flexed and externally rotated to facilitate sharp dissection of the anterior and inferior capsule off the humeral neck. A finger can be placed in the inferior recess to assess the amount of redundant capsule and the adequacy of the shift. As more capsule is mobilized and upward traction is placed on the sutures, the volume of the pouch will reduce and push the finger out indicating an adequate shift.

The inferior component in unidirectional instability is minimal, and thus, an inferior shift and the horizontal incision may be unnecessary. With a significant inferior capsular redundancy, the horizontal limb of the T in the capsule is made between the inferior and middle glenohumeral ligaments. A Fukuda retractor is then placed to visualize the glenoid (Figure 1.7). If the capsule is thin and redundant medially, a *barrel* stitch can be used to tension it as well as imbricate the capsule at the glenoid rim to serve as an additional bumper to augment a deficient labrum[49] (Figure 1.8).

Effectiveness of a shift requires anchoring of the capsule to the glenoid. When the glenohumeral ligaments and labrum are avulsed from the bone medially, they must be reattached to the glenoid rim (Figure 1.9). The Bankart lesion must be anchored to the rim before performing the capsulorraphy because the capsule must be secured to the glenoid for the shift to be effective. This can be accomplished inside out, anchoring the labrum with sutures through bone tunnels. After the glenoid rim is roughened with a curette or high-speed burr, two to three sets of holes are made adjacent to the articular surface and through the glenoid rim. Curved awls, angled curettes, and heavy towel clips may

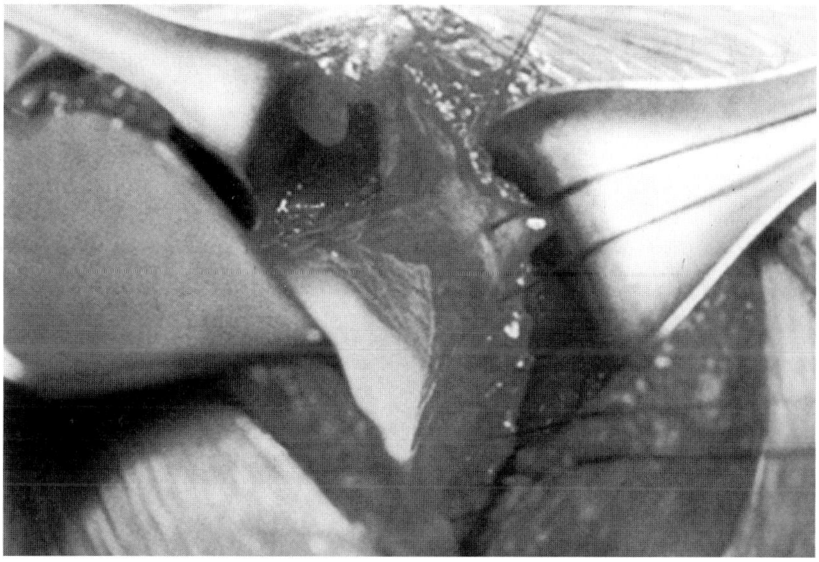

Figure 1.7. Mobilization of the capsule and placement of traction sutures in the free edge. A Fukuda retractor is placed allowing inspection of the glenoid.

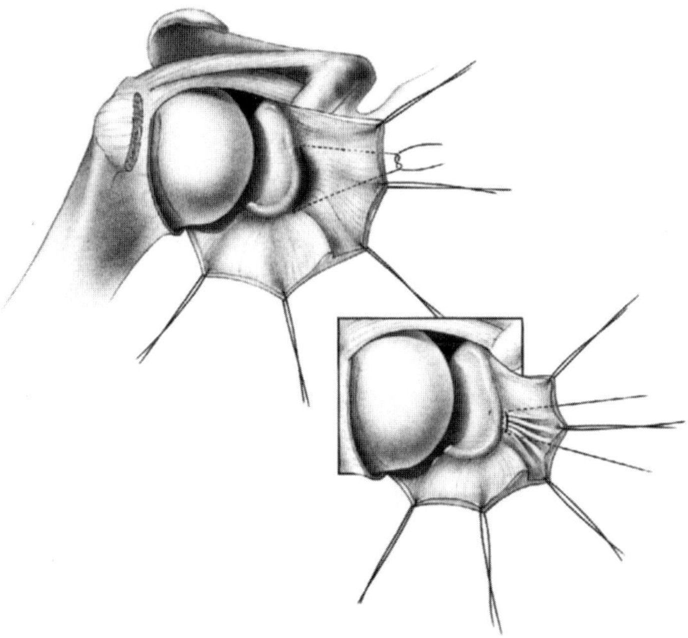

Figure 1.8. A *barrel* stitch may be used medially to bunch up tissue at the glenoid rim to compensate for a deficient labrum. (From Post M, Bigliani L, Flatow E, Pollock R. The Shoulder: Operative Technique. Lippincott Williams & Wilkins, New York. 1998. p. 184.)

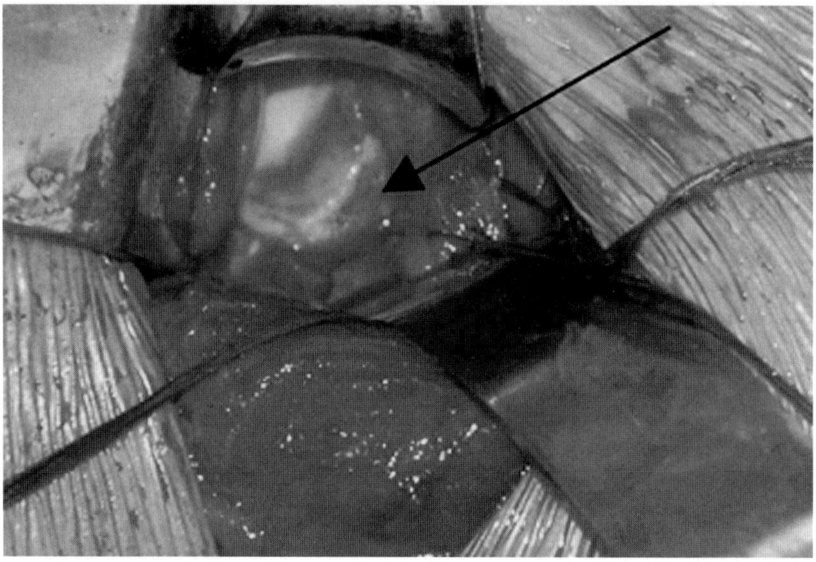

Figure 1.9. Avulsion of the glenohumeral ligaments and labrum from the glenoid rim. Solid black arrow indicates bare anterior glenoid rim.

be used to fashion the tunnels. A small CurvTek (Arthrotek, Warsaw, IN) may also be helpful in making the holes. Number 0 nonabsorbable braided sutures (e.g., Ethibond; Ethicon/Johnson & Johnson, Somerville, NJ) are passed through the tunnels. Both limbs are then brought inside out through the labrum and tied on the outside of the capsule. Alternatively, suture anchors can be used, placing them adjacent to the articular margin and careful not to insert them medially to avoid a step-off between the rim and the labrum.

Glenoid deficiency from a fracture of the rim or from repeated wear from chronic instability may contribute to the pathologic process. Defects representing less than 25% of the articular surface area may be repaired by reattaching the labrum and capsule back to the remaining glenoid rim. If a fragment of bone remains attached to the soft tissues, this can be mobilized and repaired back to the glenoid with sutures. Larger fragments can be reattached with a cannulated screw, countersinking the head of the screw within the bone. Defects larger than 25% without a reparable fragment, leaving an inverted-pear glenoid, in which the normally pear-shaped glenoid had lost enough anterior-inferior bone to assume the shape of an inverted pear,[50] should be augmented with bone. Femoral head allograft can be fashioned to reconstitute the rim. Another alternative to deepening the socket is to perform a Bristow-Laserjet procedure, transferring the coracoid tip with the attached coracobrachialis and short head of the biceps into the defect, close to the articular margin and behind the repaired capsule.[4] A cannulated screw, carefully engaging the posterior cortex of the glenoid, and a washer are used to secure the coracoid to the glenoid.

An engaging Hill-Sachs lesion may be another source of recurrent instability requiring attention for a successful repair. Preventing the head defect from engaging the glenoid rim can be accomplished in one of three ways. First, the capsular shift can be performed to tighten the anterior structures enough to restrict external rotation. This should be done with caution as previously mentioned, given the unwanted result in overhead athletes and the risk of late glenohumeral arthrosis. Second, a size-matched humeral osteoarticular allograft or a cortico-cancellous iliac graft can be utilized to fill the defect. Finally, an internal rotation proximal humeral osteotomy can be performed, albeit with significant technical difficulty and potential morbidity, shifting the defect out of the arc of motion.

The arm is positioned in at least 20 degrees of external rotation and 30 degrees of abduction and 10 degrees of flexion while securing the tissues for the capsular shift. In overhead athletes, approximately 10 degrees more abduction and external rotation may be used. Once any adherent soft tissues impeding excursion of the capsule are dissected from the capsule, the inferior flap should be shifted superiorly first, followed by the superior flap to a more inferior position. A suture may be placed medially to reinforce overlap of the two flaps. The subscapularis is then repaired as previously described followed by a layered closure and a subcuticular skin closure.

Postoperative Care

The challenge following an instability procedure is to find the delicate balance between early gradual motion and maintenance of stability. In general, patients are protected in a sling for 6 weeks with immediate active hand, wrist, and elbow motion and isometric shoulder exercises started at approximately 10 days. From 10 days to 2 weeks, gentle assisted motion is permitted with external rotation with a stick to 10 degrees and elevation to 90 degrees. From 2 to 4 weeks, motion is progressed to 30 degrees of external rotation and 140 degrees of elevation. From 4 to 6 weeks, external rotation to 40 degrees and elevation to 160 degrees are initiated in addition to light resistive exercises. Terminal elevation stretching and external rotation to 60 degrees are permitted after 6 weeks. After 3 months, when the soft tissues have adequately healed, terminal external rotation stretches are allowed. Patients can expect a return to sport at 9 to 12 months postoperatively. These are broad guidelines that should be adapted to each individual case based on intraoperative findings and frequent postoperative exams. Poor tissue quality, durability of the repair, patient reliability, and future demands on the shoulder should dictate the progression of the rehabilitation program.

Results

Good results have been achieved with most open capsulorraphy techniques to treat anterior/anterior-inferior glenohumeral instability. Thomas and Matsen[51] reported 97% good or excellent results in 63 shoulders with repair of the Bankart lesion and incising both the subscapularis and capsule. Pollock et al.[52] reported 90% successful results with an anterior-inferior capsular shift in 151 shoulders with a 5% rate of recurrent instability. Bigliani et al.[46] studied 68 shoulders in athletes who underwent an anterior-inferior capsular shift with 94% of patients with good or excellent results. Fifty-eight patients (92%) of patients returned to the major sports and 47 (75%) at the same competitive level.

References

1. Du Toit GT, Roux D. Recurrent dislocation of the shoulder: A twenty-four year study of the Johannesburg stapling operation. J Bone Joint Surg. 1956; 38A:1–12.
2. Magnuson PB, Stack JK. Recurrent dislocation of the shoulder. JAMA. 1943; 123:889–892.
3. Clarke HO. Habitual dislocation of the shoulder. J Bone Joint Surg. 1948; 30B:19–25.
4. Helfet AJ. Coracoid transplantation for recurring dislocation of the shoulder. J Bone Joint Surg. 1958;40B:198–202.
5. Weber BG, Simpson LA, Hardegger F, et al. Rotational humeral osteotomy for recurrent anterior dislocation of the shoulder associated with a large Hill-Sachs lesion. J Bone Joint Surg. 1984;66A:1443–1450.
6. Saha AK. Theory of Shoulder Mechanism: Descriptive and Applied. Springfield, IL, Charles C. Thomas, 1961.
7. Samilson RL, Prieto V. Dislocation arthropathy of the shoulder. J Bone Joint Surg. 1983;65:456–460.
8. Hawkins RJ, Angelo RL. Glenohumeral osteoarthrosis. A late complication of the Putti-Platt repair. J Bone Joint Surg. 1990;72:1193–1197.
9. Young DC, Rockwood CA Jr. Complications of a failed Bristow procedure and their management. J Bone Joint Surg. 1991;73:969–981.
10. Steinmann SR, Flatow EL, Pollock RG, et al. Evaluation and surgical treatment of failed shoulder instability repairs. Orthop Trans. 1992;16:727.
11. O'Driscoll SW, Evans DC. Long-term results of staple capsulorraphy for anterior instability of the shoulder. J Bone Joint Surg. 1993;75:249–258.
12. Blazina ME, Satzman JS. Recurrent anterior subluxation of the shoulder in athletics: a distinct entity. J Bone Joint Surg. 1969;51:1037–1038.
13. Rowe CR, Zarins B. Recurrent transient subluxation of the shoulder. J Bone Joint Surg. 1981;63:863–872.
14. Hastings DE, Coughlin LP. Recurrent subluxation of the glenohumeral joint. Am J Sports Med. 1981;9:352–355.
15. Garth WP Jr, Allman FL, Armstrong WS. Occult anterior subluxations of the shoulder in noncontact sports. Am J Sports Med. 1987;15:579–585.
16. Turkel SJ, Panio MW, Marshall JL, et al. Stabilizing mechanisms preventing anterior dislocation of the glenohumeral joint. J Bone Joint Surg. 1981; 63:1208–1217.
17. Bigliani LU, Pollock RG, Soslowsky LJ, et al. The tensile properties of the inferior glenohumeral ligament. J Orthop Res. 1992:10:187–197.
18. Neer CS II. Involuntary inferior and multidirectional instability of the shoulder: etiology, recognition, and treatment. Instr Course Lect. 1985;34:232–238.
19. Beall MS Jr, Diefenbach G, Allen A. Electromyographic biofeedback in the treatment of voluntary posterior instability of the shoulder. Am J Sports Med. 1987;15:175–178.
20. Davidson PA, Elattrache NS, Jobe CM, et al. Rotator cuff and posterior-superior glenoid labrum injury associated with increased glenohumeral motion: a new site of impingement. J Shoulder Elbow Surg. 1995;4: 384–390.
21. Rowe CR, Zarins B. Recurrent transient subluxation of the shoulder. J Bone Joint Surg. 1981;63:863–872.

22. Neviaser RJ, Neviaser TJ. Recurrent instability of the shoulder after age 40. J Shoulder Elbow Surg. 1995;4:416–418.
23. Neer CS II, Foster CR. Inferior capsular shift for involuntary inferior and multidirectional instability of the shoulder. A preliminary report. J Bone Joint Surg. 1980;62:897–908.
24. Hawkins RJ, Bokor DJ. Clinical evaluation of shoulder problems. In Rockwood CA Jr, Matsen FA III, editors. The Shoulder. Philadelphia, PA: WB Saunders, 1990:149–177.
25. Speer KP, Hannafin JA, Altchek DW, et al. An evaluation of the shoulder relocation test. Am J Sports Med. 1994;22:177–183.
26. Jobe FW, Tibone JE, Jobe CM, et al. The shoulder in sports. In Rockwood CA Jr, Matsen FA III, editors. The Shoulder. Philadelphia, PA: WB Saunders, 1990:149–177.
27. Hawkins RJ, Koppert G, Johnston G. Recurrent posterior instability (subluxation) of the shoulder. J Bone Joint Surg. 1984;66:169–174.
28. Danzig LA, Greenway G, Resnick D. The Hill-Sachs lesion. An experimental study. Am J Sports Med. 1980;8:328–332.
29. Garth WP Jr, Slappey CE, Ochs CW. Roentgenographic demonstration of instability of the shoulder: the apical oblique projection. A technical note. J Bone Joint Surg. 1984;66:1450–1453.
30. Itoi E, Lee SB, Amrami KK, et al. Quantitative assessment of classic anteroinferior bony Bankart lesions by radiography and computed tomography. Am J Sports Med. 2003;31:112–118.
31. Nyffeler RW, Jost B, Pfirrmann CW, et al. Measurement of glenoid version: conventional radiographs versus computed tomography scans. J Shoulder Elbow Surg. 2003;12:493–496.
32. Beltran J, Rosenberg ZS, Chandnani VP, et al. Glenohumeral instability: evaluation with MR arthrography. Radiographics 1997;17:657–673.
33. Shankman S, Bencardino J, Beltran J. Glenohumeral instability: evaluation using MR arthrography of the shoulder. Skeletal Radiol. 1999;28:365–382.
34. Parmar H, Jhankaria B, Maheshwari M, et al. Magnetic resonance arthrography in recurrent anterior shoulder instability as compared to arthroscopy: a prospective comparative study. J Postgrad Med. 2002;48: 270–273; discussion 273–274.
35. Cvitanic O, Tirman PF, Feller JF, et al. Using abduction and external rotation of the shoulder to increase the sensitivity of MR arthrography in revealing tears of the anterior glenoid labrum. AJR Am J Roentgenol. 1997; 169:837–844.
36. Wintzell G, Larsson H, Larsson S. Indirect MR arthrography of anterior shoulder instability in the ABER and the apprehension test positions: a prospective comparative study of two different shoulder positions during MRI using intravenous gadodiamide contrast for enhancement of the joint fluid. Skeletal Radiol. 1998;27:488–494.
37. Allmann KH, Uhl M, Gufler H, et al. Cine-MR imaging of the shoulder. Acta Radiol. 1997;38:1043–1046.
38. Rowe CR. Prognosis in dislocations of the shoulder. J Bone Joint Surg. 1956; 38:957–977.
39. Wheeler JH, Ryan JB, Arciero RA, et al. Arthroscopic versus nonoperative treatment of acute shoulder dislocations in young athletes. Arthroscopy 1989;5:213–217.
40. Simonet WT, Cofield RH. Prognosis in anterior shoulder dislocation. Am J Sports Med. 1984;12:19–24.
41. Hovelius L. Anterior dislocation of the shoulder in teen-agers and young adults. Five-year prognosis. J Bone Joint Surg Am. 1987;69:393–399.

42. Perthes G. Uber operationen bei habitueller schulterluxation. Deutsch Ztschr Chir. 1906;85:199–227.
43. Bankart ASB. Recurrent or habitual dislocation of the shoulder joint. Br Med J. 1923;2:1132–1135.
44. Neer CS II, Foster CR. Inferior capsular shift for involuntary inferior and multidirectional instability of the shoulder. A preliminary report. J Bone Joint Surg. 1980;62:897–908.
45. Pollock RG, Owens JM, Nicholson GP, et al. Anterior inferior capsular shift procedure for anterior glenohumeral instability: long-term results. Orthop Trans. 1993;17:974.
46. Bigliani LU, Kurzweil PR, Schwartzbach CC, et al. Inferior capsular shift procedure for anterior-inferior shoulder instability in athletes. Am J Sports Med. 1994;22:578–584.
47. Matsen FA, Thomas SC, Rockwood CA, et al: Glenohumeral instability. In Rockwood CA Jr., Matsen FA III, editors. The Shoulder. New York: Churchill Livingstone, 1998:717.
48. Rubenstein DL, Jobe FW, Glousman RE, et al. Anterior capsulolabral reconstruction of the shoulder in athletes. J Shoulder Elbow Surg. 1992;1:229–237.
49. Ahmad CS, Freehill MQ, Blaine TA, et al. Anteromedial capsular redundancy and labral deficiency in shoulder instability. Am J Sports Med. 2003; 31:247–252.
50. Burkhart SS, De Beer JF. Traumatic glenohumeral bone defects and their relationship to failure of arthroscopic Bankart repairs: significance of the inverted-pear glenoid and the humeral engaging Hill-Sachs lesion. Arthroscopy 2000;16:677–694.
51. Thomas SC, Matsen FA III. An approach to the repair of avulsion of the glenohumeral ligaments in the management of traumatic anterior glenohumeral instability. J Bone Joint Surg Am. 1989;71:506–513.
52. Pollock RG, Owens JM, Nicholson GP, et al. The anterior inferior capsular shift procedure for anterior glenohumeral instability. Technique and long-term results. Orthop Trans. 1993–1994;17:1109.

2

Mini-Open Rotator Cuff Repair

Jason A. Schneider and Frances Cuomo

Rotator cuff tears have long been recognized as a disabling problem of the upper extremity. Codman reportedly performed the first open rotator cuff repair in 1911.[1] However, it was not until 1972 when Neer reported the results of anterior acromioplasty in combination with cuff mobilization and repair that results substantially improved.[2] The surgical fundamentals detailed by Neer significantly improved the reliability and outcome of the surgery. These principles include the preservation or meticulous repair of the deltoid origin, adequate decompression of the subacromial space, adequate mobilization of the rotator cuff tendons with release of adhesions, secure fixation of the tendon to bone, and a closely supervised rehabilitation program.[3] Traditional open methods of rotator cuff repair have achieved good results because of these basic fundamental principles.[4–8] Neer reported on 233 rotator cuff repairs in 1988. In this series he reported that 91% resulted in an excellent or satisfactory rating.[8] Hawkins similarly reported on 100 patients. He reported that 86% of patients had no or slight pain.[7] However, the risks of postoperative stiffness, possible deltoid detachment, an inability to accurately diagnose and treat articular pathology, and significant postoperative pain continue to pose difficult problems.

The advent of shoulder arthroscopy has had a profound effect on the evolution of rotator cuff treatment. The use of arthroscopy in the shoulder has dramatically expanded since its introduction. Burman[9] and Wantanabe[10] initially described shoulder arthroscopy in the 1930s. However, shoulder arthroscopy was not commonly used until Wiley and Older developed arthroscopic techniques and applied them for diagnostic purposes in the 1980s.[11] As surgeons have become increasingly comfortable with the use of the arthroscope in the shoulder, the indications have expanded. Since the initial description of the arthroscopic subacromial decompression by Ellman, there has been a substantial trend toward the use of more minimally invasive surgery to accomplish the same results as those seen previously with the gold standard open repair.[12] Levy and associates[13] and then subsequently Paulos and Kody[14] described the arthroscopically enhanced mini-open approach to rotator cuff repair in 1990 and 1994, respectively.

The mini-open rotator cuff repair has become an increasingly popular means of addressing rotator cuff tears.[13–23] Once regarded as a new and innovative procedure performed by only a few surgeons, arthroscopically assisted mini-open repairs have quickly become common and widely accepted. This technique combines arthroscopic subacromial decompression with open tendon repair through a minimally invasive deltoid splitting technique. The procedure permits preservation of the deltoid origin during repair of the torn tendon because the decompression is performed arthroscopically. It represents a middle ground between the formal open repair and the fully arthroscopic repair.

Regardless of the technique, the general principles of rotator cuff repair remain the same. Neer's fundamental principles of rotator cuff repair must be adhered to regardless of whether the surgery is performed arthroscopically, open, or through a mini-open approach.

The major advantage of the mini-open repair is the preservation of the deltoid origin. Although the mini-open repair does not eliminate injury to the deltoid, it does significantly decrease the surgical insult. The open repair requires some form of anterior deltoid origin takedown or elevation combined with a lateral deltoid split. Despite this, the reported incidence of deltoid avulsion by the most experienced surgeon is only 0.5%.[24–26] Deltoid dehiscence is a devastating complication. The insult to the anterior deltoid is diminished in the mini-incision approach because the deltoid is only split, leaving its origin intact. As the anterior acromioplasty has already been performed arthroscopically, further anterior deltoid detachment is no longer necessary. Additionally, the open repair has been associated with more perioperative pain than the mini-open repair.[13–15,18,19,23] The increased pain of the open repair is likely secondary to the deltoid detachment required for formal open repair. This pain can hinder early rehabilitation and early motion.

A second significant advantage of the mini-open repair is that it allows glenohumeral joint inspection through the arthroscope. Therefore, associated joint pathology can not only be identified but addressed as well. Miller and Savoie evaluated 100 consecutive patients with full thickness tears of the rotator cuff. They found a 76% prevalence of intra-articular pathologic disorders.[27] Gartsman and Taverna reported a 60.5% incidence of associated intra-articular pathology. Of the patients in this study, 12.5% study had major coexisting intra-articular pathology that required operative treatment or changed postoperative rehabilitation.[28]

Although arthroscopic mini-open rotator cuff repair has provided a useful addition to the armamentarium of the shoulder surgeon, this technique is not applicable for all rotator cuff tears. Since the exposure is somewhat limited, massive and retracted rotator cuff tears are difficult to treat through a mini-open technique due to lack of exposure. Larger tears requiring more extensive releases are more easily and reliably treated through a formal open approach. Additionally, rotator cuff tears with significant subscapularis involvement are difficult to manage also due to inadequate exposure.

Surgical Technique

The procedure is performed with the patient under interscalene block regional anesthesia. The patient is placed in the beach-chair position with the head and back of the operating table elevated. A shoulder arthroscopy-positioning device is often helpful to gain adequate exposure to the posterior aspect of the shoulder. Once adequately anesthetized, an examination under anesthesia is performed to assure full range of motion. The shoulder is prepped and draped and all osseous landmarks are carefully outlined with a marking pen. This facilitates accurate portal placement.

A standard posterior portal is placed approximately 2 cm inferior to and 2 cm medial to the posterolateral corner of the acromion. If necessary, an anterior portal is created to evaluate and treat any intra-articular pathology. A spinal needle is used to facilitate proper placement of this portal and is placed in the interval below the long head of the biceps and above the subscapularis tendon. A thorough inspection of the glenohumeral joint is performed. Arthroscopy allows visualization of associated intra-articular pathology that would not be possible with open repair of small and medium-sized rotator cuff tears. Significant degenerative changes of the glenohumeral joint or fraying of the labrum and biceps tendon may be encountered and treated accordingly. After a thorough evaluation of the glenohumeral joint, the insertion of the rotator cuff tendon is closely inspected. Partial thickness tears of the rotator cuff are probed and the extent of the tear is determined. Depending on the degree of cuff involvement, partial tears may be debrided with a shaver to stimulate a healing response or merely to enhance visualization of the defect. A spinal needle can be introduced percutaneously into the region of the tear, and through it, a colored suture can be passed to mark this region for identification during bursal side inspection in the subacromial space.

The arthroscope is removed from the glenohumeral joint and is placed into the subacromial space with the use of a blunt trocar. An anterolateral portal is made 2 cm distal and posterior to the anterolateral corner of the acromion. The portal should be centered over the rotator cuff tear. The portal incision is oriented horizontally along the skin creases parallel to the lateral acromial border. With the use of electrocautery and a full radius shaver, a bursectomy is performed to allow visualization of the bursal side of the rotator cuff. An arthroscopic anterior acromioplasty is performed. A 6.0-mm arthroscopic burr is used to complete the decompression (Figure 2.1). The burr may be inserted from the anterolateral portal or the posterior portal. Only enough bone is removed to flatten the undersurface of antero-inferior acromion. The goal is to create a smooth undersurface of the acromion without rough or irregular edges and to decompress the cuff. The acromion should be viewed from the lateral portal to confirm a flat, smooth undersurface.

After the subacromial space is decompressed, attention is turned to the rotator cuff. If the cuff was previously marked because of an undersurface tear, the bursal side is closely inspected and probed to determine the thickness of the remaining tendon. If a complete tear

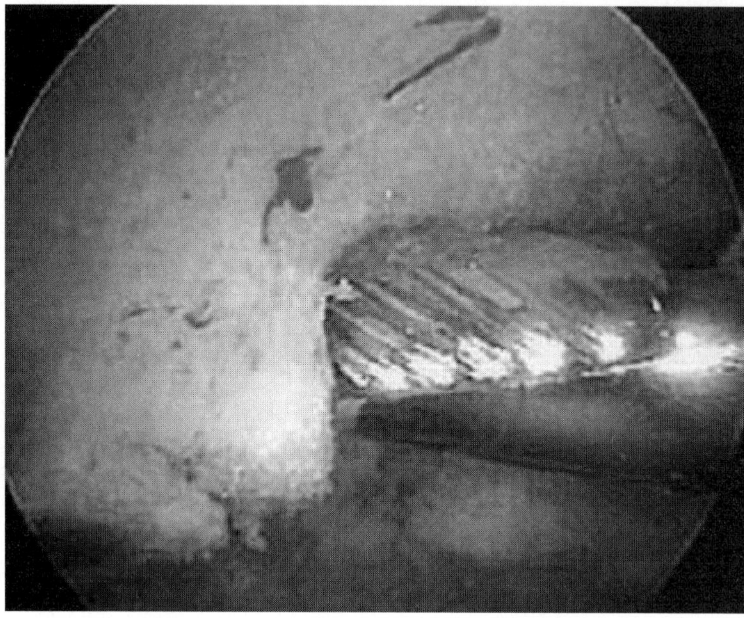

Figure 2.1. Subacromial decompression performed arthroscopically.

has been identified, the tendon edges are freshened with an arthroscopic shaver.

The arthroscope is then removed from the shoulder. The lateral portal incision is extended to a total length of 3 cm to 4 cm. Care is taken to ensure that the skin incision is horizontal and in line with Langer's lines (Figure 2.2). This allows for a more cosmetically pleasing scar. The subcutaneous tissue is undermined to expose the underlying deltoid fascia. The deltoid is split in line with its fibers, incorporating the preexisting arthroscopic puncture site in the split (Figure 2.3). The deltoid split should not extend more than 4 cm distal to the lateral edge of the acromion to avoid injury to the axillary nerve. Care is also taken while retracting the deltoid so as not to avulse the deltoid from its origin on the acromion. The acromioplasty is palpated through the split and maybe fine-tuned with a small rasp if necessary. Additional bursectomy may be performed to improve tear visualization.

Varying the rotation of the arm allows the rotator cuff tear to be positioned beneath the deltoid split. The torn edge of the rotator cuff tendon is visualized. Sutures are placed into the tendon along the periphery of the tear to assist with mobilization and repair (Figure 2.4). Extra-articular adhesions are released if not already performed arthroscopically. The goal is to mobilize the rotator cuff to obtain free excursion of the tendon to the anatomic neck with the arm at the side. Coracohumeral ligament release and intra-articular releases are performed as needed.

The greater tuberosity is visualized and the bony surface is prepared. The cortex is debrided of soft tissue and excrescences removed, but decortication is not recommended. This is supported by an elegant

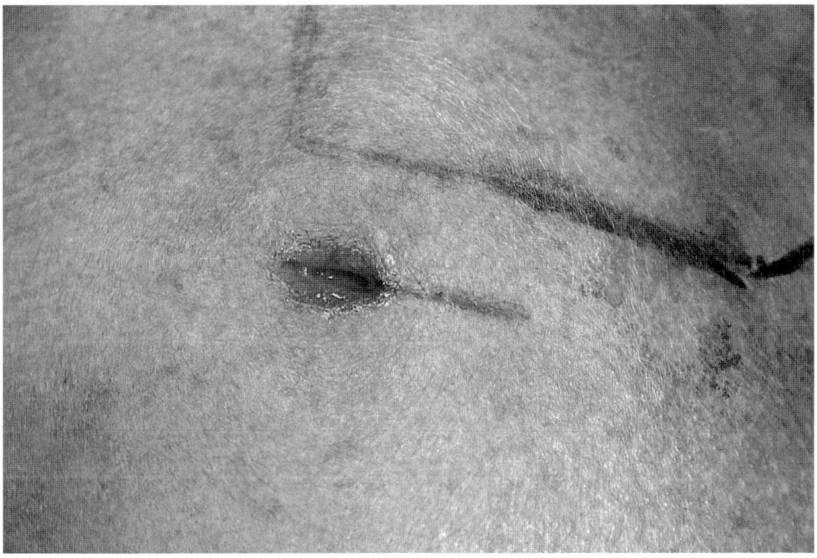

Figure 2.2. The anterolateral portal is extended within Langer's lines. The incision usually measures between 3 cm and 4 cm in length.

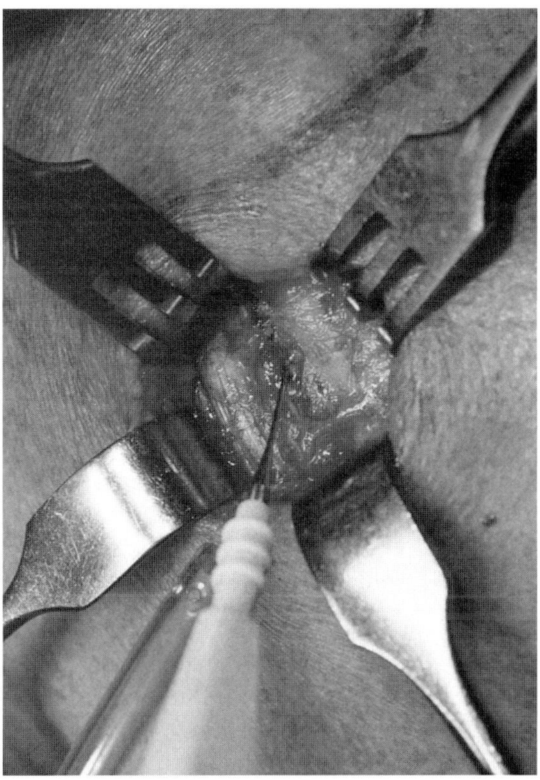

Figure 2.3. Once the subcutaneous dissection is performed, the deltoid is split in line with its fibers, incorporating the preexisting arthroscopic puncture site in the split.

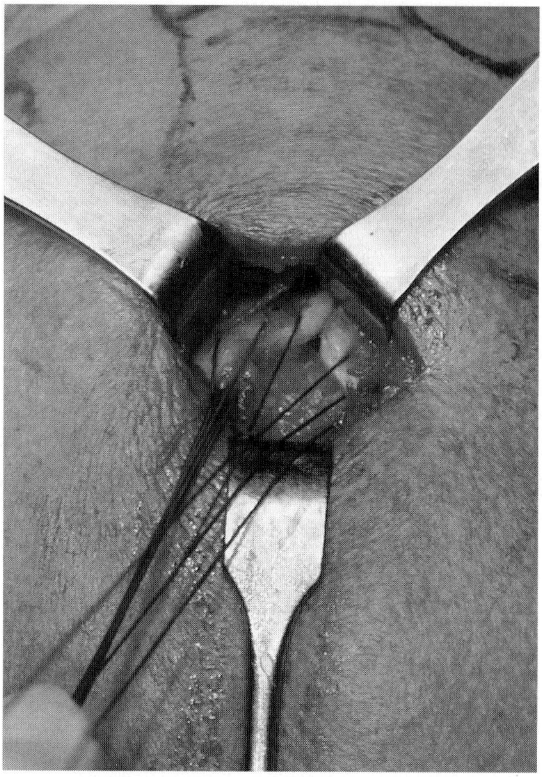

Figure 2.4. The torn edge of the rotator cuff tendon is visualized. Stay sutures are placed into the tendon along the periphery of the tear to assist with mobilization and repair.

study by St. Pierre and colleagues evaluating tendon healing to bone. The authors compared tendon healing when reattached directly to cortical bone versus tendon healing to cancellous bone through a trough. Histological analysis was indistinguishable between the cortical and cancellous specimens. The biomechanical properties between the two groups were approximately equal. The study demonstrated no significant benefit from the creation of a cancellous trough to achieve tendon-to-bone healing.[29]

Fixation of the tendon to the bone is obtained by means of either suture anchors or bone tunnels. Transosseous sutures are preferred to suture anchors in osteoporotic bone. If the bone quality is sufficient then suture anchors may be used. In either case, the rotator cuff tendon is repaired back to its insertion with multiple no. 2 nonabsorbable braided sutures (Figure 2.5). The repair should be performed with the arm at the patient's side. The arm is then taken through a range of motion to test for the safe zone to guide therapy.

The wound is irrigated and the deltoid fascia is meticulously reapproximated with nonabsorbable suture (Figure 2.6). The skin is closed with a running subcuticular suture, and a sterile dressing is applied.

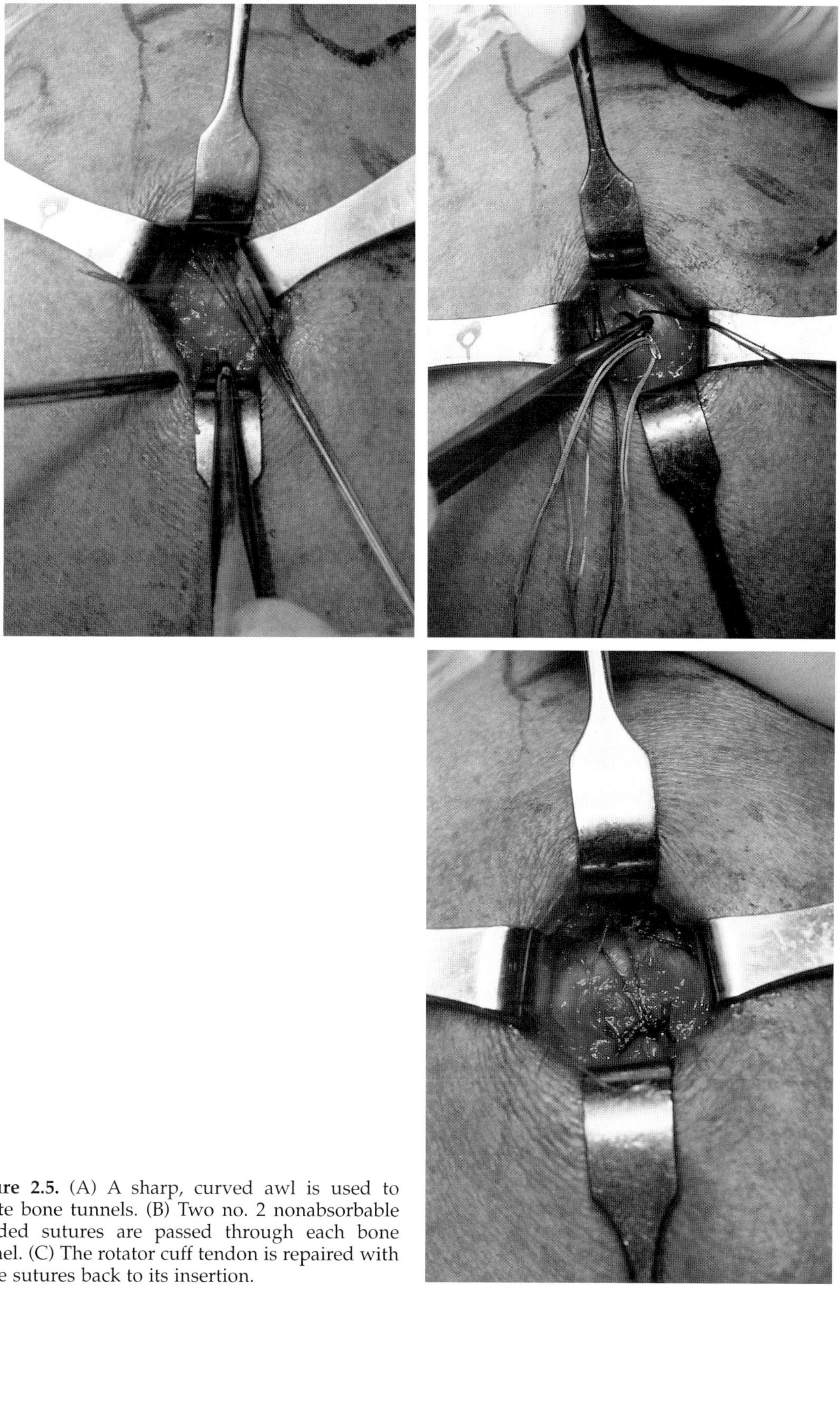

A B C

Figure 2.5. (A) A sharp, curved awl is used to create bone tunnels. (B) Two no. 2 nonabsorbable braided sutures are passed through each bone tunnel. (C) The rotator cuff tendon is repaired with these sutures back to its insertion.

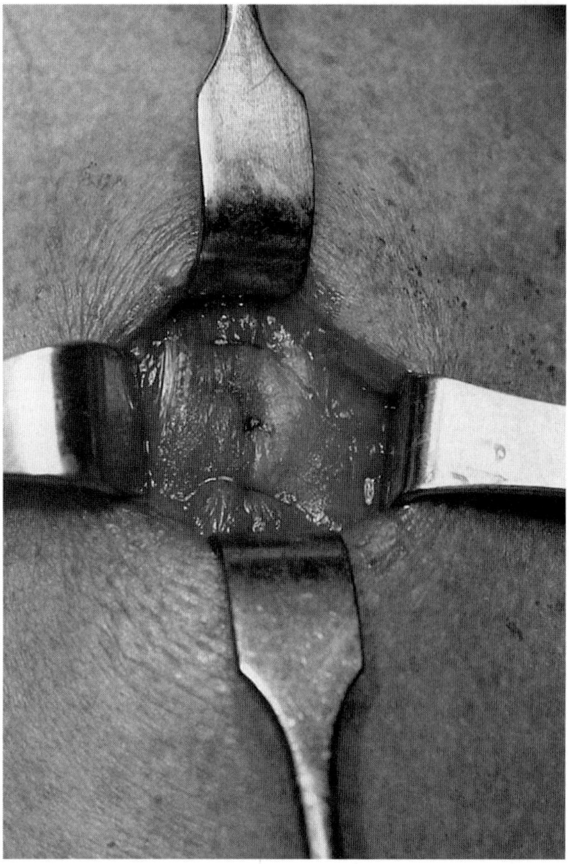

Figure 2.6. The deltoid fascia is meticulously reapproximated with nonabsorbable suture.

The shoulder is placed in a sling, and transported to the recovery room where immediate passive range of motion exercises are initiated.

Postoperative Protocol/Rehabilitation

Patients are discharged home either the same day of surgery or the next morning. Passive range of motion (PROM) exercises are initiated the same day of surgery including passive forward elevation, passive external rotation, and pendulum exercises. Internal rotation and active range of motion (AROM) exercises are prohibited. Elbow and hand exercises are also employed at this time. Exercises are performed 4 to 5 times daily on their own in addition to formal therapy several times a week. At 6 weeks postoperatively and when the tendon is deemed to be healed, the sling is discontinued and PROM exercises are advanced. Active assisted range of motion (AAROM) exercises are also initiated at this time progressing to AROM. Strengthening may begin at 8–12 weeks depending on the tear size and the quality of the tissue and repair. Larger tears are progressed more slowly. A progressive resistance and dynamic strengthening program is continued. All patients are encouraged to continue with a rotator cuff strengthening program as well as stretching for one full year after the repair.

Results

The outcome of mini-open repair in general has been good and comparable to long-term results seen in open rotator cuff repair series.[13–15,17–19,22,23,30,31] In 1990, Levy initially reported on 25 patients with a minimum of 1 year follow-up. Based on the UCLA shoulder rating, 96% of the patients were satisfied with the procedure and 80% of the patients were rated as good or excellent.[13]

The first long-term study of patients treated with the mini-incision technique was presented by Paulos and Kody in 1994. Eighteen patients were followed for an average of 46 months with 88% good to excellent results. Pain and function scores significantly improved with 94% of the patients reporting satisfaction with their results.[14]

Warner and associates reported on 24 patients who were carefully selected for the mini-open technique based on strict preoperative selection criteria. The preoperative criteria included refractory pain, good ROM and strength, absences of superior humeral head migration, and MRI evidence of minimally retracted tear. Seven of the 24 patients required conversion to an open approach to mobilize retracted and friable tendon tissue in a complex tear configuration. The remaining 17 patients underwent transosseosus rotator cuff repair through a mini-open approach. The average post-operative ASES score was 96 out of 100. The authors concluded that through careful selection mini-open rotator cuff repair could achieve excellent results.[22]

Baker and Liu compared formal open and arthroscopically assisted mini-open rotator cuff repairs in 37 patients. The open repair group comprised 20 shoulders with an average follow-up of 3.3 years; the arthroscopically assisted repair group consisted of 17 shoulders with an average follow-up of 3.2 years. Overall, the open repair group had 80% good to excellent results and 88% patient satisfaction. The arthroscopically assisted mini-open group had 85% good to excellent results and 92% patient satisfaction. The functional outcome between the two groups did not significantly differ; however, the mini-open group was hospitalized fewer days and returned to previous activity an average of 1 month earlier.[15]

Hata et al. in 2001 reported on comparison of 22 mini-open rotator cuff repairs and 36 formal open repairs. Results of the mini-open repair were as good as those of conventional open repairs for small, moderate, and large tears of the rotator cuff. No significant difference was seen between the UCLA shoulder scores of the two groups 1 year after the repair. However, active forward elevation in the mini-open group was significantly greater than in the control group 3 and 6 months after surgery. The authors also concluded that the mini-open repair patients were able to return to sports and social activities earlier than the formal open repair patients.[32]

Summary

The arthroscopically assisted mini-open approach has proven to be an effective means of treating rotator cuff tears. It has become a popular and accepted procedure with proven clinical results.[13–23] It combines the benefits of arthroscopic subacromial decompression with the benefits of open rotator cuff repair. Importantly, it has potential to diminish deltoid injury, which can translate into less perioperative pain and an easier functional recovery when the principles of patient selection and technique are adhered to meticulously.

References

1. Codman EA. Complete rupture of the supraspinatus tendon: Operative treatment with report of two successful cases. Boston Med Surg J. 1911; 164:708–710.
2. Neer CS II. Anterior acromioplasty for the chronic impingement syndrome in the shoulder: A preliminary report. J Bone Joint Surg Am. 1972;54:41–50.
3. Neer CS II, ed. Shoulder reconstruction. Philadelphia: WB Saunders; 1990:41–142.
4. Bigliani L, Cordasco F, McIlveen S, et al. Operative treatment of massive rotator cuff tears: long term results. J Shoulder Elbow Surg. 1992;1:120–130.
5. Gazielly DF, Gleyze P, Montagnon C. Functional and anatomical results after rotator cuff repair. Clin Orthop. 1994;304:43–53.
6. Gupta R, Leggin BG, Iannotti JP. Results of surgical repair of full thickness tears of the rotator cuff. Orthop Clin North Am. 1997;28:241–248.
7. Hawkins RJ, Misamore GW, Hobelka PE. Surgery for full-thickness rotator cuff tears. J Bone Joint Surg Am. 1985;67:1349–1355.
8. Neer CS II, Flatow EL, Lech O. Tears of the rotator cuff. Long term results of anterior ancromioplasty and repair. Orthop Trans. 1988;12:735.
9. Burman MS. Arthroscopy or the direct visualization of joints: An experimental cadaver study. J Bone Joint Surg Am. 1931;13:669–695.
10. Wantanabe M. Arthroscopy of the shoulder joint. In: Wantanabe M, ed. Arthroscopy of Small Joints. Tokyo: Igaku-Shoin; 1985:45–56.
11. Wiley AM, Older MB. Shoulder arthroscopy: investigations with a fibrooptic instrument. Am J Sports Med. 1980;8:18.
12. Ellman H, Kay SP. Arthroscopic subacromial decompression for chronic impingement. Two to five year results. J Bone Joint Surg Br. 1991;73:395–398.
13. Levy HJ, Uribe JW, Delaney LG. Arthroscopic assisted rotator cuff repair: preliminary results. Arthroscopy 1990;6:55–60.
14. Paulos LE, Kody MH. Arthroscopically enhanced "miniapproach" to rotator cuff repair. Am J Sports Med. 1994;22:19–25.
15. Baker CL, Liu SH. Comparison of open and arthroscopically assisted rotator cuff repairs. Am J Sports Med. 1995;23:99–104.
16. Blevins FT, Warren RF, Cavo C, et al. Arthroscopic assisted rotator cuff repair: results using a mini-open deltoid splitting approach. Arthroscopy 1996;12: 50–59.
17. Hersch JC, Sgaglione NA. Arthroscopically assisted mini-open rotator cuff repairs: functional outcome at 2- to 7- year follow-up. Am J Sports Med. 2000; 28:301–311.
18. Liu SH, Baker CL. Arthroscopically assisted rotator cuff repair: correlation of functional results with integrity of the cuff. Arthroscopy 1994;10:54–60.

19. Liu SH. Arthroscopically assisted rotator cuff repair. J Bone Joint Surg Br. 1994; 76:592–595.
20. Park JY, Levine WN, Marra G, et al. Portal-extension approach for the repair of small and medium rotator cuff tears. Am J Sports Med. 2000;28: 312–316.
21. Pollock RG, Flatow EL. The rotator cuff: Full-thickness tears: Mini-open repair. Orthop Clin North Am. 1997;28:169–177.
22. Warner JJ, Goitz RJ, Irrgang JJ, Groff YJ. Arthroscopic-assisted rotator cuff repair: patient selection and treatment outcome. J Shoulder Elbow Surg 1997;6:463–472.
23. Weber SC, Schaefer R. "Mini-open" versus traditional open repair in the management of small and moderate size tears of the rotator cuff (abstract). Arthroscopy 1993;9:365–366.
24. Karas EH, Iannotti JP. Failed repair of the rotator cuff: evaluation and treatment of complications. Instr Course Lect. 1998;47:87–95.
25. Mansat P, Cofield RH, Kersten TE, et al. Complications of rotator cuff repair. Orthop Clin North Am. 1997;28:205–213
26. Yamaguchi, K. Complications of rotator cuff repair. Tech Orthop. 1997;12: 33–41.
27. Miller C, Savoie FH. Glenohumeral abnormalities associated with full-thickness tears of the rotator cuff. Orthop Rev. 1994;23:159–162.
28. Gartsman GM, Taverna E. The incidence of glenohumeral joint abnormalities associated with full thickness, reparable rotator cuff tears. Arthroscopy 1997;13:450–455.
29. St. Pierre P, Olson EJ, Elliott JJ, et al. Tendon-healing to cortical bone compared with healing to cancellous trough. A biomechanical and histological evaluation in goats. J Bone Joint Surg. 1995;77:1858–1866.
30. Posada A, Uribe JW, Hechtman KS, et al. Mini-deltoid splitting rotator cuff repair: do results deteriorate with time? Arthroscopy 2000;16:137–141.
31. Shinners TJ, Noordsij PG, Orwin JF. Arthroscopically assisted mini-open rotator cuff repair. Arthroscopy 2002;18:21–26.
32. Hata Y, Saitoh S, Murakami N, et al. A less invasive surgery for rotator cuff tear: mini-open repair. J Shoulder Elbow Surg. 2001;10:11–16.

3

Mini-Incision Fixation of Proximal Humeral Four-Part Fractures

Jim Hsu and Leesa M. Galatz

Proximal humerus fractures are notoriously difficult to treat. The surrounding rotator cuff musculature makes intraoperative assessment of the reduction of fractures, especially those involving the articular surface, difficult to assess. Even fractures fixed with open reduction and internal fixation often require intraoperative fluoroscopic guidance to ensure appropriate anatomic reduction. The anatomic relationship between the articular surface and the surrounding rotator cuff has a critical influence on the final result. Furthermore, fixation is a challenge to maintain as the rotator cuff exerts strong deforming forces on the tuberosities, which are often of poor bone quality and do not hold hardware well. In spite of this, many unstable proximal humerus fractures are treated successfully with established methods of open reduction and internal fixation.

Four-part proximal humerus fractures as classified by Neer,[1,2] are particularly problematic. Historically, they have a very high rate of avascular necrosis following fixation. Because of this, Neer recommended hemiarthroplasty for the treatment of these fractures. However, a subgroup of 4-part proximal humerus fractures, the 4-part valgus impacted fracture, is readily amenable to reduction and fixation. Neer did not specify this fracture in his initial classification system. In the more recent AO/ASIS classification, however, the valgus impacted humeral head fracture is regarded as a separate type of fracture.[3] The valgus impacted 4-part fracture is an ideal fracture for minimally invasive fixation, and it is the focus of this chapter.

There has been a surge of interest in minimally invasive techniques in many different subspecialty areas of orthopedics. The recent trauma literature contains several reports of percutaneous fixation of the femur, tibia and tibial pilon fractures.[4–6] Principles of preserving blood supply and minimizing soft tissue stripping are receiving increased attention in fracture fixation. With respect to the treatment of proximal humerus fractures, there have been a few reports in the past several years of successful percutaneous reduction and fixation.[7–9] In selected fractures, percutaneous pinning allows preservation of the intact soft tissue sleeve and periosteal blood supply while obtaining and maintaining a stable reduction. Other potential advantages include smaller incisions, less dissection and less scarring. A minimally invasive approach minimizes trauma to the rotator cuff and deltoid, and with experience can decrease operative time. While still a difficult, technically demanding procedure, percutaneous pinning of valgus-impacted 4-part proximal humerus fractures shows considerable potential. This chapter discusses the unique characteristics of valgus-impacted fractures and outlines in detail the minimally invasive fixation technique.

Historical Perspective

Percutaneous pinning has been used in a variety of subtypes of proximal humerus fractures (Table 3.1). Böhler[10] originally described a method of closed reduction and pinning for the treatment of epiphyseal fractures of the proximal end of the humerus in adolescents. This technique has been modified over the years and applied to treat proximal humerus fractures more commonly seen in the older population. In 1991, Jakob[11] reported on the treatment of 19 valgus-impacted 4-part proximal humerus fractures, 5 of which were treated closed. This is the first description of elevation of the valgus-impacted articular fragment with minimal soft tissue dissection to preserve remaining blood supply to the proximal humerus. The valgus-impacted 4-part fracture configuration became recognized as one in which there was a significantly lower rate of avascular necrosis compared to other 4-part fractures. In 1995 Resch[12] reported a series of 22 patients with open reduction and internal fixation of the valgus-impacted proximal humerus fracture, further solidifying the understanding of the fracture as one that does not require hemiarthroplasty. In fact, the results of these studies showed better results after fixation than the historical results after hemiarthroplasty.

In 1992 Jaberg et al.[7] reported on percutaneous stabilization of 54 displaced proximal humerus fractures of varying types. In this series closed reduction was performed and the fractures were stabilized with K wires placed in both antegrade and retrograde fashion. Resch et al.[8] later reported on percutaneous fixation of 3-part and 4-part proximal humerus fractures. The authors described using a pointed hook retractor percutaneously in the subacromial space for reduction of greater tuberosity fragments and elevation of the humeral head in the valgus-impacted 4-part fractures.

Table 3.1. Fractures amenable to percutaneous pinning

2-part	Surgical neck Greater tuberosity * Lesser tuberosities
3-part	Surgical neck/greater tuberosity * Surgical neck/lesser tuberosity
4-part	Valgus impacted

* Without associated posterior dislocation.

Anatomic Considerations

Four-part valgus-impacted humerus fractures have been described as "impacted with inferior subluxation,"[13] "impacted and little displaced fractures,"[3] and minimally displaced fractures.[14] Fourteen percent of all humeral head fractures are valgus impacted. The articular segment is impacted into the metaphysis, causing avulsion of both the greater and the lesser tuberosities with a line of fracture through the anatomic neck (Figure 3.1A and B). The blood supply to the articular segment via the tuberosities is therefore disrupted. The main source of vascularization for the humeral head, the ascending anterolateral branch of the anterior humeral circumflex artery,[15,16] is interrupted at its point of entry into the humeral head in the area of the intertubercular groove. The only remaining blood supply is medially via the periosteum. Numerous vessels ascend along the inferior capsule and periosteum from both the anterior and posterior humeral circumflex arteries to the calcar region of the medial portion of the anatomic neck. Any lateral displacement of the articular fragment damages the periosteal hinge and consequently interrupts this last remaining source of vascularization. Therefore, a true valgus-impacted humeral head fracture will be impacted such that the medial hinge is intact. Any lateral displacement of the head segment has been associated with a higher rate of avascular necrosis.[12]

Indications for Percutaneous Pinning

Successful outcome after operative treatment of unstable proximal humerus fractures, regardless of approach or choice of hardware,

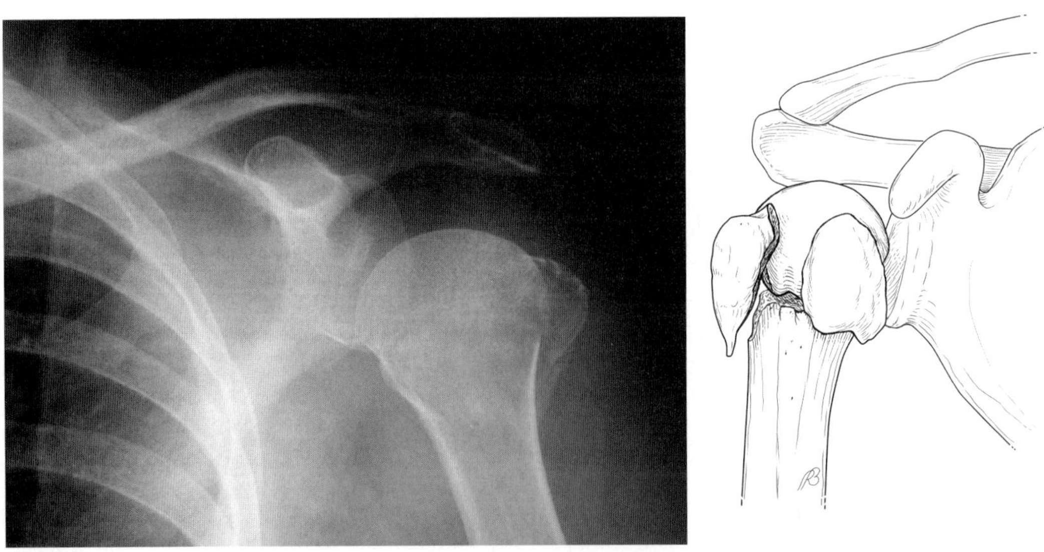

A B

Figure 3.1. (A) This AP radiograph of a valgus-impacted 4-part fracture demonstrates the intact medial periosteal hinge with avulsion and lateral displacement of the greater tuberosity. (B) This valgus-impacted 4-part fracture drawing also demonstrates the otherwise superimposed lesser tuberosity fragment fracture, making this a true 4-part fracture.

Table 3.2. Conditions for successful pinning

Good bone stock
Intact medial calcar
Substantial greater tuberosity fragment
Stable reduction under fluoroscopy after pinning
Reliable, cooperative patient

depends on three critical factors: (1) anatomic reduction, (2) stable fixation, and (3) careful management of soft tissues. Plate fixation offers a reliably stable construct in patients with good bone quality. The surgical approach and plate application require more extensive soft tissue stripping, which may contribute to the problem of devascularization and subsequent avascular necrosis. Intramedullary rods with cerclage wires are another alternative and have been shown to be a biomechanically stable construct.[17] However, mechanical impingement in the subacromial space remains a potential problem.

Percutaneous pinning offers an excellent alternative to the open approach in selected fractures (Table 3.2). An anatomic reduction and stable fixation are just as important in this procedure. Patients must have good bone stock to ensure secure pin fixation. The displaced greater tuberosity fragment requiring reduction and fixation must be large and substantial enough to hold 1 or 2 screws. An intact medial calcar region is important for stability after reduction of the proximal humerus. This is the portion that must be intact in the valgus-impacted humeral head fracture to preserve remaining vascularity.

Patient compliance is critical. Therefore, patient selection plays an important role. Postoperative rehabilitation is more conservative than after an open procedure. Patients are generally immobilized for the first couple of weeks. Patients must undergo close surveillance and consistent follow-up in order to prevent complications related to pin migration, either antegrade or retrograde, and to detect any unexpected early loss of fixation.

Percutaneous pinning is contraindicated in (1) patients with poor bone stock, (2) fracture in which there is a comminuted proximal shaft fragment, especially in the medial calcar region, (3) displaced 4-part fractures (other than the valgus-impacted configuration) in elderly people requiring hemiarthroplasty, (4) non-compliant patients or patients unable or unwilling to comply with strict follow-up and rehabilitation limitations, and (5) fractures with displaced greater tuberosity fragments that are too comminuted or small for hardware fixation.

Patient Evaluation

Patient evaluation begins with a complete history and physical examination. The mechanism of injury should be noted and all associated injuries thoroughly evaluated. Most proximal humerus fractures are the result of low energy falls in elderly patients. Another subset of fractures results from high energy injuries in the younger population. A thorough neurovascular examination should be performed prior to any attempt at percutaneous pinning. The patient's social situation should be assessed in order to discern whether the patient is appropriate in terms of complying with rehabilitation and close follow-up. Patients should be advised that one of the disadvantages of this procedure is that the pins may be uncomfortable in the subcutaneous position. They require subsequent removal as either an office or short operative procedure.

Radiographic evaluation consists of 4 standard views: an anteroposterior view of the shoulder, an anteroposterior view of the scapula, axillary view and a scapular Y. This combination of radiographs is helpful in evaluating posterior displacement of greater tuberosity fragments as well as anterior displacement of the shaft fragment. These x-rays are usually sufficient. A CT scan can be considered if further radiographic evaluation is desirable. Three-dimensional reconstructions are rarely necessary. Studies help evaluate the suitability of the particular fracture for percutaneous reduction and fixation.

Elderly people with significant osteopenia and non-compliant patients may be better candidates for open reduction and internal fixation, a procedure that can potentially lead to more secure fixation biomechanically. Less concern exists over loss of fixation and pin migration. Preoperative consent should include possible conversion to an open procedure if the fracture cannot be adequately reduced and held with percutaneous fixation.

Surgical Procedure

Patient Positioning

Patient position must allow unencumbered access to the shoulder, both for easy visualization under fluoroscopy and for pin placement (Figure 3.2). The patient is placed on a radiolucent operating room table with the head in a head holder such that the shoulder is proximal and lateral to the edge of the table. Adequate visualization of the shoulder under fluoroscopy should be confirmed before prepping and draping. The procedure can be performed with the patient in the supine position; however, raising the head of the bed 15 degrees to 20 degrees is often helpful for orientation and instrumentation. A mechanical arm holder is used for positioning the arm during the procedure. The holder can be useful for placing traction on the arm when necessary. The C-arm fluoroscope is positioned at the head of the bed, parallel to the patient, leaving the area lateral to the shoulder open for access and pin placement. Alternatively, the C-arm can be angled perpendicular to the patient; however, it is much more difficult to get an axillary view with the C-arm in this position. The monitor is placed on the opposite side of the patient for easy visualization by the surgeon. We recommend not using an adhesive, plastic drape directly on the skin at the operative site because it can become adherent to the pins inadvertently during insertion and may be introduced into the wound. The shoulder should be draped to accommodate conversion to an open procedure, should it be necessary.

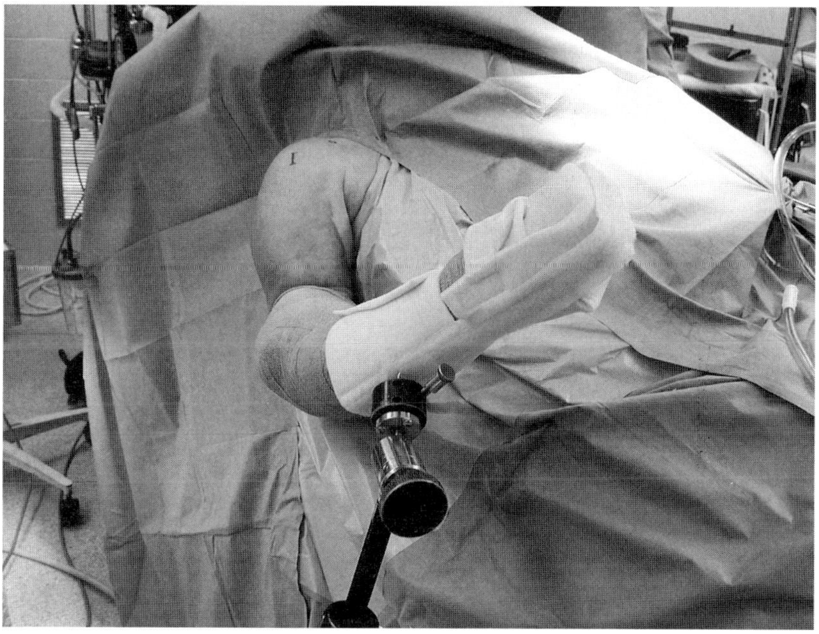

Figure 3.2. Patient positioning allows for unencumbered access to anterior, posterior and lateral shoulder for easy visualization on a radiolucent table as well as pin placement. The reduction portal is drawn in its location approximately 1–2 cm distal to the anterolateral corner of the acromion.

Percutaneous Reduction

Bony landmarks are outlined on the skin, specifically the acromion, clavicle and coracoid. A small 1-cm to 2-cm incision is made 2 to 3 cm distal to the anterolateral corner of the acromion. Formation of this "reduction portal" facilitates reduction of the fracture percutaneously prior to pin fixation (Figure 3.3). The reduction portal is positioned distal to the anterolateral corner of the acromion at the level of the surgical neck of the humerus, posterior and lateral to the biceps tendon. The fracture between the greater and the lesser tuberosities lies approximately $^{1}/_{2}$-1 cm posterior to the biceps groove. Localizing the reduction portal over the split between the tuberosities enables elevation of the head fragment by placing the instrument through the natural fracture line.

The deltoid is gently and bluntly spread in order to avoid possible injury to the anterior branch of the axillary nerve in this location. A blunt-tipped elevator or a small bone tamp is placed through the reduction portal at the level of the surgical neck through the split in the tuberosities and under the lateral aspect of the humeral head (Figure 3.4). Position is checked under fluoroscopy. The bone tamp or elevator is tapped with a mallet, elevating the head into the reduced position, restoring the normal angle between the humeral shaft and the articular surface of the humeral head. Characteristically, in a valgus-impacted proximal humerus fracture, once the head fragment is reduced anatomically the tuberosities naturally fall into the reduced position. Occasionally, the lesser tuberosity may still be displaced

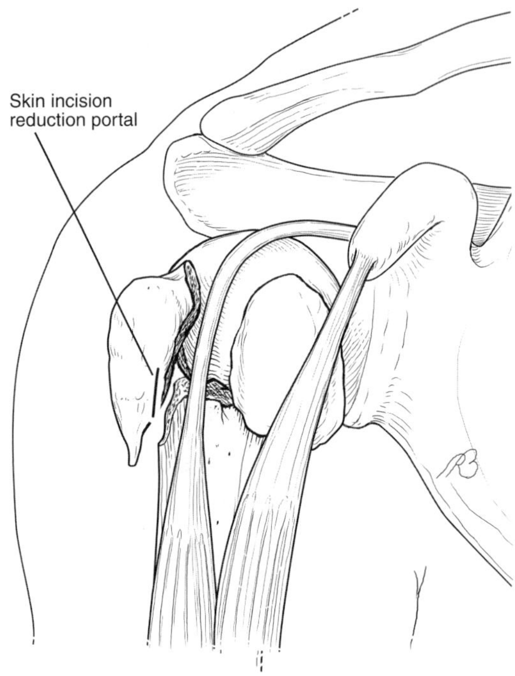

Figure 3.3. The reduction portal is positioned distal to the anterolateral corner of the acromion at the level of the surgical neck of the humerus. This allows for easy instrumentation between the greater and the lesser tuberosity for reducing the fracture.

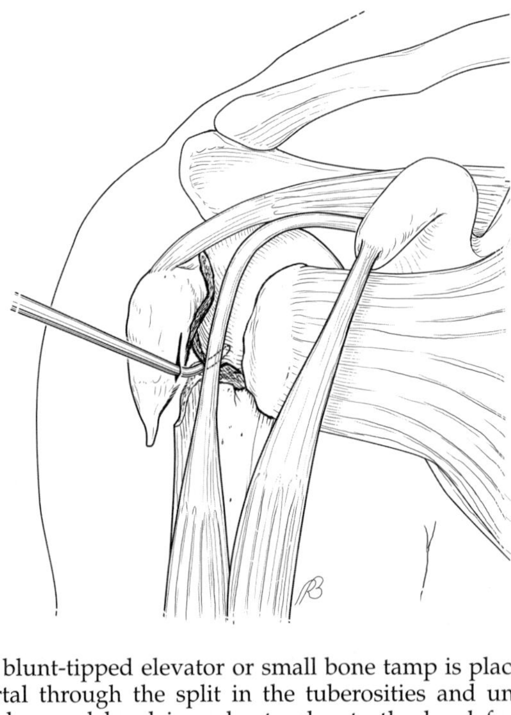

Figure 3.4. A blunt-tipped elevator or small bone tamp is placed through the reduction portal through the split in the tuberosities and under the lateral aspect of the humeral head in order to elevate the head fragment into an anatomic position.

medially and can potentially require lateral traction via a small hook in the subdeltoid space to bring it into anatomic position. Final reduction is confirmed using fluoroscopic imaging.

A potential pitfall includes overly aggressive impaction with the mallet, leading to loss of cancellous bone in the head fragment and potential fracture. Valgus-impacted fractures can only be reduced using this technique before healing has taken place. Ideally, it is recommended in the first 2 weeks after the fracture. Beyond that timepoint, more aggressive manipulation may be required in order to mobilize the head fragment.

Instrumentation

Instrumentation includes 2.5-mm or 2.7-mm terminally threaded pins. Terminally threaded K wires or alternatively, the guidewires from the Synthes (Synthes, Paoli, PA) 7.3-mm cannulated screw set can be used. Fully threaded pins are not used to protect the soft tissues. Terminal threads are desirable in order to prevent migration. Pins are inserted through very small incisions. Optimally, a drill guide should be used. A drill guide can be obtained from a small fragment fracture set. Alternatively, a drill guide used for arthroscopic anchor insertion can be useful.

Two to 3 retrograde pins are placed from the shaft into the head fragment. The pins should enter the skin distal to the site where the pins actually enter the bone in order to obtain the correct angle so that the pins do not cut out posteriorly before gaining fixation in the head fragment (Figure 3.5). The direction of the pins is generally anterolateral to posteromedial because of the anatomic retroversion of the humeral head. Pins should not be placed directly in the coronal plane because of the normal retroversion of the humeral head. This results in pins cutting out anteriorly. The starting points of the pins should not be too close to one another to avoid a stress riser in the lateral cortex. Additionally, the pins should be multi-directional in order to stabilize the construct. Two to 3 pins parallel to one another will act as a single point of fixation, allowing rotation.

The tuberosities are then secured. Pins or cannulated screws can be used. We prefer fixation with cannulated screws because the ends of the pins protrude through the deltoid and can cause irreparable muscle damage. Pins, if used, must be removed before starting early range of motion exercises for this reason. We prefer 4.5-mm cannulated screws to secure the greater tuberosity. The 4.5-mm screws have a substantial guidewire and come in adequate lengths. The guidewire is placed under fluoroscopic guidance through the greater tuberosity approximately 1 cm below the rotator cuff insertion, engaging the medial cortex of the shaft fragment (Figure 3.6). A screw with a washer is used, but one must be careful not to over-tighten the screw as the compression with the washer can potentially fracture the greater tuberosity. Ideally two screws are placed. The second screw can be a cancellous screw directed into the articular fragment. Often with one antegrade screw and two retrograde pins, there is not enough room in the metaphysis for a second antegrade screw from the greater tuberosity.

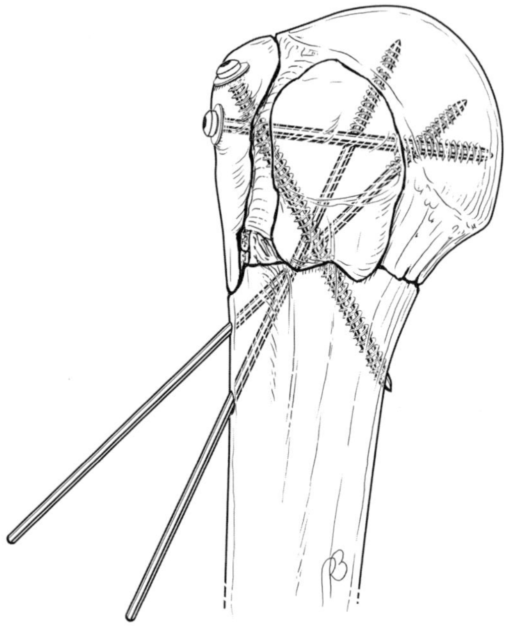

Figure 3.5. The pins are placed in an anterolateral to posteromedial position because of the anatomic retroversion of the humeral head. Screws should be placed lateral and distal enough to avoid mechanical impingement symptoms in the subacromial space.

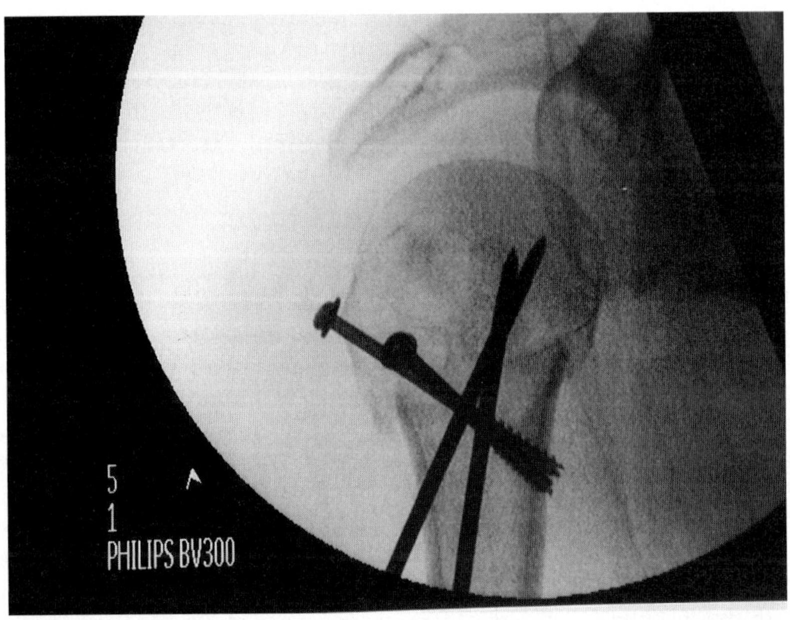

Figure 3.6. The pins and screws are placed under fluoroscopic guidance. Reduction of the fracture as well as hardware placement can be checked using continuous fluoroscopy or spot views in multiple positions.

Fixation of the lesser tuberosity is debatable. Once the humeral head and greater tuberosity are reduced and fixed, the lesser tuberosity is nearly always in anatomic position. If there is excessive medial displacement, a hook retractor can be used through the reduction portal in the subdeltoid space to move the fragment laterally and a percutaneous cannulated screw can be placed from the anterior to posterior direction to secure the lesser tuberosity. We generally prefer to leave the lesser tuberosity in the reduced position without additional fixation. It has not been found to result in any functional disability postoperatively.

After percutaneous fixation, the pins are cut below the skin. This reduces the chance of superficial pin tract infection. All of these small incisions are closed using interrupted nylon suture.

Postoperative Management

Following the procedure, the affected extremity is immobilized in a sling for approximately 3 weeks. Active wrist, elbow and hand range-of-motion exercises are encouraged. Radiographs are obtained 1, 3, and 6 weeks postoperatively. If the fracture is thought to be stable, pendulum exercises can be initiated immediately; however, in many cases, pendulum exercises, passive forward flexion in the scapular plane and external rotation are not started for 3 weeks provided the fracture remains stable. Active assisted and active range-of-motion exercises are initiated at 6 weeks if there are signs of fracture healing. Progression to light strengthening is as tolerated at that point. The pins are removed 4 to 6 weeks postoperatively. In a very unstable fracture configuration, it is optimal to leave the pins in for 6 weeks; however, loosening may necessitate earlier removal. The pins are removed either as an office procedure or in the operating room under local anesthesia, depending on patient and surgeon preference.

Results

Jakob et al.[11] first presented his results of the treatment of 19 valgus-impacted 4-part proximal humerus fractures. Five of these were treated closed. He reported an avascular necrosis rate of 26%. Jaberg et al.[7] reported the results of 48 fractures fixed with percutaneous stabilization of unstable fractures of the proximal humerus fracture. This series had 29 fractures of the surgical neck, 3 of the anatomic neck, eight 3-part fractures, five 4-part fractures, and 3 fracture dislocations. They had 38 good to excellent results, 10 fair and 4 poor. One patient with a 2-part fracture had avascular necrosis at approximately 11 months postoperatively. Eight had localized transient avascular necrosis of the small portion of the humeral head, which did not necessitate humeral head replacement.

Resch et al.[12] published his results of percutaneous pinning of nine 3-part fractures and eighteen 4-part fractures. None of the 3-part fractures went on to avascular necrosis, and all had a good or very good result. There was an 11% incidence of avascular necrosis in the 4-part fractures. Those with anatomical reconstructions did very well. Five of these patients had 4-part fractures with significant lateral displacement at a humeral head. One of these required revision one week after surgery, and one went on to late avascular necrosis. Soete et al.[18] recommended against percutaneous pinning for the treatment of 4-part proximal humerus fracture because of avascular necrosis and unsatisfactory reduction. These were not all valgus-impacted proximal humerus fractures, however.

Complications

The most worrisome complication of percutaneous pinning is nerve injury. Nerves at risk are primarily the axillary, musculocutaneous, and to a lesser extent the radial nerve. The axillary nerve courses posteriorly through the quadrangular space to the undersurface of the deltoid and is located approximately 3 cm to 5 cm distal to the lateral border of the acromion. When making the anterolateral reduction portal, the deltoid should be gently and bluntly spread in order to avoid any nerve traction. This incision is generally superior to the zone where the nerve is located; however, one should still be cautious during this portion of the procedure. The axillary nerve is also at risk when placing screws through the greater tuberosity. If the screws are placed more inferior along the greater tuberosity, a drill guide can be inserted more superiorly and gently advanced distally in order to keep the nerve from the path of the drill.

An anatomic study of percutaneous pinning of the proximal part of the humerus[19] demonstrated that the proximal lateral retrograde pins were located a mean distance of 3 mm from the anterior branch of the axillary nerve. The screws through the tuberosity were located a mean distance of 6 mm and 7 mm from the axillary nerve and the posterior humeral circumflex artery. While they are at risk during placement, these structures are easily protected if the screws are placed in careful fashion. The anterior pin was located adjacent to the long head of the biceps tendon, 11 mm from the cephalic vein, and could potentially be near the musculocutaneous nerve.[19] These findings emphasize the importance of using a drill guide. The radial nerve will not be injured as long as the retrograde pins are inserted proximal to the deltoid insertion.

The most common complication is pin migration. Most commonly, the pins back out and become prominent under the skin. Proximal migration into the joint is possible. Percutaneous pinning requires very close follow-up and strict patient compliance. Serious complications of pin migration are prevented by following patients with radiographs at regular intervals. Loss of fixation may occur as with any type of fracture fixation. In some situations this can be treated with repeat percutaneous pinning. However, if it is believed that the fracture is in an unstable configuration and further loss of fixation may occur, open reduction and internal fixation is recommended. Malunion may result. This is usually well tolerated if the tuberosities are well reduced in relation to the humeral head. Displacement at the surgical neck is well tolerated in comparison to that of the tuberosities.

Superficial infections of the pins have been reported. Jaberg et al.[7] reported 7 superficial pin tract infections which were treated with local debridement and antibiotics. There was one deep infection in a diabetic patient. In his series the pins were left through the skin. Because of this risk, we prefer to cut the pins deep to the skin.

Conclusion

Percutaneous pinning of proximal humerus fractures requires a thorough 3-dimensional understanding of proximal humeral anatomy. Placement of the pins can be difficult and dangerous if the pins exit the bone incorrectly or penetrate nearby neurovascular structures. Assessment of reduction and stability can be challenging. The surgeon must be able to use the 2-dimensional image obtained on fluoroscopy to assess a 3-dimensional reduction. Success of this procedure is also dependent upon patient selection. Only fractures which can be stably reduced with pins are appropriate for this procedure. The 4-part valgus-impacted proximal humerus fracture is generally very stable after reduction and is easily amenable to this type of treatment. Excessive comminution of the proximal shaft, especially the medial calcar area, indicates a fracture, which may require open treatment with more secure fixation. The surgeon should always be prepared to convert to an open reduction and internal fixation if percutaneous pinning becomes difficult or impossible. In spite of the above concerns, successful percutaneous pinning in an appropriate patient offers significant advantages over open treatment in a valgus-impacted 4-part proximal humerus fracture. Benefits include less dissection and the ability to take advantage of the intact soft tissue sleeve, which exists in these proximal humerus fractures. The procedure is shorter in terms of operative time and results in less blood loss. Additional advantages may include less scar formation and possibly accelerated rehabilitation. As our experience with percutaneous pinning increases and we become more familiar with this technique, we will likely see expanding indications for percutaneous pinning.

References

1. Neer CS II. Displaced proximal humeral fractures. II. Treatment of three-part and four-part displacement. J Bone Joint Surg Am. 1970;52(6):1090–1103.
2. Neer CS II. Displaced proximal humeral fractures. I. Classification and evaluation. J Bone Joint Surg Am. 1970;52(6):1077–1089.
3. Jakob RP, Kristiansen T, Mayo K, et al. Classification and aspects of treatment of fractures of the proximal humerus. In: Bateman J, Welsh R, eds. Surgery of the Shoulder. Philadelphia: B. C. Decker; 1984.
4. Probe RA. Minimally invasive fixation of tibial pilon fractures. Oper Tech Orthop. 2001;11(3):205–217.
5. Kanlic EM, Pesantez RF, Pachon CM. Minimally invasive plate osteosynthesis of the femur. Oper Tech Orthop. 2001;11(3):156–167.
6. Morgan S, Jeray K. Minimally invasive plate osteosynthesis in fractures of the tibia. Oper Tech Orthop. 2001;11(3):195–204.

7. Jaberg H, Warner JJP, Jakob RP. Percutaneous stabilization of unstable fractures of the humerus. J. Bone Joint Surg Am. 1992;74-A(4):508–515.
8. Resch H, Povacz P, Frohlich R, et al. Percutaneous fixation of three- and four-part fractures of the proximal humerus. J Bone Joint Surg Br. 1997; 79(2):295–300.
9. Chen CY, Chao EK, Tu YK, et al. Closed management and percutaneous fixation of unstable proximal humerus fractures. J Trauma. 1998; 45(6): 1039–1045.
10. Bohler J. Perkutane osteosynthese mit dem Rontgenbildrier-Starker. Wiener Klin Wochenschr. 1962;74:485–487.
11. Jakob RP, Miniaci A, Anson PS, et al. Four-part valgus impacted fractures of the proximal humerus. J Bone Joint Surg Br. 1991;73(2):295–298.
12. Resch H, Beck E, Bayley I. Reconstruction of the valgus-impacted humeral head fracture. J Shoulder Elbow Surg. 1995;4:73–80.
13. deAnquin CE, deAnquin CA. Prosthetic replacement in the treatment of serious fractures of the proximal humerus. In: Bayley I, Lessel L, eds. Shoulder Surgery. Berlin: Springer-Verlag; 1982:207–217.
14. Stableforth PG. Four-part fractures of the neck of the humerus. J Bone Joint Surg Br. 1984;66(1):104–108.
15. Laing PG. The arterial supply of the adult humerus. J. Bone Joint Surg Am. 1956; 38A:1105–1116.
16. Gerber C, Schneeberger AG, Vinh TS. The arterial vascularization of the humeral head. An anatomical study. J Bone Joint Surg Am. 1990; 72(10):1486–1494.
17. Wheeler DL, Colville MR. Biomechanical comparison of intramedullary and percutaneous pin fixation for proximal humeral fracture fixation. J Orthop Trauma. 1997;11(5):363–367.
18. Soete P, Clayson P, Costenoble V. Transitory percutaneous pinning in fractures of the proximal humerus. J Shoulder Elbow Surg. 1999;8(6):569–573.
19. Rowles DJ, McGrory JE. Percutaneous pinning of the proximal part of the humerus. An anatomic study. J Bone Joint Surg Am. 2001;83-A(11): 1695–1699.

4

Minimally Invasive Approach for Shoulder Arthroplasty

Theodore Blaine, Ilya Voloshin, Kevin Setter, and Louis U. Bigliani

Minimally invasive surgical techniques in joint arthroplasty have received increased enthusiasm in the past decade. In addition to the obvious advantages in cosmesis and patient satisfaction with smaller incisions, minimally invasive approaches may potentially result in less trauma to soft tissues and may improve recovery rate and patient outcomes. While considerable advances have been made in minimally invasive surgery for the hip and knee, minimally invasive arthroplasty procedures for the shoulder have not yet been described.

This chapter describes our experience with minimally invasive shoulder arthroplasty (SA). There are some potential advantages of minimally invasive surgery specifically for the shoulder. The average age of patients undergoing SA is younger when compared with hip and knee arthroplasty.[1] The minimally invasive approach to SA is even more attractive from a cosmetic and functional standpoint in this patient population. The shoulder is a more socially exposed joint than knee and hip. Cosmesis around the shoulder is an important issue for many patients. This younger cohort tends to be very active and have high expectations regarding postoperative function. This leads to a potential for a greater possibility for revision surgery. Minimal disruption of soft tissue and a potential for a faster recovery are very attractive potential benefits of MIS. However, precise placement of prosthetic components and meticulous soft tissue balancing are extremely important and should not be compromised by the length of incision. If extensive releases of surrounding musculature are required, minimally invasive approach may not be feasible. Careful patient selection for the minimally invasive approach to SA is crucial at this stage of the development of this technique.

Techniques

Minimally invasive approaches, techniques and instrumentation for SA are still evolving at this time. Clinical results utilizing minimally invasive techniques have yet to be determined. The goals are to decrease trauma to surrounding soft tissues, accelerate postoperative rehabilitation, and decrease perioperative complications. Currently, there are two techniques available to achieve the necessary exposure. The use of these techniques is based upon the pathology, the severity of disease, instrumentation, and surgeon experience.

Surgical Approaches

Concealed Axillary Approach

While the typical skin incision for shoulder arthroplasty begins at the coracoid process and extends laterally toward the humerus and the insertion of the deltoid at the deltoid tuberosity, a more cosmetic concealed axillary incision has been described by the author (LUB).[2] The traditional incision measures 10cm to 15cm in length compared to the shorter and more cosmetic (7-cm) concealed axillary incision (Figure 4.1). This incision is used mostly in SA for avascular necrosis (AVN) of the humeral head and for arthritic disorders of the glenohumeral joint. In fracture cases this incision may not provide enough exposure to address the tuberosities. The subcutaneous dissection involves elevating skin flaps medially and laterally to expose the deltopectoral inter-

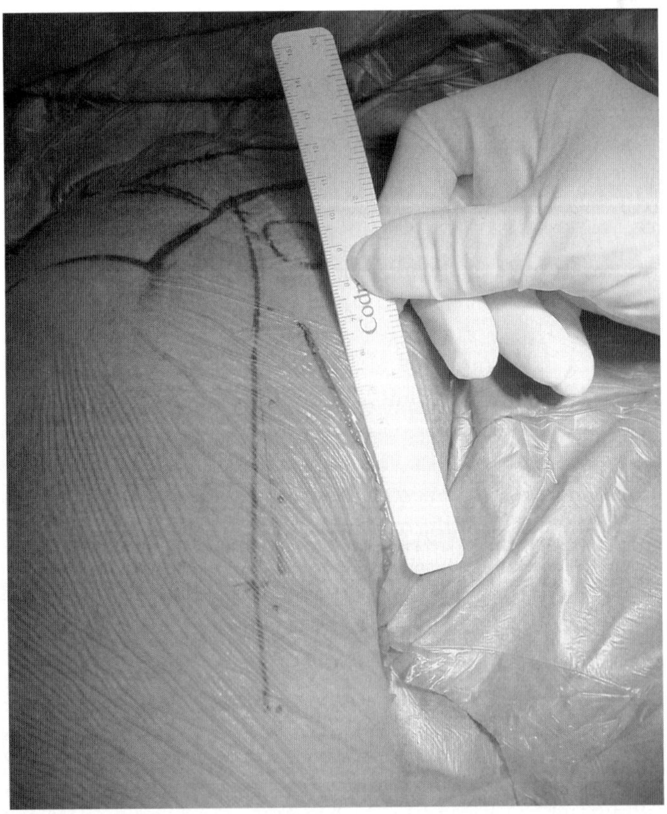

Figure 4.1. Incision used for axillary approach during total shoulder arthroplasty.

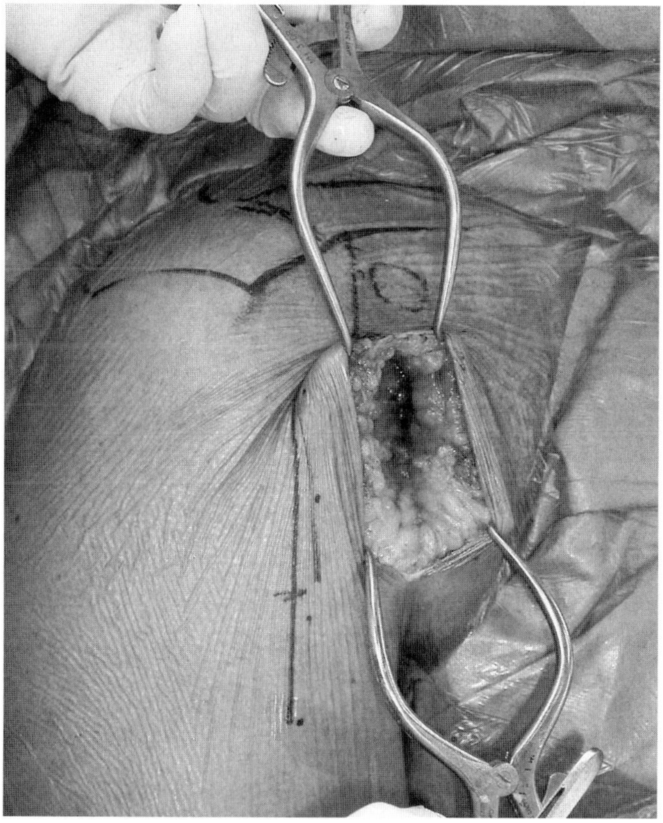

Figure 4.2. Full thickness skin flaps are elevated providing a mobile window for increased exposure.

val (Figure 4.2). The pectoralis major is retracted medially, and the deltoid with the cephalic vein is retracted laterally (Figure 4.3). The clavipectoral fascia is then identified and incised just lateral to the conjoint tendon (Figure 4.4). The conjoint tendon is retracted medially (Figure 4.5). The biceps tendon is generally preserved unless significantly damaged. The leading edge of the CA ligament is then resected improving superior visualization of the rotator interval (Figure 4.6). A complete anterior bursectomy is then performed allowing excellent exposure and clear identification of the subscapularis. The upper border of the subscapularis is identified by finding the rotator interval. The lower border is heralded by the anterior circumflex artery and its two venea commitantes. These vessels are then coagulated using the needle tipped bovie, or tied depending on their girth. Further exposure is based on the pathology present and proceeds as indicated in the ensuing sections of this chapter.

Mini-Incision Approach

Based on cadaveric studies and our own clinical experience, we have found that the current instrumentation used for shoulder arthroplasty tends to exit the skin in a two-inch (5-cm) arc centered and just lateral

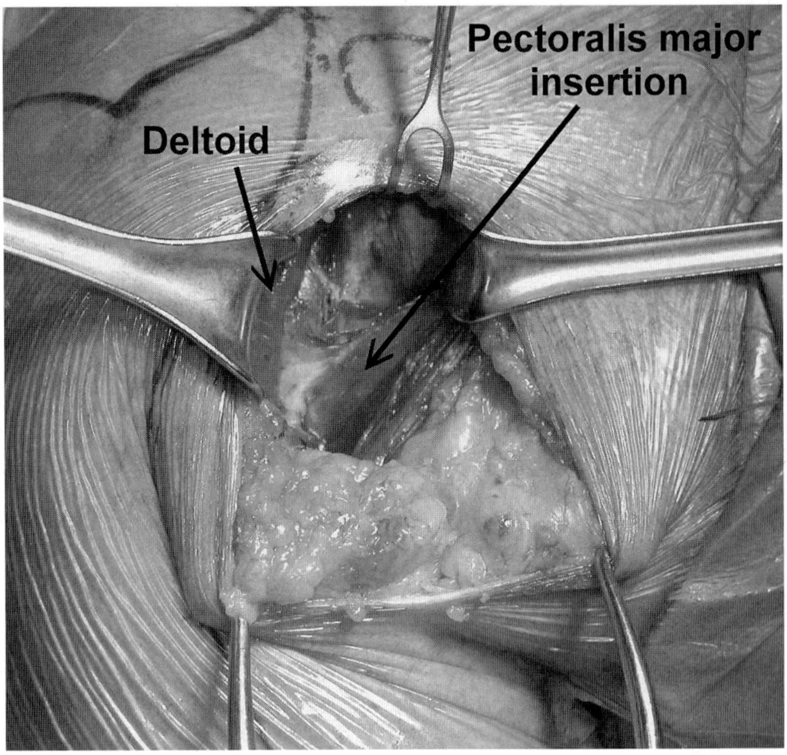

Figure 4.3. The upper 0.5 cm to 1 cm of the pectoralis major tendon may be released for improved exposure. It is tagged and repaired anatomically at the end of the procedure.

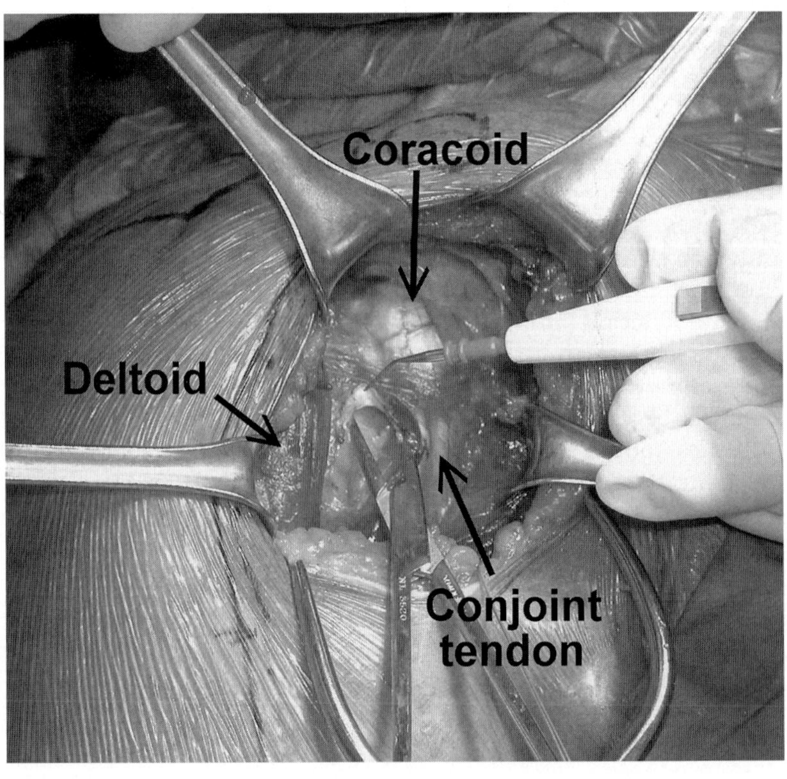

Figure 4.4. The clavipectoral fascia is incised lateral to the conjoint tendon.

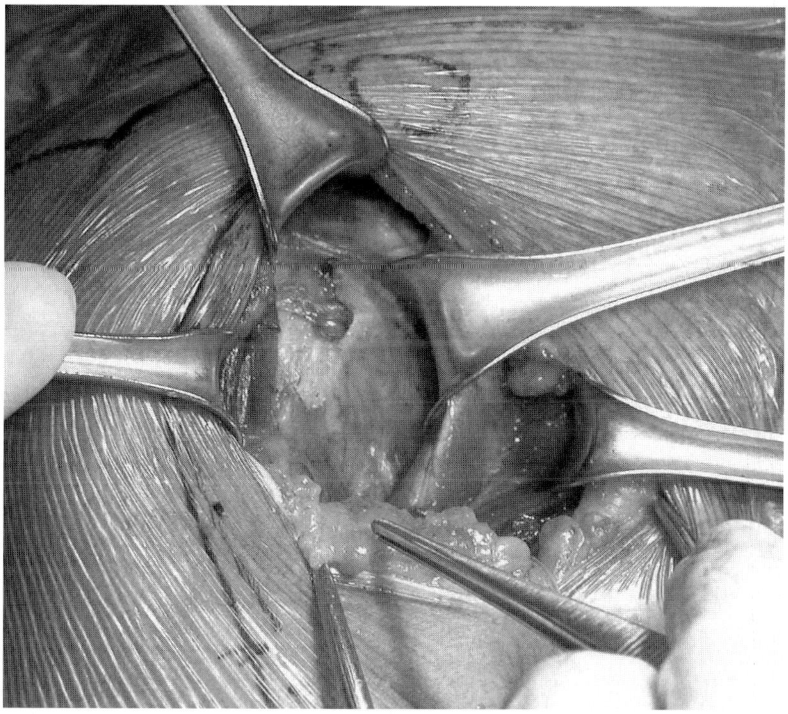

Figure 4.5. The conjoint tendon is retracted laterally exposing the bursa overlying the subscapularis.

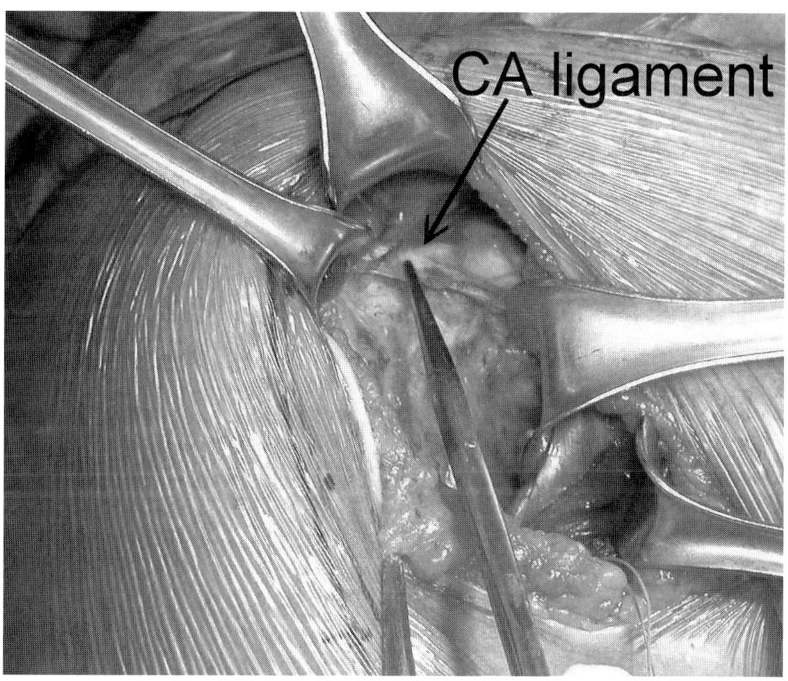

Figure 4.6. The anteriolateral leading edge of the coracoacromial (CA) ligament is resected for increased superior exposure.

to the coracoid process. Furthermore, we and others have also found that the average diameter of the humeral head at the surgical neck is approximately 49 mm.[3,4] Based on these findings, we believe that the skin incision for shoulder arthroplasty must be at least 5 cm (2 in.) to allow placement of a humeral head component in shoulder arthroplasty, but should not need necessarily to be any larger. One of the authors (TAB) has therefore devised a skin incision that is centered just lateral to the coracoid process. This incision can be used in SA for a variety of diagnoses. The location of the incision allows better access to tuberosities in fracture cases and provides adequate glenoid exposure in arthritic disorders. The incision measures approximately 2 in., just enough to deliver the humeral head from the wound (Figure 4.7). The placement of the starting incision is crucial for this approach. It has to be superior enough to provide direct access to the humeral canal for humeral preparation and placement of the prosthesis as well as adequate exposure of the glenoid.

The deltopectoral interval is identified and incised in a similar manner to the traditional anterior approach. Subcutaneous dissection is necessary along the deltopectoral interval superiorly and inferiorly for adequate exposure (Figure 4.8). Care is taken to protect the attachment of the deltoid to the clavicle and acromion. The cephalic vein is generally retracted with the deltoid muscle secondary to the fact that there are more contributories superiorly from the deltoid than inferi-

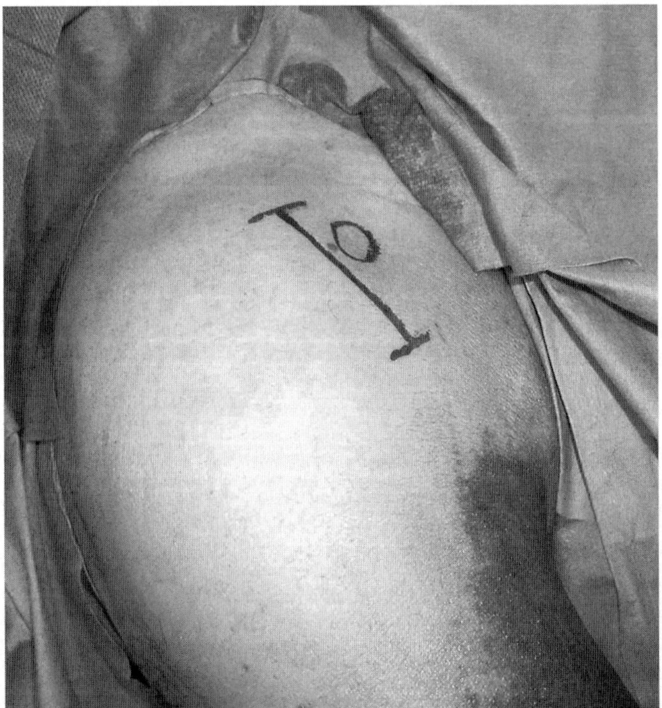

Figure 4.7. Alternate incision used for minimally invasive approach for total shoulder arthroplasty or hemiarthroplasty for fracture.

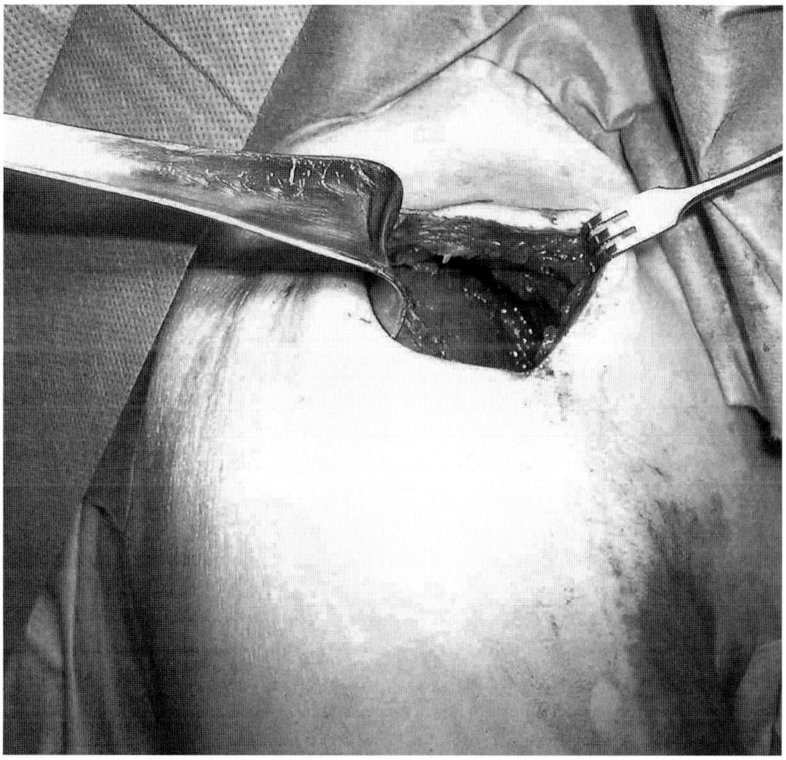

Figure 4.8. Full thickness flaps provide a mobile window for easy exposure of the deltopectoral interval.

orly from the pectoralis. The pectoralis major is retracted medially, and the deltoid with the cephalic vein is retracted laterally. The rest of the exposure to the subscapularis muscle is similar to the concealed axillary approach. Further exposure is based on the pathology present and proceeds as follows.

Four-Part Proximal Humerus Fractures: Multiple reports in the literature advocated hemiarthroplasty for treatment of the four-part proximal humerus fractures.[5–11] One of the great challenges in treating proximal humerus fractures with hemiarthroplasty is to achieve anatomic healing of the tuberosities.[12,13] On occasion, it is also difficult to determine the appropriate height for placement of the humeral component. In the setting of hemiarthroplasty for fractures treatment, a minimally invasive approach needs to provide adequate exposure for secure tuberosity fixation as well as minimal soft tissue dissection to preserve the biological environment to foster bone healing. New innovative technological advances in prosthetic design aid the surgeon in achieving these goals. These include a less bulky design to the proximal aspect of the prosthesis as well as coating the proximal aspect of the humerus with biologically friendly substances, such as tantalum.[14] Generally, the musculature around the shoulder in proximal humerus fractures is healthy and has excellent excursion, obviating the need for extensive surgical releases. Lack of stiffness combined with new technology for placement of the prosthesis and fixation of the tuberosities makes the minimally invasive approach an excellent option for these patients.

The approach for hemiarthroplasty in proximal humerus fracture involves a small skin incision centered just lateral to the coracoid (see Figure 4.7). The incision measures approximately 2 inches, just enough to deliver the humeral head from the wound (Figure 4.9). The placement of the starting incision is crucial for this approach. It has to be superior enough to provide direct access to the humeral canal for humeral preparation and placement of the prosthesis as well as adequate exposure of the tuberosities. An initial approach to the subscapularis muscle is performed as mentioned previously.

In the fracture setting, the subdeltoid bursa is generally not adherent to surrounding tissue and extensive releases are not necessary. The tuberosities and humeral head are identified. Tag stitches are placed through the rotator tendons and tuberosities to gain control over the fragments. The biceps tendon is generally preserved unless significantly damaged. The biceps tendon is often useful in helping to judge and guide the height of the prosthesis. If significant damage is present, the biceps is tenodesed in the biceps groove using suture soft tissue fixation after prosthesis placement.

Meticulous dissection and exposure should provide adequate visualization of all the parts of the fracture. The humeral head is delivered out of the wound and the glenoid is inspected for any pathology. The

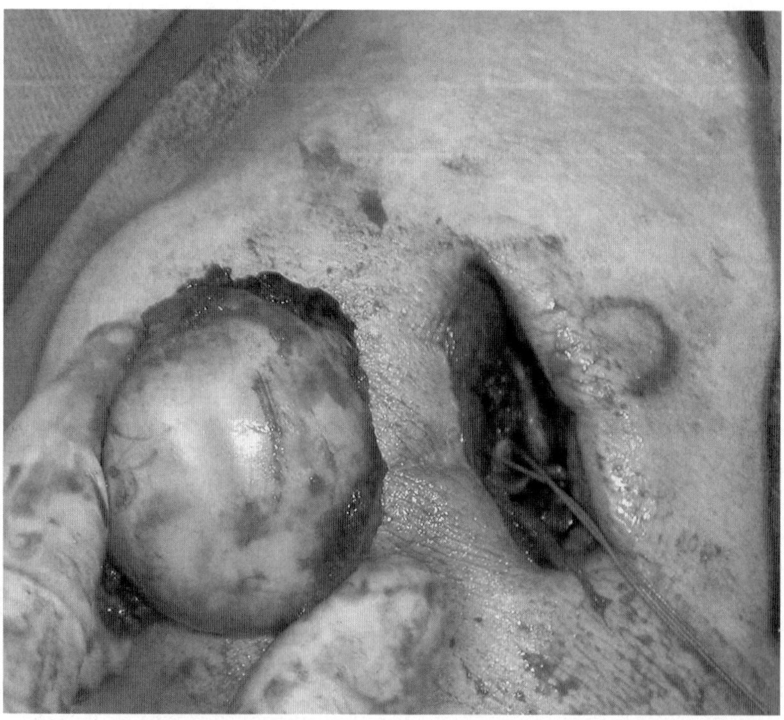

Figure 4.9. The fractured head can easily be removed from the incision.

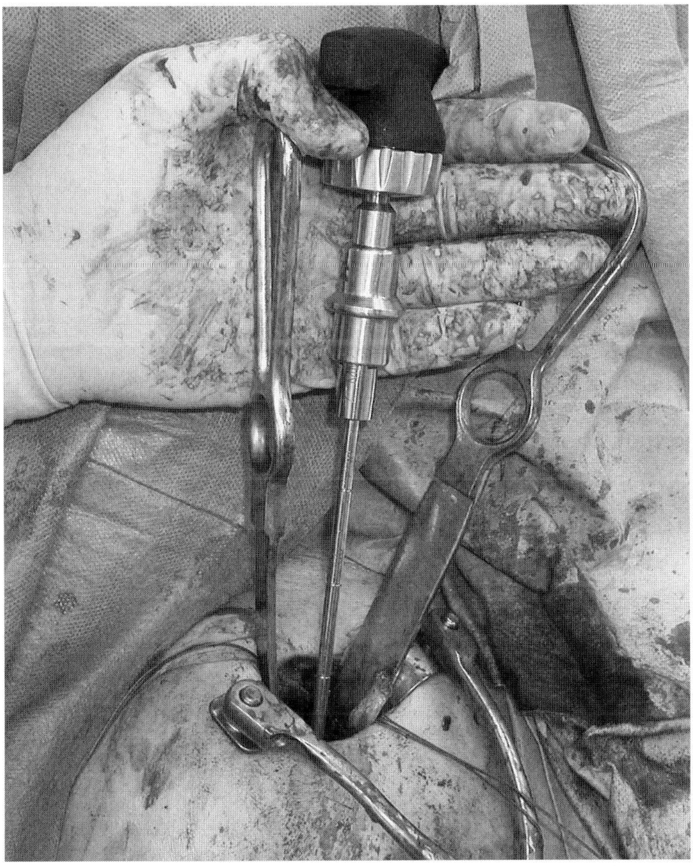

Figure 4.10. This incision allows a straight shot down the humeral shaft.

next step in the process is humeral preparation. Correct placement of the initial skin incision is crucial for having adequate exposure to the tuberosities superiorly and humeral canal inferiorly. A direct shot of the humeral canal for reaming has to be achieved. Usually, the arm needs to be slightly extended and externally rotated to achieve satisfactory visualization. An arm positioner (Tenet Medical Engineering, Calgary, Alberta, Canada) can be extremely helpful in this regard. The humerus is reamed in a standard fashion to achieve good interference fit (Figure 4.10). Trials for the humeral prosthesis are used to determine proper version, head size, and height (Figure 4.11).

New technological advances have been made to assist in determining the proper height of the prosthesis during the minimally invasive approach. Canal sponges of appropriate size are fitted over the provisional stems to assist in testing the prosthesis and to steady the provisional in the humeral canal preventing spinning and pistoning during trial reductions (Figure 4.12). Fin clamps available in three different sizes have been developed to mark the appropriate determined height on the provisional stems and on the actual prosthetic component (Figure 4.13). Once the height is determined with the provisional, a fin clamp of appropriate size is secured to the fin and the

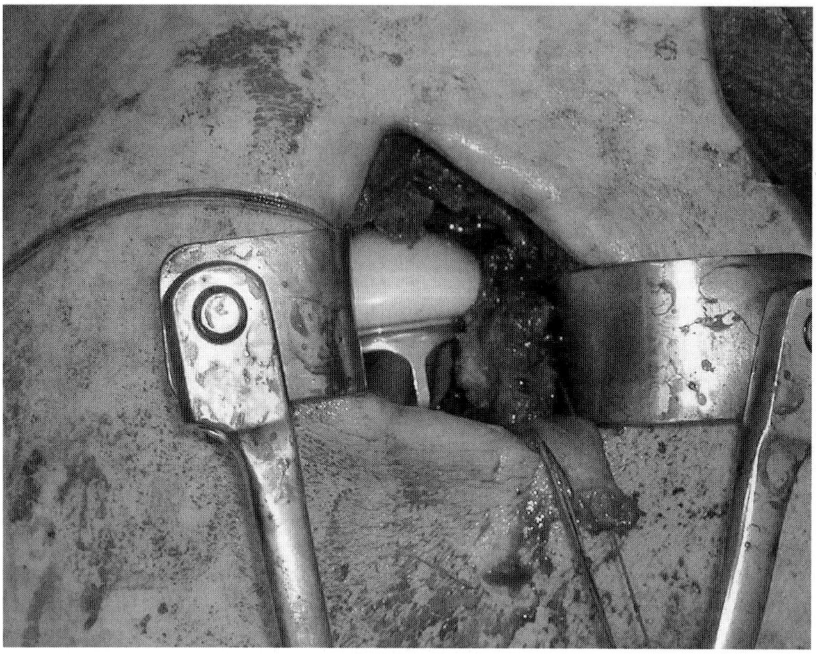

Figure 4.11. With the provisional prosthesis in place, prosthetic height and version can be inspected.

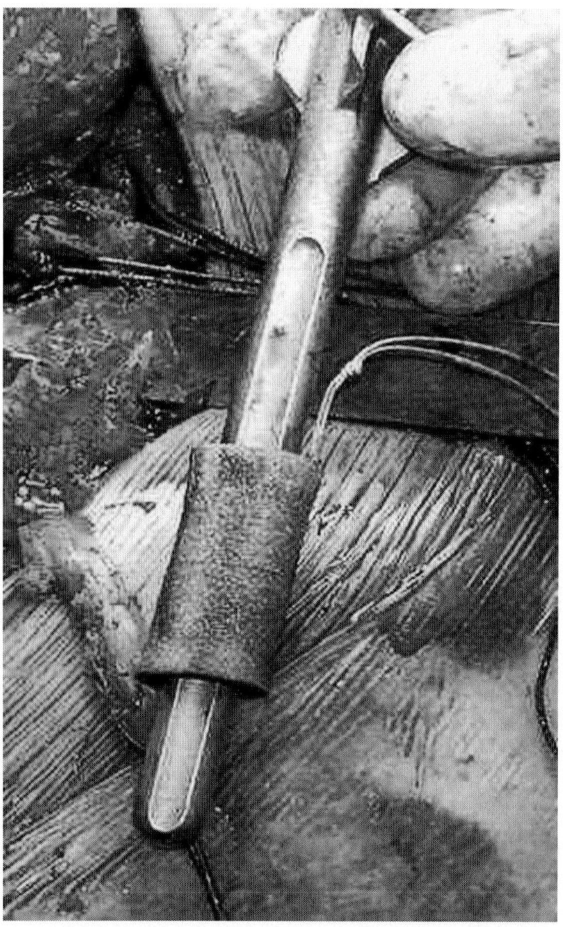

Figure 4.12. Special fracture sponges can be used on the prosthetic shaft to help hold the provisional in place while testing the prosthesis.

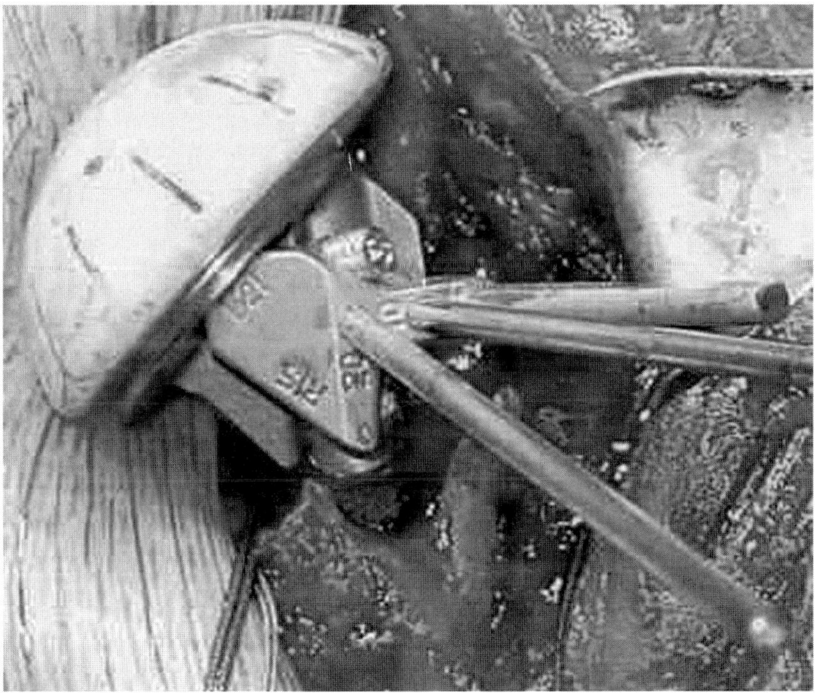

Figure 4.13. Fin clamps can be attached to the provisional stem. These clamps assist with determining the proper prosthetic height and version. Version rods can be attached to the clamp, and prosthetic version can be referenced from the epicondylar axis.

determined height can be assessed without the need for supporting the provisional. This limits the need for supporting the provisional component at the proper height and reduces the need for extra space and exposure during the trial process. Alignment pins can also be attached directly to the fin clamp, which avoids the need for placing the inserter back on the trial to judge the version of the component. Sutures are passed around the tuberosities to assist in reduction around the provisional. This step is critical to ensure that final reduction and fixation of the tuberosities will be appropriate after placement of the component. Once the proper height is confirmed and stability of the glenohumeral articulation is checked, the provisional is removed and the same fin clamp is secured to the implanted prosthesis to ensure exact placement and recreation of anatomic height as determined from the trial process (Figure 4.14). Prior to the placement of the prosthesis, drill holes in the shaft are made and sutures are passed for future tuberosity fixation. The prosthesis is cemented or press-fitted into the humeral canal with height guided by the fin clamp. The version can be guided by alignment rods that fit onto the clamp or prosthesis handle (Figure 4.15). The low profile of this instrumentation allows excellent visualization to perform these steps without the need for extra exposure that is usually required. The appropriate sized humeral head is placed to recreate normal anatomic relationships in the proximal humerus.

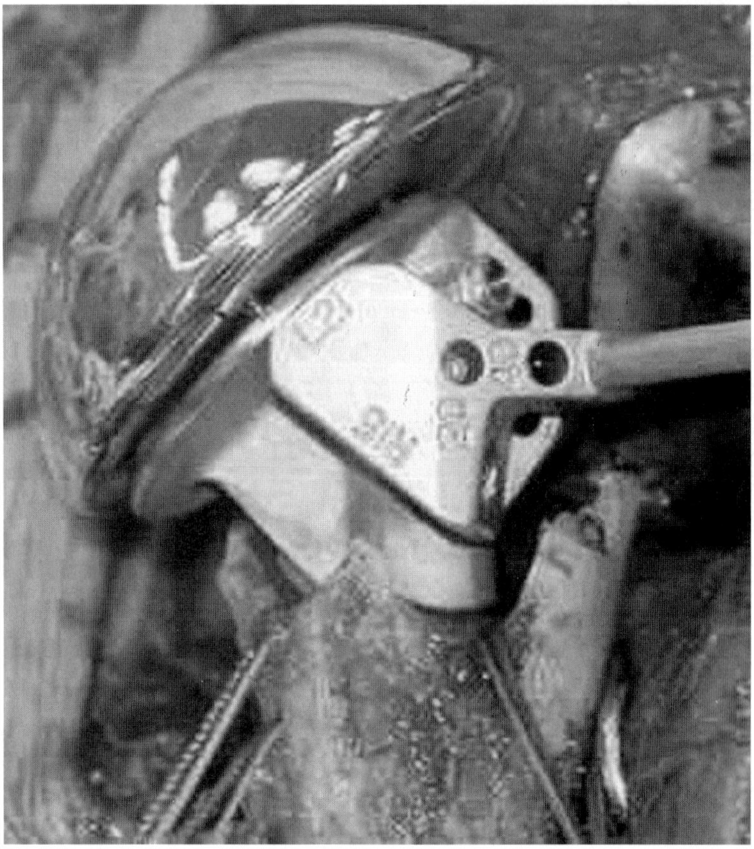

Figure 4.14. The fin clamps can also be attached to the final prosthesis matching component version and height with that of the desired provisional.

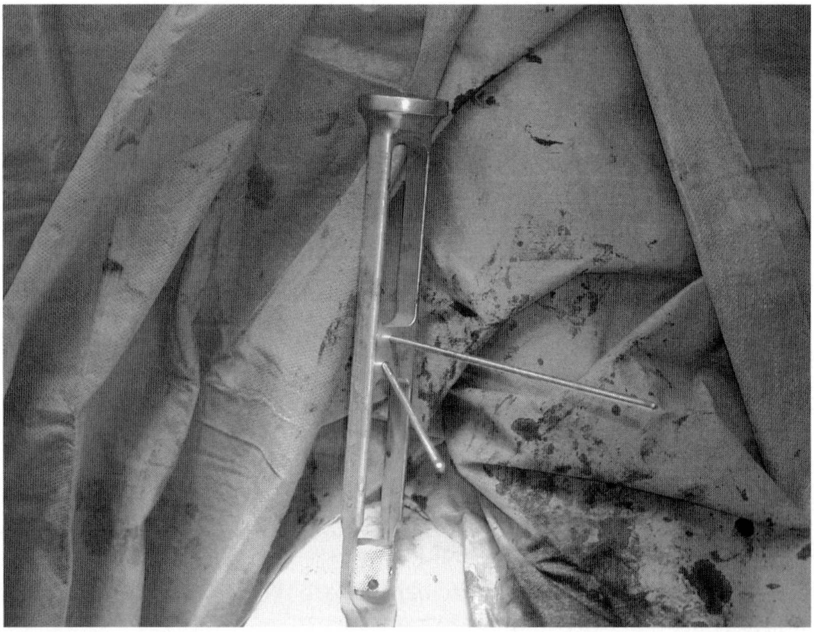

Figure 4.15. Alignment pins can be attached to the insertion device to assist with component version.

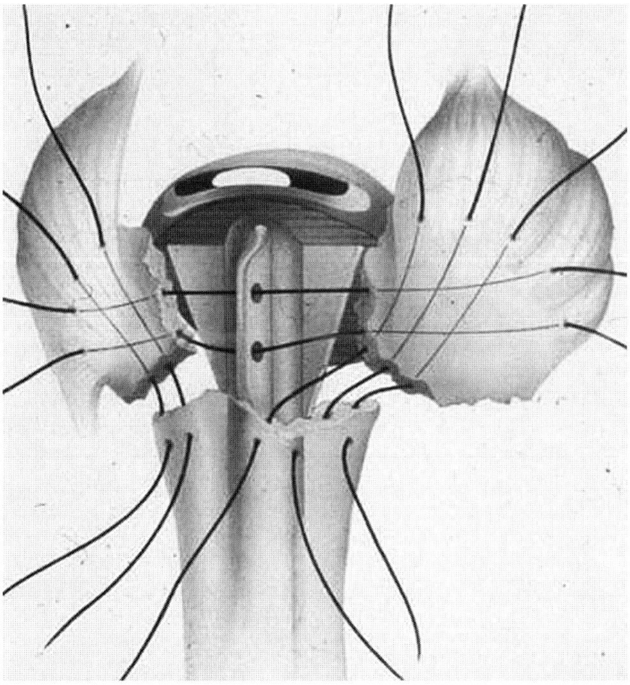

Figure 4.16. The tuberosities are repaired to the shaft through drill holes.

Trabecular metal (TM) is a new innovative technology that is presently being tested for use with glenoid and proximal humerus fixation. Initial studies demonstrate increased bone in growth into TM prosthesis.[14] This valuable feature can be used in proximal humerus fractures to augment the healing of tuberosities to the prosthesis and the shaft of the humerus. Our initial clinical experience with this technology in shoulder fractures has been extremely satisfying. As mentioned previously, fixation and healing of the tuberosities are some of the most challenging aspects of arthroplasty for proximal humerus fractures. Secure fixation is a necessity. Standard suture fixation of the tuberosities is performed (Figures 4.16 and 4.17). The passive range of motion is gently tested after the repair. This helps determine postoperative therapy limits. The wound is closed in the usual fashion, and a drain is placed if necessary.

Avascular Necrosis

While total shoulder arthroplasty has had superior results to hemiarthroplasty in patients with glenohumeral arthritis in several recent series, there are some cases in which hemiarthroplasty is the procedure of choice. These include avascular necrosis (Cruess stages I-III, and sometimes IV) in which the glenoid is not significantly involved.[15,16] The minimally invasive approach in a setting of avascular necrosis can use either a concealed axillary incision or an incision centered just lateral to the coracoid.

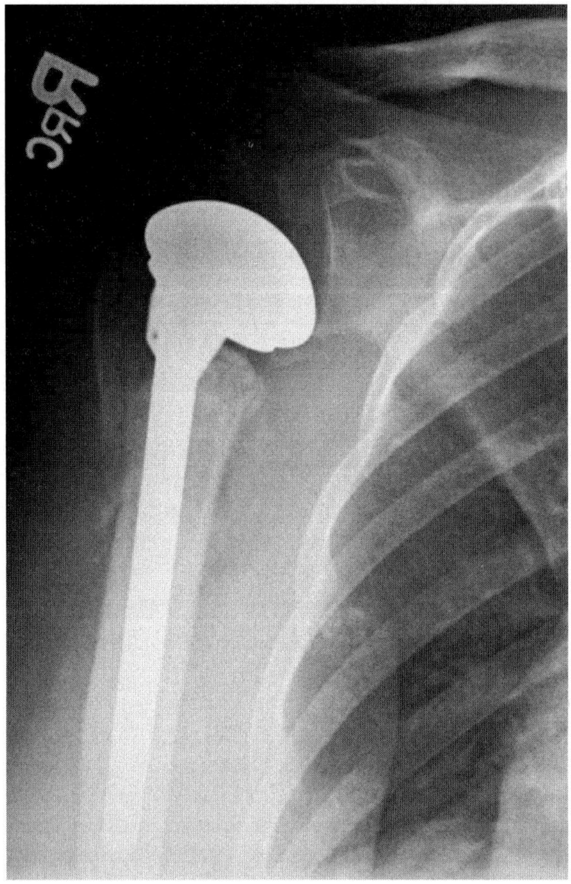

Figure 4.17. AP radiograph of a four-part proximal humerus fracture treated with hemiarthroplasty.

The deltopectoral interval is developed and entered in a similar fashion. After exposure to the subscapularis muscle is achieved, the muscle is detached directly off the lesser tuberosity, superiorly, starting at the rotator interval. The tendon is incised as lateral as possible, just medial to the bicep tendon. The rotator interval is also released all the way to the base of the coracoid. Care is taken not to disrupt the biceps tendon. The subscapularis needs to be detached just enough to deliver the humeral head from the wound. Inferiorly, the subscapularis insertion may be preserved. The preparation of the humerus is performed in the usual fashion. A direct shot for humeral reaming is easier when the incision is centered lateral to the coracoid. The trial process is similar to the one during standard approach. Correct alignment of the component is crucial and one has to have adequate visualization. Incision should be enlarged if the visualization is poor. Bone tunnels are made and sutures are passed for future subscapularis repair. After placement of the humeral component, the upper part of the subscapularis is repaired securely to the lesser tuberosity. The rotator interval is left opened to prevent stiffness in external rotation. Closure of the wound is performed in the usual fashion.

Glenohumeral Arthritis

Many patients undergoing shoulder arthroplasty for arthritis have substantial contractures that require extensive releases and exposure to properly address the pathology; in these cases, mini incisions may not be adequate and this judgment needs to be made by the surgeon. In general, patients with large osteophytes (greater than 1 cm) and limited range of motion require a traditional approach for osteophyte excision, appropriate soft tissue release, and adequate exposure. Large or muscular patients also require the traditional approach for adequate exposure. Generally, in small female patients with satisfactory range of motion (FF of 100 degrees and ER of 20 degrees and IR to L3) and small osteophytes, a minimally invasive approach is a reasonable option. Decreased soft tissue disruption and limited detachment of subscapularis muscle during this approach are beneficial in terms of restoration of subscapularis function and accelerated rehabilitation postoperatively.

In general, the literature reports superior range of motion and better pain relief achieved in patients undergoing total shoulder arthroplasty versus hemiarthroplasty for osteoarthritis.[17,18] Glenoid pathology in the setting of shoulder arthroplasty usually requires resurfacing of the glenoid component.

Again, either a concealed axillary incision or the incision lateral to the coracoid can be used. The deltopectoral interval is developed and entered in a similar fashion. After exposure to the subscapularis muscle is achieved, the muscle is detached directly off the lesser tuberosity, superiorly, starting at the rotator interval (Figure 4.18). The tendon is

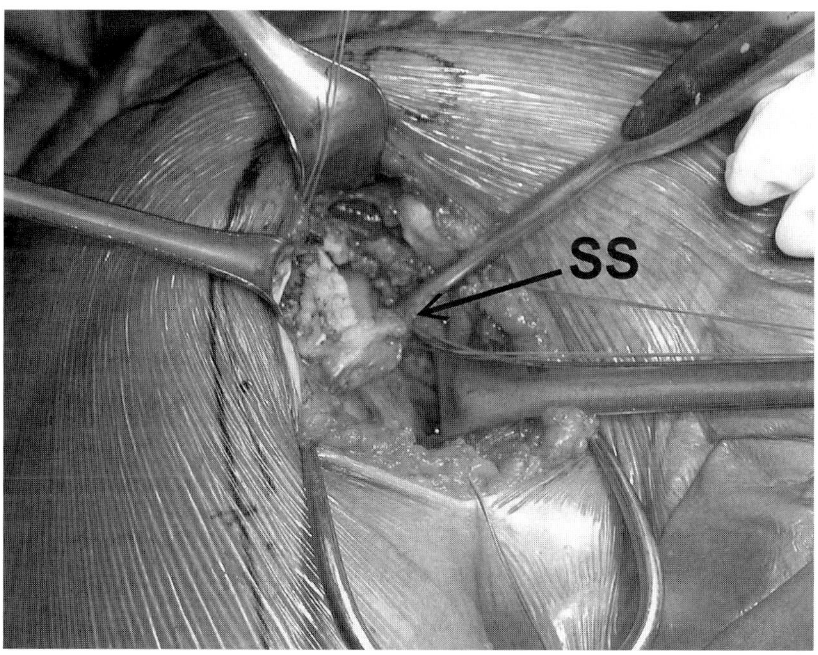

Figure 4.18. After exposure to the subscapularis (SS) muscle, the muscle is detached directly off the lesser tuberosity, superiorly, starting at the rotator interval.

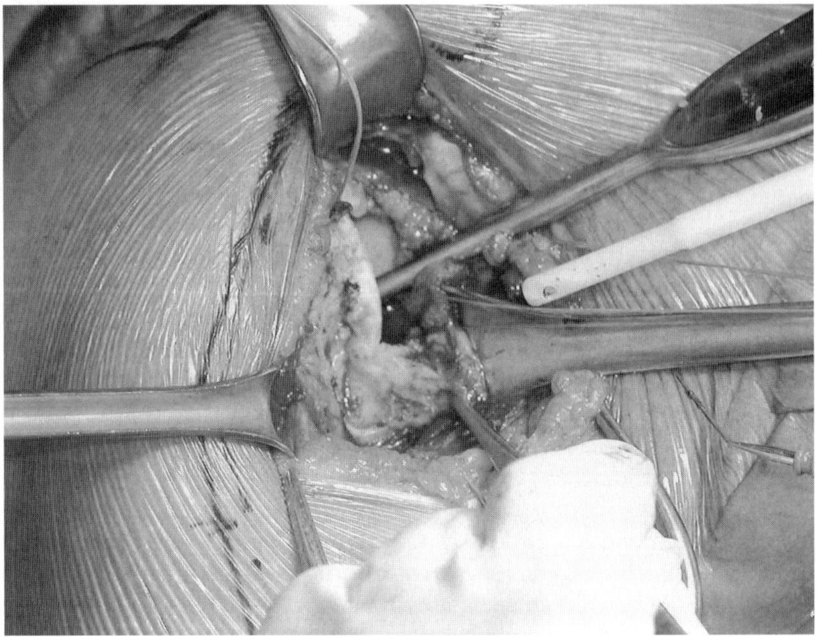

Figure 4.19. The subscapularis is removed from the lesser tuberosity enough to expose and remove the humeral head.

incised as lateral as possible, just medial to the bicep tendon. The rotator interval is also released all the way to the base of the coracoid. Care is taken not to disrupt the biceps tendon. The subscapularis needs to be detached just enough to deliver the humeral head from the wound. Inferiorly, the subscapularis insertion may be preserved (Figure 4.19). The preparation of the humerus is performed in the usual fashion (Figures 4.20 and 4.21). The trial process is similar to the one during standard approach. Correct alignment of the component is crucial and one has to have adequate visualization; the incision should be enlarged if the visualization is poor. Bone tunnels are made and sutures are passed for future subscapularis repair (Figure 4.22). Attention is directed to the glenoid exposure (see following discussion). After placement of the humeral component, the upper part of the subscapularis is repaired securely to the lesser tuberosity (Figure 4.23). The rotator interval is left open to prevent stiffness in external rotation. Closure of the wound is performed in the usual fashion (Figure 4.24).

The concealed axillary incision in elective TSA for arthritis allows better exposure for any necessary releases of subdeltoid and subacromial spaces as well as around the subscapularis muscle. However, exposure for humeral canal preparation can be challenging. The approach with incision centered just lateral to the coracoid provides better exposure for the humeral reaming; however, less exposure may be obtained for necessary releases.

Figure 4.20. An intramedullary alignment guide is used to make the humeral osteotomy.

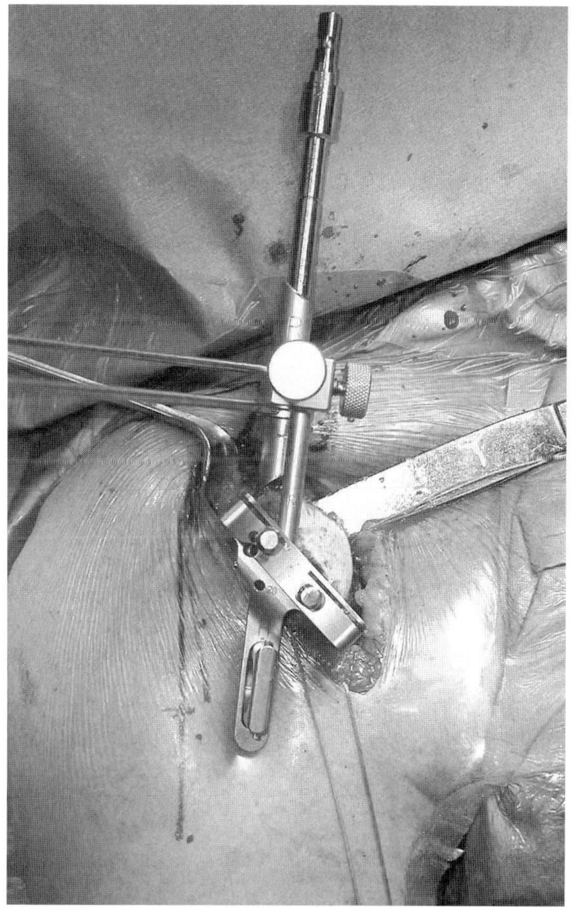

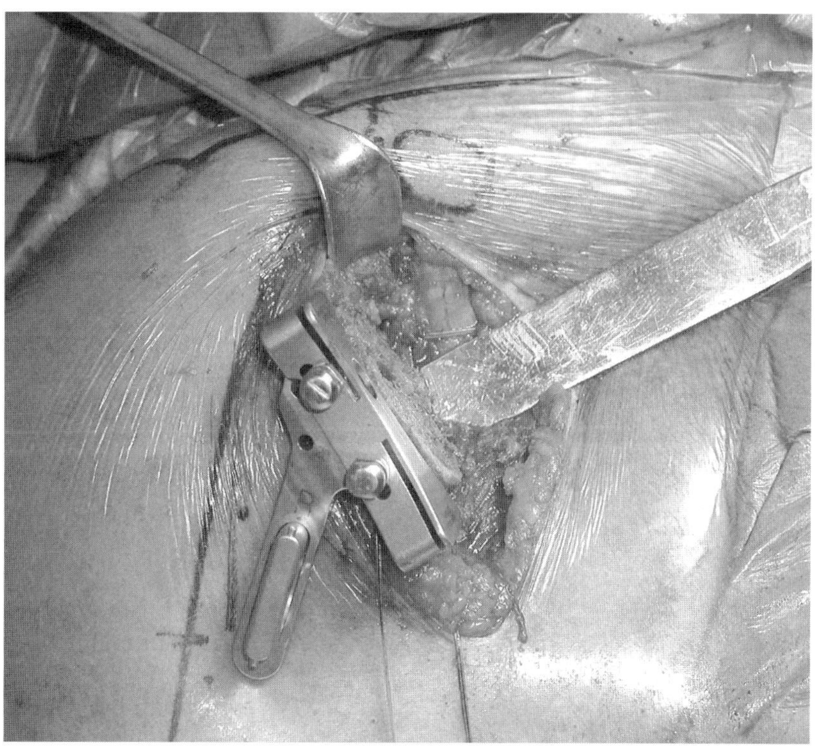

Figure 4.21. The cutting guide is used to make the osteotomy.

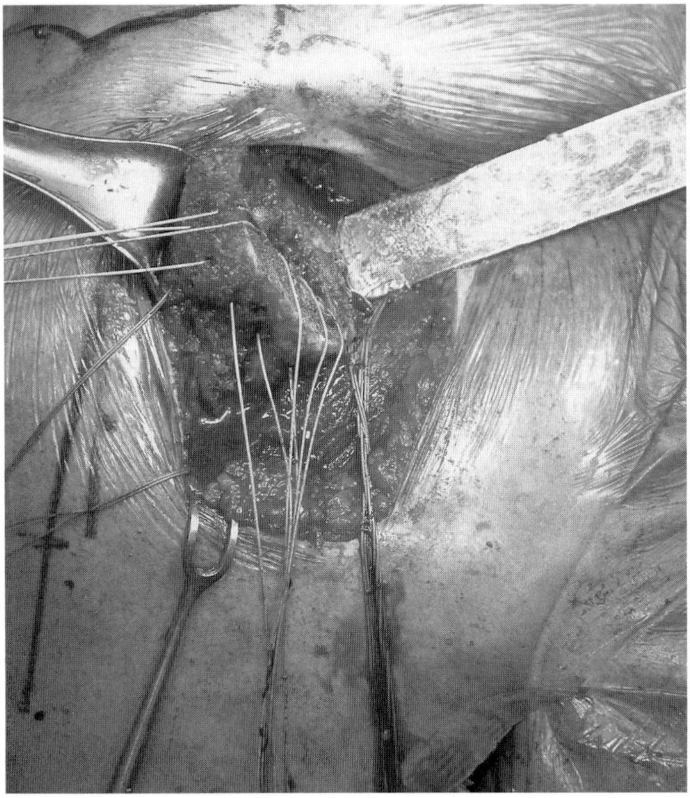

Figure 4.22. Drill holes are made in the proximal humerus providing a wide bony bridge for repair of the subscapularis.

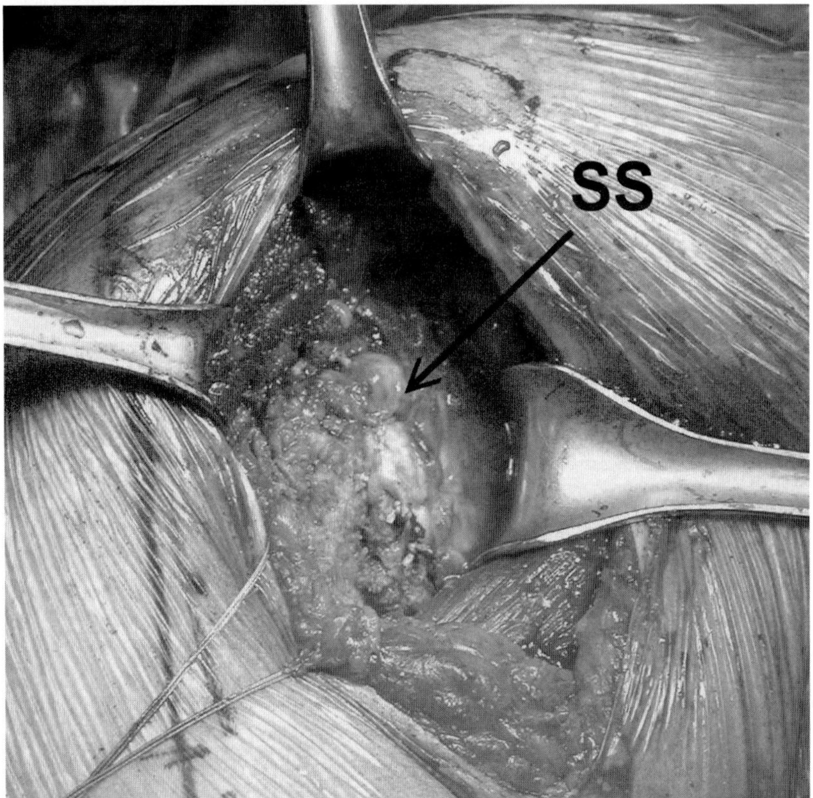

Figure 4.23. The subscapularis (SS) is repaired with non-absorbable sutures.

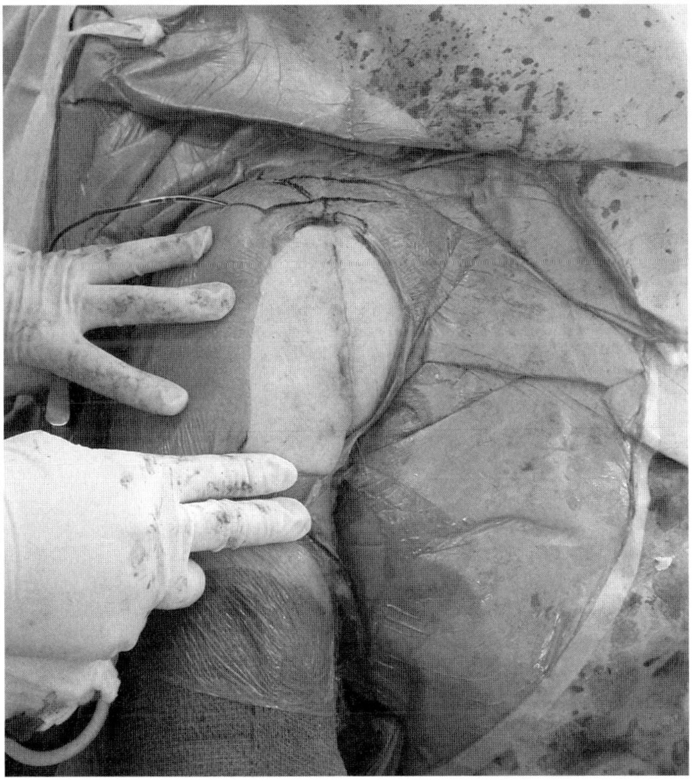

Figure 4.24. A layered closure is performed. A drain is routinely used.

Glenoid Exposure in Total Shoulder Arthroplasty

Glenoid exposure can be challenging even through the traditional incision; therefore, careful patient selection for a minimally invasive approach for total shoulder arthroplasty is required. Proper preparation of the glenoid and placement of the component is crucial. The minimally invasive approach is appropriate in thin patients with good range of motion. After proper humeral preparation, as described previously, a Fukuda retractor is placed to assess the glenoid. This helps retract the humerus lateral and posterior (Figure 4.25). The provisional humeral stem is left in the canal during glenoid exposure and preparation. This helps to protect the integrity of the humeral stem during retraction.

To achieve adequate exposure to the glenoid, capsular release superiorly, anteriorly, and inferiorly around the glenoid is performed. Care is taken to protect the axillary nerve by staying directly on the humeral neck inferiorly and retracting the inferior capsule in an inferior direction with a Darrach. For routine total shoulder arthroplasty in which instability is not a problem and the rotator cuff is usually intact, an anterior capsulectomy may be performed to improve exposure. This should not proceed however below the 6 o'clock position (inferior glenoid) to avoid injury to the axillary nerve. A special spiked Darrach

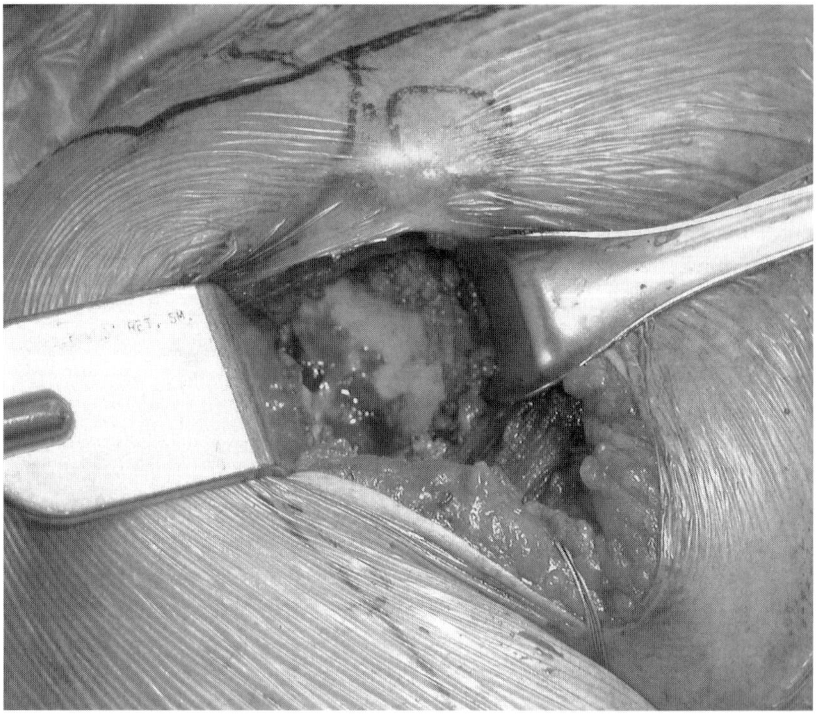

Figure 4.25. A Fukuda retractor is used to facilitate posterior glenoid exposure.

retractor is placed anteriorly for adequate visualization. In thin patients with good range of motion and minimal glenoid deformity this is usually enough for adequate visualization and reaming of the glenoid. The glenoid is prepared in the usual fashion with reaming to achieve concentric stable fit of the glenoid component in appropriate version (Figures 4.26 through 4.31). Pegged or keeled glenoid components may be used. In one study, pegged glenoids were found to have superior fixation to keeled.[19] However, the pegged component requires a larger glenoid vault and the keeled glenoid may be more appropriate in patients with a small native glenoid. Cement is pressurized in the pegged or keeled vault (Figure 4.32). Once the glenoid component is placed, attention is turned back to the humerus. The humeral component and the humeral head are placed as described above. The wound is closed in the usual fashion.

Postoperative Care

Postoperative care is a critical component of managing patients after minimally invasive shoulder arthroplasty. Because of decreased soft tissue damage patients tend to have faster recovery time. Despite the patient's eagerness to get back to functional activities, standard postoperative rehabilitation program must be followed at this early stage of implementation of this technique.[20] The amount of time that is required for soft tissue healing is still the same regardless of the approach.

Figure 4.26. A scraper is used to remove excess cartilage from the glenoid surface.

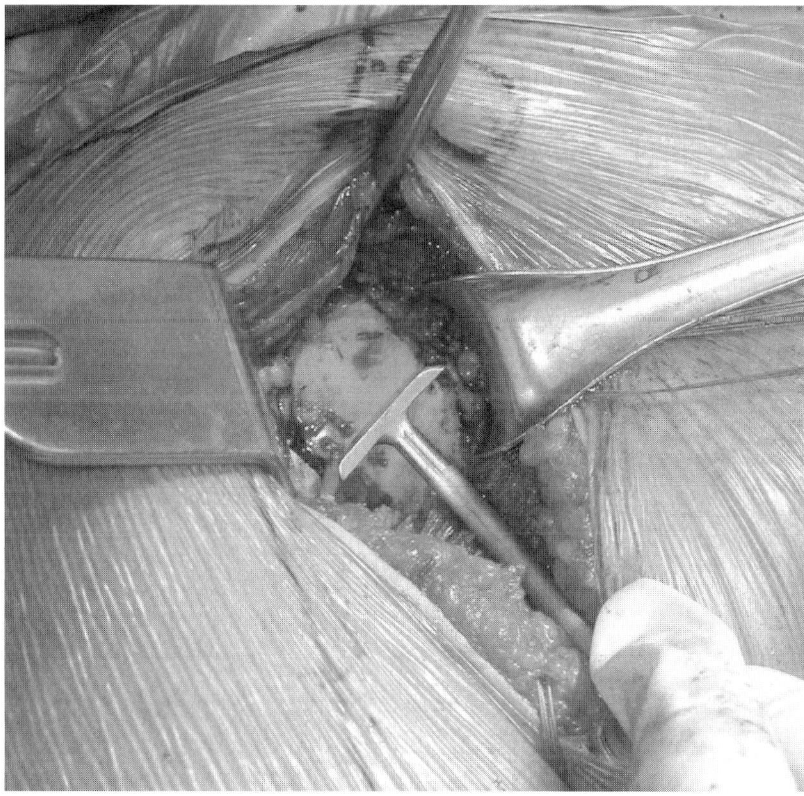

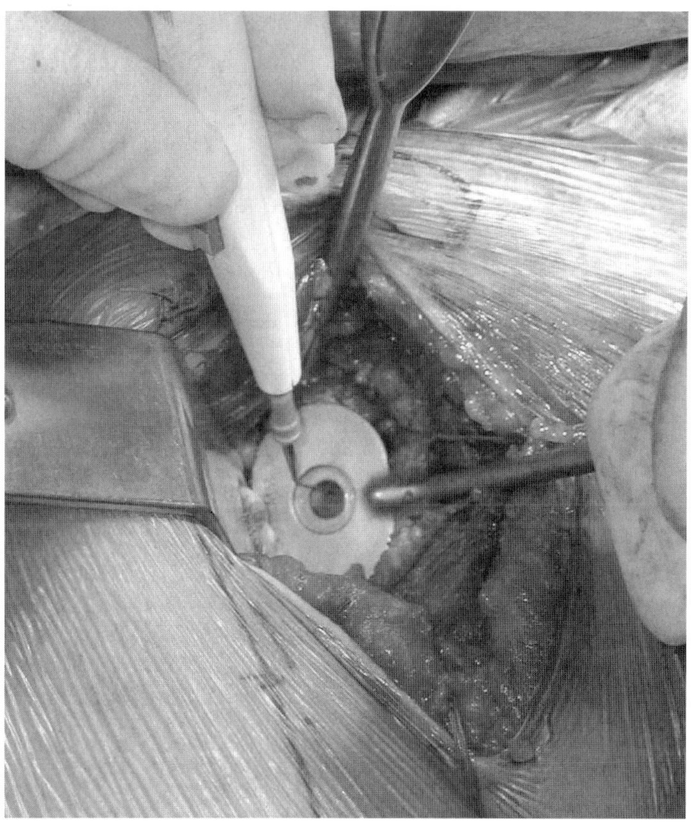

A

Figure 4.27. (A) The center of the glenoid is marked with a bovie. (B) A centering guide is used to drill the centering hole.

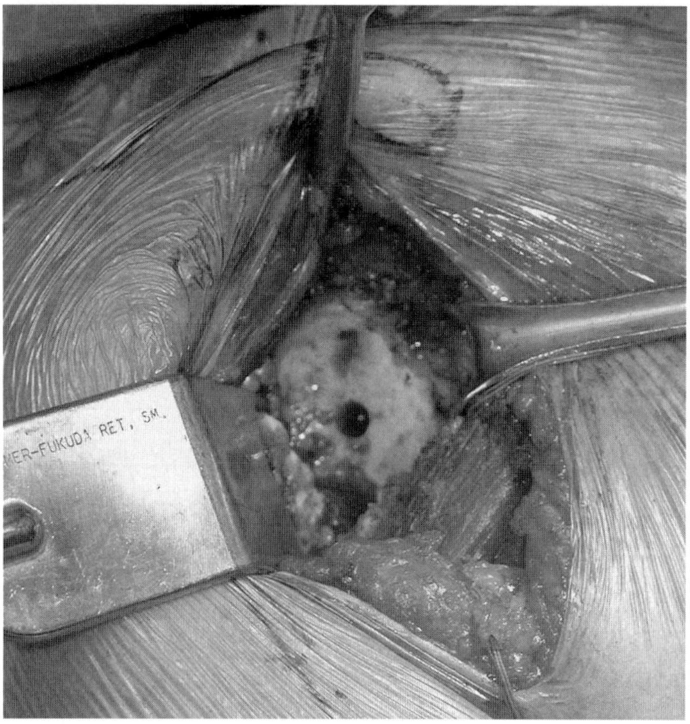

B

Figure 4.27. *Continued*

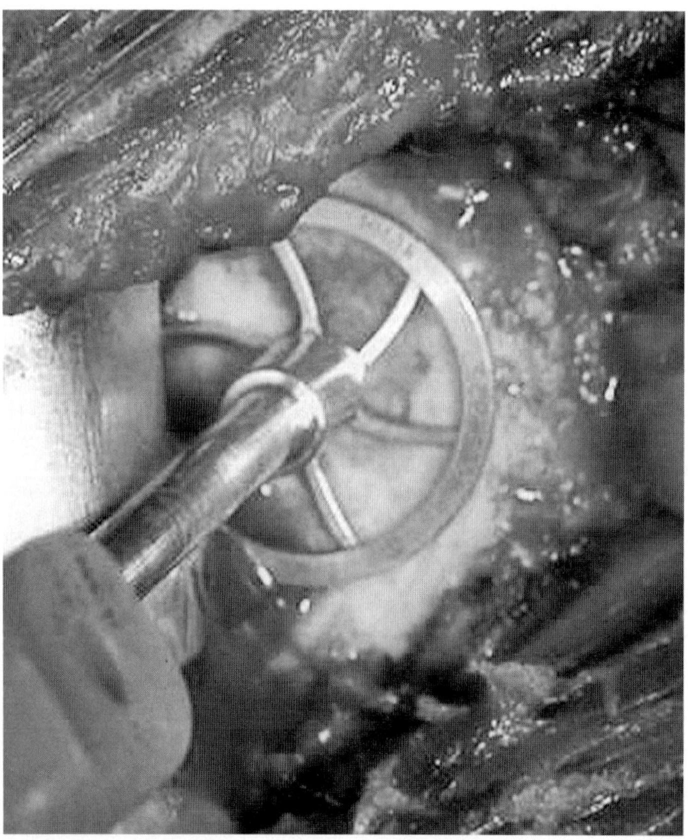

Figure 4.28. An open-faced reamer allows a better view of the glenoid while reaming.

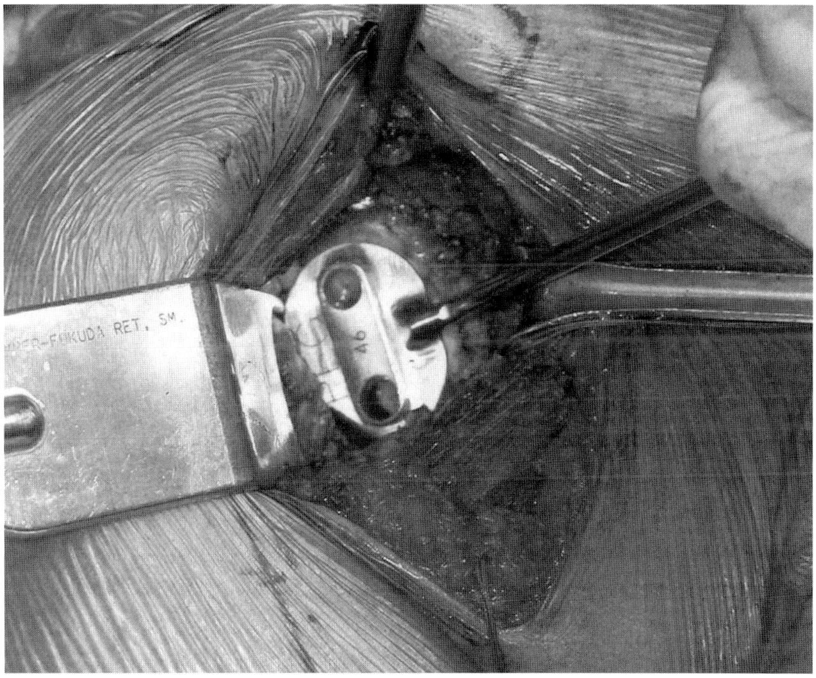

Figure 4.29. The appropriate sized glenoid guide is used to drill the superior and inferior holes for the pegged component.

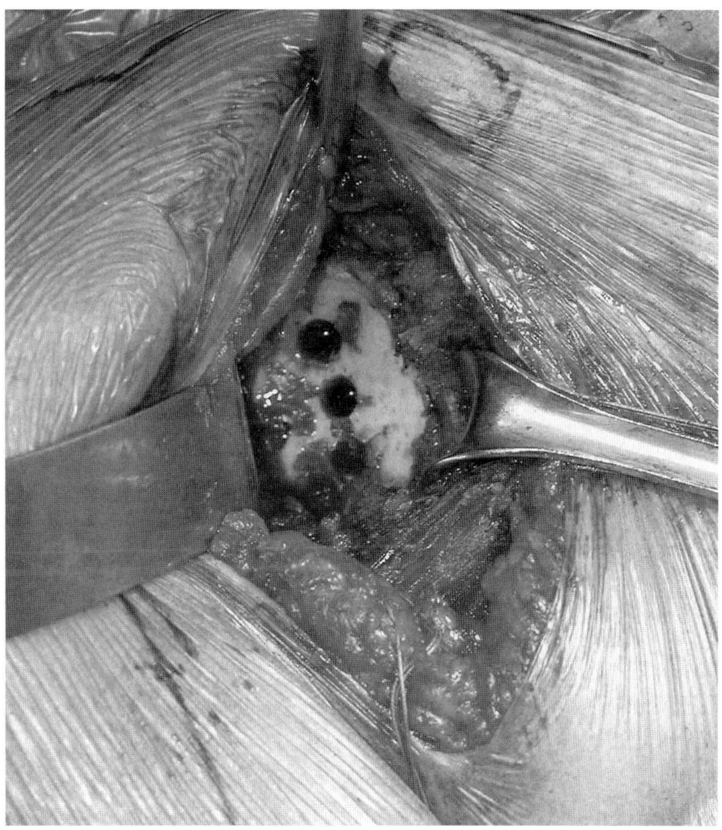

Figure 4.30. The three peg holes are impacted to removed and remaining bone to facilitate complete implant seating.

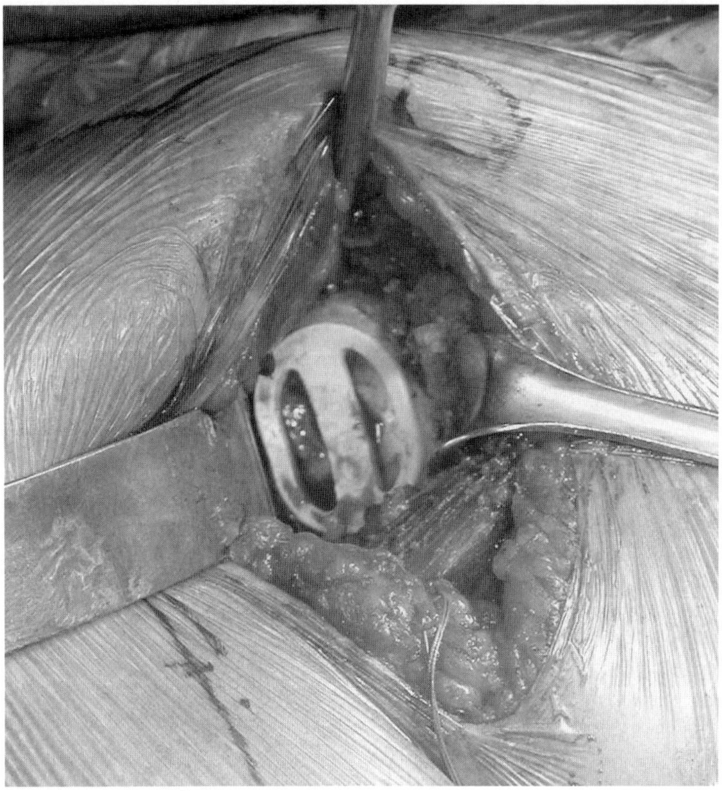

Figure 4.31. The open-faced provisional glenoid prosthesis is tested. It is checked for completeness of seating and toggling.

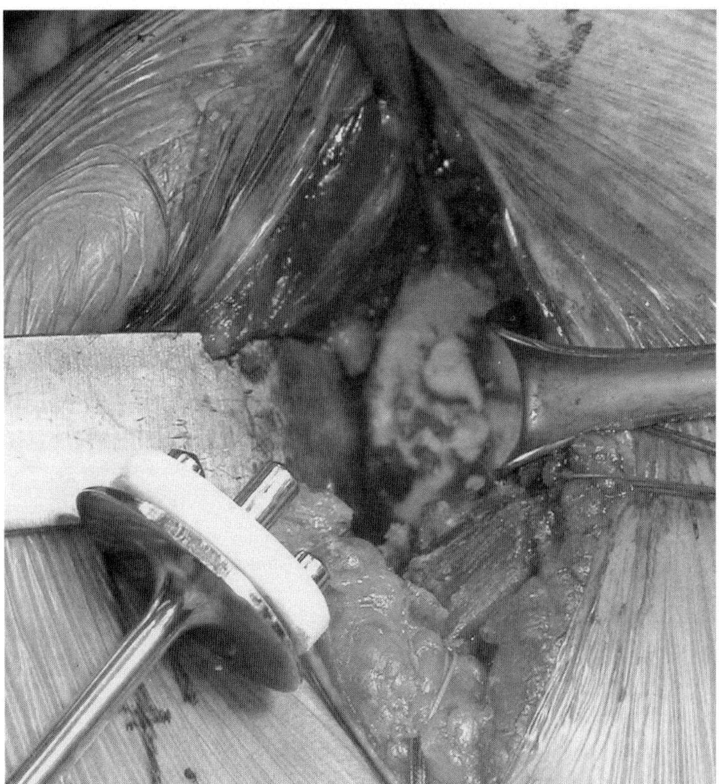

Figure 4.32. Cement is pressurized into the peg holes.

Conclusion

Minimally invasive approaches for shoulder arthroplasty may offer improved patient cosmesis, faster recovery, and less soft tissue trauma; however, surgeons need to weigh these benefits in the context of the potential risks of these procedures. Proximity of the neurovascular structures, glenoid exposure, and proper positioning of the implants with fewer landmarks available for reference make this technique very challenging; surgeons must anticipate a relatively steep learning curve. As these techniques continue to develop, however, and patient demand increases, the development of new instrumentation (retractors, cutting guides, component insertion/removal instruments and computer-guided navigation) may ultimately make minimally invasive shoulder arthroplasty the preferred technique. Early results using currently available instruments and techniques have been encouraging and support the further advancement of minimally invasive approaches to shoulder arthroplasty.

References

1. Wirth MA, Rockwood CA Jr. Complications of total shoulder-replacement arthroplasty. J Bone Joint Surg Am. 1996;78(4):603–616.
2. Bigliani L, Flatow E. Total Shoulder Arthroplasty: A Technical Manual. New York: Springer-Verlag; 2004.
3. Iannotti JP, Gabriel JP, Schneck SL, et al. The normal glenohumeral relationships. An anatomical study of one hundred and forty shoulders. J Bone Joint Surg Am. 1992;74(4):491–500.
4. Blaine T, et al. Presentation, American Shoulder and Elbow Surgeons. Focus; 2003.
5. Tanner MW, Cofield RH. Prosthetic arthroplasty for fractures and fracture-dislocations of the proximal humerus. Clin Orthop. 1983;179:116–128.
6. Neer CS II. Displaced proximal humeral fractures. I. Classification and evaluation. J Bone Joint Surg Am. 1970;52(6):1077–1089.
7. Bosch U, Skutek M, Fremerey RW, et al. Outcome after primary and secondary hemiarthroplasty in elderly patients with fractures of the proximal humerus. J Shoulder Elbow Surg. 1998;7(5):479–484.
8. Frich LH, Sojbjerg JO, Sneppen O. Shoulder arthroplasty in complex acute and chronic proximal humeral fractures. Orthopedics. 1991;14(9):949–954.
9. Goldman RT, Koval KJ, Cuomo F, et al. Functional outcome after humeral head replacement for acute three- and four-part proximal humeral fractures. J Shoulder Elbow Surg. 1995;4(2):81–86.
10. Hawkins RJ, Switlyk P. Acute prosthetic replacement for severe fractures of the proximal humerus. Clin Orthop. 1993;289:56–60.
11. Moeckel BH, Dines SM, Warren RS, et al. Modular hemiarthroplasty for fractures of the proximal part of the humerus. J Bone Joint Surg Am. 1992; 74(6):884–889.
12. Boileau P, Trojani C, Walch G, et al. Shoulder arthroplasty for the treatment of the sequelae of fractures of the proximal humerus. J Shoulder Elbow Surg. 2001;10(4):299–308.
13. Boileau P, Krishnan SG, Tini L, et al. Tuberosity malposition and migration: reasons for poor outcomes after hemiarthroplasty for displaced fractures of the proximal humerus. J Shoulder Elbow Surg. 2002;11(5):401–412.

14. Bobyn JD, Toh KK, Hacking SA, et al. Tissue response to porous tantalum acetabular cups: a canine model. J Arthroplasty. 1999;14(3):347–354.
15. Cruess, RL. Steroid-induced avascular necrosis of the head of the humerus. Natural history and management. J Bone Joint Surg Br. 1976;58(3):313–317.
16. David, H.G., Bridgman SA, Davies SC, et al. The shoulder in sickle-cell disease. J Bone Joint Surg Br. 1993;75(4):538–545.
17. Orfaly RM, Rockwood CA Jr, Esenyel CZ, et al. A prospective functional outcome study of shoulder arthroplasty for osteoarthritis with an intact rotator cuff. J Shoulder Elbow Surg. 2003;12(3):214–21.
18. Gartsman GM, Roddey TS, Hammerman SM. Shoulder arthroplasty with or without resurfacing of the glenoid in patients who have osteoarthritis. J Bone Joint Surg Am. 2000;82(1):26–34.
19. Connor PM, et al. Presentation. AAOS: Dallas, TX; 2002.
20. Hughes M, Neer CS II. Glenohumeral joint replacement and postoperative rehabilitation. Phys Ther. 1975;55(8):850–858.

5

Mini-Incision Medial Collateral Ligament Reconstruction of the Elbow

Steven J. Thornton, Andrew Willis, and David W. Altchek

The anterior bundle of the medial collateral ligament (MCL) of the elbow is the primary restraint to valgus load. It has been well documented that baseball pitchers are prone to injury of this structure secondary to the repetitive valgus loads subjected to the elbow with overhead pitching.[1–4] Although originally described in javelin throwers,[5] this injury is now almost exclusively seen in throwing athletes with baseball pitchers being the most prevalent patients (Figure 5.1). In addition to these athletes, injury to the MCL has also been shown in wrestlers, tennis players, professional football players, and arm wrestlers.[1,5–7] Symptomatic valgus instability can arise in these athletes after injury to the MCL, thus necessitating operative intervention. Although injury to the medial collateral ligament in the nonthrowing athlete can have excellent results with nonoperative intervention,[8,9] the overhead throwing athlete may find an injury to the medial collateral ligament of the elbow to be a career-ending event if surgical intervention is not employed.

Biomechanics and Anatomy

The medial collateral ligament complex is composed of an anterior bundle, a posterior bundle, and a transverse bundle (Figure 5.2).[10] The anterior bundle has been shown to be the primary restraint to valgus stress at the elbow.[11–15] Injury to the anterior bundle can cause instability of the elbow with subsequent disabling pain in overhead throwing athletes.[9,16–19] The humeral origin of both the anterior and posterior bundles is the medial epicondyle. The anterior bundle originates from the anteroinferior aspect of the medial epicondyle[10,20–22] and inserts at the sublime tubercle of the ulna.[10,22,23] On average, the anterior bundle occupies two-thirds of the width of the medial epicondyle in the coronal plane.[22] It averages 4.7 mm in width and 27 mm in length.[21] The posterior bundle is triangular, smaller, and fanlike in nature; it originates from the posteroinferior aspect of the medial epicondyle and attaches to the medial olecranon margin.[14]

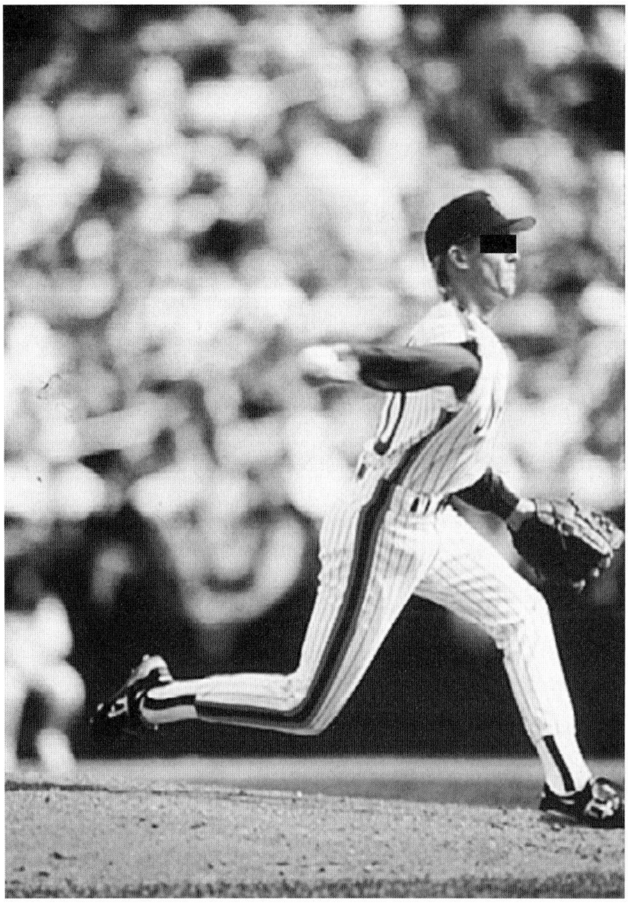

Figure 5.1. Professional baseball pitcher. Extreme valgus loads are placed across the elbow during the baseball pitch.

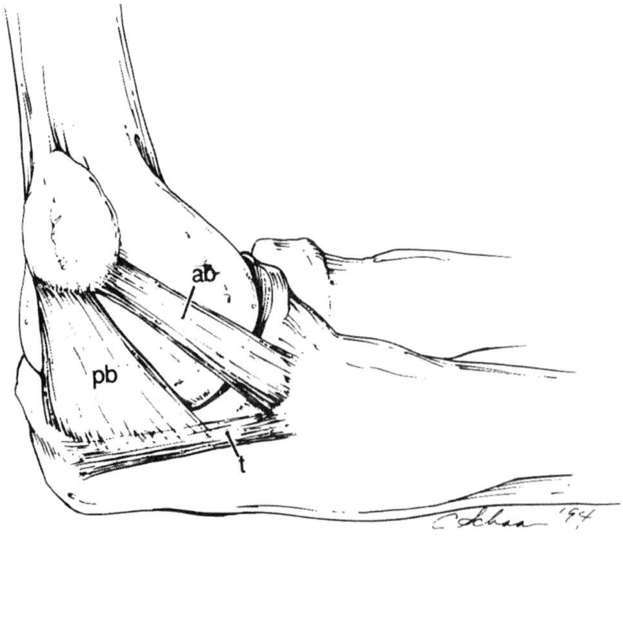

Figure 5.2. Medial ulnar collateral ligament complex. The anterior bundle of the ulnar collateral ligament is the primary stabilizer to valgus stress. (From Field, Callaway, O'Brien, et al.,[25] by permission of Am J Sports Med.)

The anterior bundle has separate bands that function as a cam tightening in a reciprocal fashion as the elbow is flexed and extended.[14,21,24] In a cadaveric study, Callaway et al.[10] performed sequential cutting of the medial collateral ligament while a valgus torque was applied. The anterior band of the anterior bundle was the primary restraint to valgus rotation at 30, 60, and 90 degrees of flexion. The posterior band of the anterior bundle was a co-primary restraint with the anterior band at 120 degrees. In a separate study, Field and Altchek[25] evaluated the laxity seen with MCL injury when viewed through the arthroscope. They found that ulnohumeral joint opening was not visualized in any specimen until complete sectioning of the anterior bundle was performed. However, only 1 mm or 2 mm of joint opening was present with complete transection of the anterior bundle emphasizing the subtle exam findings in these athletes. It was shown that the maximum amount of valgus laxity was seen best at 60 degrees to 75 degrees of flexion.

The flexor carpi ulnaris (FCU) is the predominant muscle overlying the medial collateral ligament.[26] It is the most posterior structure of the flexor-pronator mass, which places it directly overlying the anterior bundle of the medial collateral ligament. Thus, the FCU is optimally positioned to provide direct support to the MCL in regard to valgus stability. Preservation of the FCU is important during reconstruction of the MCL to maintain one of the secondary restraints to valgus stress. The ulnar nerve lies in close proximity to the MCL as well. It courses from a point posterior to the medial intermuscular septum above the medial epicondyle toward the anterior aspect of the medial elbow. Once it passes anterior to the intermuscular septum, the ulnar nerve then courses posterior to the medial epicondyle within the cubital tunnel. It then progresses distally to a point just posterior to the sublime tubercle. At this point, the ulnar nerve dives into the flexor carpi ulnaris which it innervates. It is important to be familiar with the anatomy of this vulnerable structure during the medial collateral ligament reconstruction in order to avoid an iatrogenic injury.

History and Physical Examination

In the evaluation of overhead athletes with medial sided elbow complaints, it is important to first obtain a detailed history. Questions should be posed as to the chronicity of the symptoms as well as its effect on the overhead activity. Issues regarding velocity, accuracy, and stamina are important to the throwing athlete and should therefore be addressed. It is important to note that many of these athletes modify their pitching techniques to compensate for the pain; however, these patients will not be able to reach their maximal throwing velocity secondary to the altered mechanics being implemented. The phase of throwing in which the pain occurs is another important aspect. Conway et al. have shown that nearly 85% of athletes with medial elbow instability complain of discomfort during the acceleration phase of throwing, in contrast to less than 25% of athletes who experience pain during the deceleration phase.[1] This same study also showed that up to 40% of patients with medial collateral ligament injuries may be associated with ulnar neuritis.[1] Therefore, a history of ulnar nerve symptoms should be ascertained as well as information pertaining to the position in which these symptoms are most prevalent.

Patients present either with an acute event or an acute on chronic episode. In an acute event, the patient reports having heard a pop, and subsequently experienced acute medial pain without the ability to continue pitching. In an acute on chronic event, the patient will have experienced an innocuous onset of medial sided elbow pain over an extended period of time with overhead throwing. This would preclude the acute event as described previously with an inability to continue with full velocity pitching.

Both passive and active range of motion of the elbow should be documented. Range of motion is frequently diminished in these athletes with loss of extension. During the range of motion testing, attention should be turned to the detection of any crepitus, pain, or mechanical blocks. Patients with valgus overload will frequently develop posteromedial osteophytes that will present as a bony block to full extension. A possible loose body may also present with similar findings.

Direct palpation of the origin of the medial collateral ligament is unreliable secondary to the overlying flexor-pronator mass and ulnar nerve. However, an attempt should be made to elicit discomfort in this region with palpation. The ulnar nerve should be palpated to assess for ulnar neuritis or subluxation of the nerve resulting in paresthesias. A Tinel's test should always be assessed. The medial epicondylar insertion of the flexor pronator mass should also be palpated for tenderness. If the flexor pronator tendon is involved, pain will be reproduced with resisted forearm pronation. This resisted maneuver will help differentiate a MCL injury from a flexor pronator tendonitis.

Posterior impingement secondary to posteromedial olecranon osteophytes should be assessed. This is accomplished through the valgus extension overload test.[18] The examiner uses one hand to apply a valgus force across the elbow while stabilizing the joint with the opposite hand. The forearm is placed in a pronated position and the elbow is then quickly brought to full extension while the valgus load is applied. A positive test is indicated by pain in the posteromedial aspect of the elbow.

Specific testing of the MCL includes the following: (1) valgus stress test, (2) O'Brien's milking test, (3) arthroscopic stress test, and (4) O'Driscoll's moving valgus stress test. When performing the valgus stress test, the patient is placed in a seated position. The physician secures the patient's forearm near the wrist by placing the wrist and hand of the patient between the examiner's arm and torso. The elbow is then flexed to 30° so that the olecranon will become unlocked from its fossa. Though it has been shown biomechanically that flexion angles greater than 30 degrees will make instability of the MCL more apparent, it is difficult to adequately stabilize the humerus at these angles to apply the valgus load. To apply a valgus force through the elbow, one of the examiner's hands acts as a post on the lateral aspect of the elbow.

This hand facilitates the valgus force necessary to elicit pain or instability, as well as stabilizes humeral rotation. The other hand is placed over the MCL to palpate for tenderness in the area while the valgus stress is applied (Figure 5.3). If the patient complains of increased medial sided elbow pain or if valgus instability is present, then the test result is considered positive. However, it must be noted that the amount of instability present in these cases is often too small to be picked up by this maneuver. Thus, pain is the predominant alert for a MCL injury with this test.

O'Brien has described the milking maneuver to help diagnose those tears that remained in continuity and therefore did not demonstrate gross instability. This is performed by grasping the thumb of the patient's injured extremity and applying a radially directed force. The elbow is then placed in a flexed position at 70 degrees to 90 degrees. A valgus stress is applied across the MCL as the elbow is flexed by pulling radially on the patient's thumb. The patient complains of discomfort if a partial injury is present. O'Driscoll has described the moving valgus stress test. This test is performed by positioning the shoulder in an

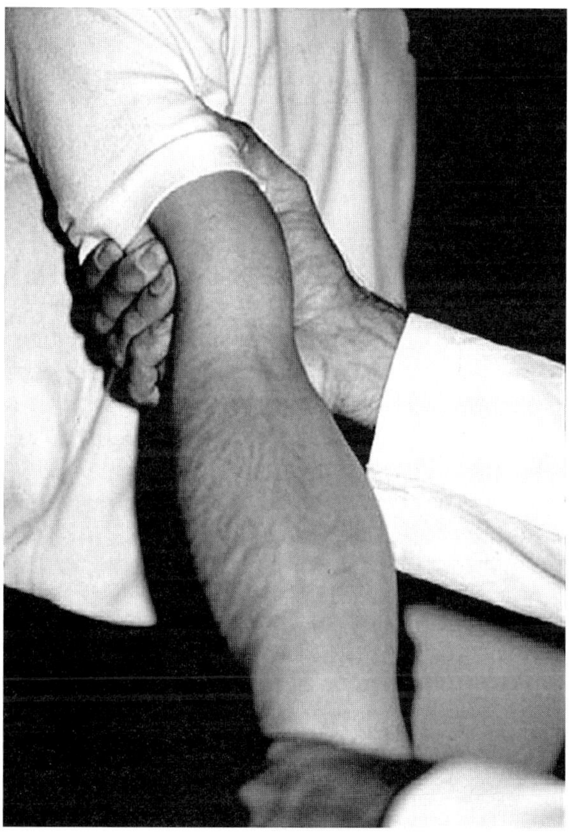

Figure 5.3. Valgus stress test. While one hand of the examiner supports the elbow, valgus stress is applied with the elbow in approximately 30 degrees of flexion. Tenderness to palpation over the ulnar collateral ligament as well as valgus laxity are assessed.

abducted and externally rotated position, and then placing a valgus stress across the elbow as the patient quickly flexes and extends the elbow. Similar to other diagnostic tests, the patient will complain of pain if an injury to the MCL is present.

The arthroscopic stress test, as described by Timmerman et al.,[18] can be used to help increase the sensitivity of the valgus stress test on gross physical examination. The anterolateral portal is used to view the medial joint line arthroscopically for evidence of ulnohumeral joint opening. This test is performed by placing a valgus load across the joint while the elbow is flexed at 70 degrees. Field and Altchek[27] performed a series of cadaveric dissections to evaluate the use of the arthroscopic valgus instability test. After complete sectioning of the anterior bundle, they found 1 mm to 2 mm of medial ulnohumeral joint laxity present with a valgus force placed across the elbow. When the entire MCL complex was sectioned, 4 mm to 10 mm of opening was noted. The greatest degree of opening was seen at 60 degrees to 75 degrees of elbow flexion with the forearm in a pronated position. Additionally, ulnohumeral cartilage wear and potential loose bodies as well as posteromedial olecranon osteophytes can be inspected with the arthroscope. It is for these reasons that we recommend all patients having a MCL reconstruction to receive an elbow arthroscopy performed at the time of surgery. The use of the arthroscope during this procedure is discussed in more detail in the technique section.

Imaging

Plain radiographs remain the primary tool for initial evaluation of the elbow. Routine anteroposterior (AP), lateral, and oblique views should be obtained. These standard radiographic views may reveal calcifications in the MCL, medial spurs on the humerus and ulna at the joint line, spurs on the posterior olecranon tip, or loose bodies present in the olecranon fossa (Figure 5.4). Stress radiographs have been suggested to aid in the diagnosis of medial collateral ligament tears as well.[28,29]

MRI has also been advocated for use in the evaluation of the MCL. Mirowitz and London[30] showed that MRI was useful for depiction of the presence and severity of a MCL abnormality, but they had surgical confirmation in only 6 of 11 throwing athletes. The sensitivity of MRI in detecting partial MCL tears has been shown to be increased by injecting the elbow joint with saline before imaging. In a series of 40 throwing athletes, Schwartz et al.[31] showed that the use of saline-enhanced MR arthrography revealed 24 of 26 individuals with MCL tears which were confirmed at the time of surgery. Sensitivity of complete tears was 95%, and 86% for partial tears in these 26 patients.

At Hospital for Special Surgery, the use of 3-dimensional volumetric gradient-echo and fast spin-echo techniques enables thin-section (<3 mm) imaging of the elbow, thus improving visualization of partial tears of the medial collateral ligament and obviating the need for contrast injection.[32,33] Partial tears can be seen on MRI as areas of focal interruption that do not extend through the full thickness of the ligament.

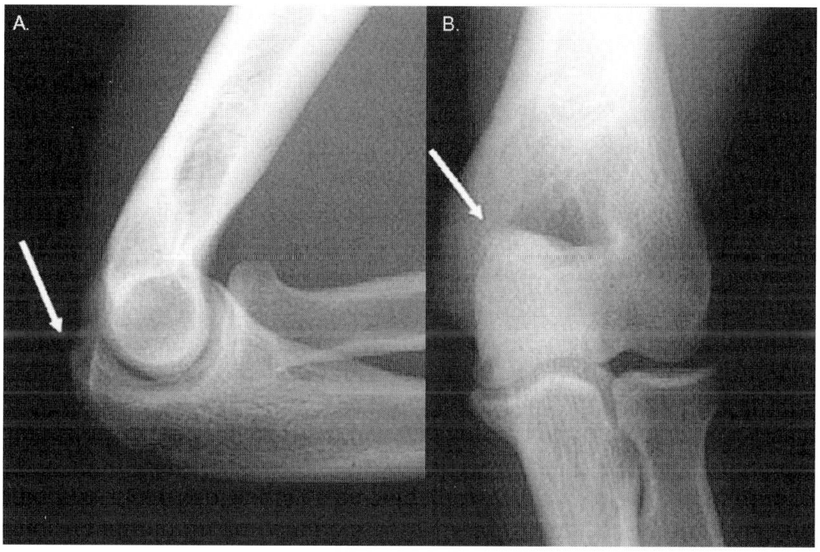

Figure 5.4. Radiographs of elbow. (A) Lateral radiograph showing prominent osteophyte noted at tip of olecranon. (B) Anteroposterior radiograph showing a small posteromedial osteophyte of olecranon.

Complete tears can be seen on coronal MR images as increased signal intensity and focal disruption of the normally hypointense, vertically oriented ligament (Figure 5.5). In chronic ligament injuries without tears, the MCL will appear thickened without focal discontinuity, but

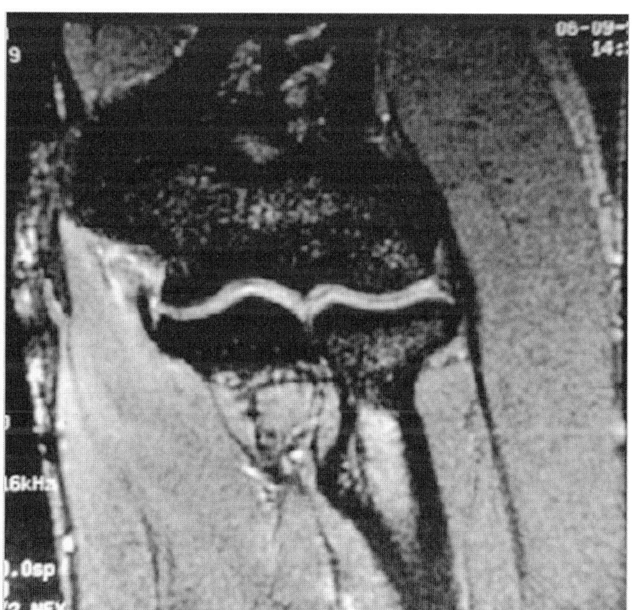

Figure 5.5. Coronal MRI image of elbow. Increased signal intensity and focal disruption is noted at the ulnar collateral ligament indicative of a complete tear.

with global increased signal intensity. Because arthroscopic evaluation of the MCL is limited in its ability to visualize the anterior bundle and humeral or ulnar insertions,[25] MRI is an effective technique for distinguishing ligament tears from flexor or pronator tendinopathy. In addition, ulnar neuritis may be observed with enlargement and increased signal intensity in the nerve. Osteochondral impaction injuries to the radiocapitellar joint may also be seen, which emphasizes the importance of obtaining appropriate cartilage pulse sequencing.

Whereas complete disruption of the MCL will often result in clinically apparent valgus instability, partial disruption may not. Diagnosis of both partial tears and complete tears is important because athletes with partial tears may undergo MCL reconstruction if rehabilitation and conservative treatments have failed. An athlete will more quickly return to competition if an early diagnosis of a partial tear of the MCL is noted and appropriate surgical reconstruction implemented. Thus, at initial presentation, we recommend that all throwing athletes undergo both plain films and MRI with appropriate pulse sequences, as standard MRI techniques may yield unrewarding images.

Surgical Technique: The Docking Procedure

Early experience at HSS with the Jobe procedure led to concerns over the morbidity of the original procedure. These concerns included (1) adequate tensioning of the graft at the time of final fixation, (2) potential complications from detachment of the flexor origin, (3) potential complications from the placement of three drill holes in a limited area, and (4) the strength of suture fixation of the free tendon graft as the graft was not placed in an osseous tunnel. Other studies had shown the high rate of complications associated with ulnar nerve transposition,[1,3] and the routine transfer of the ulnar nerve was questioned. Also, the results of anatomic and EMG studies suggest that the flexor mass contributes greatly to the dynamic stability of the elbow.[17,26] Therefore, an attempt should be made to limit dissection of the flexor pronator mass. In 1996, Altchek began to look at alternative methods to reconstruct the MCL which resulted in several modifications of the Jobe procedure. This procedure was named the docking technique as the graft was docked within an osseous tunnel at the time of final fixation[34] as opposed to reliance on suture fixation alone.

In a series of 15 fresh-frozen cadaveric dissections at HSS, Smith et al.[35] described the "safe zone" for a flexor carpi ulnaris muscle splitting incision thereby preserving the origin of the flexor pronator mass. They demonstrated that the anterior band of the MCL can easily be exposed for reconstruction without taking down the origin of the flexor pronator mass and without transposing the ulnar nerve. This approach offers several advantages. First, repair of the flexor mass is unnecessary which lessens operative time. Second, the morbidity associated with pain and rehabilitation may be lessened, as this approach is less traumatic. Third, the anterior bundle of the MCL lies directly beneath the flexor carpi ulnaris and not under the anterior portion of the common flexor mass. As an internervous plane exists in the flexor muscle group between the flexor carpi ulnaris muscle and the flexor digitorum superficialis, this provides a suitable avenue for a muscle-splitting approach. Fourth, the ulnar nerve does not directly overlie the anterior bundle of the MCL, but rather crosses the bundle near its attachment at the sublime tubercle of the ulna.[10] This allows one to safely retract the ulnar nerve posteriorly without necessitating an anterior transposition. Finally, the dissections of this study found that there was consistently an area of musculature where no innervating branches crossed. This watershed area is safe as long as the muscle split is not extended more than 1 cm to 3 cm past the sublime tubercle. This provides ample space to drill the bony tunnels in the proximal ulna as originally described by Jobe.[3]

We routinely perform an arthroscopic evaluation both anteriorly and posteriorly of all patients prior to reconstruction. Secondary to the mechanics of valgus extension overload, it is not unusual for these patients to demonstrate intraarticular pathology. In a recent study by Altchek and colleagues,[34] 45% (13 of 29 patients) of chronic MCL insufficiency patients undergoing reconstruction had arthroscopically treatable lesions, particularly impingement lesions such as fragmented spurring. In this same study, it was also noted that detection of the lesions on preoperative imaging studies occurred in only 8 of 13 cases. As a significant number of patients present with arthroscopically treatable lesions, we feel that a complete arthroscopic examination is important.

The goals of the docking technique are as follows:

1. To perform a tendon graft reconstruction of the MCL through a muscle-splitting "safe zone" approach.
2. To avoid an obligatory transposition of the ulnar nerve.
3. To routinely arthroscopically assess and treat intraarticular pathology, particularly posteromedially.
4. To place the tendon graft in bone tunnels.
5. To reduce the number of humeral drill holes from three, as has previously been described,[3] to a single hole in the hope of reducing both the initial morbidity as well as possible complication of epicondylar fracture.
6. To simplify graft tensioning and improve fixation methods.

At HSS, the procedure is generally performed with axillary block anesthesia. After being blocked, a tourniquet is placed on the upper arm and the patient remains supine on the operating table while the hand and arm are prepared and draped in the usual sterile manner. Using a McConnell arm holder (McConnell Orthopedic Manufacturing Company, Greenville, TX), the surgeon places the humerus and forearm in a position such that the forearm is across the chest. This position allows the arthroscopy to be performed in a position that mimics the prone position (Figure 5.6).

The arthroscope is introduced through an anterolateral portal into the anterior compartment. A diagnostic arthroscopy is performed of the anterior compartment, evaluating the articular surfaces and the synovium as well as identifying loose bodies. A valgus stress test is then

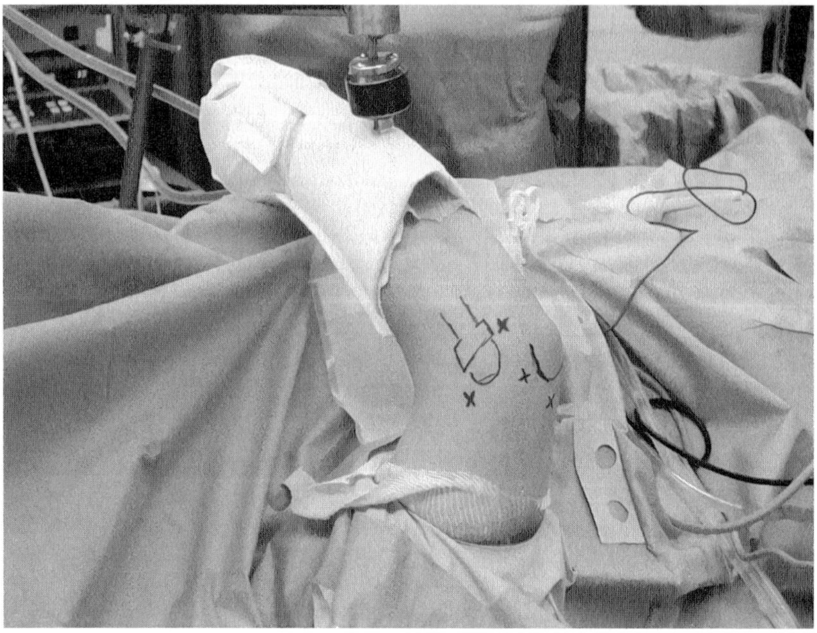

Figure 5.6. Supine position of patient. Patient is placed in a supine position for elbow arthroscopy. The McConnell arm holder allows the elbow to be positioned in a manner to mimic the prone position.

applied with the elbow placed at 90 degrees of flexion and the forearm in a pronated position to evaluate the competence of the medial collateral ligament. In the normal elbow, a maximum of 1 mm to 2 mm of medial opening will be observed. If laxity of more than 3 mm of opening between the coronoid and the medial humerus is observed, then the MCL is considered incompetent.

After completing the anterior compartment arthroscopy, attention is then turned to the posterior compartment of the elbow. The arthroscope is removed leaving the cannula in the anterior portal. The inflow is then introduced through this cannula. When the joint is distended, a posterolateral portal is created and the arthroscope is inserted into the posterior compartment. The medial, lateral, and central olecranon is evaluated for the presence of spurs. The humeral fossa is evaluated for spurs or loose bodies. The medial humeral condyle is evaluated for articular injury. Finally, the posterior radiocapitellar joint is evaluated by advancing the arthroscope down the lateral gutter. If an operative procedure is necessary, such as a spur removal, a transtriceps portal is created through the center of the tendon at the level of the olecranon tip. The most common problem is a fragmented spur on the medial border of the olecranon. These spurs may not be evident on preoperative radiographs. In addition, loose bodies can be present in or about the radiocapitellar joint. If a loose body is visualized here, it is usually necessary to create a new portal through the anconeus directly into this region of the joint.

Once the arthroscopy has been completed, the arm is released from the arm holder and placed on the hand table below. If a reconstruction is planned, the graft is harvested at this juncture. The most commonly used graft is the ipsilateral palmaris longus. The palmaris longus tendon has been shown to fail at higher loads with nearly four times the ultimate strength as compared with the anterior band of the medial collateral ligament.[14] It is imperative to document the presence of a palmaris longus tendon preoperatively. If it is not present, then the contralateral palmaris tendon or the gracilis may be used. The palmaris longus is harvested through a 5-mm to 1-cm incision placed in the distal wrist crease. Rather than multiple incisions, we use a tendon stripper specially made for this use. At the time of harvest, we place a no. 1 braided nonabsorbable suture using a no. 1 Ethibond Excel OS-2 needle (Ethicon, Inc., a Johnson & Johnson Company, Westwood, MA) in a Krackow fashion in one end of the tendon (Figure 5.7). After harvest, the tendon is placed in a moist sponge on the back table.

To expose the MCL, the arm is exsanguinated and the tourniquet is inflated. A 5-cm to 7-cm incision is created from the distal third of the intermuscular septum across the medial epicondyle to a point 2 cm beyond the sublime tubercle of the ulna (Figure 5.8). While exposing the fascia of the flexor pronator, take care to identify and preserve the antebrachial cutaneous branch of the median nerve, which frequently crosses the operative field. The posterior raphe of the flexor carpi ulnaris is incised longitudinally in line with the fibers of the fascia, and the underlying flexor muscle is bluntly split exposing the underlying ligament. Once the ligament has been exposed, a deep, blunt, self-retaining retractor is placed to maintain exposure (Figure 5.9A). The anterior bundle of the MCL is incised longitudinally, exposing the joint. At this point, MCL laxity can be confirmed by observing the separation of the joint surfaces by 3 mm or more with valgus stress (Figure 5.9B).

The tunnel positions for the ulna are exposed. The posterior tunnel requires that the surgeon subperiosteally expose the ulna 4 mm to 5 mm

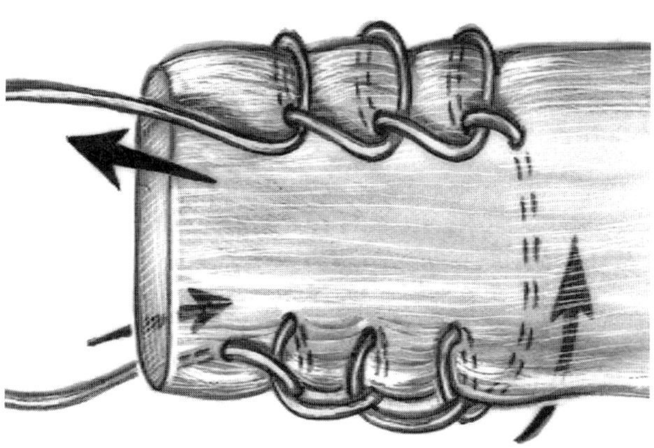

Figure 5.7. Krackow stitch. Placement of Krackow stitch using a no. 1 Ethibond placed in the end of the palmaris graft.

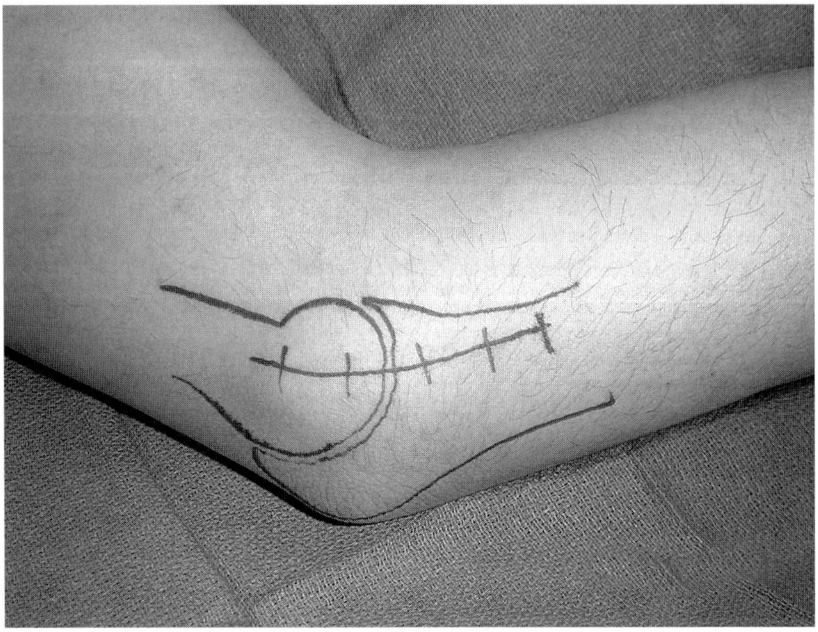

Figure 5.8. Skin incision. A 5-cm to 7-cm incision is centered over the medial epicondyle and extended just distal to the approximate position of the sublime tubercle. Care is taken to preserve the medial antebrachial cutaneous nerve.

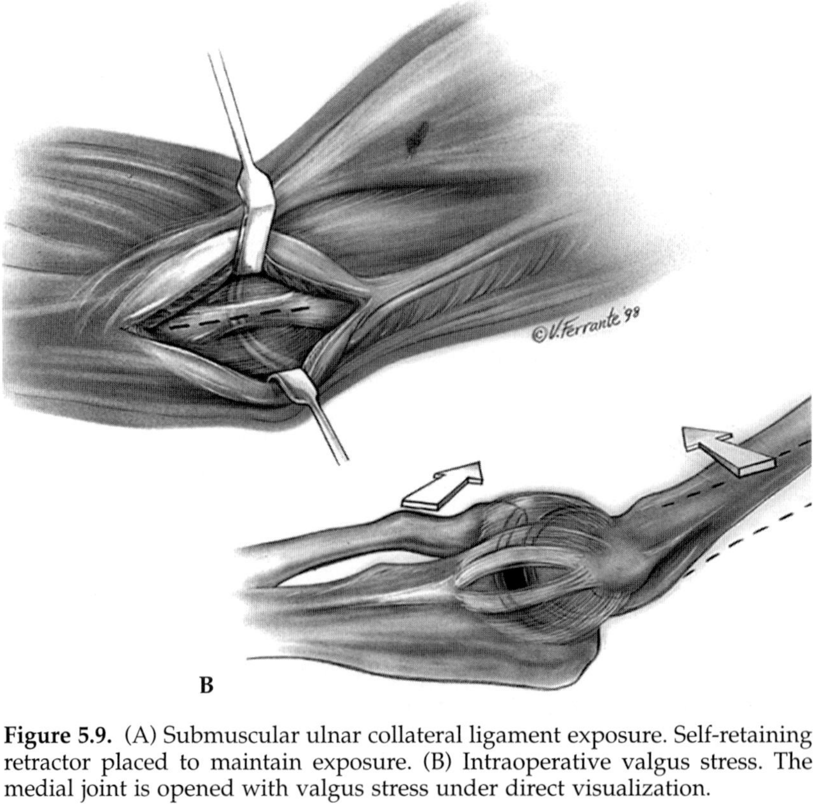

A

B

Figure 5.9. (A) Submuscular ulnar collateral ligament exposure. Self-retaining retractor placed to maintain exposure. (B) Intraoperative valgus stress. The medial joint is opened with valgus stress under direct visualization.

posterior to the sublime tubercle while meticulously protecting the ulnar nerve. If the nerve is seen to subluxate anteriorly such that it cannot be adequately protected, a transposition of the ulnar nerve may be performed. Using a no. 3 burr, tunnels are made anterior and posterior to the sublime tubercle such that a 2-cm bridge exists between them. The tunnels are connected using a small, curved curette, taking care not to violate the bony bridge (Figure 5.10A). A no. 1 Ethibond Excel OS-2 needle is then used to pass a looped 2-0 suture. The humeral tunnel position is located in the anterior half of the medial epicondyle in the anterior position of the existing MCL. Using a no. 4 burr, a longitudinal tunnel is created up the axis of the medial epicondyle to a depth of 15 mm (Figure 5.10B). The upper border of the epicondyle, just anterior to the intramuscular septum, is then exposed. Using a dental drill with a small bit, two small exit punctures separated by 5 m to 1 cm are created to allow suture passage from the primary humeral tunnel (Figure 5.10B). A suture passer is used from each of the two exit punctures to pass a looped suture, to be used for later graft passage. With the elbow reduced, the horizontal incision in the MCL is repaired using a 2-0 absorbable suture (Figure 5.11).

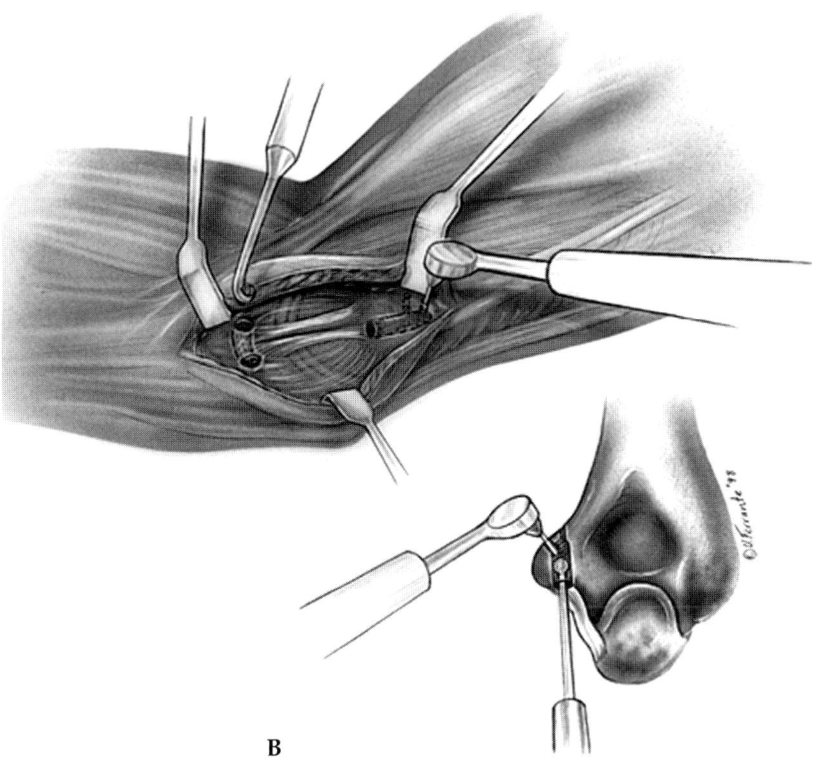

A

B

Figure 5.10. (A) Creation of ulnar tunnels. A curved curette is used to connect the ulnar tunnels. (B) Creation of the humeral tunnel. A 4-mm burr creates a longitudinal bony tunnel in the medial epicondyle. A dental burr provides puncture holes for passage of suture from within the humeral tunnel.

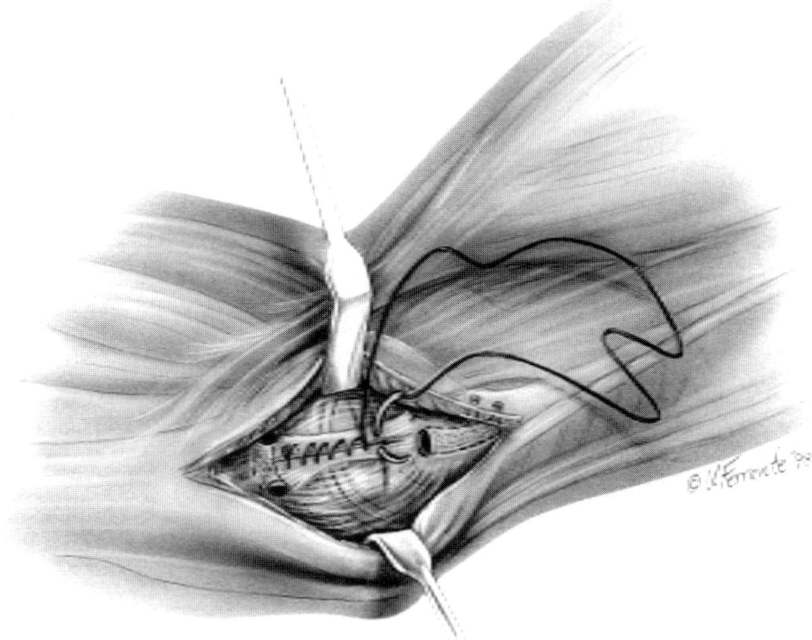

Figure 5.11. Native ligament repair. Suture repair of the longitudinal incision of the medial collateral ligament using absorbable suture.

The graft is then passed through the ulnar tunnel from anterior to posterior (Figure 5.12). The limb of the graft that has sutures already placed is then passed into the humeral tunnel with the sutures pulled exiting one of the small superior humeral punctures. With this first limb of the graft securely docked in the humerus, the elbow is reduced with forearm supination and gentle varus stress. While tension is maintained on the graft, the elbow is ranged from flexion to extension to eliminate potential creep within the graft. The final length of the graft is then measured by placing the free end of the graft adjacent to the humeral tunnel and visually estimating the length of the graft that will allow the graft to be tensioned within the humeral tunnel (Figure 5.13). This point is marked with dye and a no. 1 braided nonabsorbable suture is placed in a Krackow fashion. The excess graft is excised immediately above the Krackow stitch. This end of the graft is then docked securely in the humeral tunnel, with the sutures exiting the small puncture holes.

Final graft tensioning is performed by again placing the elbow through a full range of motion with varus stress placed on the elbow. Once the surgeon is satisfied with graft tension, the two sets of graft sutures are tied over the bony bridge on the humeral epicondyle (Figure 5.14). The tourniquet is deflated and the wound is copiously irrigated. Closure is performed by approximating the flexor carpi ulnaris fascia and subcutaneous and subcuticular tissues. The elbow is then placed in a plaster splint at 60 degrees of flexion and neutral rotation with the hand and wrist free.

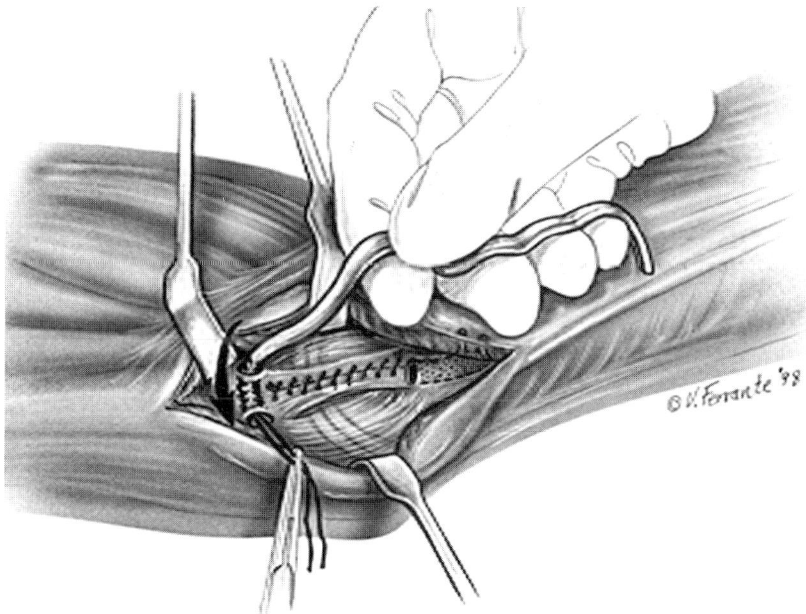

Figure 5.12. Passage of the graft. The palmaris longus graft is placed from an anterior to posterior direction in the ulnar tunnel.

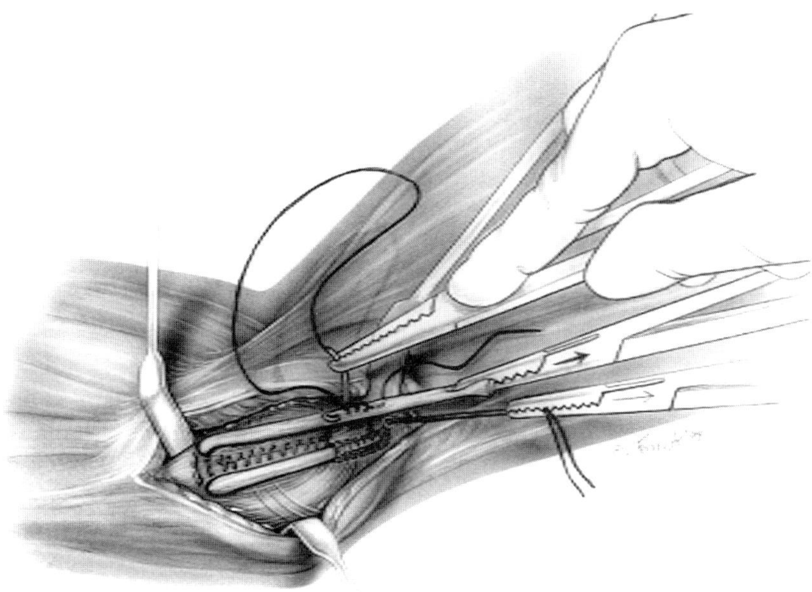

Figure 5.13. Tensioning of the graft. The anterior limb of the graft is passed into the humeral tunnel. The graft is tensioned with the forearm supinated and while a varus stress is applied.

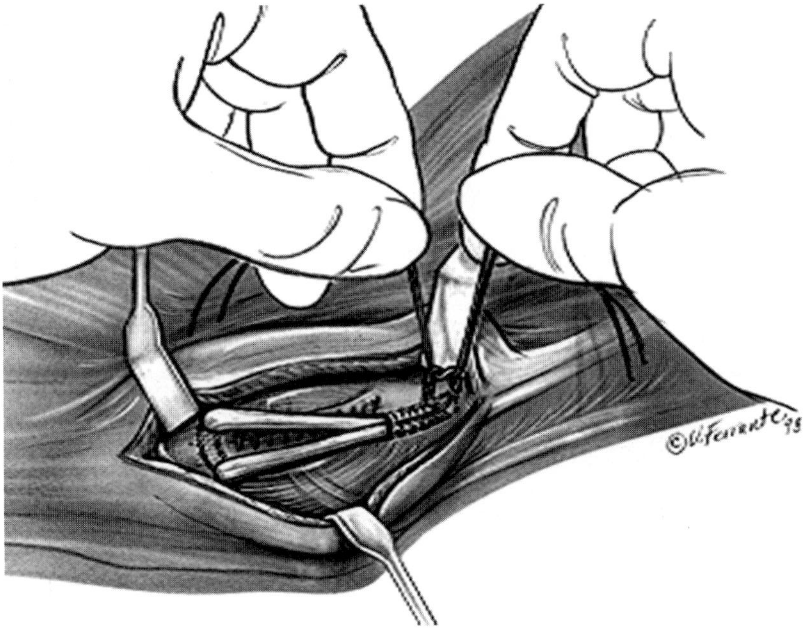

Figure 5.14. Suture fixation. The two sets of graft sutures are tied over the bony bridge.

Postoperative Mangement

The arm is maintained in the postoperative splint for the first week. After this period, the sutures are removed and the elbow is placed in a hinged elbow brace. Initially, motion is allowed between 45 degrees of extension and 90 degrees of flexion. Distal range of motion is encouraged as well, including gentle wrist flexion and extension and hand grip exercises. However, the patient is warned against any pronation. Over the next 5 weeks, elbow range of motion is gradually advanced to full.

At the 6-week postoperative period, formal physical therapy is initiated. The emphasis at this point is to correct residual losses of elbow motion and to gradually strengthen the forearm and shoulder musculature. The physical therapist should be instructed to avoid any valgus load across the elbow during this phase of rehabilitation. At the 12-week postoperative period, the strengthening program is advanced, and activities such as bench pressing light to moderate weights are allowed. At 4 months, a throwing program is initiated, beginning with short tossing. Dillman et al.[36] have shown the high forces that occur across the elbow with throwing, thus necessitating the slow advance of the throwing regimen during the postoperative period. At 6 months, pitching from flat ground is started with the anticipation of pitching from the mound at 7 months. In general, players do not pitch in competitive situations until the ninth month when the shoulder, elbow, and the forearm are pain-free during the throwing motion and have returned to normal strength. This allows for mature biologic healing of the graft into the bone tunnels.

Results

Conway et al.[1] conducted the first outcome study on the original procedure, as described by Jobe,[3] which included detachment of the flexor-pronator mass and routine transposition of the ulnar nerve. Even though 95% of these athletes were able to return to play, only 68% were able to return to either their prior or a higher level of competition. In addition, 15 of 71 patients were observed to develop postoperative ulnar nerve neuropathies. This was thought to be unacceptable and stirred further study into alternatives to this technique.

Thompson et al.[7] were the first to report on outcomes after a muscle-splitting approach. Eighty-three athletes underwent a MCL reconstruction with a muscle-splitting approach without transposition of the ulnar nerve. In their technique, the traditional suture fixation of the graft to itself was utilized. Of these 83 patients, thirty-three were followed for at least 2 years. The surgical result was excellent in 27 of 33 patients (82%), good in 4 (12%), and fair in 2 (6%). These results improved to 93% excellent results if those patients who had had a prior procedure were excluded. The mean time of return to competition was 13 months in this subset of 33 patients.

Altchek and colleagues[34] have recently reported on 36 consecutive MCL reconstructions using the docking technique with an average follow-up of 3.3 years. Thirty-three of 36 patients (92%) returned to or exceeded their previous level of competition for at least 1 year, meeting the Conway-Jobe classification criteria of "excellent." All 22 professional or collegiate athletes enrolled in the study returned to or exceeded their previous competition level.

Summary

The modifications described in the docking technique have resulted in excellent outcomes for athletes at all levels of play, and has proven to be a reliable method of reconstruction of the MCL. We feel that technical issues such as graft fixation and tensioning, as well as potential ulnar nerve complications, are addressed with the technique described. Furthermore, the potential complication of tunnel fracture is lessened with the use of fewer tunnels and thus without the need of a bony bridge at the medial epicondyle. These modifications allow for a minimally invasive approach to the reconstruction of the MCL with excellent results.

References

1. Conway JE, Jobe FW, Glousman RE, Pink M. Medial instability of the elbow in throwing athletes. Treatment by repair or reconstruction of the ulnar collateral ligament. J Bone Joint Surg Am. 1992;74(1):67–83.
2. Hamilton CD, Glousman RE, Jobe FW, Brault J, Pink M, Perry J. Dynamic stability of the elbow: electromyographic analysis of the flexor pronator group and the extensor group in pitchers with valgus instability. J Shoulder Elbow Surg. 1996;5(5):347–354.

3. Jobe FW, Stark H, Lombardo SJ. Reconstruction of the ulnar collateral ligament in athletes. J Bone Joint Surg Am. 1986;68(8):1158–1163.
4. Tullos HS, Erwin WD, Woods GW, Wukasch DC, Cooley DA, King JW. Unusual lesions of the pitching arm. Clin Orthop. 1972;88:169–182.
5. Waris W. Elbow injuries of javelin-throwers. Acta Chir Scand. 1946;93: 563–575.
6. Kenter K, Behr CT, Warren RF, O'Brien SJ, Barnes R. Acute elbow injuries in the National Football League. J Shoulder Elbow Surg. 2000;9(1):1–5.
7. Thompson WH, Jobe FW, Yocum LA, Pink MM. Ulnar collateral ligament reconstruction in athletes: muscle-splitting approach without transposition of the ulnar nerve. J Shoulder Elbow Surg. 2001;10(2):152–157.
8. Kenter K, Behr CT, Warren RF, O'Brien SJ, Barnes R. Acute elbow injuries in the National Football League. J Shoulder Elbow Surg. 2000;9(1):1–5.
9. Miller CD, Savoie FH III. Valgus Extension Injuries of the Elbow in the Throwing Athlete. J Am Acad Orthop Surg. 1994;2(5):261–269.
10. Callaway GH, Field LD, Deng XH, Torzilli PA, O'Brien SJ, Altchek DW, et al. Biomechanical evaluation of the medial collateral ligament of the elbow. J Bone Joint Surg Am. 1997;79(8):1223–1231.
11. Hotchkiss RN, Weiland AJ. Valgus stability of the elbow. J Orthop Res. 1987;5(3):372–377.
12. Morrey BF, An KN. Articular and ligamentous contributions to the stability of the elbow joint. Am J Sports Med. 1983;11(5):315–319.
13. Morrey BF, Tanaka S, An KN. Valgus stability of the elbow. A definition of primary and secondary constraints. Clin Orthop. 1991;(265):187–195.
14. Regan WD, Korinek SL, Morrey BF, An KN. Biomechanical study of ligaments around the elbow joint. Clin Orthop. 1991;(271):170–179.
15. Sojbjerg JO, Ovesen J, Nielsen S. Experimental elbow instability after transection of the medial collateral ligament. Clin Orthop. 1987;(218):186–190.
16. Andrews JR, Whiteside JA. Common elbow problems in the athlete. J Orthop Sports Phys Ther. 1993;17(6):289–295.
17. Glousman RE, Barron J, Jobe FW, Perry J, Pink M. An electromyographic analysis of the elbow in normal and injured pitchers with medial collateral ligament insufficiency. Am J Sports Med. 1992;20(3):311–317.
18. Timmerman LA, Schwartz ML, Andrews JR. Preoperative evaluation of the ulnar collateral ligament by magnetic resonance imaging and computed tomography arthrography. Evaluation in 25 baseball players with surgical confirmation. Am J Sports Med. 1994;22(1):26–31.
19. Wilson FD, Andrews JR, Blackburn TA, McCluskey G. Valgus extension overload in the pitching elbow. Am J Sports Med. 1983;11(2):83–88.
20. Fuss FK. The ulnar collateral ligament of the human elbow joint. Anatomy, function and biomechanics. J Anat. 1991;175:203–212.
21. Morrey BF, An KN. Functional anatomy of the ligaments of the elbow. Clin Orthop. 1985;(201):84–90.
22. O'Driscoll SW, Jaloszynski R, Morrey BF, An KN. Origin of the medial ulnar collateral ligament. J Hand Surg Am. 1992;17(1):164–168.
23. Timmerman LA, Andrews JR. Undersurface tear of the ulnar collateral ligament in baseball players. A newly recognized lesion. Am J Sports Med. 1994;22(1):33–36.
24. Schwab GH, Bennett JB, Woods GW, Tullos HS. Biomechanics of elbow instability: the role of the medial collateral ligament. Clin Orthop. 1980; (146):42–52.
25. Field LD, Callaway GH, O'Brien SJ, Altchek DW. Arthroscopic assessment of the medial collateral ligament complex of the elbow. Am J Sports Med. 1995;23(4):396–400.

26. Davidson PA, Pink M, Perry J, Jobe FW. Functional anatomy of the flexor pronator muscle group in relation to the medial collateral ligament of the elbow. Am J Sports Med. 1995;23(2):245–250.
27. Field LD, Altchek DW. Evaluation of the arthroscopic valgus instability test of the elbow. Am J Sports Med. 1996;24(2):177–181.
28. Ellenbecker TS, Mattalino AJ, Elam EA, Caplinger RA. Medial elbow joint laxity in professional baseball pitchers. A bilateral comparison using stress radiography. Am J Sports Med. 1998;26(3):420–424.
29. Rijke AM, Goitz HT, McCue FC, Andrews JR, Berr SS. Stress radiography of the medial elbow ligaments. Radiology. 1994;191(1):213–216.
30. Mirowitz SA, London SL. Ulnar collateral ligament injury in baseball pitchers: MR imaging evaluation. Radiology. 1992;185(2):573–576.
31. Schwartz ML, al Zahrani S, Morwessel RM, Andrews JR. Ulnar collateral ligament injury in the throwing athlete: evaluation with saline-enhanced MR arthrography. Radiology. 1995;197(1):297–299.
32. Gaary EA, Potter HG, Altchek DW. Medial elbow pain in the throwing athlete: MR imaging evaluation. AJR Am J Roentgenol. 1997;168(3):795–800.
33. Potter HG. Imaging of posttraumatic and soft tissue dysfunction of the elbow. Clin Orthop. 2000;(370):9–18.
34. Rohrbough JT, Altchek DW, Hyman J, Williams RJ III, Botts JD. Medial collateral ligament reconstruction of the elbow using the docking technique. Am J Sports Med. 2002;30(4):541–548.
35. Smith GR, Altchek DW, Pagnani MJ, Keeley JR. A muscle-splitting approach to the ulnar collateral ligament of the elbow. Neuroanatomy and operative technique. Am J Sports Med. 1996;24(5):575–580.
36. Dillman CJ, Fleisig GS, Andrews JR. Biomechanics of pitching with emphasis upon shoulder kinematics. J Orthop Sports Phys Ther. 1993;18(2): 402–408.

6

Mini-Incision Distal Biceps Tendon Repair

Jason A. Schneider and Peter D. McCann

Stark first described distal biceps tendon rupture in 1843.[1] The earliest reports of surgical repair was in 1897 by Johnson and later in 1898 by Acquaviva.[1,2] Fischer and Shepanek in 1956[3] and Meherin and Kilgore in 1960[4] reported on a single incision for reattachment of the biceps to the radial tuberosity. This was shown to significantly improve flexion and supination strength, but extensive exposure was required and subsequently several cases of radial nerve palsy were reported. In 1961, Boyd and Anderson described a two-incision technique to limit the extent of the anterior dissection.[5] This technique was designed to avoid radial nerve injury and to access the bicipital tuberosity more easily. Unfortunately, this resulted in several reports of postoperative radioulnar synostosis.[2,6–9] Morrey described a muscle splitting modification that avoided subperiosteal elevation off the ulna in an attempt to reduce the incidence of radioulnar synostosis.[2,8,9] Despite the modification, debate exists over the risk of heterotopic ossification and subsequent limitation of forearm rotation after a two-incision technique.[9,10]

Recently, fixation of distal biceps tendon ruptures using suture anchors and a limited anterior incision has been reported.[11–13] The use of bone sutures allows for limited exposure of the bicipital tuberosity, eliminating the need for a posterior incision.[9,11,12] It is believed that the limited exposure would decrease the risk of radial nerve injury or heterotopic ossification. Mini-incision techniques have become popular in recent years in the fields of hip and knee arthroplasty. The purported advantages of the minimal approach include decreased perioperative morbidity and satisfaction of patient demand for a more cosmetic approach. Similar advantages apply to the mini-incision approach in patients undergoing distal biceps tendon repairs.

Etiology

Distal biceps tendon ruptures are rare, accounting for only 3% of all biceps brachii ruptures and are typically seen in men between the ages of 40 to 60 years of age.[2,6,11,12] There are only a few reports of this injury occurring in women.[1,16] The dominant arm is more commonly affected.[2,12,15] The injury usually occurs during an unexpected forceful eccentric muscle contraction against a partially flexed elbow. Typically, a patient loses control of an object and during the attempt to regain control of the object a sudden eccentric muscle contraction occurs which results in tendon failure. The tendon usually avulses from the bicipital tuberosity, although ruptures within the tendon substance and the musculotendinous junction have been reported. The bicipital aponeurosis may or may not rupture acutely.

The pathogenesis of distal biceps tendon ruptures is poorly understood. Degenerative and mechanical processes have been implicated as well as tendon hypovascularity.[17,18] In 1956, Davis and Yassine proposed that local inflammation and impingement at the bicipital tuberosity are possible contributing mechanisms.[17] The space available for the biceps tendon between the radius and ulna has been shown to change depending on the forearm position. The space available for the biceps tendon between the radial tuberosity and the ulna significantly decreases in pronation. Dynamic computed tomography of the proximal radioulnar space revealed a 50% reduction in the radioulnar joint at the radial tuberosity from full supination to full pronation.[18] This fact along with inflammation and irritation of the tendon may predispose the distal tendon to rupture.[17,18] Tendon hypovascularity and intrinsic degeneration may also be factors contributing to tendon ruptures in some patients.[2,18] Seiler evaluated the vascularity of the distal biceps tendon using light microscopy, multiplanar injection, and Spalteholz vascular injection. A hypovascular zone was found to exist in the distal biceps tendon just proximal to its insertion into the bicipital tuberosity.[18]

History and Physical Examination

Patients often reported an unexpected extension force applied to a flexed arm. The majority of patients who experience a distal biceps tendon rupture report a discrete popping or tearing sensation in the antecubital fossa combined with immediate and sharp pain. The intense pain subsequently subsides and is replaced with a dull aching pain. Ecchymosis and swelling is initially visible in the antecubital fossa. Local tenderness and pain is present in the acute phase. The rest pain eventually dissipates, but the patient often notes persistent weakness and endurance fatigue. Often the patient reports difficulty opening doors, using a screwdriver, or performing repetitive movements with the affected arm. The patient often notes asymmetry of the biceps contour, with proximal retraction and loss of resting tone in the muscle belly.

Clinically, the physician also notes a proximal retraction of the biceps muscle. There is local tenderness and a palpable loss of continuity of the biceps tendon in the antecubital fossa. With elbow flexion, the muscle contracts proximally with an obvious alteration of the muscle contour. The biceps tendon will no longer be taut in the antecubital fossa, and may be palpable under the skin more proximally. Range of

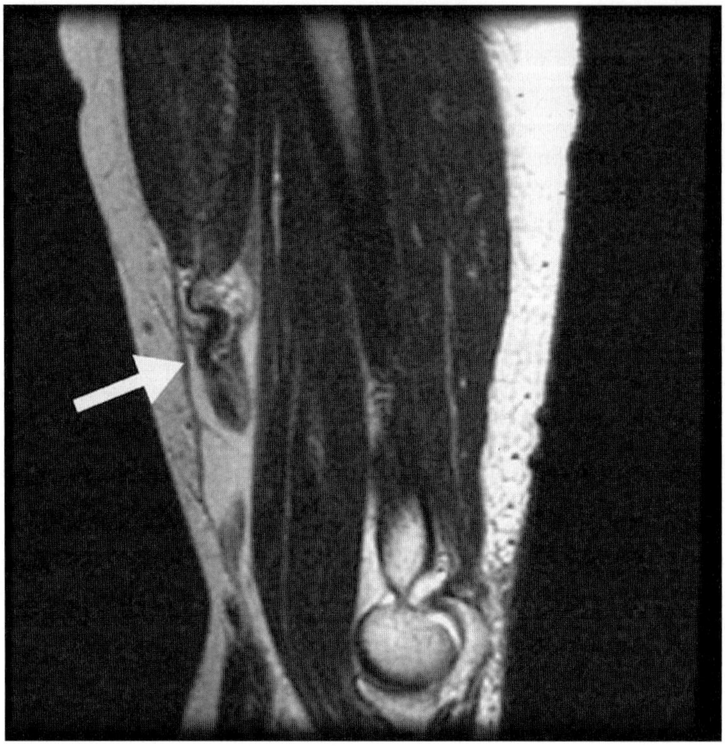

Figure 6.1. T1-weighted sagittal image of a complete rupture of the distal biceps tendon. The biceps tendon is retracted proximally (arrow).

motion is often not altered, except in the early phase secondary to pain. Supination and flexion strength are decreased when compared to the contralateral side.

The diagnosis of complete distal biceps tendon rupture can usually be established by history and physical exam alone. Radiographs are typically unremarkable but are recommended to rule out avulsion fractures or irregularity of the bicipital tuberosity. Occasionally the radiographs will show a small avulsion fleck from the tuberosity. Magnetic resonance imaging (MRI) may be considered to confirm the diagnosis of a distal biceps rupture (Figure 6.1). An MRI is indicated if the diagnosis is in question secondary to extensive swelling obscuring the antecubital fossa in acute injuries or to differentiate a complete tear from a partial tear.

Surgical Indication

Most authors recommend operative repair of distal biceps tendon ruptures in active individuals to restore optimal function.[2,8,12,13,19,20] Nonoperative management of distal biceps tendon rupture has been shown to result in a significant decrease in supination endurance and elbow flexion strength.[6,8,19] Morrey reported a mean loss of 40% supination strength and 30% of flexion strength when patients are treated nonoperatively.[2,8] Baker and coworkers compared operative versus nonoperative treatment. They observed that nonoperative treatment resulted in weakness in elbow flexion and forearm supination. Such weakness was clinically evident in several activities, such as the use of a screwdriver or swinging a baseball bat.[6] Tenodesis to the brachialis resulted in approximately 50% loss of supination strength but near normal flexion strength.[8] Rantanen and Orava presented a series of 19 avulsions of the distal biceps tendon with and average follow-up of 3 years. Ninety percent of the patients treated with an anatomic reinsertion had good to excellent results compared with only 60% for nonanatomic repairs and 14% for nonoperative treatment. From this data the authors concluded that anatomic reinsertion of the avulsed distal biceps tendon to the radius is the preferred treatment.[20]

Technique

Our mini-incision technique for distal biceps repair uses a single 3-cm anterior incision. The incision is made along the ulnar border of the brachioradialis muscle. The incision begins just distal to the elbow flexion crease and proceeds distally. The lateral antebrachial cutaneous nerve is identified and protected (Figure 6.2).

Generous subcutaneous flaps are elevated to permit both proximal and distal exposure. Establishing such flaps is essential to move the

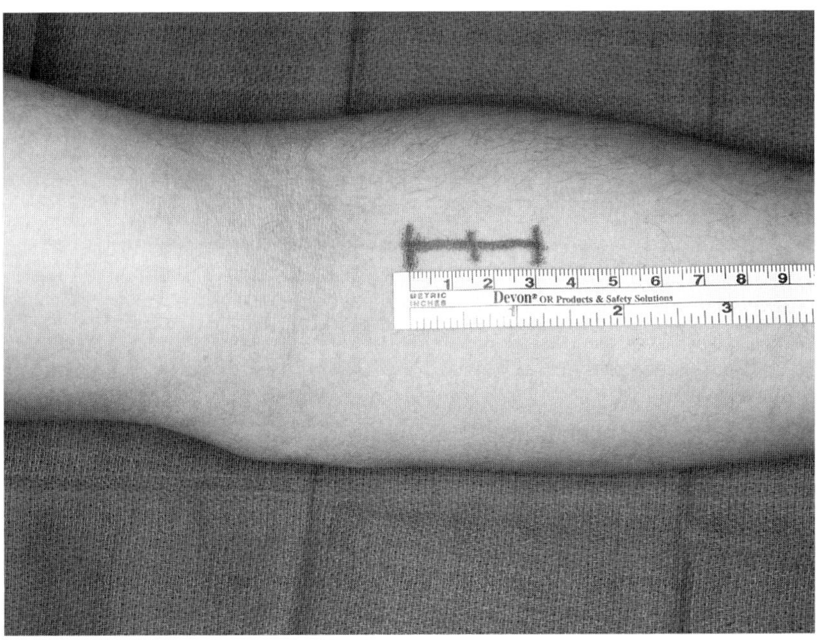

Figure 6.2. The authors' preferred incision for a single 3-cm mini-incision anterior approach. The incision is made along the ulnar border of the brachioradialis muscle. The incision begins just distal to the elbow flexion crease and proceeds distally.

mini-incision proximally and distally. Elbow flexion and proximal retraction of the subcutaneous flap delivers the biceps tendon stump into the field and, conversely, elbow extension and distal retraction of the subcutaneous flap allow easy access to the region of the bicipital tuberosity on the radius.

The retracted distal biceps tendon is identified and retrieved. It is located in the distal arm just superficial to the brachialis fascia. The tendon and muscle are freed from any adhesions. Care is taken to completely release any adhesions around the muscle and tendon units in order to allow for proper excursion.

After the biceps tendon is retrieved, dissection then proceeds distally towards the radial tuberosity. The dissection proceeds along the ulnar border of the brachioradialis, through the interval between the pronator teres and the brachioradialis. In acute cases, the empty biceps tendon sheath can frequently be followed distally to the tuberosity by blunt dissection. Care is taken to ligate the leash of recurrent radial vessels commonly encountered. Maximum supination of the forearm is maintained to keep the posterior interosseous nerve lateral to the operative field.

With maximal forearm supination, the bicipital tuberosity is identified at the distal and medial aspect of the wound. The tuberosity is exposed and any remnant of the biceps tendon insertion is removed. The cortex is lightly roughened, but decortication is not recommended. An elegant study by St. Pierre and colleagues evaluated tendon healing to bone. They compared tendon healing directly to cortical bone versus tendon healing to cancellous bone through a trough. Histological analysis was indistinguishable between the cortical and cancellous specimens. The biomechanical properties between the two groups were approximately equal. The study demonstrated no significant benefit from the creation of a cancellous trough to achieve tendon-to-bone healing. The implication of this study for biceps tendon repairs is that a cancellous trough is not necessary and that suture anchor repair of tendon to roughened cortical bone is sufficient.[21]

After the cortex is roughened, two suture anchors with preloaded no. 2 braided nonabsorbable suture are placed into the bicipital tuberosity approximately 1 cm apart. One anchor is placed distally and one proximally along the radial ridge of the tuberosity (Figure 6.3).

After the tuberosity is prepared, the biceps tendon is manually reduced to the radial tuberosity. This is done to ensure that the muscle contour of the arm can be restored as well as ensuring that the tendon can be reduced without excessive tension. The arm is flexed approximately 30 degrees to 45 degrees during reduction of the biceps tendon. After ensuring that the tendon can be reduced without excessive tension, the tendon is then sharply debrided to healthy appearing tissue. The distal portion of the ruptured biceps tendon is frequently thickened and degenerated. Up to 1 cm of the tendon can be safely debrided.

One limb of the no. 2 Ethibond suture from each anchor is woven through the tendon distal to proximally and then proximally to distally using a modified Krackow stitch (Figure 6.4). Care is taken not to

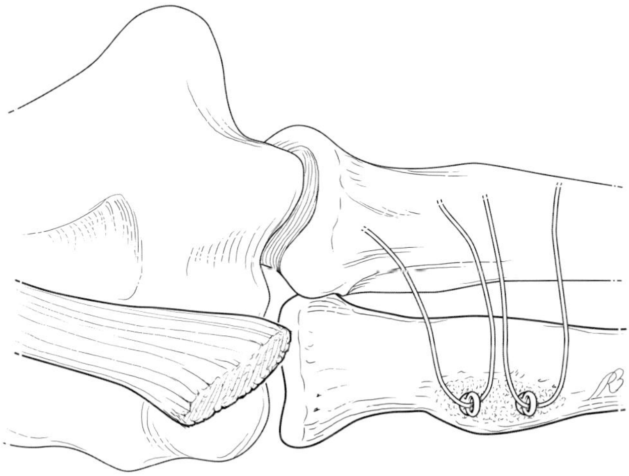

Figure 6.3. Two suture anchors with pre-loaded no. 2 braided nonabsorbable suture are placed into the bicipital tuberosity approximately 1 cm apart.

inadvertently cut the no. 2 Ethibond during the Krackow weave. The forearm is fully supinated and flexed to approximately 75 degrees. The tendon is then manually guided to the tuberosity with forceps and the slack is removed from each suture by pulling on the free limb of

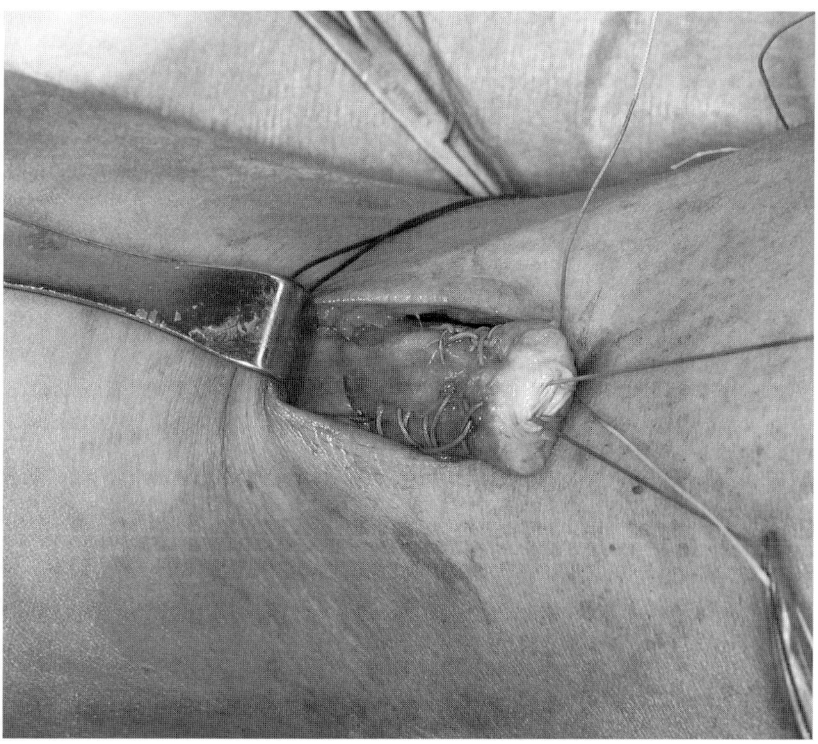

Figure 6.4. One limb of the no. 2 Ethibond suture from each anchor is woven through the tendon using a modified Krackow stitch.

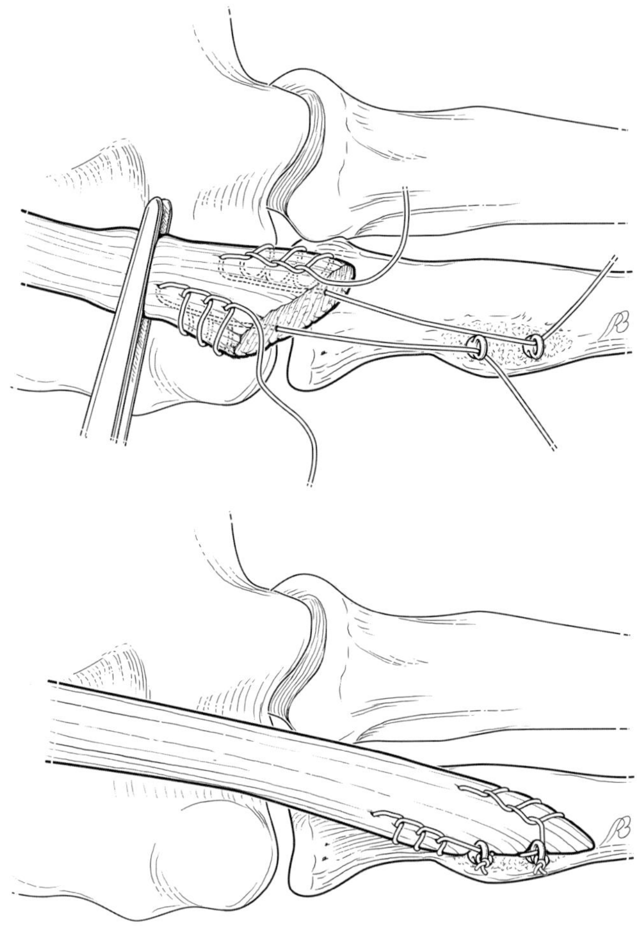

A

B

Figure 6.5. (A) The tendon is then manually guided to the tuberosity with forceps and the slack is removed from each suture by pulling on the free limb of the suture passing through the anchor. (B) The tendon is anatomically and securely reduced to the bicipital tuberosity.

the suture passing through the anchor. The sutures are then sequentially tied. Care is taken to ensure that all slack is removed from the sutures and that the tendon is anatomically and securely reduced to the bicipital tuberosity (Figure 6.5).

Following repair of the distal biceps tendon, the elbow is slowly extended to evaluate the security of the repair. The repaired tendon should be under firm tension at 45 degrees of elbow flexion (Figure 6.6). The tourniquet is deflated and hemostasis is obtained. The wound is copiously irrigated and the subcutaneous layer approximated with 2-0 vicryl suture. The skin is closed with 3-0 subcuticular prolene. The arm is placed in a well-padded posterior splint with the elbow flexed 90 degrees. The wrist is not incorporated in the splint. A postoperative lateral radiograph is obtained in the recovery room to evaluate the position of the suture anchors (Figure 6.7).

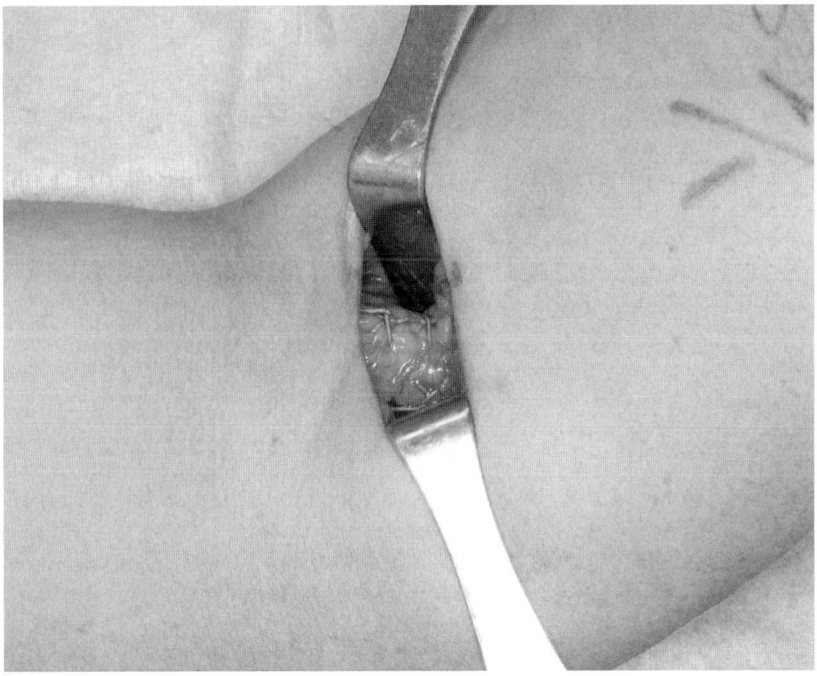

Figure 6.6. An intraoperative photograph showing the repaired tendon under firm tension at approximately 45 degrees of elbow flexion.

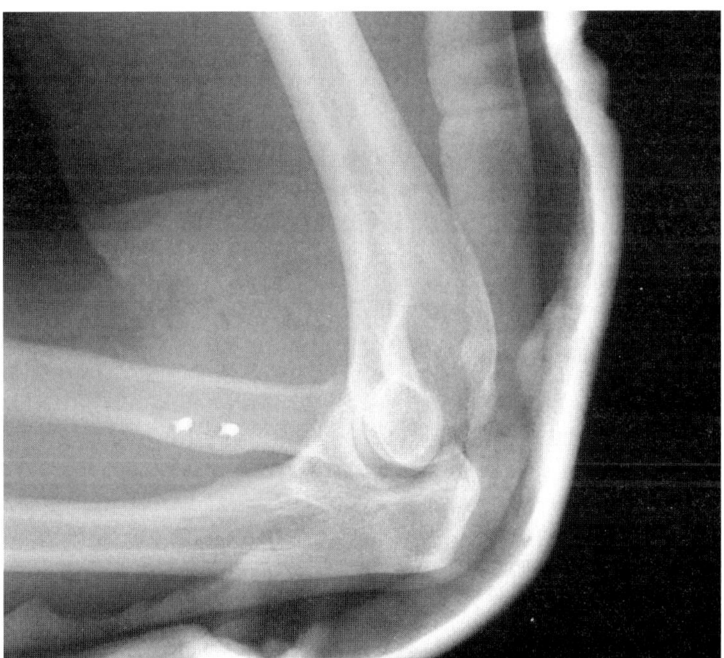

Figure 6.7. A lateral radiograph demonstrating proper placement of the two suture anchors within the bicipital tuberosity approximately 1 cm apart.

Rehabilitation

Postoperative rehabilitation is based on the injury acuity, security of repair, quality of tissue, and patient reliability. The patient is placed in a long arm splint in the operating room with the forearm in neutral rotation. The hand and wrist are kept free. The security of the repair is sufficient to allow the patient to use the hand for activities of daily living. Approximately 14 days after surgery, the patient is seen in the office and the skin suture is removed. A long arm cast is applied, maintaining the arm in 90 degrees of flexion. Once again, the wrist is kept free. The use of the hand is encouraged. The patient is kept immobilized for approximately 6 weeks from the time of surgery (Table 6.1). After the 6 weeks of immobilization, the cast is removed. Self-assisted range of motion exercises are started, and the patient is encouraged to continue to use the arm for activities of daily living. No lifting more then a few pounds is permitted during this 6-week period, and no formal physical therapy is prescribed. After 6 weeks of assisted range of motion exercises, the patient is reevaluated. If full range of motion has not been achieved, formal ROM exercises are begun with a physical therapist. Light strengthening exercises are begun at this stage as well and continue for 6 weeks. Progressive strengthening continues for an additional 6 weeks up to 6 months postoperatively, at which time full, unrestricted activity is allowed.

Complications

Radial nerve injuries after biceps tendon repair with the use of a single anterior incision have been reported.[4,14,22] These, however, are older series in which a more extensive volar approach was used. These palsies typically resolve completely, although permanent radial nerve injury has been reported.[4] There have been no reported cases of injury to the radial or posterior interosseous nerve with the more recent volar approach using suture anchors.[9,11,12,13,23] This is attributed to the less extensive soft tissue dissection and retraction. Injury to the lateral antebrachial cutaneous nerve has been reported with a single anterior incision or the 2-incision technique.[9,10,23] Injury to the lateral antebrachial coetaneous nerve can be minimized by careful dissection and protection of the nerve. Heterotopic ossification, a complication primarily associated with the 2-incision approach has only been reported once in series using a single anterior approach.[23] Failure of the repair and recurrent rupture of the biceps tendon has not been reported.[9,11,12,13,23]

Table 6.1. Rehabilitation protocol

6 weeks immobilization
6 weeks self-assisted ROM exercises
6 weeks light strengthening exercises
6 weeks of progressive strengthening
Full, unrestricted activity begins postoperatively at 6 months.

Summary

Rupture of the distal biceps tendon occurs when an unexpected extension force is applied against a contracting biceps muscle. A thorough history and physical examination is usually all that is needed to make the diagnosis. Operative treatment with anatomic repair of the distal biceps tendon is the treatment of choice for active individuals desiring full functional restoration of flexion and supination strength. Injury to the radial nerve can be avoided by careful surgical technique. Heterotopic ossification can be avoided by using a single anterior incision and minimal exposure of the radial tuberosity. The use of suture anchors facilitates a minimal incision. We recommend operative repair with suture anchors via a single minimally invasive anterior incision.

References

1. McReynolds IS. Avulsion of the insertion of the biceps brachii tendon and its treatment. J Bone Joint Surg Am. 1963;45:1780–1781.
2. Morrey BF. Tendon injuries about the elbow. In: Morrey BF, ed. The Elbow and Its Disorders. 3rd ed. Philadelphia, PA: WB Saunders; 2000:468–478.
3. Fischer WR, Shepanek LA. Avulsion of the insertion of the biceps brachii. Report of a case. J Bone Joint Surg Am. 1956:38:158–159.
4. Meherin JM, Kilgore ES. The treatment of ruptures of the distal biceps brachii tendon. Am J Surg. 1960;99:636–640.
5. Boyd HB, Anderson LD. A method for reinsertion of the distal biceps tendon. J Bone Joint Surg Am. 1961;43:1041–1043.
6. Baker BE, Bierwagen D. Rupture of the distal tendon of the biceps brachii. Operative versus nonoperative. J Bone Joint Surg Am. 1985;67:414–417.
7. Failla JM, Amadio PC, Morrey BF, et al. Proximal radioulnar synostosis after repair of distal biceps brachii rupture by the two-incision technique. Report of four cases. Clin Orthop. 1990;253:133–136.
8. Morrey BF, Askew LJ, An KN, et al. Rupture of the distal tendon of the biceps brachii. A biomechanical study. J Bone Joint Surg Am. 1985;67: 418–421.
9. Sotereanos DG, Perce TD, Varitimidis SE. A simplified method for repair of distal biceps tendon ruptures. J Shoulder Elbow Surg. 2000; 9:227–233.
10. Kelly EW, Morrey BF, O'Driscoll SW. Complications of repair of the distal biceps tendon with the modified two-incision technique. J Bone Joint Surg Am. 2000;82:1575–81.
11. Lintner S, Fischer T. Repair of the distal biceps tendon using suture anchors and an anterior approach. Clin Orthop. 1996;322:116–119.
12. Morrison KD, Hunt TR. Comparing and contrasting methods for tenodesis of the ruptured distal biceps tendon. Hand Clin. 2002;18:169–178.
13. Strauch RJ, Michelson H, Rosenwater MP. Repair of rupture of the distal tendon of the biceps brachii. Review of the literature and report of three cases treated with a single anterior incision and suture anchors. Am J Orthop. 1997;26:151–156
14. Norman WH. Repair of avulsion of insertion of biceps brachii tendon. Clin Orthop. 1985;193:189–194.
15. Safran MR, Graham SM. Distal biceps tendon ruptures: incidence, demographics, and the effect of smoking. Clin Orthop. 2002;404:275–283.

16. Toczylowski HM, Balint CR, Steiner ME, et al. Complete rupture of the distal biceps brachii tendon in female patients: A report of 2 cases. J Shoulder Elbow Surg. 2002;11:516–518.
17. Davis WM, Yassine Z. An etiologic factor in tear of the distal tendon of the biceps brachii. Report of two cases. J Bone Joint Surg Am. 1956;38: 1365–1368.
18. Seiler JF, Parker LM, Chamberland PD, et al. The distal biceps tendon. Two potential mechanisms involved in its rupture: Arterial supply and mechanical impingement. J Shoulder Elbow Surg. 1995;4:149–156.
19. Pearl ML, Bessos PT, Wong K. Strength deficits related to distal biceps tendon rupture and repair: A case report. Am J Sports Med. 1998;26: 295–296.
20. Rantanen J, Orava S. Rupture of the distal biceps tendon. A report of 19 patients treated with anatomic reinsertion and meta-analysis of 147 cases found in the literature. Am J Sports Med. 1999;27:128–132.
21. St. Pierre P, Olsen EJ, Elliot JJ, et al. Tendon healing to cortical bone compared to healing to cancellous trough. J Bone J Surg Am. 1995;77:1858–1866.
22. Boucher PR, Morton KS. Rupture of the distal biceps brachii tendon. J Trauma. 1991;271:143–148.
23. El-Hawary R, MacDermid JC, Faber KJ. Distal biceps tendon repair: Comparison of surgical techniques. J Hand Surg Am. 2003;28:496–502.

Section II

The Hip

7

A Technique for the Anterolateral Approach to MIS Total Hip Replacement

Richard A. Berger

An anterolateral mini-incision approach to total hip arthroplasty (THA) can be preformed on most patients. Patients with retained hardware, such as a dynamic hip screw, which must be removed with a longer incision, and patients with Crowe 4 hip dysplasia that requires a subtrochanteric osteotomy should not be done with this approach. As the surgeon embarks to learn how to preform a mini-incision total hip arthroplasty, start with a longer incision and gradually shorten the skin incision with improved confidence and skill. Incisions smaller than 4.5 in. require specialized retractors and instrumentation, which is now readily available. As with all new techniques, start with patients who are thinner, less muscular, have minimal deformity, and few osteophytes. Later, improved confidence and skill will allow the surgeon to expand the indications of mini-incision THA to almost all patients. Again, gradually decrease the incision size until you have achieved a true mini-incision THA (2.5 in. to 3.5 in.) on almost all patients. It is important to note that a mini-incision THA is not simply a standard approach done through a small incision; instead, it is a modified approach that transects less muscle and tendon in addition to a small incision. The following is a detailed description of how to perform an anterolateral mini-incision total hip arthroplasty.

Surgical Technique

Preoperative planning and templating is very important. This is particularly true in the case of a mini-incision total hip arthroplasty in which visualization of extra-articular landmarks is limited. The objective of preoperative planning is to enable you to gather anatomic parameters that allow accurate intraoperative placement of the femoral and acetabular implants. Optimal femoral and acetabular component fit, the level of the femoral neck cut, the prosthetic neck length, and the femoral component offset can be evaluated through preoperative radiographic analysis. While the overall goal of total hip arthroplasty is to restore the original anatomic length and offset of the patient, occasionally this must become secondary to assuring good stability and tissue tension, particularly in the collapsed or very deformed hip.

Exposure

The patient is placed in the lateral position. Some form of rigid pelvis-stabilizing device, other than a beanbag, should be used. Most pelvis stabilizing devices flex or roll the pelvis forward; it is important to compensate for this by tilting the table posteriorly. Use a drape with a leg-holding bag, or create a bag with a sterile sheet, to hold the leg when it is placed anteriorly.

Once the patient is prepped and draped, mark the most proximal border of the greater trochanter, and the anteroposterior midline of the greater trochanter (Figure 7.1). In heavy patients, a 22-gauge spinal needle can be used to palpate the bone through the soft tissue. Along the anteroposterior midline of the greater trochanter midline, make a mark 3/4 in. distal to the tip of the greater trochanter. This identifies the midpoint of the incision. With the usual anterolateral approach to the hip, the incision is in line with the femur. As the surgeon reduces the incision length, the incision should be angled from anterior and inferior to posterior and superior. As the incision reduces to 2.5 in. to 3.0 in., make the incision approximately 20 degrees to 30 degrees to the long axis of the femur, beginning anterior and inferior, and extending superiorly and posteriorly approximately 2.5 in. to 3.0 in. so it passes through the marked point. Half the incision should be anterior and inferior to the mark 3/4 in. distal to the tip of the greater trochanter, and half should be superior and posterior. (In heavier patients slightly more of the incision should be posterior and it should be closer to the 30 degree orientation.)

Divide the subcutaneous fat down to the fascia. Use a Cobb elevator to expose the fascia lata about 1 cm on either side of the incision, facilitating closure. Incise the fascia lata in an orientation halfway between its fibers and the skin incision, about 15 degrees to 20 degrees to the axis of the femoral shaft. This aids closure. As the fascial incision is made, a small portion of the gluteus maximus muscle may be encountered (Figure 7.2). Use the electrocautery to open the gluteus maximus muscle posteriorly and superiorly within its fibers.

The trochanteric bursa will be exposed. If the bursa is thickened, slide a finger anteriorly and posteriorly to loosen the bursa and expose the greater trochanter and gluteus medius muscle. Place a Charnley retractor transversely across the incision. Place the anterior arm of the retractor first, then the posterior arm. It is important to use a specialized long arm retractor, which has been modified from the standard Charnley retractors. The arms of a standard Charnley retractor will not engage the frame for mini-incision without significant tension on the incision. Do not overtighten the Charnley retractor, as this will diminish the exposure and cause skin compromise.

Find the anterior tip of the greater trochanter; this is the point where the abductor is usually entered for a standard anterolateral approach that removes about 50% of the abductor off the trochanter. From the tip of the trochanter, slide anteriorly to the anterior ridge of the trochanter;

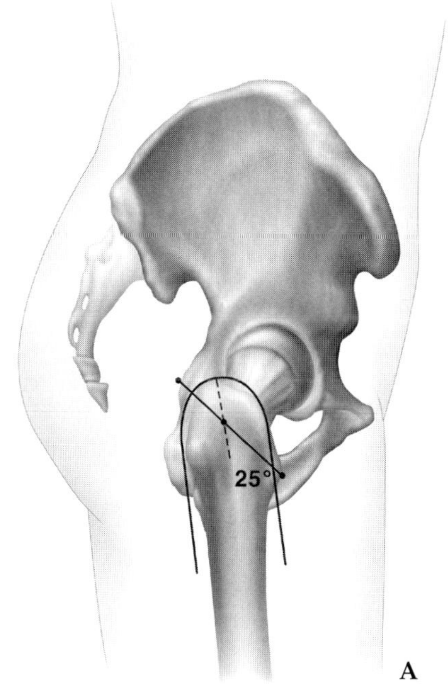

A

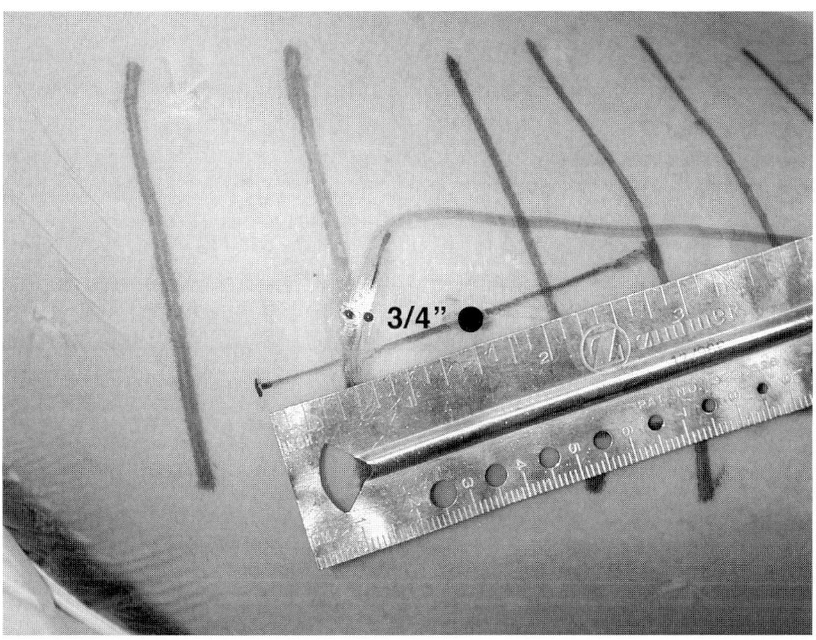

B

Figure 7.1. The incision. (A) The placement and orientation of the skin incision for a mini-incision. (B) The skin incision on the patient. The center point of the incision is marked $\frac{3}{4}$ in. distal to the tip of the trochanter and in the midline of the femur.

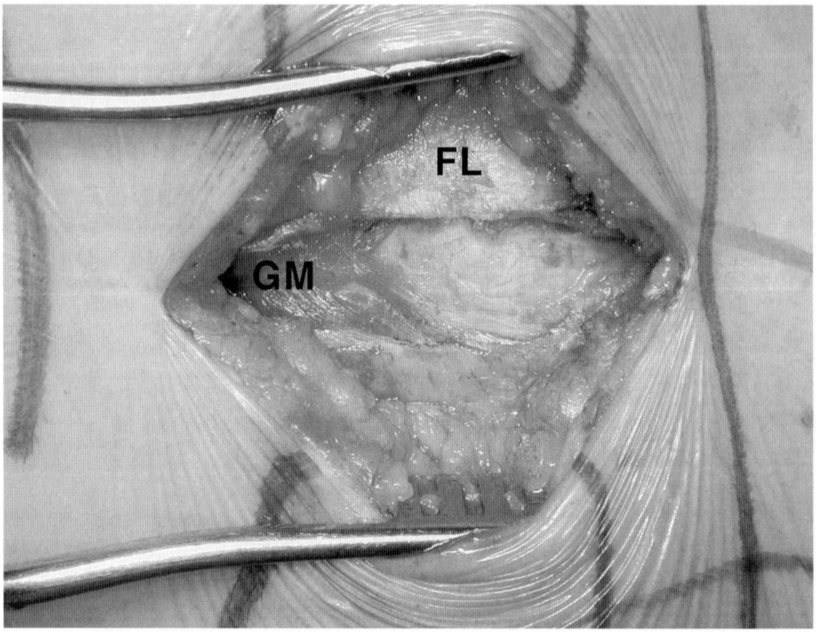

Figure 7.2. The incision through the fascia lata (FL). The fibers of the gluteus maximus (GM) are seen prior to being split.

the confluence of the anterior and superior trochanter (Figure 7.3). With this point, only about 20% to 25% of the abductor is taken off the trochanter. Find this ridge and insert a pair of curved Mayo scissors in the recess of the gluteus medius muscle in line with its fibers until the gluteus minimus muscle is felt with the tip of the scissors. This divides the anterior 20% to 25% of the gluteus medius muscle. Insert two Army-Navy retractors to retract the gluteus medius muscle and expose the gluteus minimus tendon, which will be oblique to the opening in the gluteus medius muscle (Figure 7.4). Next, make an L-shaped incision in the gluteus minimus tendon, beginning the incision proximally in line with the fibers and extending it to the incision in the gluteus medius muscle. Then transect approximately 0.5 cm of the gluteus minimus tendon in line with the gluteus medius muscle (Figure 7.5). This separates the anterior 20% to 25% of the gluteus medius and minimus muscle. Then remove the Army-Navy retractors.

Place the leg in slight external rotation. Use electrocautery to detach the fascia over the vastus ridge where it blends with the gluteus medius tendon. You do not need to violate the vastus muscle. Following the contour of the greater trochanter, proximally transect the gluteus medius tendon. Leave the posterior half of the tendon attached to the greater trochanter, and the anterior half attached to the muscle (Figure 7.6). While slowly externally rotating the hip, use electrocautery to detach the anterior 20% to 25% of the gluteus medius and gluteus minimus muscles from the greater trochanter. Distally, find the interval between the capsule and the gluteus minimus tendon over the

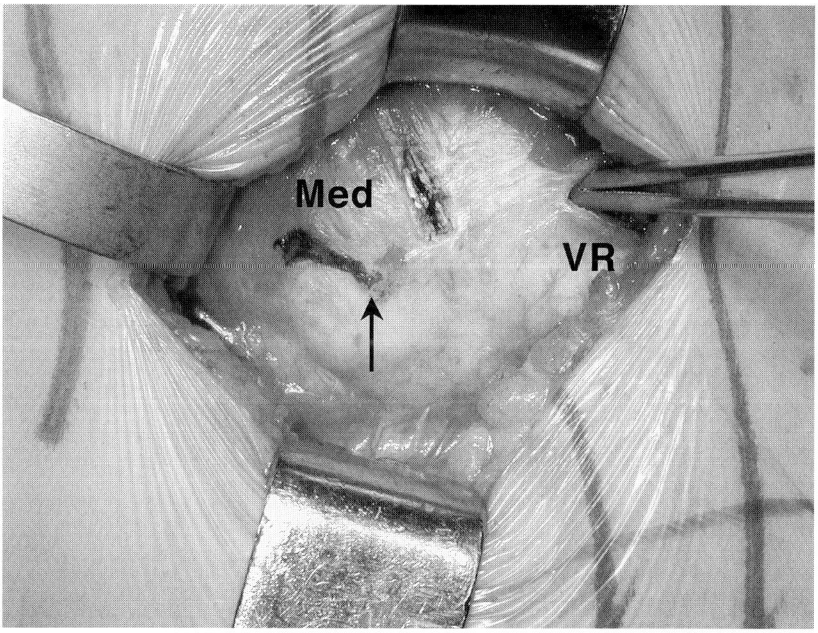

Figure 7.3. The greater trochanter. The forceps show the location of the vastus ridge (VR). The arrow marks the location of the tip of the trochanter where the abductor is typically incised for a standard anterolateral approach (marked). The incision in the gluteus medius (Med) corresponding to 25% for the abductor is shown with the electric cautery.

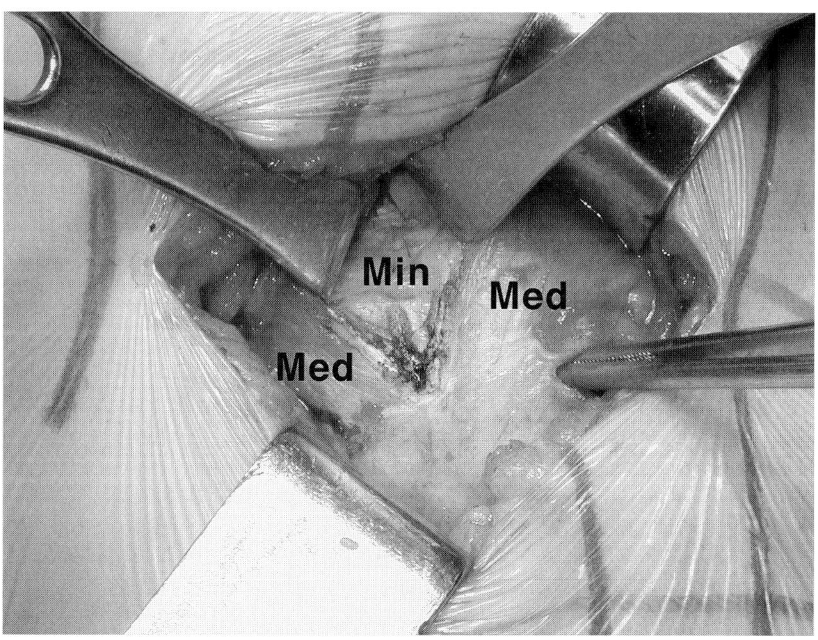

Figure 7.4. The gluteus medius (Med) split, separating the anterior 25% from the posterior 75%. The gluteus minimus (Min) is shown beneath. The forceps shows the location of the vastus ridge.

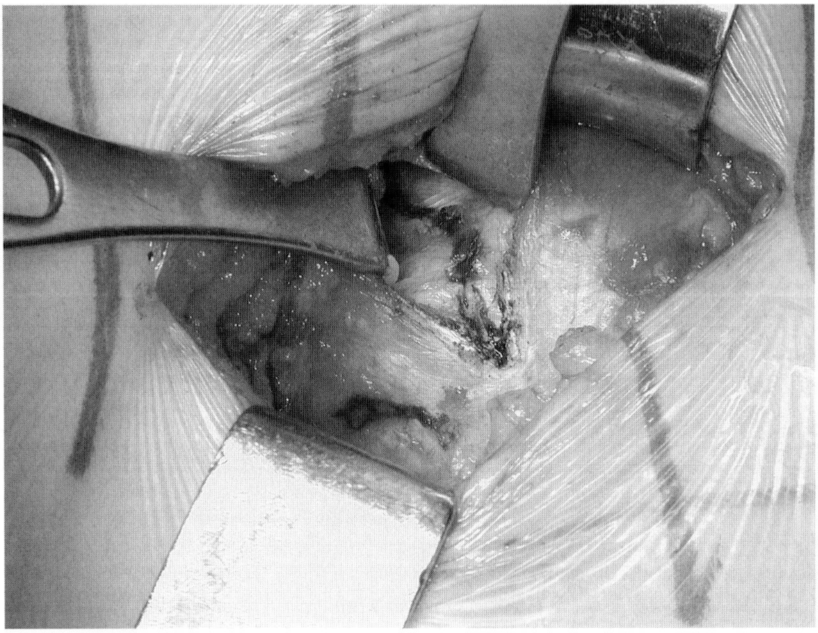

Figure 7.5. The location of the split in the gluteus minimus is shown.

bursa of the quadriceps muscle. Open this interval and follow it proximally; insert a single point large retractor. The tendon will likely be confluent to the capsule. Use electrocautery to separate the gluteus minimus tendon from the capsule. Move the single point large retrac-

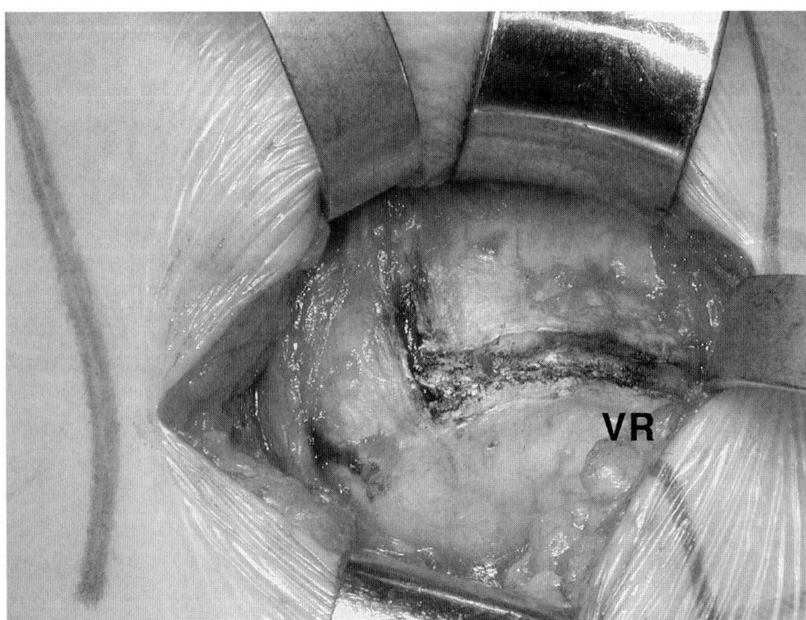

Figure 7.6. The anterior 25% of the gluteus medius and gluteus minimus taken off the trochanter from the vastus ridge (VR) to the split in the gluteus.

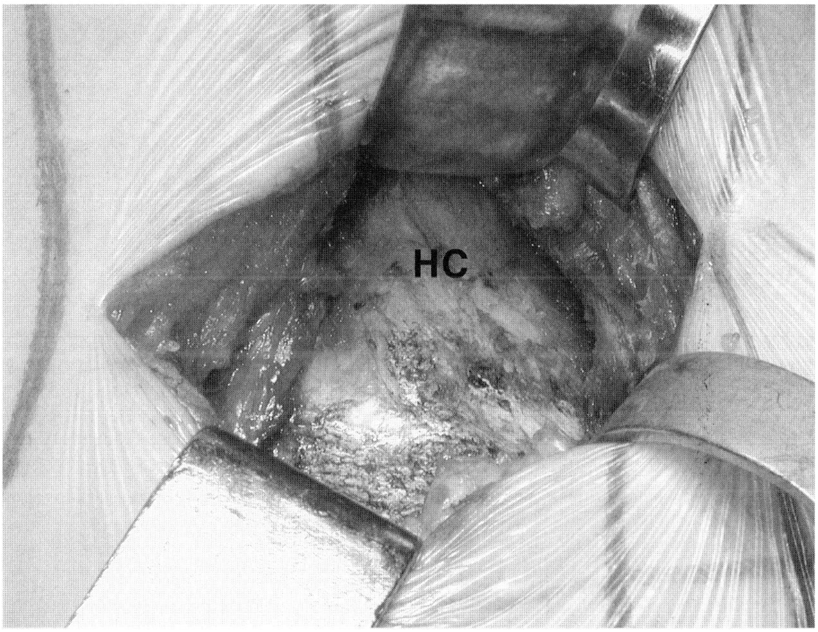

Figure 7.7. The hip capsule (HC) exposed, with the abductors retracted anteriorly.

tor anteriorly and cephalad, placing it on the superior/anterior rim of the acetabulum. This exposes the capsule (Figure 7.7). Additionally, a small portion of the quadriceps muscle may be detached from the capsule with the electrocautery. The release can extend as far anteriorly and inferiorly as necessary to expose the anteroinferior capsule. Abduction, flexion, and externally rotating the leg can facilitate this process. Avoid invading the muscle; this will cause bleeding.

When the anterior capsule is exposed, excise the anterior/inferior portion of the capsule. Then fully extend and slightly externally rotate the limb. Excise the anterior/superior capsule to expose the femoral head. About one quarter of the capsule can be excised. Check to be sure that the anterior capsule is freed inferiorly, along the femoral neck, to allow the femoral head to be dislocated. Alternatively, the capsule may be retained and simply incised.

Establish landmarks and obtain measurements before dislocating the hip so that, after reconstruction, a comparison of leg length and femoral shaft offset can be obtained. From this comparison, adjustments can be made to achieve the goals established during preoperative planning. There are several methods to measure leg length, dependent on individual surgeon preference.

Apply traction and insert a hip-skid retractor in the joint space. This will aid in dislocating the hip. Remove all the retractors and insert a bone hook around the femoral neck. The hip should be flexed to only 45 degrees with slight adduction; in this position the assistant should externally rotate the leg as the surgeon applies the anterior and lateral traction with the bone hook. This will dislocate hip without injury to the remaining abductor (Figure 7.8).

This technique of only detaching about 20% to 25% of the abductor off the trochanter improves rehabilitation and postoperative limp. However, there are two points in this procedure when the additional preserved abductor can be injured or torn; these points are during dislocation and femoral preparation. The most common time of abductor injury is during dislocation. If the hip is flexed more than 45 degrees with significant external rotation to dislocate the hip the abductor can be stretched and the anterior portion will be torn. Limiting hip flexion to 45 degrees and using a bone hook will prevent this problem. The second time of abductor injury is during femoral canal preparation; hyper-external rotation during femoral preparation will prevent abductor injury.

After dislocation it is usually easier to make a provisional neck cut high on the neck to remove the bulk of the femoral head. This facilitates seeing the lesser trochanter and making the actual femoral neck cut. Some of the inferior capsule can be released to expose the lesser trochanter if necessary. Make the final neck cut from the level of the lesser trochanter as determined from the preoperative templating. An osteotomy guide may be used. To prevent possible damage to the greater trochanter, stop the cut as the saw approaches the greater trochanter. Remove the saw and use a sagittal saw to finish the cut superiorly. Excise the posterior synovium, and remove the final neck segment. Remove the Charnley retractor.

To retract the femur posteriorly, a large two-point retractor is used to straddle the ischium approximately 1 cm posterior to the posterior wall of the acetabulum (Figure 7.9). Special retractors (Mini-incision instrument set, Zimmer) with built-in fiberoptic lights are helpful. To

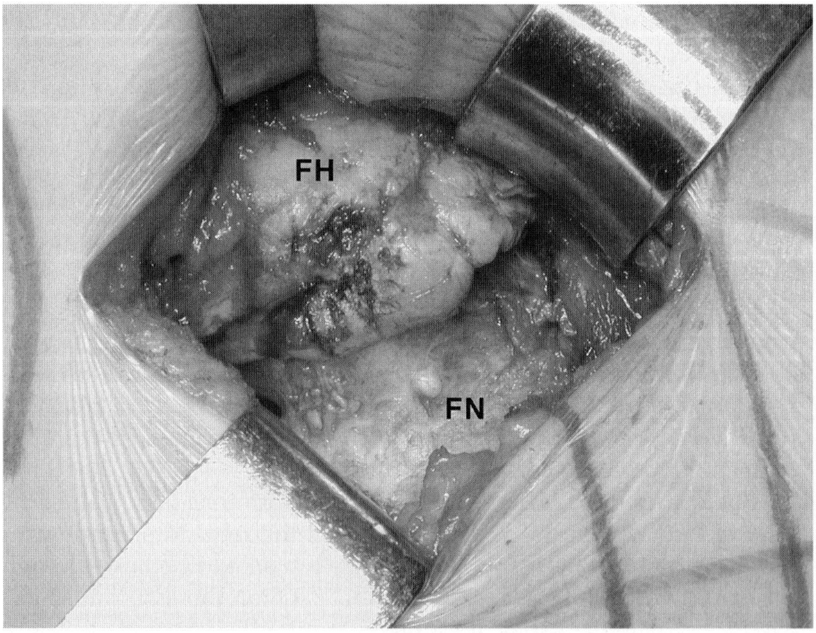

Figure 7.8. The femoral head (FH) and femoral neck (FN) after the hip has been dislocated.

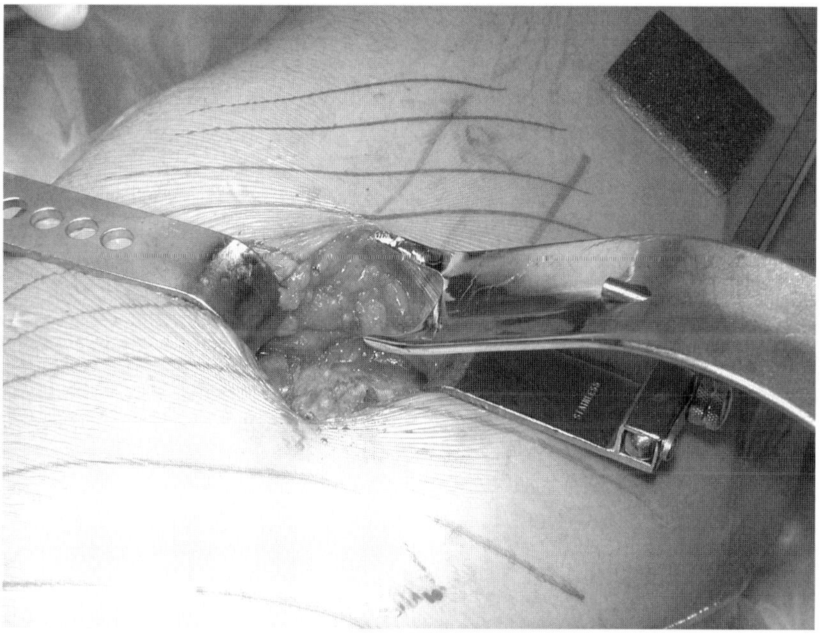

Figure 7.9. The posterior lit retractor with two points to straddle the ischium.

facilitate placement of this retractor, the hip is flexed to 45 degrees, abducted to 25 degrees, and externally rotated to 30 degrees. This retractor is placed intracapsular, which retracts the capsule and avoids sciatic nerve injury. A few gentle taps set the retractor and holds it in place. The assistant should avoid vigorous retraction, as this will dislodge the retractor or injure the skin.

Approximately 180 degrees to the ischium, place the single point large retractor through the interval between the capsule and the anterosuperior acetabulum. Use this retractor to hold the anterior portions of the gluteus medius and gluteus minimus muscles anteriorly (Figure 7.10). Insert the curved Hohmann retractor (Mini-incision instrument set, Zimmer) over the anteroinferior rim of the acetabulum to hold the anterior capsule and iliopsoas tendon anteriorly. The fiberoptic lights in these retractors augment visualization (Figure 7.11). Additional remaining anterior or inferior capsule may be resected if needed; however, be careful to avoid the peritenon of the iliopsoas tendon anteriorly and the gluteus minimus posteriorly. Then resect the acetabular labrum circumferentially. Osteophyte resection may be performed before or after the acetabular shell has been inserted. It is often easier to remove osteophytes once the component has been inserted. Use a curved osteotome. Remove the Hohmann retractor and leave the two opposing large retractors.

Preparation of the Acetabulum

A specially designed Low-Profile acetabular reamer (Mini-incision instrument set, Zimmer) facilitates passing the reams between the

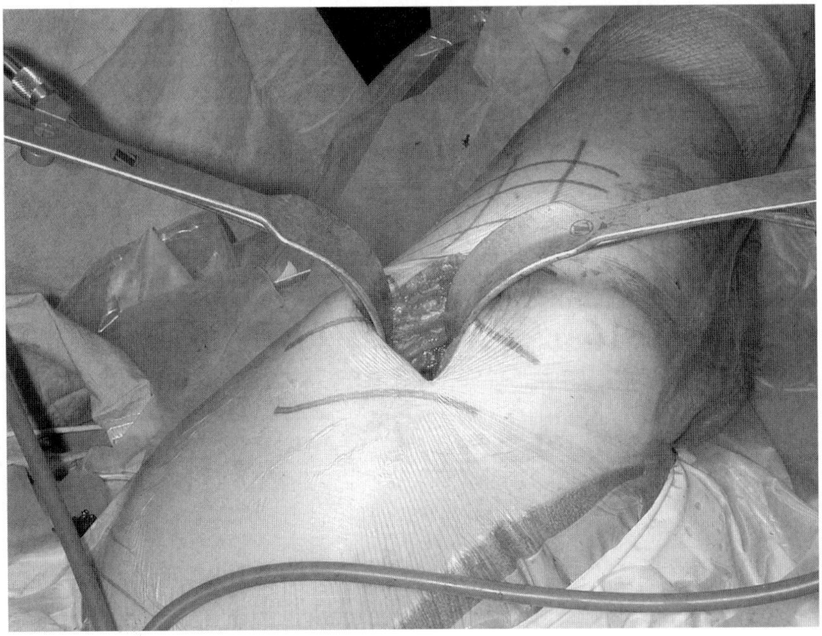

Figure 7.10. The anterior and posterior retractors around the acetabulum.

opposing retractors (Figure 7.12). Begin reaming the acetabulum with the largest Low-Profile acetabular reamer that will fit into the acetabulum. These reamers are designed to be used in this manner. They have square teeth that are aggressive. The shells of the Low-Profile acetab-

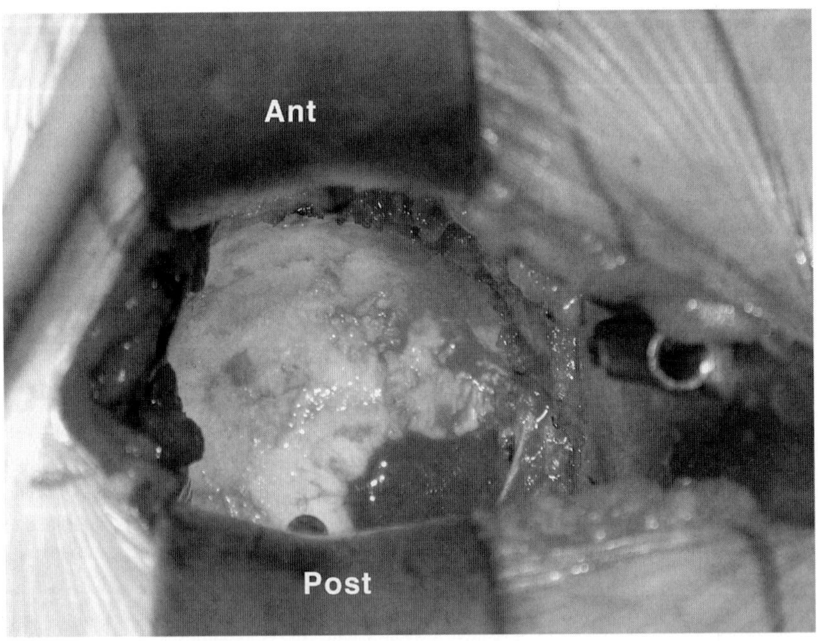

Figure 7.11. The acetabulum. Note the lit retractors illuminating the acetabulum anteriorly (Ant) and posteriorly (Post).

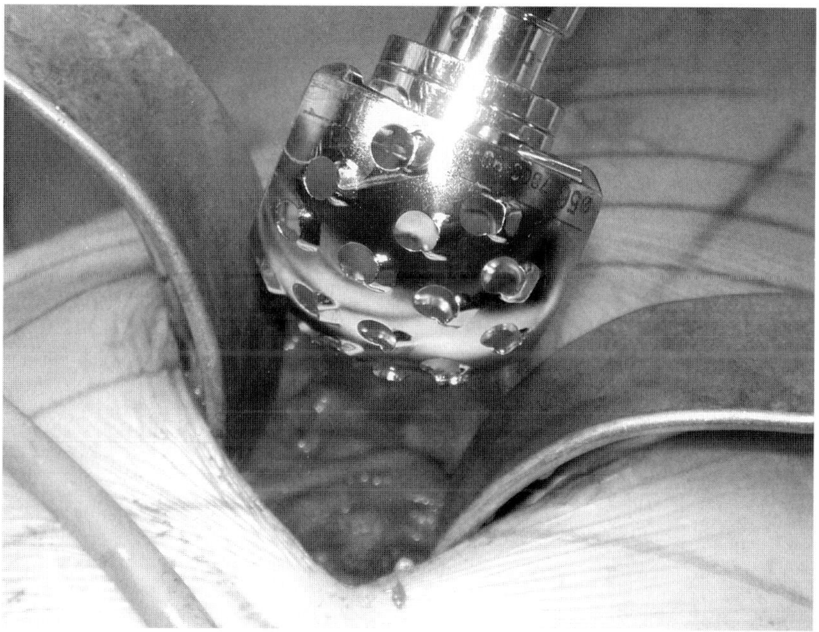

Figure 7.12. The Low-Profile reamer. Note how the cutout shape facilitates the reamer into the acetabulum.

ular reamers are more than hemispherical. The perimeter edge extends an additional 15 degrees beyond the level of a hemisphere. This reams peripheral osteophytes facilitating the acetabular component being fully seated. Moreover, this design (more than a full hemisphere), is forgiving; the reamer can be up to 15 degrees off the acetabular component axis and still ream a perfect hemisphere for the final acetabular component's position. The acetabulum is generally reamed to 2 mm less than the size of the selected acetabular component.

Check to make sure the patient is correctly positioned on the table. Connect the final prosthesis to the offset shell inserter (Mini-incision instrument set, Zimmer) (Figure 7.13). This offset design avoids vertical cup placement, which is common in mini-incision total hip replacement. Insert the shell into the prepared acetabulum. The alignment frame achieves 45 degrees abduction and 20 degrees forward flexion (Figure 7.13). Impact the cup in place, assuring the shell is fully seated (Figure 7.14). Acetabular screws may be used for additional fixation. If osteophytes are present and overhanging they should be removed. The polyethylene liner is inserted. Remove retractors around the acetabulum.

Preparation of the Femur

Position the long femoral elevator (Mini-incision instrument set, Zimmer) on the lateral greater trochanter, lateral to the abductors. This elevates the proximal femur out of the wound and protects the proximal pole of the incision (Figure 7.15). Placing the leg into the sterile bag anteriorly, the hip is positioned in flexion, adduction, and

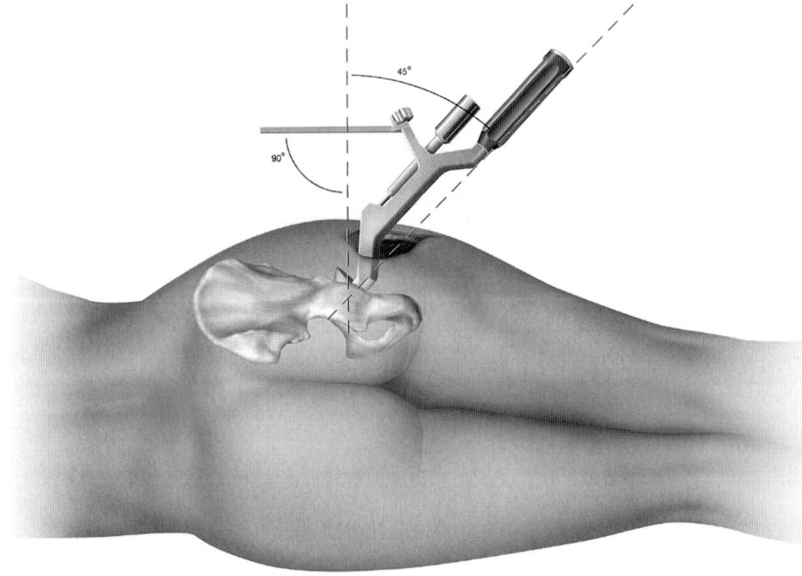

Figure 7.13. The acetabular component positioner. Note how the dogleg positioner goes around the skin to achieve proper component placement. (By permission of Zimmer, Inc., Warsaw, IN.)

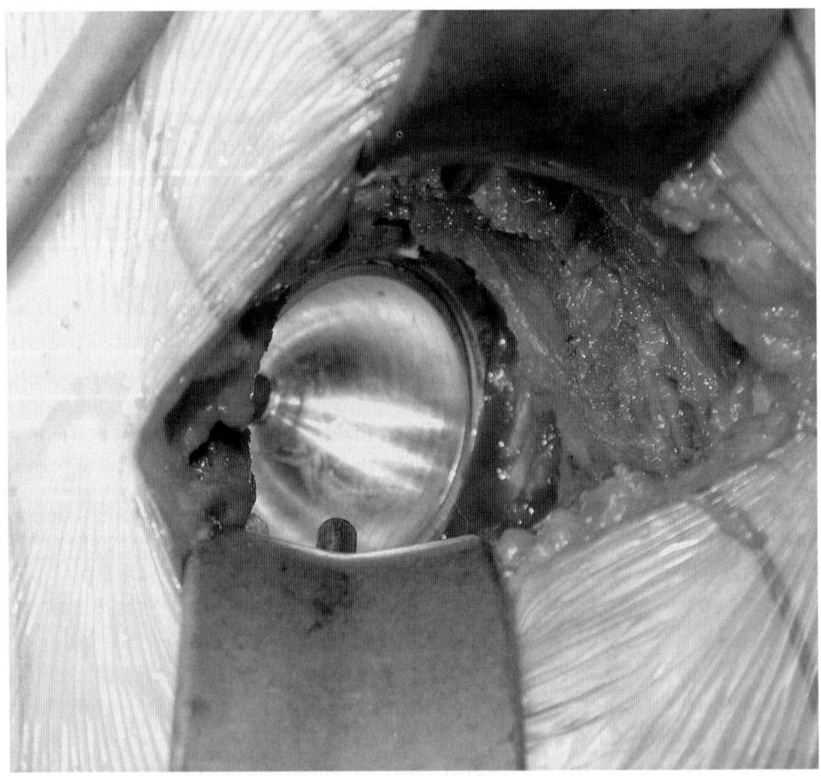

Figure 7.14. The acetabular component in place with the retractors lighting the component.

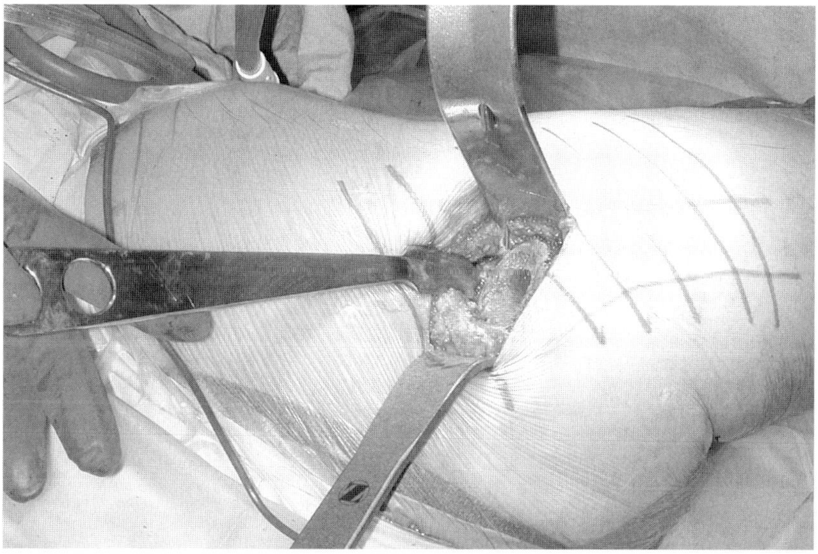

Figure 7.15. Placement of the retractor around the femur.

hyperexternal rotation (approximately 135 degrees). Place the double point large lit retractor (Mini-incision instrument set, Zimmer) over the medial border of the calcar. This keep the proximal metaphysis exposed and well lit. Last, place a straight Hohmann retractor in the piriformis fossa to hold and protect the abductors posteriorly (Figure 7.15). As noted earlier, the hyperexternal rotation of the hip moves the abductor posteriorly, thereby avoiding injury or maceration of the abductor during femoral canal preparation.

A box osteotome and tapered awl is used to gain access to the canal. Side cutting reamers (Mini-incision instrument set, Zimmer) can be used to remove the medial portion of the lateral trochanter to avoid varus alignment. The smooth bullet tip of this side cutting reamer is designed to engage in the upper diaphysis to assure neutral alignment of the component. A straight rasp handle during rasping minimizes impingement of the handle with the proximal pole of the skin incision. In addition, there is a tendency for the proximal pole of the incision to apply an anteverting force onto the rasp handle, which is minimized with the straight rasp handle. To facilitate control of the handle, a bar can be inserted into one of the three holes in the handle. These holes (0, 7.5, and 15 degrees) can also be used to check anteversion. The femoral canal is prepared for the intended prosthesis by matching the rasp to the anteversion of the metaphysis (Figure 7.16). While a cementless tapered design will be shown, any design can be used with this approach: cemented, proximally coated, splined, or fully coated.

Specially designed provisional neck and provisional head, which can be inserted from the side, facilitates the trial reduction (Mini-incision instrument set, Zimmer). Insert the provisional head and neck and perform a trial reduction. Check the leg length and offset of the femur

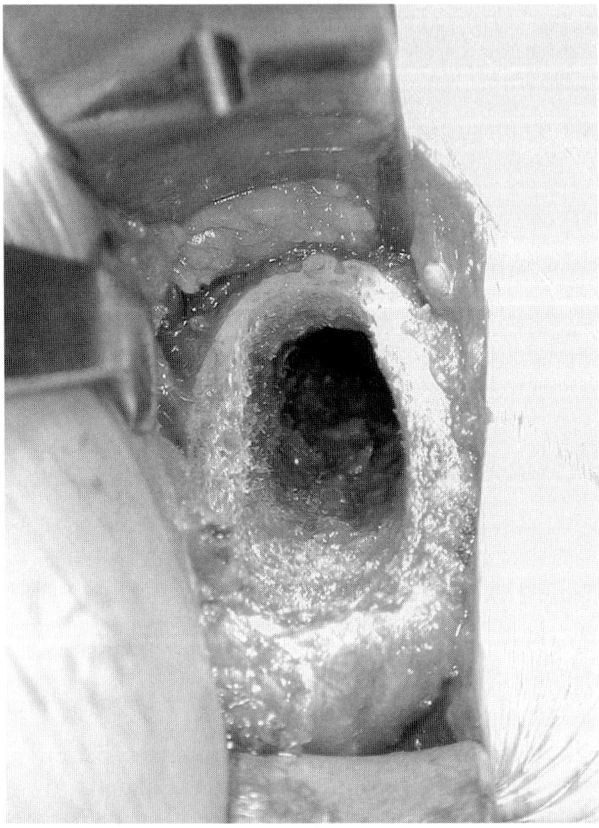

Figure 7.16. The view of the femur with the anterolateral mini-incision.

by referencing the lengths measured before the hip was dislocated. Adjust the neck length by changing the femoral head provisionals to achieve the desired result. When satisfactory leg length, offset, range of motion, and stability have been achieved, dislocate the hip. Remove the rasp and insert the femoral component (Figure 7.17). Insert the femoral component until the prosthesis is fully seated or until the implant will no longer advance (Figure 7.18).

Use the provisional head inserter to sequentially seat the side-loading slotted provisional heads on the femoral neck until appropriate leg length, joint tension, and joint stability have been achieved. Seat the actual head that corresponds to the trail head selected (Figure 7.19). Reduce the hip, and assess leg length, range of motion, and stability and abductor tension for the final time (Figure 7.20).

Closure is important to maintain muscle function and expedite recovery. To facilitate closure, replace the Charnley retractor and internally rotate and abduct the hip. Predrill the lateral trochanter; do not drill through to the anterior portion. Insert two heavy Mersilene sutures from lateral to anterior. Pass the Mersilene sutures under the gluteus minimus and gluteus medius muscles. Place one or two non-absorbable sutures through the gluteus minimus muscle, closing it to

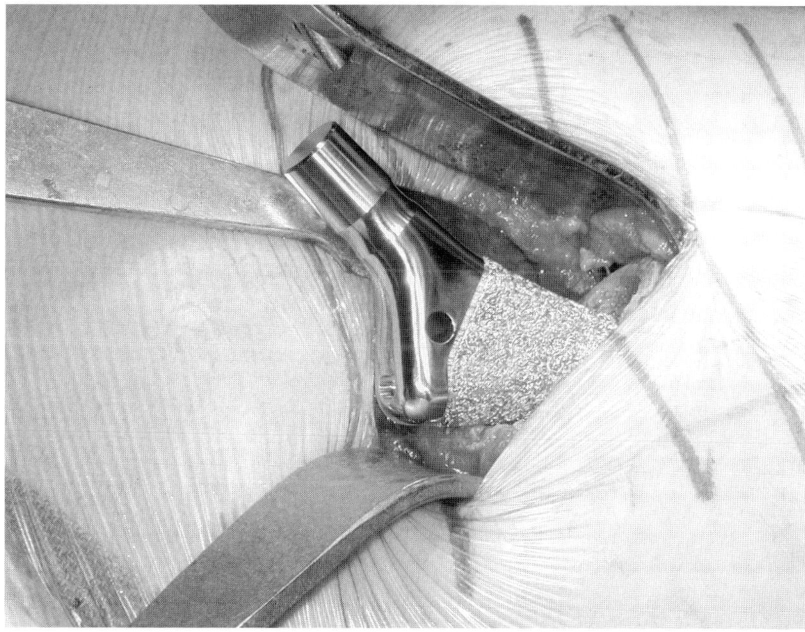

Figure 7.17. The femoral component entering the femoral canal.

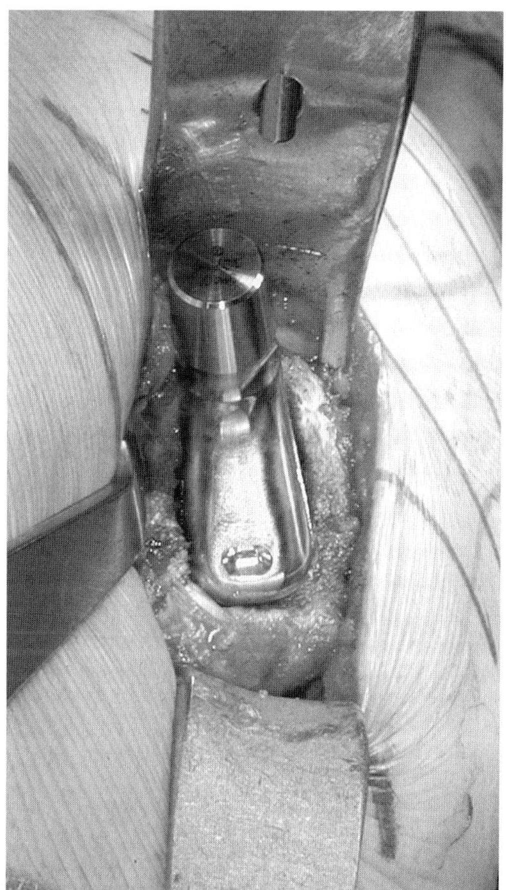

Figure 7.18. The femoral component fully seated.

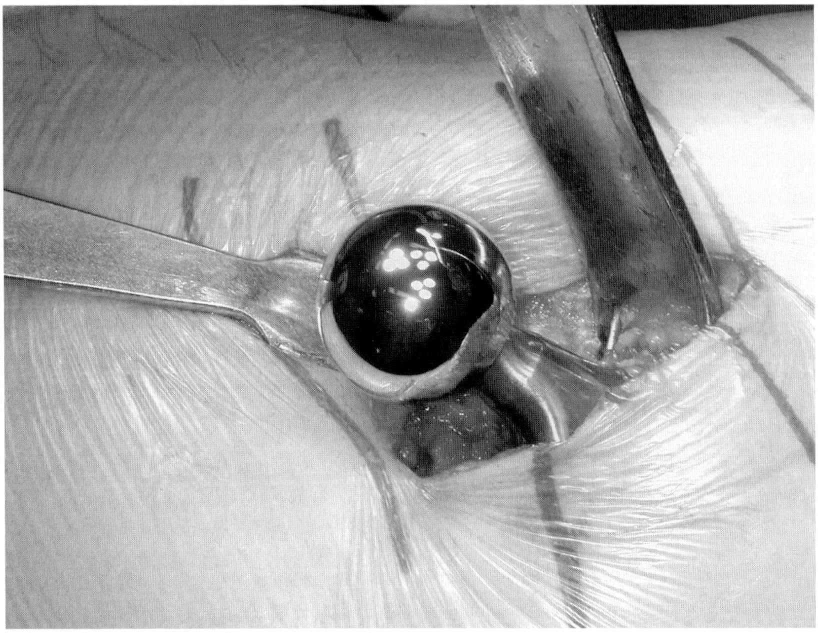

Figure 7.19. The femoral component with the head attached.

itself (Figure 7.21). Next, tie the Mersilene sutures tightly to return the gluteus minimus and gluteus medius muscles back to the trochanteric bed. Last, use number 1 Ethibond sutures to perform an end-to-end anastomosis of the gluteus medius tendon. This completely and securely reattached the gluteus minimus and gluteus medius back to the greater trochanter (Figure 7.22).

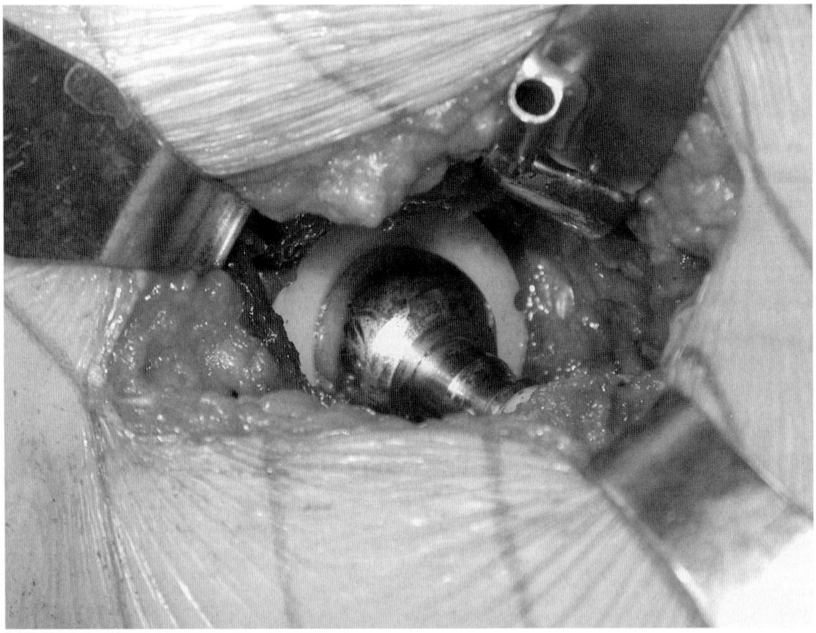

Figure 7.20. The femoral component located within the acetabular component.

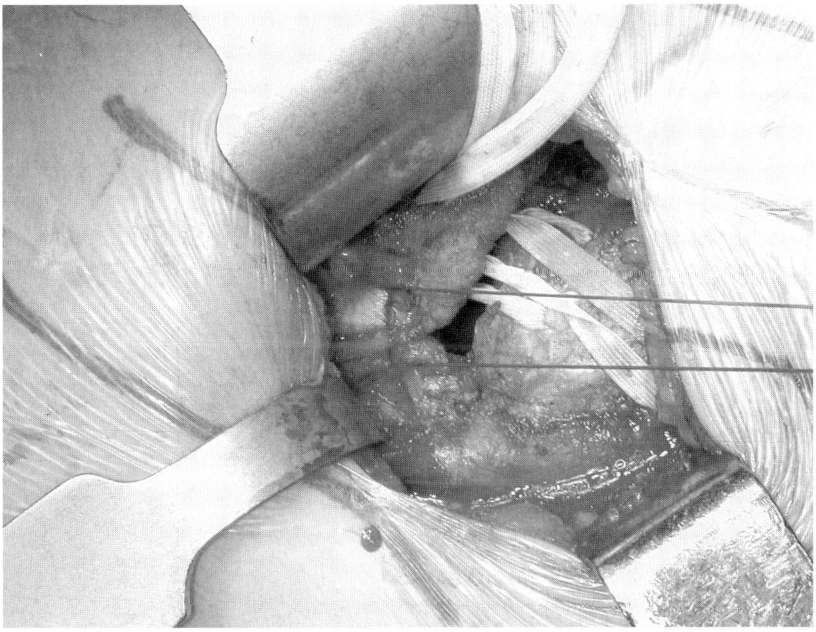

Figure 7.21. The gluteus minimus tendon closed with a nonabsorbable suture. Also shown are the two Mersilene sutures through the trochanter around the gluteus medius and gluteus minimus.

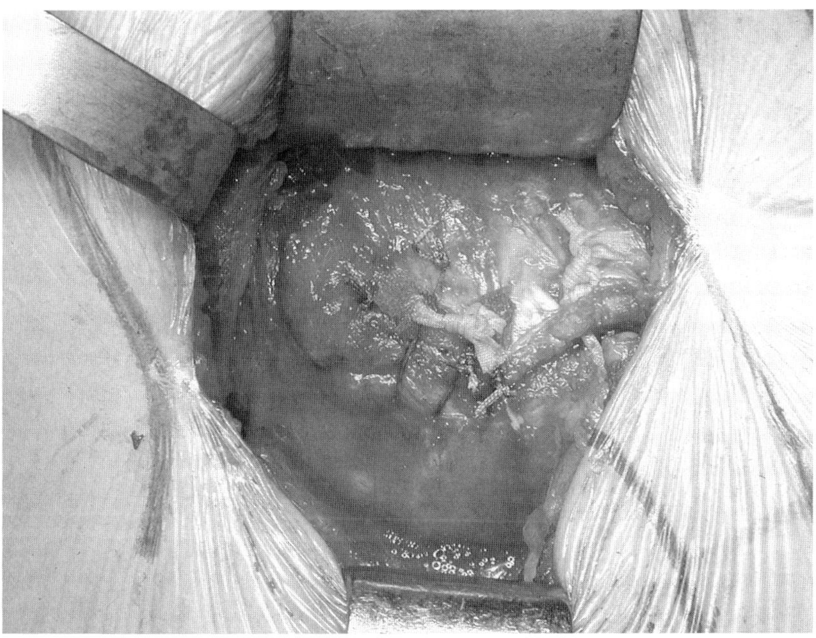

Figure 7.22. The gluteus medius and gluteus minimus completely closed back to the trochanter.

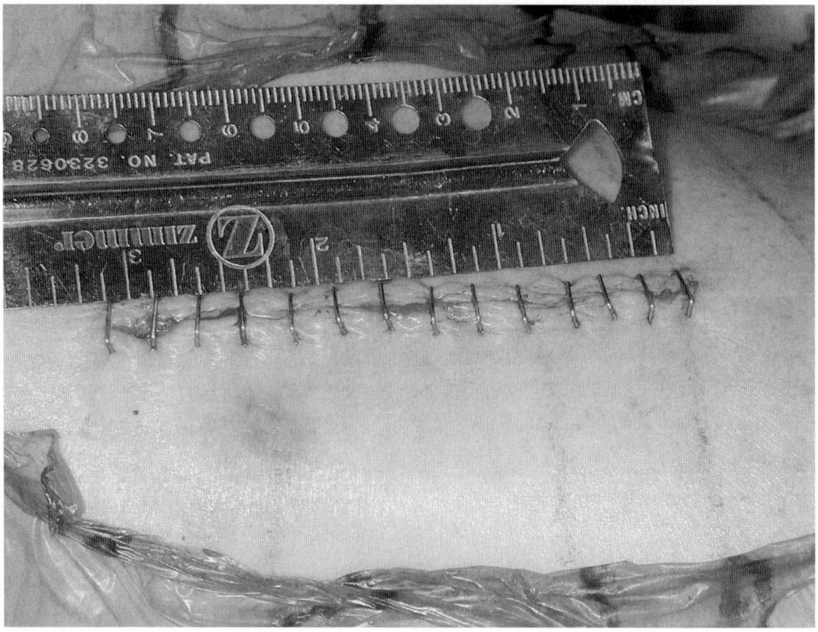

Figure 7.23. The final closure of the 3-in. incision.

Remove the Charnley retractor. With the hip slightly abducted, close the fascia lata using nonabsorbable sutures. Then close the remaining layers with 2.0 Vicryl, followed by staples or subcuticular closure (Figure 7.23). Apply a sterile dressing.

Conclusion

The mini-incision exposure can be used in most primary total hip arthroplasty (THA) patients. As the surgeon begins to perform mini-incision total hip arthroplasty, gradually shorten the skin incision with improved confidence and skill. A true mini-incision THA (2.5 in. to 3.5 in.) requires specialized retractors and instrumentation such as the mini-incision set. Following the technique presented here will not only result in a smaller incision, but also will transect less muscle and tendon. This less invasive approach can result in a shorter length of stay, less pain, fewer rehabilitation transfers, quicker recovery, and better cosmesis. All of these combine to produce a more satisfied THA patient.

8

The Anterior Approach for Total Hip Replacement: Background and Operative Technique

Joel M. Matta

This technique follows the Heuter approach, which was first described in the German orthopedic literature in the 1930s. The approach can also be called the Short Smith-Peterson because it follows the interval of the Smith-Petersen distal to the anterior superior iliac spine.

The first hip arthroplasty performed through this approach was by Robert Judet in 1947 at Garches Hospital in Paris and a Judet acrylic prosthesis was implanted.[1] The surgery was facilitated by operating on the Judet table with the patient in the supine position. The Judet table was originally designed by Henri Judet, an orthopedic surgeon and Robert Judet's father. The reasons for Judet's choice of this approach for hip arthroplasty are several: (1) The hip is an anterior joint, closer to the skin anterior than posterior; (2) The approach follows the anatomic interval between the zones of enervation of the superior and inferior gluteal nerves lateral and the femoral nerve medial; (3) The approach exposes the hip without detachment of muscle from the bone.

Today Thierry Judet, the son of Robert Judet continues to use this approach as well as the Judet table for hip arthroplasty. Prof. Thierry Judet, Chief of Orthopedics at Garches, has used this approach and table for over 20 years and more than 2000 cases.[2] It has been the preferred technique for primary and revision hip arthroplasty at Garches since 1947. It has been used for a great variety of prostheses including the Judet acrylic, the Judet uncemented, conventional cemented, partial femoral head resurfacing and total hip surface replacement. The original approach was slightly longer and extended onto the iliac crest and also more distally. The tensor fascia lata muscle was partly detached from the crest. Over time the incision has to a degree shrunk but the interval remains the same.

While this history of the anterior approach for THA has been little known in the orthopedic world, the history of Charnley's experience is widely known.[3,4] Charnley implanted the first consistently successful THA in the 1960s. He also positioned the patient supine, though using a more standard flat topped operating table with the leg draped free and manipulated by a scrubbed assistant. This approach necessitated a trochanteric osteotomy. Because of recognized complications of this osteotomy, the posterior approach was later adopted by many surgeons with the patient necessarily positioned in the lateral position. Because of problems with hip dislocation, however, following the posterior approach, some surgeons later adopted the anterolateral Harding approach. The downside of the Harding approach, however, has been the necessity of detachment of the gluteus minimus and a portion of the gluteus medius from the greater trochanter, which can lead to a delay in functional recovery.

The anterior approach, however, preserves posterior structures that are important for preventing dislocation while preserving important muscle attachments to the greater trochanter. It is obvious that lack of disturbance of the minimus and medius insertions facilitates recovery of a normal gait. The surgeon should also consider the role of the gluteus maximus and tensor fascia lata muscles as abductors and pelvic stabilizers. These two muscles insert on the fascia lata/iliotibial band which joins them and together form a deltoid of the hip (Figure 8.1). Lack of disturbance of this hip deltoid is a further benefit of the anterior approach.

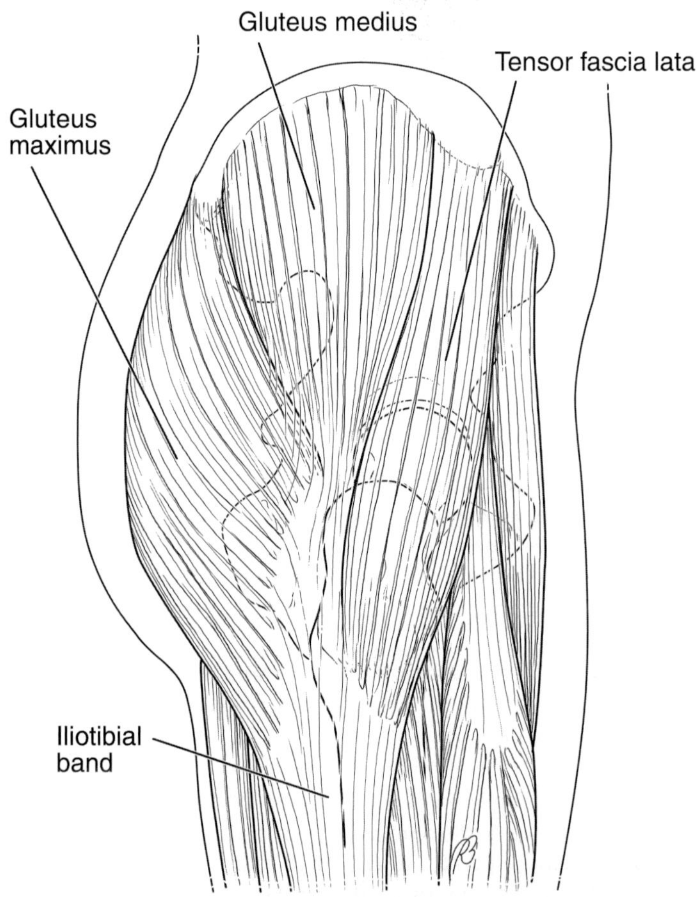

Figure 8.1. Lateral view of the hip deltoid; the gluteus maximus, and tensor fascia lata muscles and their insertion on the iliotibial tract.

The author first saw this THA technique in 1981 on a visit with Emile Letournel in Paris to study acetabular and pelvic fracture surgery. Letournel had been Robert Judet's resident. The patient was placed supine on the Judet table. The leg was not draped free but the foot placed in a boot and manipulated by a mobile spar that was operated by an unscrubbed assistant. I recall being quite impressed but a little confused and I did not pursue this technique. My main interest at the time was pelvic and acetabular fracture treatment and when I performed THA I continued to use the posterior approach. In 1996, I was approached by a patient who had had one hip replaced by this technique in France but now lived in the United States and required replacement of the other hip. He was very enthusiastic about the anterior approach because of the lack of muscle disturbance and the rapid recovery he had experienced and requested that I replace his other hip by the same technique. This led me to reconsider the value of this technique and its potential benefits of reduced dislocation risk and enhanced recovery rate. At the time, I frequently used the Judet table for acetabular fracture surgery. I replaced this man's hip using the anterior approach on the Judet table and began my own series of patients. I proceeded slowly at first with only 20 to 30 cases per year but I now use this approach frequently and for all primary hip arthroplasties.

Regarding minimally invasive procedures, it is more important what the surgeon does under the skin than the specific length of the incision. Stretching, contusing and abrading tissue are not minimally invasive. The main advantage of this approach is that it is not necessary to detach or split any muscle from the pelvis or the femur and the hip deltoid is not disturbed. The result is that there is an immediate stability of the hip that obviates the need for dislocation precautions. Also, there is a rapid recovery of function. Another advantage of the technique with the patient supine on the OSI PROfx table is the use of the image intensifier for immediate information regarding acetabular position and femoral length and offset. Accuracy of component position and leg length is thereby enhanced. The supine position that is preferred for this approach facilitates the accuracy of acetabular position as well as assessment of leg length.

For surgeons not familiar with THA through the anterior approach, it is easy to appreciate the straightforward acetabular access. The femoral access, however, is less easy to conceptualize. The femoral access is greatly enhanced by a special orthopedic table. The original table designed and used in France was the Judet/Tasserit table. Today the PROfx table is the new and improved surgical tool. With the patient positioned supine the leg is not draped free but is attached to a mobile strut that can apply traction, rotate the leg, and angulate the leg in all directions. External rotation of the leg to 90 degrees and hyperextension of the hip to 30 degrees allows femoral preparation and prosthesis insertion in a somewhat anterior to posterior direction. The table also elevates the proximal femur to enhance access. The anterior approach is the approach used for acetabular component insertion with the minimally invasive 2 incision technique. With use of the table however, a second posterior incision becomes unnecessary.

Either cemented or uncemented components can be implanted through this approach. Femoral components that require straight reamers, however, are more difficult to place and not as applicable to this approach.

The author has used this approach for primary THA for the past 8 years and now uses it for all primary cases unless there is an acetabular posterior defect that requires posterior graft and plate fixation.

The question is often asked: Is the Judet/Tasserit or PROfx table necessary for use of this approach. Kristaps Keggi of Waterbury, CT, has used the anterior approach (Heuter) for more than 3000 hip replacements while operating on a standard table.[5] It is Keggi's practice, however, to frequently use secondary incisions for acetabular and/or femoral preparation. Although it is possible to use the anterior approach without the table, the table obviates the need for secondary incisions. Additionally, it is my impression that femoral access is significantly more difficult without the PROfx table. Improving the femoral access not only eliminates secondary incisions but also reduces muscle trauma that can result from forceful retraction. Keggi's approach also involves splitting the medial portion of the tensor fascia lata muscle and a frequent necessity for debriding portions of damaged sections of the tensor at the conclusion of the procedure.

The image intensifier improves the accuracy of acetabular position as well as leg length and offset. Image time averages 50 seconds. The surgeon experiences negligible x-ray exposure if he or she stands one meter away while imaging. If the surgeon prefers, the operation can be performed without the image intensifier utilizing the normal measures for assessing leg length (preoperative templates, prosthesis relation to femoral landmarks, soft tissue tension, and patella palpation).

Most small incision surgery techniques advocated are only for selected patients. The most common criterion is a body mass index (weight in kg/height in meters) of less than 35. I use the anterior approach for all patients; certainly high BMI patients are more difficult but incisions over 10 cm are infrequent and 12 cm is almost always the maximum necessary. Small incision surgery of obese patients through the anterior approach is possible partly because the subcutaneous fat over the anterolateral proximal thigh does not increase in thickness as dramatically as it does posteriorly or laterally.

As we endeavor to minimize the soft tissue invasion, it is useful to consider which patients need the most help in dislocation prevention and functional rehab, the thin and fit patient or the obese and deconditioned patient?

Surgical Technique

After administration of general or regional anesthesia, the patient is placed in the supine position on the PROfx table (Figure 8.2). A perineal post is used and the feet placed in the traction boots. It is normal to use a leg support for the leg that will not be operated and no leg support for the hip to be operated. The hip that will not be operated is

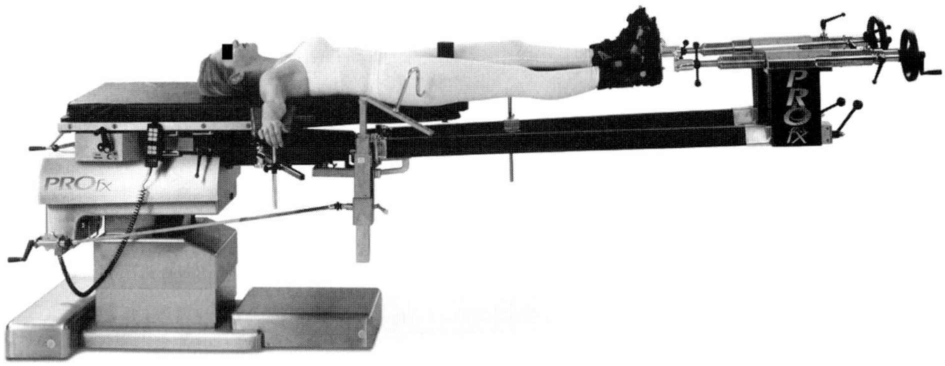

Figure 8.2. Patient positioning, supine on PROfx table (Union City, CA), femur jack and femur hook attached. (OSI, Subsidiary of The Mizuho Group, Union City, CA.)

placed in neutral rotation, extension and abduction-adduction to serve as a radiographic reference for the operated side. The jack that will raise and lower the femoral hook is placed near the side of the patient so that the hook bracket will lie roughly parallel to the long axis of the patient. Avoiding external rotation of the hip to be operated will make the external landmarks of the hip more reliable and enhance the landmark of the natural bulge of the tensor fascia lata muscle. The table should be leveled with the table level button on the hand control. It is normal for the patient's arms to be placed roughly perpendicular outward and not over the chest. Pneumatic compression *boots* are applied to the legs for intraoperative DVT prophylaxis.

The normal team consists of the surgeon, his assistant, the anesthesiologist, the scrub nurse, circulating nurse/table operator and x-ray tech. The following description refers to actions that may be taken by the surgeon, his assistant or the operator of the PROfx table.

Though the incision is normally small (8 cm to 10 cm), the author drapes a relatively wide area from just proximal to the iliac crest to the junction of the middle and distal thirds of the thigh. Draping a relatively wide area around the incision enhances the sterility by making the vinyl skin covering less likely to detach and thereby allow mobility of the drape edges. Also, the wider draping allows additional extensile access if necessary. Following draping with paper drapes, the surgeon makes a hole in the drapes overlying the table jack post. The square tubular receptacle of the hook bracket is placed through the drape hole and over the post. The hole is sealed with a vinyl drape.

The normal incision starts 2 cm posterior and slightly distal to the anterior superior iliac spine. This straight incision extends in a distal and slightly posterior direction to a point 2 cm to 3 cm anterior to the greater trochanter (Figure 8.3). On thinner patients the bulge of the tensor fascia lata muscle marks the center of the line of the incision. After incision of the skin and subcutaneous the tensor can be seen through the translucent fascia lata. Incise the fascial lata over the tensor and continue the fascial incision slightly distal and proximal beyond the ends of the skin incision (Figure 8.4).

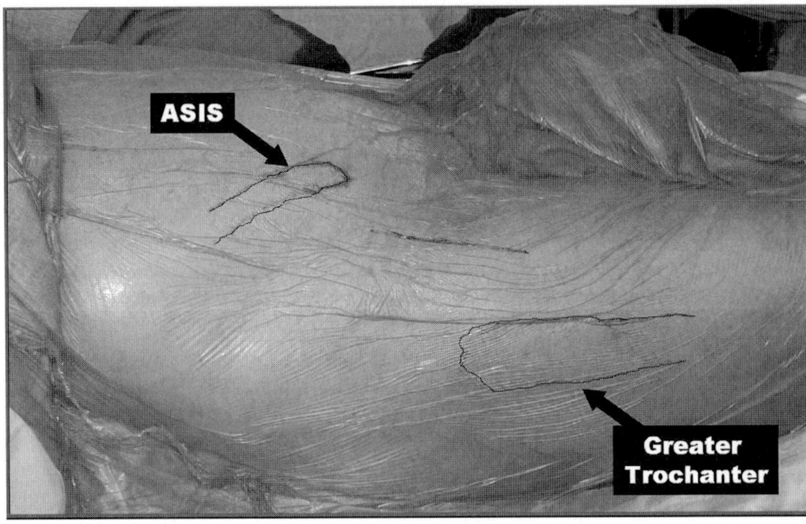

Figure 8.3. An 8-cm incision for the right hip and its relation to the anterior superior iliac spine (ASIS) and the greater trochanter.

Lift the fascia lata off the medial portion of the tensor and follow the interval medial to the tensor in a posterior and proximal direction. Dissection by feel is most efficient at this point and the lateral hip capsule can be easily palpated. Place a Cobra retractor along the lateral hip capsule and retract the sartorius and rectus femoris muscles medially with a Hibbs retractor. It is easy to make the mistake of perforating and incompletely retracting the gluteus minimus muscle with the Cobra, so check for this. If the retractors are properly placed the reflected head

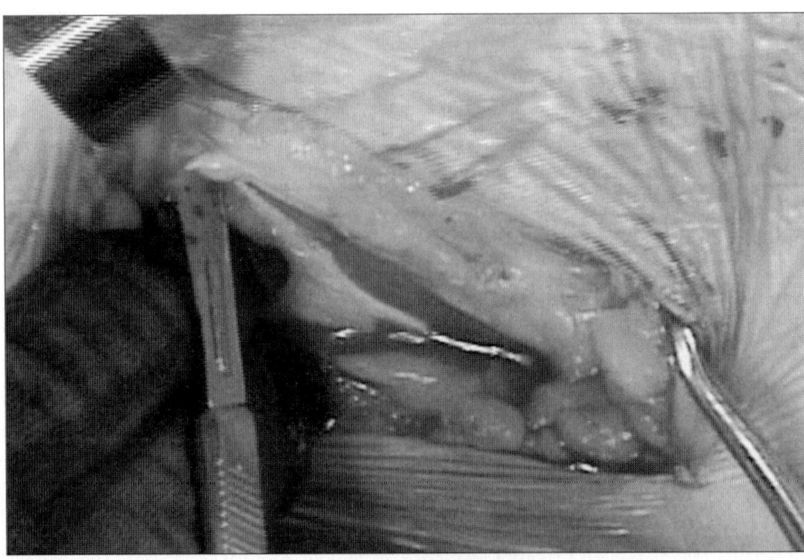

Figure 8.4. Incision of skin, subcutaneous and fascia lata over tensor fascia lata muscle.

of the rectus that follows the lateral acetabular rim will be visible. A small periosteal elevator placed just distal to the reflected head and directed medial and distal elevates the iliopsoas and rectus femoris muscles from the anterior capsule. The elevator opens the path for a second Cobra retractor to be placed on the medial hip capsule.

The medial and lateral retraction of the Cobras brings the lateral femoral circumflex vessels into view as they cross the distal portion of the wound. These vessels are clamped, cauterized and transected. Further distal splitting of the aponeurosis that overlies the anterior capsule and at times excision of a fat pad enhances exposure of the capsule and the origin of the vastus lateralis muscle. I perform an anterior capsulototomy with an L-shaped cut (Figure 8.5). The capsulototomy begins at the antero-lateral acetabular rim and courses distally and laterally along the anterolateral neck ending at the junction of the anterolateral neck and greater trochanter. From there the capsule is detached from the anterior intertrochanteric line in a lateral to medial direction. The corner of the flap is tagged with a suture and a reciprocal tag suture is placed on the lateral capsule just proximal to the greater trochanter. Alternatively, the anterior capsule can be excised. The Cobra retractors are now placed inside the capsule around the medial and lateral neck. It is important to be able to see the junction of the lateral neck and greater trochanter.

A narrow Hohmann's retractor is now placed on the antero-lateral acetabular rim. With this exposure the antero-lateral labrum is excised and sometimes an associated osteophyte. Distal traction on the extremity will create a small gap between the femoral head and the roof of the acetabulum. A femoral head skid is placed into this gap and rotated to a medial position. The traction is partially released. As the extrem-

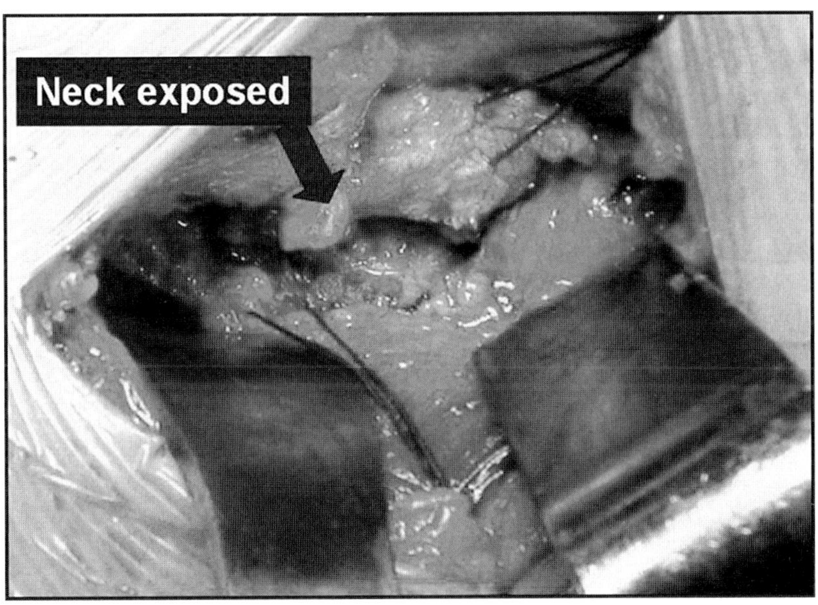

Figure 8.5. Following L-shaped anterior capsulotomy.

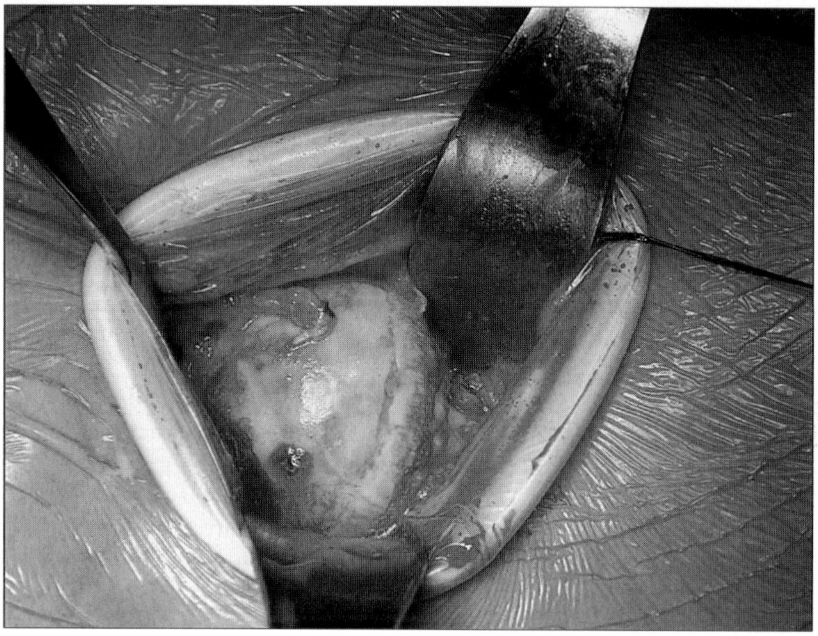

Figure 8.6. Femoral head and medial neck following anterior dislocation.

ity and hip are externally rotated and leverage applied to the skid, the hip is dislocated anteriorly and the femur externally rotated 90 degrees (Figure 8.6). External rotation of the femur is accomplished by rotation of the leg spar rotation wheel and aided by the scrubbed assistant grasping the distal femoral condyles. If the patient is very osteoporotic, undue force from the rotation wheel can fracture the tibia or ankle. To ease dislocation and reduce extremity torque, I prefer a femoral head corkscrew. After the skid has been placed medial to the head the hip is gently externally rotated. If dislocation does not occur easily, I place a 4.5-mm drill hole in the lateral femoral head in an anterior to posterior direction followed by insertion of the femoral head corkscrew into the hole. An anterior pull and external rotation force through the corkscrew will facilitate dislocation. If the hip is unusually difficult to dislocate, check for adequate capsular release and osteophyte excision and extend the hip slightly.

After dislocation, place the tip of a narrow Hohmann retractor distal to the lesser trochanter and beneath the vastus lateralis origin. Transect the capsule on the medial neck parallel to the neck and expose the lesser trochanter and posterior neck. During exposure of the posterior and medial neck, keep in mind that Hohmann retraction of the vastus protects the enervation of this muscle which comes from medial and at a surprisingly proximal location. Happily, however, this muscle is typically also enervated more distally. Reapply traction, internally rotate and reduce the hip.

Replace the cobra retractors around the medial and lateral neck and retract the vastus origin and distal tensor with a Hibbs. Cut the femoral neck with a reciprocating saw at the desired level and angle. The junction of the lateral shoulder of the neck and greater trochanter is used as the indicator for the level of the cut, and to place the lateral portion of the cut slightly distal to this point. Cut the medial portion of the neck first and take care to not cut the greater trochanter with the saw. The neck cut is completed with an osteotome placed in the sagittal plane that divides the lateral neck from the medial greater trochanter (Figure 8.7). The level of the neck cut is a little more difficult to judge than from posterior. I have experimented with cutting guides but now simply

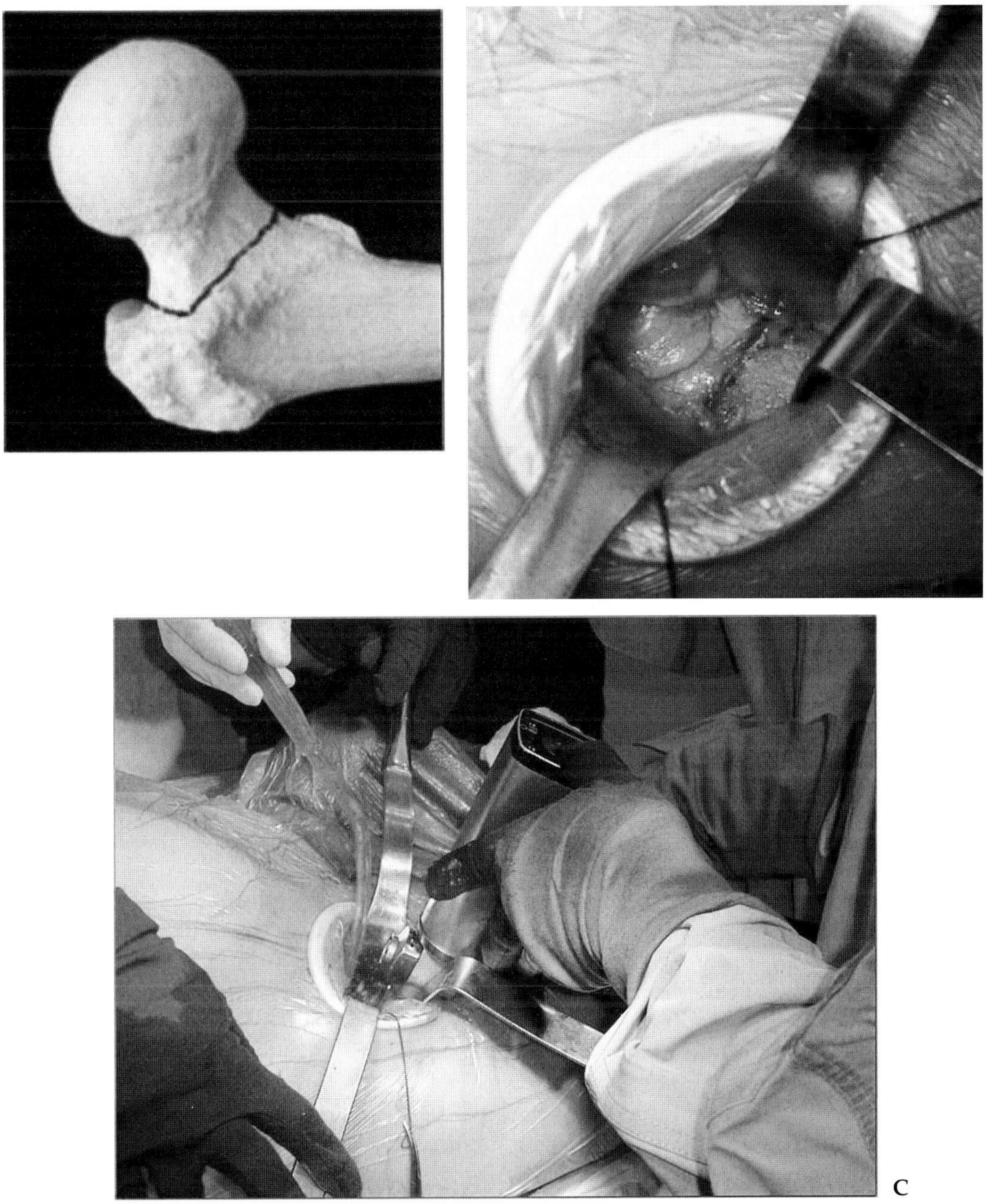

A B C

Figure 8.7. (A) Line of normal neck cut. (B) Line of neck cut seen on anterior femoral neck. (C) Cutting neck with oscillating saw.

eyeball the cut. Drill a 4.5-mm diameter hole into the anterior head and then insert the femoral head corkscrew if this step was not performed previously. Extract the head.

The original technique of Robert Judet (still used by Thierry Judet) is to cut the neck with the hip dislocated. The level of the cut is in this case judged by the level of the lesser trochanter. This technique introduces some danger of continuing the cut into the greater trochanter. The cut is completed by an osteotome to the supero-lateral neck.

I began this technique by cutting the neck in situ and then extracting the head. The advantage is that it avoids the dislocation step. The disadvantage is that the head is more difficult to extract and at times the head must be sectioned to remove it. The dislocation step increases the rotational mobility of the femur and thereby enhances femoral exposure for broaching and prosthesis insertion.

Throughout the procedure the surgeon will find that the tensor fascia lata muscle is potentially vulnerable to injury. Take care not to lever too hard on this muscle with retractors. During cutting of the neck the relatively dull side of the oscillating saw blade will cut the muscle if it contacts it. Levering the femoral head skid through wide angles can also lacerate the muscle. As the cut femoral neck is extracted the sharp bony edge can also lacerate the muscle and a Rongeur is used to round the neck cut or at least take care to protect the muscle with the Hibbs during extraction. Attention to this muscle needs to continue during the acetabular reaming and insertion and femoral broaching phases. If an initial injury to the muscle fibers is avoided, the muscle seems to hold up well through the procedure. On the other hand, an early laceration to the surface of the tensor seems to hurt its capability to resist further damage. The PROfx table, however, makes preservation of the soft tissues easier by its external and internal control of the femur and thereby makes leverage against the soft tissues less necessary.

The acetabulum is now visualized and prepared (Figure 8.8). External rotation of the femur of about 30 degrees usually facilitates acetabular exposure. A bent Hohmann retractor is used over the anterior rim of the acetabulum to retract the anterior muscles. Take care to place the tip of this retractor on bone and not into the anterior soft tissues. A Cobra retractor is placed with the tip initially on the postero-superior rim and subsequently on the mid-posterior rim. Excise the labrum circumferentially. Transection of the most prominent band of inferior capsule will facilitate later placement of the acetabular liner. Begin reaming under direct vision and later check with the image intensifier to confirm depth of reaming and adequate circumference (Figure 8.9). The indicators of torque and acetabular appearance are also used.

The acetabular prosthesis is inserted with a curved inserter (Figure 8.10). The image intensifier allows the surgeon to watch the position and progressive seating of the prosthesis. Prior to using image control, confirm that the pelvis is level with a midline image view. Symmetry of the obturator foramina or centering of the coccyx to the symphysis confirms a level pelvis. If the pelvis is not level the table can be tilted to compensate as needed. The liner is inserted in the normal fashion. During acetabular shell insertion, extension and adduction of the limb

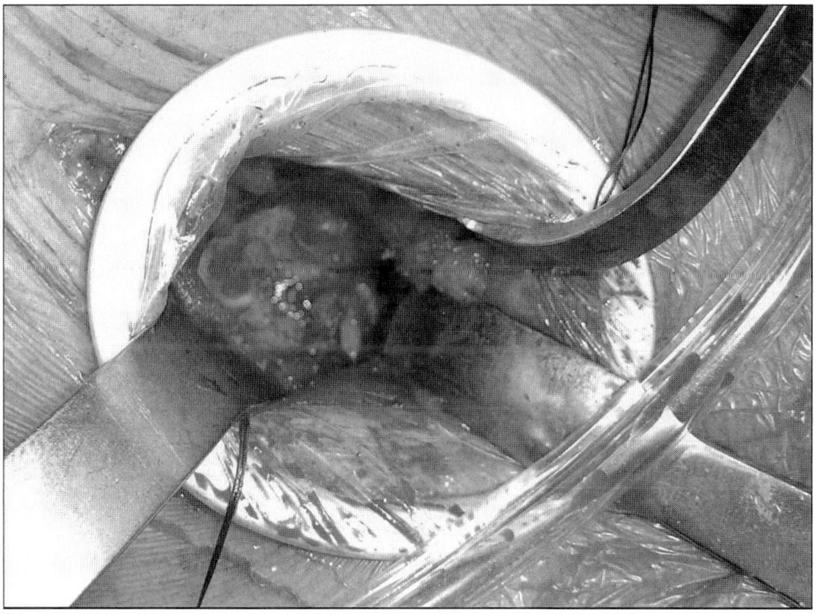

Figure 8.8. View of acetabulum prior to reaming.

can reduce interference between the distal portion of the incision and the straight inserter.

Following acetabular insertion, the gross traction control on the table is released and the femur internally rotated to neutral. The vastus ridge is palpated and the femoral hook placed just distal to this and around the posterior femur (Figure 8.11). The hook is attached to the most convenient hole on the bracket. The femur is now externally rotated 90 degrees and the hip hyperextended and adducted. This position is

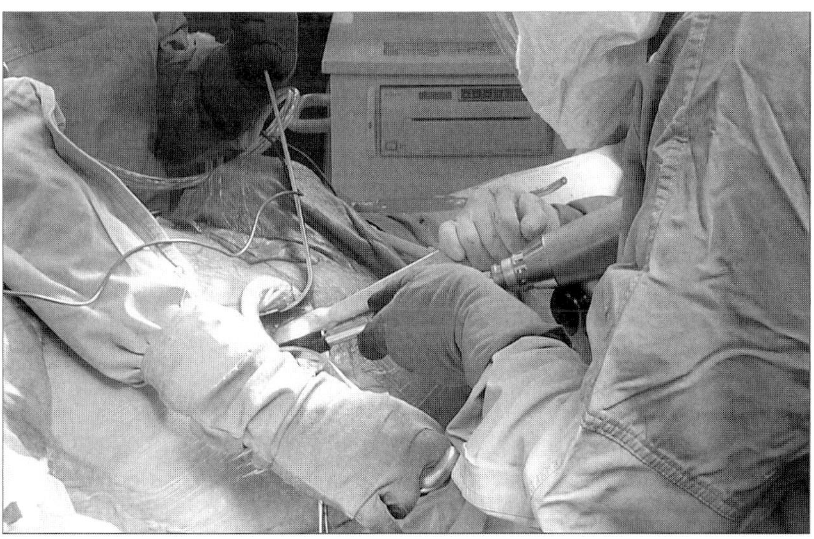

Figure 8.9. Acetabulum reaming under direct vision.

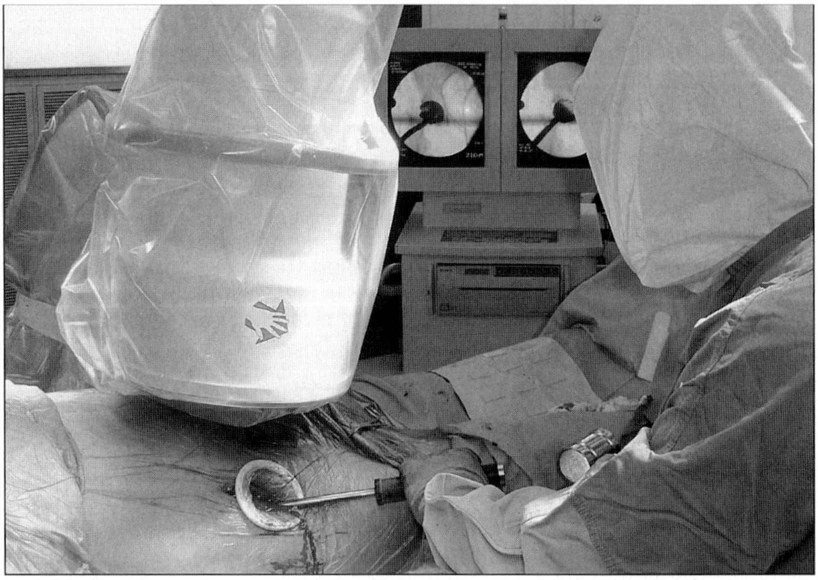

Figure 8.10. Image intensifier check of acetabular reaming and acetabular shell position during insertion.

achieved by rotating the wheel at the end of the leg spar, dropping the leg spar to the floor and adducting it (Figure 8.12). Remember to release the gross traction lock to minimize the chance of a hyperextension stretch to the femoral nerve.

For proximal femoral exposure, a long-handled Cobra is used with the tip on the posterior femoral neck and placing the tip of a trochanteric retractor over the tip of the trochanter. It is now necessary to visualize the medial aspect of the greater trochanter and obtain some femoral mobility that allows the femur to come slightly lateral and anterior. The proximal femur is now raised by the femoral hook until the tissues come under moderate tension (Figure 8.13). It is important to feel the tension by manually lifting the hook up and down as the jack raises the hook. You should be able to manually lift the femur higher than the level the hook has raised it to. Too much tension can cause a fracture of the greater trochanter. Following this initial maneuver the posterior ridge of the greater trochanter usually lies posterior to the posterior rim of the acetabulum. The femur needs to be mobile enough so that lateral and anterior displacement brings the posterior edge of the trochanter lateral and anterior to the posterior rim of the acetabulum. The lateral capsule with its tag suture will be seen lateral to the lateral neck remnant and attaching to it. In most cases the necessity to bring the femur more lateral and anterior leads the surgeon to detach the lateral capsule from its neck attachment. Following this detachment the lateral capsular flap will lie medial to the posterior neck and greater trochanter.

Replace the trochanteric retractor closer to the tip of the trochanter so that it retracts the gluteus minimus and medius and also the piriformis and obturator internus tendons. The medius tendon appears inside out and its white undersurface is seen at the posterior superior corner of the greater trochanter. The obturator externus tendon insertion is found at the point we normally term the piriformis fossa. The piriformis and obturator internus tendons insert on the mid-portion of the tip of the greater trochanter. Manually check the mobility of the femur by pulling on the hook and if it is mobile enough, raise the jack to support the femur in a more anterior position. Depending on the requirements for femoral mobility, the surgeon may choose to release one or more of the short external rotator tendons. It is most important to preserve the tendon insertion of the obturator externus because this tendon has a medial

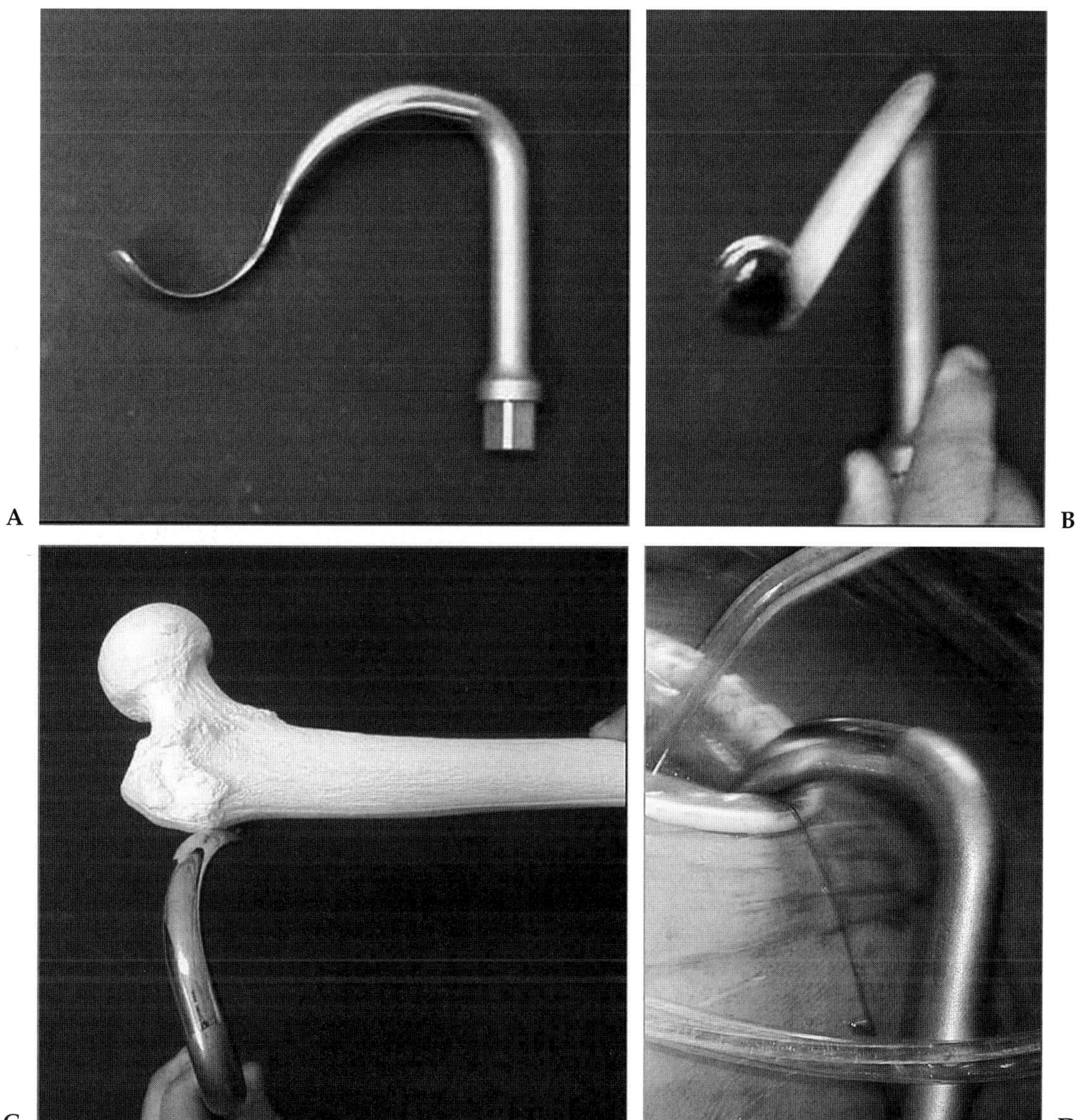

Figure 8.11. (A) Support hook for the proximal femur. (B) A 90-degree rotation view of the support hook. (C) Femoral location for the support hook. (D) Support hook after placement around the proximal femur.

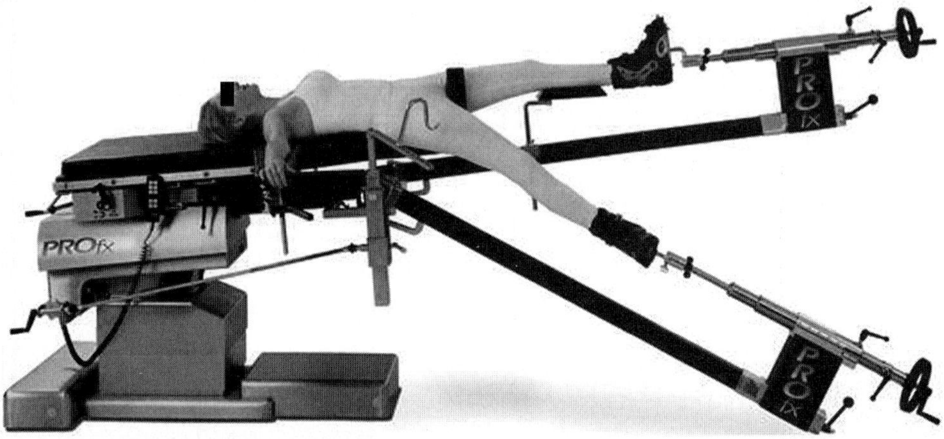

Figure 8.12. PROfx table positioned for femoral preparation. Hip is hyperextended, adducted, and femur externally rotated 90 degrees. Support hook is posterior to the femur. Trendelenburg position of table top can be used as needed. (OSI, Subsidiary of The Mizuho Group, Union City, CA.)

direction pull on the proximal femur and thereby is an important active stabilizer of the hip against dislocation.

Also many prostheses such as the Zimmer Alloclassic, which the author has used, require some cutting into the medial aspect of the trochanter for broach and prosthesis insertion and this cutting can enter an area of external rotator tendon insertion. The proximal lateral promi-

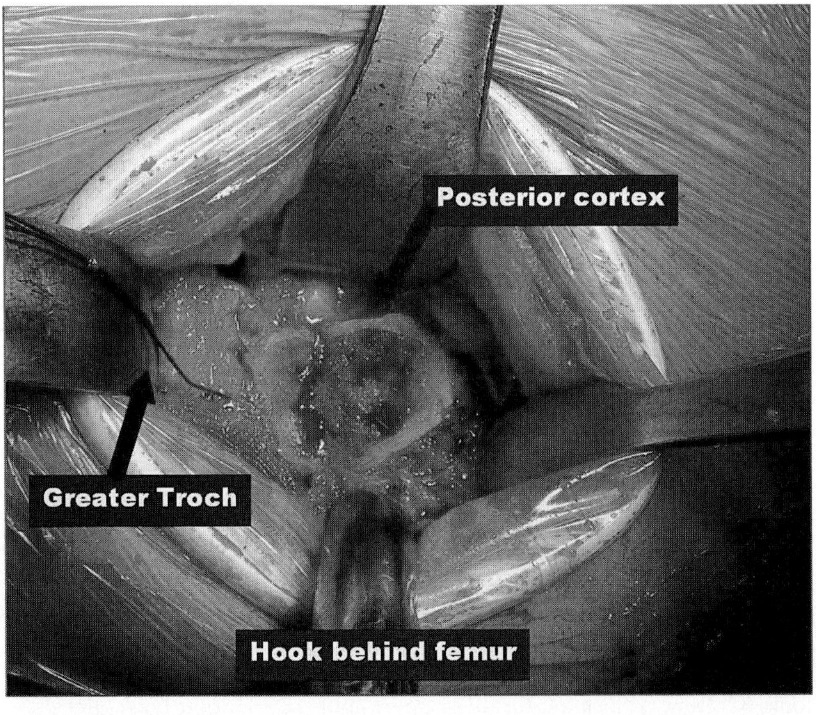

Figure 8.13. View of the proximal femur following placing the table in the femoral preparation position.

nence also increases the risk of fracture of the greater trochanter. I currently prefer prostheses with a reduced proximal lateral shoulder that are thereby less aggressive to the greater trochanter. I normally use the DePuy Corail; however, a number of other cemented and uncemented prostheses are also applicable.

With the femur in position for broaching, I use a rongeur to excise the remnant of the lateral neck. The cancellous bone of the canal is opened with a rongeur or curette. The tip of the first broach enters the medial canal near the calcar and posterior femoral cortex (Figure 8.14).

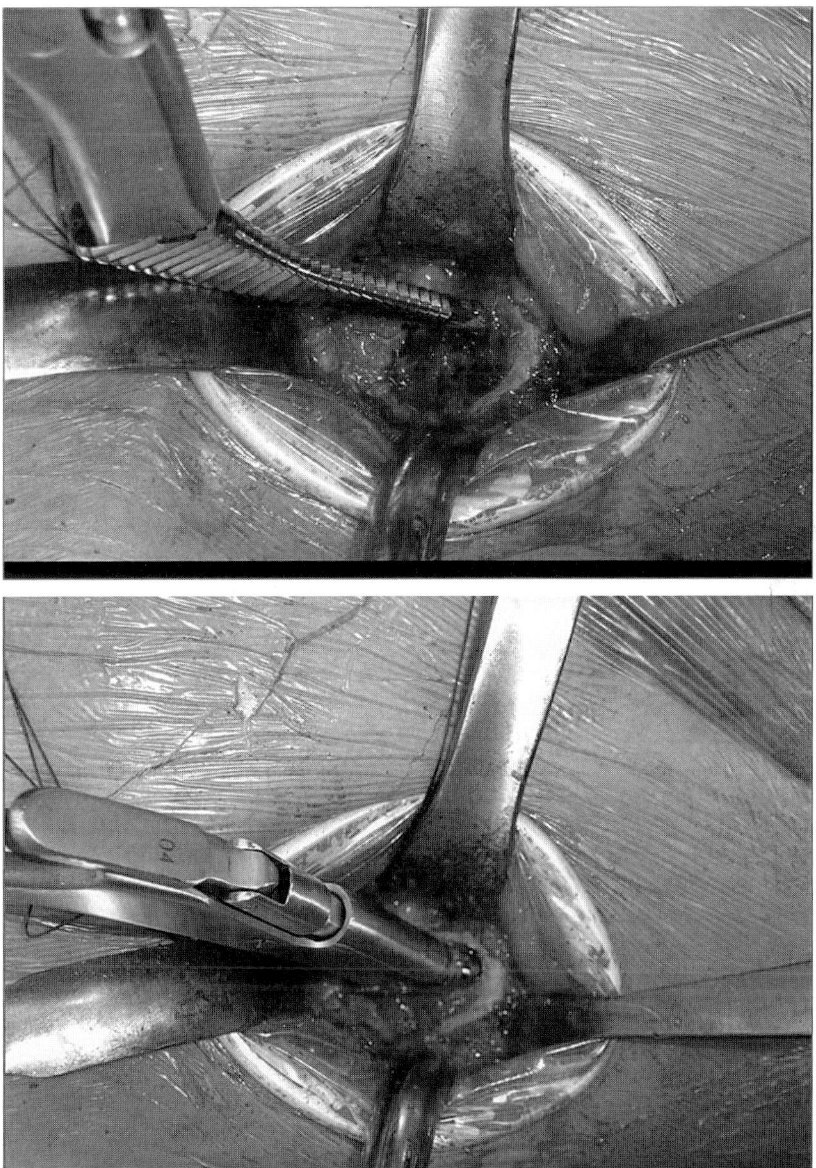

A

B

Figure 8.14. (A) Initial broach insertion into the proximal femur with the broach tip starting near the calcar and along the posterior cortex. (B) Seating of the initial Corail broach parallel to the posterior cortex.

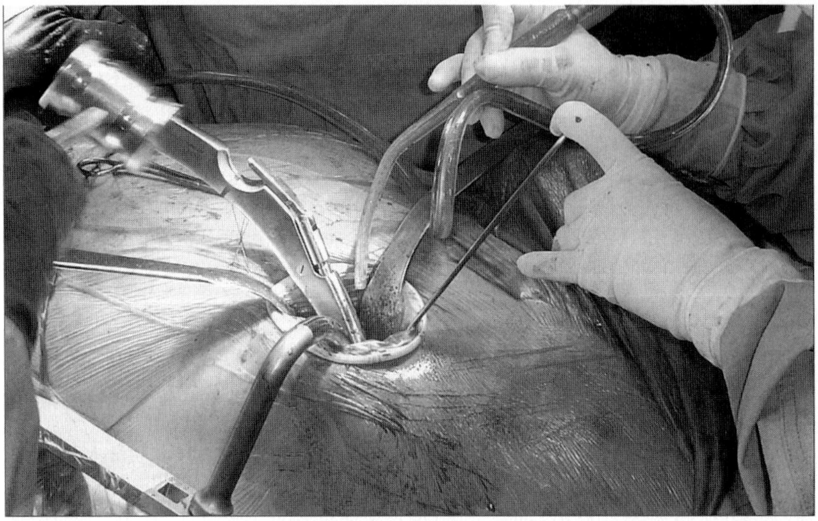

Figure 8.15. Clearance of anterior soft tissues by the offset and curved Corail broach handle.

It is possible to perforate either the posterior or lateral femoral cortex and the initial entry should guard against this. If in doubt, use the image to confirm the broach position. After the first several broaches it is often useful to open the lateral metaphysis by removing cancellous bone with a curette. This curetting helps prevent a varus positioning of the prosthesis. Proper anteversion of the broach can be assessed by several landmarks. Palpate the patella to determine femoral rotation. The neck cut also indicates proper anteversion. The plane of broach/ prosthesis anteversion should be roughly parallel to the plane of the posterior neck cortex and converge toward the plane of the anterior neck cortex (Figure 8.15).

When the broaching is complete, a trial reduction is made with the neck length estimated from the preoperative template. The femur hook jack is lowered and the hook removed. The hip is flexed to the neutral position, traction applied and the hip is reduced with simultaneous internal rotation and a push on the femoral head. The traction is released and image views of the two hips compared. The opposite hip image is placed on the right screen and the operated hip image on the left. If the length and offset does not need obvious adjustment, the author typically instructs the x-ray technician to print both images on transparencies. Then these two transparencies can be compared by overlying them on the x-ray view box. If the length and offset are not correct, appropriate adjustments are made (change in neck length, further seating of broach, or insertion of next size broach). The fit of the broach in the femoral shaft is viewed to check for alignment and fill. When comparing image views of the two hips, it is best to have both hips in comparable positions as far as flexion, abduction-adduction, and rotation. These position adjustments are easily made with the PROfx table.

When overlying the transparencies of the two hips to judge leg length and offset, first align the two femurs. For equal leg length, the image of the proximal extent of the acetabular prosthesis should extend slightly proximal to the image of the opposite femoral head to account for the loss of joint space and reaming into the roof. After superimposition of the femurs it is also useful to compare the pelvic landmarks (assuming comparable hip positions) (Figure 8.16). At times you are left with questions as to what is best. The opposite hip may be a total hip that was made too long. Should you now make this new THA too long

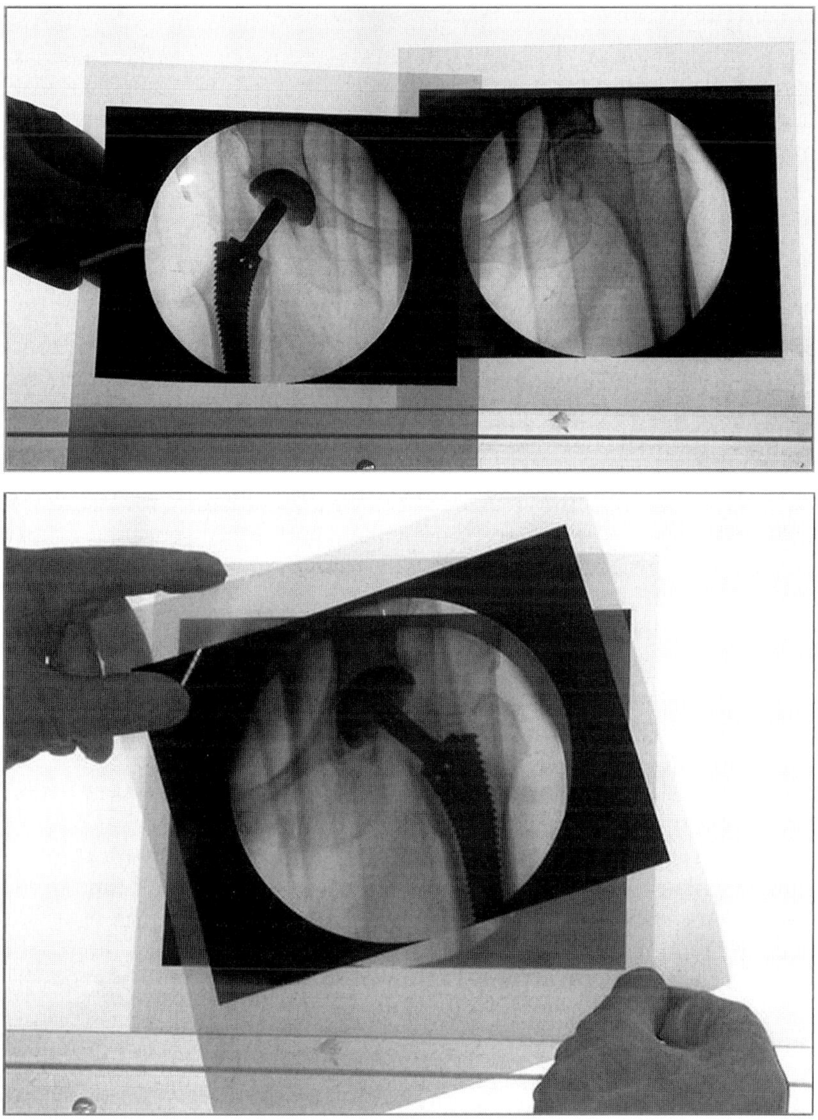

A

B

Figure 8.16. (A) X-ray prints of the right hip with trial femoral components and a normal left hip. (B) Assessment of leg length and femoral offset: Right hip transparency with trial components is flipped and placed over the left hip transparency.

or restore it to its previous anatomic length? Careful assessment of the preoperative x-rays may show a congenital length discrepancy such as in dysplasia. How much should you lengthen? Alternatively the preoperative leg lengths may be equal, indicating that the arthritic hip was once longer before loss of the cartilage space and bony wear of the head equalized the leg length. Is it then proper to restore the length to the previous inequality? If the opposite side is arthritic and slightly shortened but asymptomatic, should you make the THA slightly longer and anticipate that the patient will soon desire the other side to be done?

During the trial phase I check for hip stability in extension and external rotation. The traction is released. I watch the hip rotate as the table operator maximally externally rotates the hip. In the majority of cases he will be unable to dislocate it with this maneuver. I rarely check for posterior stability but this can be checked by an unscrubbed assistant unhooking the traction boot from the table and flexing and internally rotating the hip. Check for impingement with osteophytes and excise appropriately. Soft tissue tension can also be checked by manually pulling in the normal manner.

After the decision is made for the femoral prosthesis the femoral hook is replaced behind the proximal femur, traction applied and the hip dislocated with external rotation and often a bone hook around the femoral neck. The femur is then placed in the preparation position (90 degree external rotation, hyperextension, adduction, and proximal elevation). The femoral prosthesis is then inserted in the normal fashion (Figure 8.17). The appropriate length permanent head can be placed at that time or a second trial performed if desired. With the hip flexed to neutral the acetabulum is visualized prior to reduction to ensure that it is clear of bone or cement fragments. Another transparency printed with the image intensifier confirms leg length and offset and serves as the immediate postoperative x-ray. Prior to discharge, x-rays will be obtained in the radiology department.

A check is made for bleeding and the wound irrigated. The closure is simple. The fascia lata is closed with a running suture, followed by subcutaneous and skin. I prefer deep and subcutaneous hemovacs.

Following surgery the patient does not follow antidislocation precautions. He is encouraged to bear weight immediately and use his hip as symptoms permit.

This series of 450 anterior approaches is unselected and consecutive. The surgeries were performed on the Judet/Tasserit table until 2003. Beginning in 2003 the PROfx table became available and is now preferred. The average age is 71 and ranges from 28 to 90. The average operative time is 1.3 hours. Average blood loss is 350 cc. The average hospital time is 4 days and the most frequent is 3 days. There were 2 early anterior dislocations that were reduced closed and did not recur or require revision. There was one deep infection. The median time to doing some ambulation without external support is 10 days. The median time for doing all ambulation without external support is 3 weeks. It is my impression that pain is reduced and the recovery rate greatly enhanced.

Besides benefiting the patient, a goal of surgical technique development should be to make the technique as easy and reproducible as

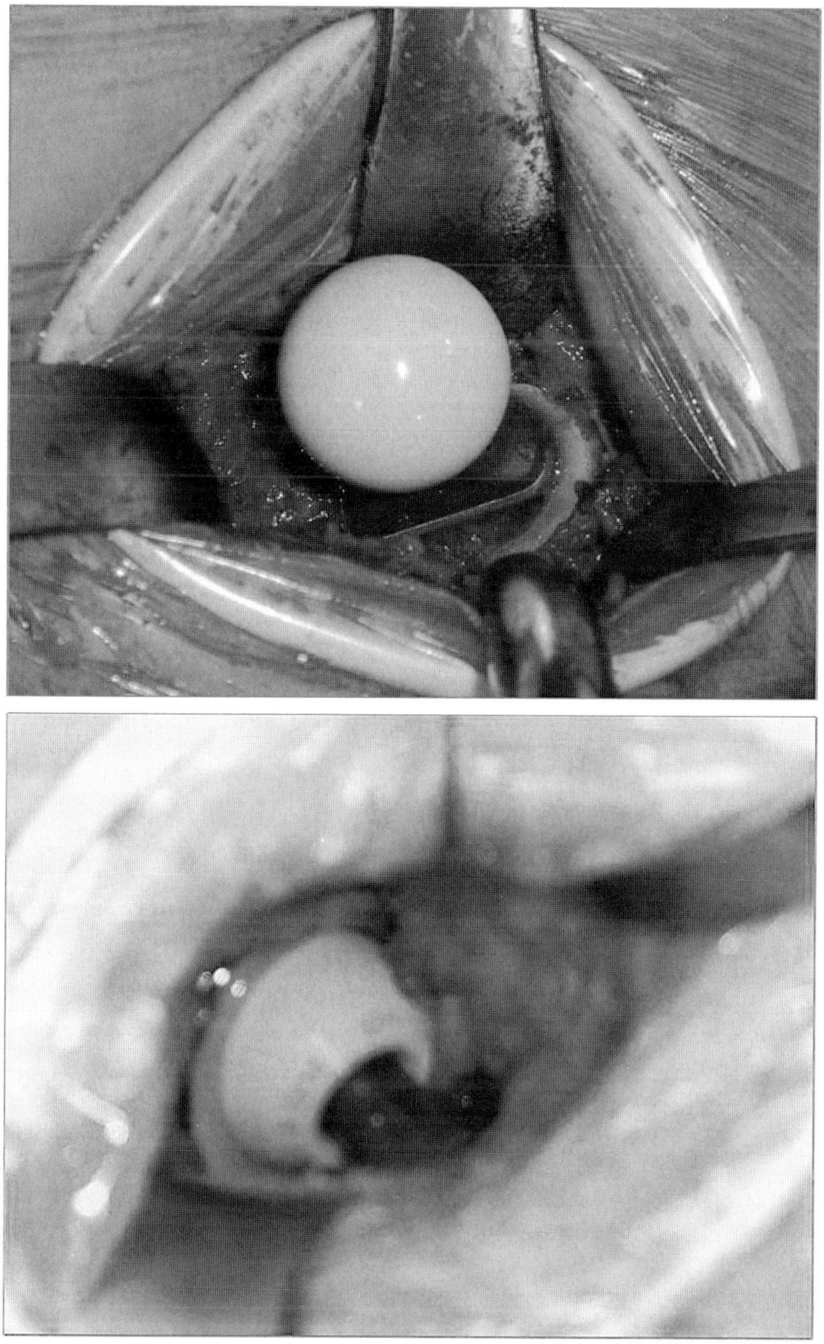

A

B

Figure 8.17. (A) Corail stem with ceramic head following insertion. (B) Following reduction of the head into the acetabular liner.

possible. It is my belief that this minimally invasive technique is easier than the majority of small incision techniques and can be performed by many surgeons with reproducible results and a low complication rate.

References

1. Judet R, Judet J. Technique and results with the acrylic femoral head prosthesis. J Bone Joint Surg Br. May 1952;34-B(2):173–80.
2. Siguier T, Siguier M, Judet T, Charnley G, Brumpt B. Partial resurfacing arthroplasty of the femoral head in avascular necrosis. Methods, indications, and results. Clin Orthop. May 2001;(386):85–92.
3. Charnley J. Total prosthetic replacement of the hip. Reconstr Surg Traumatol. 1969;11:9–19.
4. Charnley J. The long-term results of low-friction arthroplasty of the hip performed as a primary intervention. J Bone Joint Surg Br. February 1972; 54(1):61–76.
5. Kennon RE, Keggi JM, Wetmore RS, Zatorski LE, Huo MH, Keggi KJ. Total hip arthroplasty through a minimally invasive anterior surgical approach. J Bone Joint Surg Am. 2003;85-A (suppl 4):39–48.
6. Matta JM. Bilateral THA. Orthopedics. November 2002;25(11):1224.
7. Beaule PE, Griffin DB, Matta JM. The Levine Anterior Approach for Total Hip Replacement as the Treatment for an Acute Acetabular Fracture. J Orthop Trauma. October 2004;18(9):623–629.

9

Posterolateral Minimal Incision for Total Hip Replacement: Technique and Early Results

Mark A. Hartzband

Development of a minimal incision posterolateral approach to total hip arthroplasty began in 1996. As experience was gained, incision length was progressively shortened. It became clear that modification of instruments would be required to facilitate arthroplasty through incisions of less than 10 cm. This approach involves more than simply a shorter skin incision. It incorporates minimal soft tissue dissection and eliminates portions of surgical exposure unnecessary for accurate and reproducible acetabular and femoral preparation. It is a technique that can be utilized in perhaps 95% of primary total hip arthroplasties.

Between January 1998 and July 2002, the author performed 1489 cases of minimal incision posterolateral total hip arthroplasties. Initially incision length of less than or equal to 10 cm was used to define the surgical procedure as a minimal incision approach. Of the 1489 cases, 670 patients had incisions less than 8.5 cm. Several different prostheses have been used with this approach. Hybrid and fully coated noncemented total hip components have been implanted without difficulty. For the past 5 years, the majority of the operations have been performed using a noncemented, proximally coated, tapered titanium stem (Fiber Metal Taper, Zimmer Inc., Warsaw, IN). A modular acetabular component has been used throughout the author's surgical experience.

Surgical Technique

Patient selection is important, particularly during the early experience with minimal incision total hip arthroplasty. As the surgeon develops a level of comfort with the technique, it can be used in the vast majority of primary total hip candidates. A varus neck angle accompanied by a general lack of muscular development tends to facilitate the approach. As such, women may be better candidates as one starts to learn the technique. Long valgus femoral necks, particularly in muscular men, make a minimal incision total hip arthroplasty more difficult. As in all posterior approaches to the hip, significant external rotation contracture makes for a more difficult exposure. Incision size should be progressively decreased in an intelligent fashion until a truly minimal posterolateral incision has been achieved.

It is critical to keep in mind that the primary goal of any joint replacement is to create a biomechanically and structurally sound arthroplasty with excellent prosthesis position and durable interfaces. If during the course of a procedure the surgeon is presented with circumstances that require extension of the incision to ensure that adequate exposure and proper component orientation is achieved, the incision should be lengthened without hesitation. The ease of extending the approach when necessary is a major advantage of this technique.

Patient Positioning and Landmarks

The patient is initially positioned in the lateral decubitus position with the surgical side up. It is critical that the patient be held firmly in the decubitus position with any one of several readily available hip holding devices that allow for free flexion of the operative limb and accurate assessment of pelvic position and orientation. A carpenter's level is applied to the operating table to ensure that it is horizontal with respect to the floor. The level then is applied to the hip holding device so as to ensure that the patient is horizontal and, most importantly, that the pelvis is perpendicular to the floor. Any degree of forward roll of the pelvis severely compromises exposure of the acetabulum in a minimal incision posterolateral approach. It is important to keep in mind that most of the standard pelvic holding devices apply up to 20 degrees of flexion to the pelvis and therefore require a corresponding modification in acetabular component position so as to obtain appropriate acetabular anteversion.

As in all total hip arthroplasties, the most accurate method of obtaining proper leg lengths is by meticulous preoperative templating of the anterior/posterior (AP) and lateral views of the patient's pelvis. The importance of preoperative templating cannot be overly stressed, particularly when performing a minimally invasive total hip arthroplasty. Standard intraoperative neck cutting guides may be easily used through minimally invasive total hip incisions. Any one of several available intraoperative leg length confirmation systems may be utilized with this approach as well.

Once the patient is draped, the landmarks for the incision are marked (Figure 9.1A and B). In minimal incision total hip arthroplasty, correct placement of the incision has major repercussions on the ease with which the procedure is performed. The true high point of the pelvis (i.e., the point at which the lumbar paraspinal muscles meet the lateral border of the posterolateral ileum) generally can be palpated in patients who are candidates for minimally invasive total hip arthroplasty. This point is marked and a second point approximately two fingerbreadths posterior to the high point of the pelvis and directed toward the center of the greater trochanter, is marked. This line generally represents a good approximation of the acetabular anteversion angle. The proximal most border of the greater trochanter is then identified. If difficulty

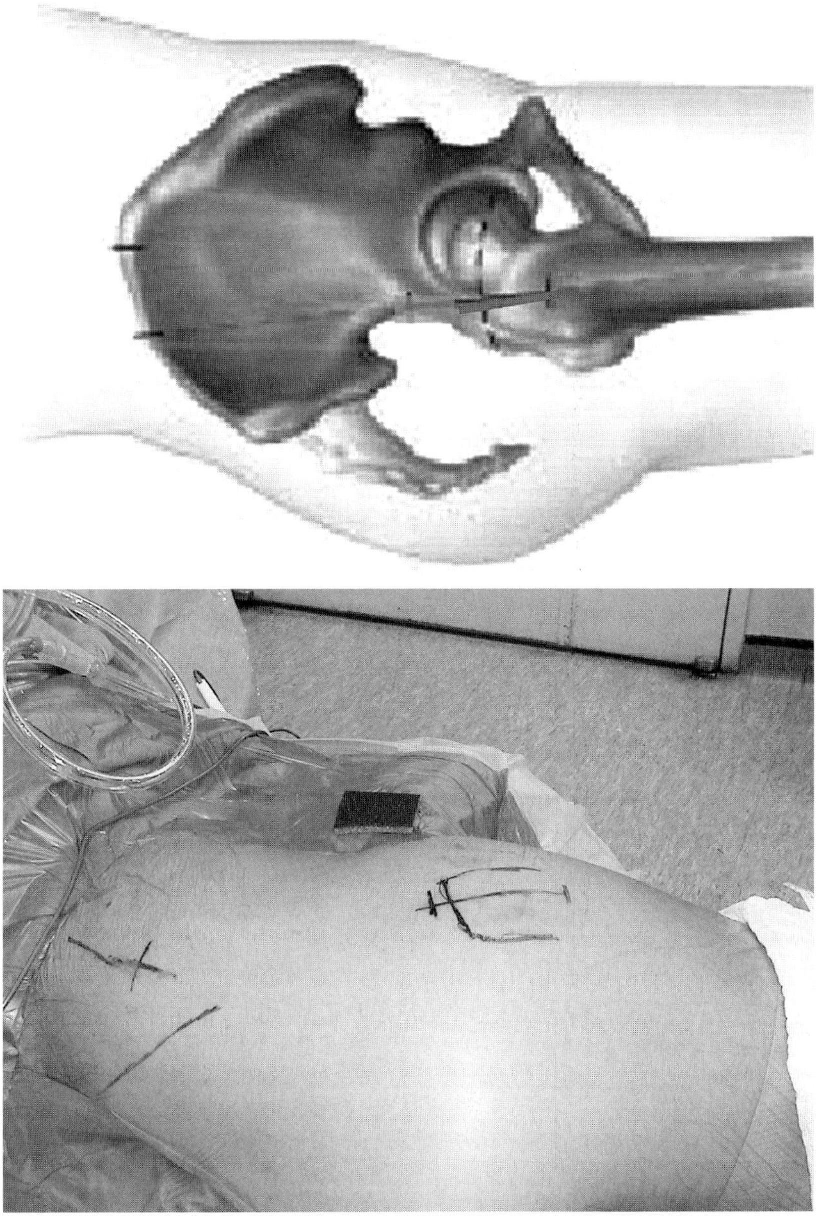

A

B

Figure 9.1. (A and B) Landmarks and location of minimal incision for total hip arthroplasty. (A, by permission of Zimmer, Inc., Warsaw, IN.)

is encountered in identifying the proximal border of the greater trochanter, a 3.5-in. spinal needle may be used to palpate and confirm the precise location of the greater trochanter. A slightly oblique incision is marked, directed parallel to the anteversion angle previously marked. This incision is typically oblique and directed posteriorly 10 degrees to 20 degrees with respect to the long axis of the femur, measuring 7 cm to 8 cm in length with approximately 80% of the incision distal to the most proximal border of the greater trochanter. The incision is centered slightly (approximately 5 mm) posterior to the midline of the proximal femur. It is moved posteriorly as the thickness of the lateral adipose tissue increases. Excessive translation of the incision posteriorly (at or beyond the posterior border of the greater trochanter) is to be avoided as this will greatly compromise visualization of the anterior portion of the acetabulum.

With experience, the location of the incision can be modified based on the patient's skeletal anatomy and body habitus. In patients who have more adipose tissue, the incision is moved proximally approximately 1 cm so that femoral canal machining can be performed without undue tension on the proximal angle of the incision. In patients with Crowe I-II type hips or significant lateral subluxation from degenerative joint disease, the incision is translated distally. In the case of a substantial lateral subluxation, the entire incision may extend distally from the most proximal border of the greater trochanter.

The mobile window is an integral concept in minimal incision total hip arthroplasty regardless of approach. It requires a properly located and oriented incision as well as instruments that maximize both mobility and visualization through this mobile window.

Patient Exposure

Once the skin incision has been made, the subcutaneous tissue is divided in the line of the incision. The gluteus maximus fascia and fascia lata are identified and incised in the direction of their fibers. The gluteus maximus muscle is bluntly split. The sciatic nerve is identified and protected. The fascia lata may occasionally be incised for a distance of 5 cm to 10 mm distal to the distal pole of the skin incision. Proximal extension of the fascial incision beyond the proximal pole of the skin incision rarely is required. A modified rectangular Charnley retractor with extended blades is then placed into the wound. The anterior blade of the retractor has been lengthened so as to facilitate its use in small incision surgery. More importantly, the blades of the Charnley retractor have been shortened to maximize visualization of deep structures.

The lower extremity is held in neutral extension, gravity adduction, and forced internal rotation. The short external rotator tendons are divided with electrocautery at their insertion into the piriformis fossa (Figure 9.2). Bending the tip of the cautery will facilitate division of the rotators and capsule at their bony insertion. The short external rotators are deliberately not mobilized from pericapsular fat or capsule during this portion of the dissection. By not separating external rotators from capsule the tendons of the piriformis and the conjoined tendon tend to remain adherent to the edge of the capsular flap and thereby facilitate closure of this layer at the conclusion of the procedure. The superior border of the piriformis is identified, and a Cobb elevator is placed along its superior border and then slid anteriorly to separate the gluteus minimus from hip capsule. The piriformis tendon is then divided at the piriformis fossa and a radial capsulotomy is performed along the superior border of the piriformis to the acetabular rim. Next

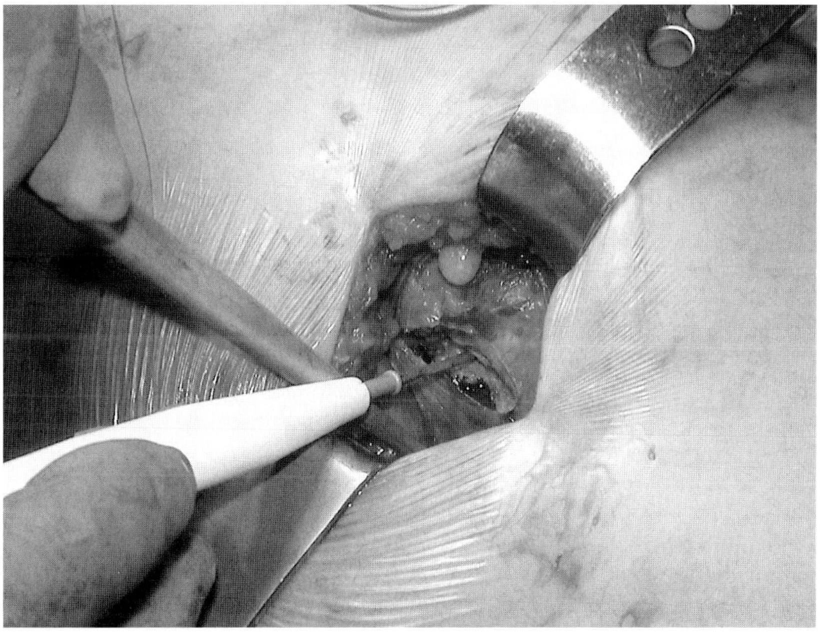

Figure 9.2. Development of posterior capsular flap.

the superior capsule is incised with a long scalpel blade under protection of the previously placed Cobb elevator to the zenith of the acetabulum (for a right hip this is from the 10 o'clock to the 12 o'clock position). With division of this posterosuperior portion of capsule, a dramatic increase in posterior laxity will be noted.

The hip is gently dislocated in slight flexion (approximately 15 degrees), adduction and internal rotation (Figure 9.3A). In many cases, 5 mm to 10 mm of quadratus femoris must be incised so as to expose the lesser trochanter. Extension of the hip then aids in visualization of the lesser trochanter. With the lesser trochanter exposed, a femoral neck cut is marked. The vertical distance from the tip of the greater trochanter or the shoulder of the femoral neck is also a valuable guide to assist in proper location of the neck osteotomy. It is best to identify the level of the neck cut by careful preoperative templating. There is ample room to apply a traditional neck-cutting guide if desired. The neck cut then is made using a reciprocating saw with teeth on only one side (Figure 9.3B). This is a critical instrument for use in the procedure, because its design protects against inadvertent injury to the posterior structures, particularly the sciatic nerve. As the femoral neck is cut from the medial calcar toward the greater trochanter, it is important that the first assistant gradually flex the hip to bring the greater trochanter into view and to avoid notching of the greater trochanter. The vertical limb of the neck cut then is made, extending distally along the piriformis fossa and medial border of the greater trochanter.

Once the femoral neck cut has been made, the hip is further extended. In doing so, the femoral head fragment generally rotates into flexion,

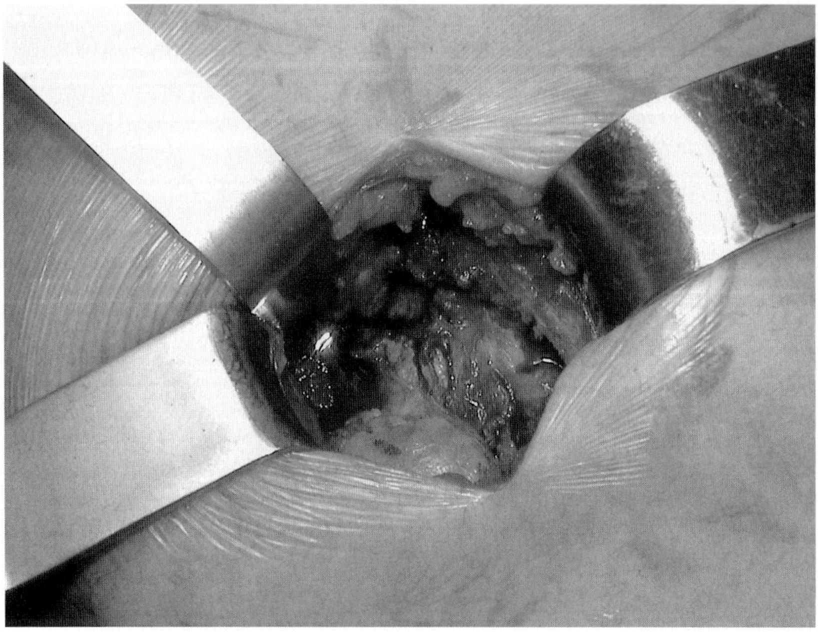

A

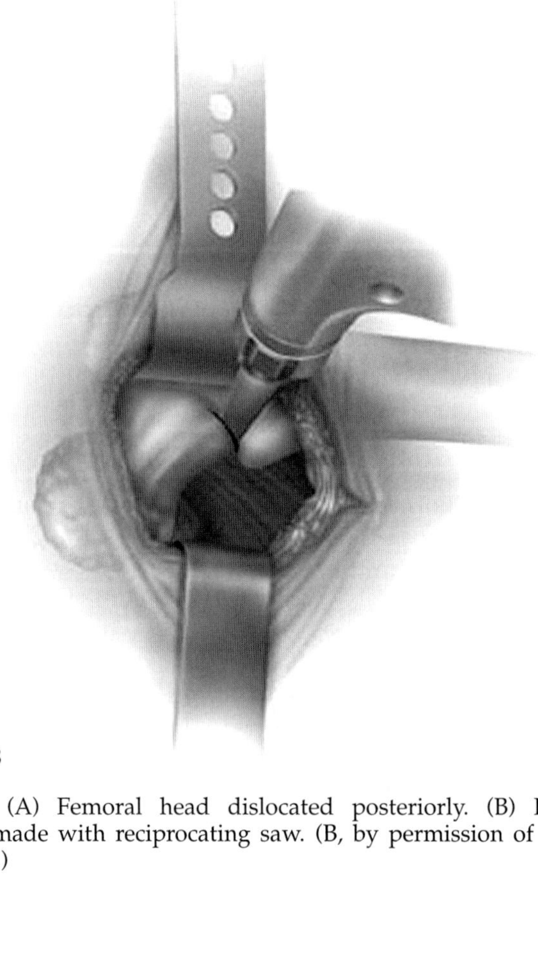

B

Figure 9.3. (A) Femoral head dislocated posteriorly. (B) Femoral neck osteotomy made with reciprocating saw. (B, by permission of Zimmer, Inc., Warsaw, IN.)

exposing the cut cancellous surface of the neck, which is easily grasped with a bone holding clamp and removed. If difficulty is encountered while removing the femoral head (for example, removing a very large diameter femoral head through a small length incision), removal of the Charnley retractor will allow even the largest of femoral heads to be removed. Once the femoral head has been removed and the height of the femoral neck cut has been confirmed, the limb is returned to a neutral position. A Kocher clamp is placed on the internal aspect of the posterior capsular flap at the posterior superior corner of the posterior capsular incision. This clamp is maintained throughout the acetabular preparation phase of the procedure so as to facilitate posterior acetabular exposure.

It is important to understand that all parts of the hip should be visualized easily throughout this procedure, but not necessarily at the same instant. This is the concept of a mobile window. The anterior two thirds of the acetabulum are visible with the limb in one position, whereas the limb position must be modified to facilitate exposure of the posterior third of the acetabulum. One of several curved, self-illuminated anterior retractors is placed into the acetabulum and brought up along the anterior acetabular wall. It then is pushed through the anterior capsule so as to retract the proximal femoral metaphysis anteriorly (Figure 9.4A and B). In large, muscular men, difficulty may be encountered in retracting the proximal femur anteriorly. In these cases, an anterior capsulotomy is performed by directing a scalpel blade under direct vision, beginning at the superior pole of the hip capsular incision and continuing anteriorly and progressively distally until adequate capsular relaxation has been obtained. Generally, by the time an additional 90 degrees of hip capsule has been incised, the femur can be retracted easily anteriorly. Overzealous retraction of the proximal femur should not be necessary if the incision is properly located, the limb and retractors are properly positioned and the capsular tissues have been adequately released. It is critical to achieve adequate anterior retraction of the femur for later stages of acetabular preparation.

The pulvinar is excised using a large curette or rongeur. If a substantial shelf osteophyte exists, a large curette or osteotome is used to identify the true medial wall. The medial wall osteophyte, when it exists, is keyholed distally to the level of the transverse acetabular ligament. If there is a significant inferior acetabular osteophyte extending over or obliterating the transverse acetabular ligament and the inferior introitus to the acetabulum, it should be removed at this time with rongeurs or osteotomes. A large, self-illuminated, blunt Homan retractor bent to 45 degrees is then directed from within the acetabulum, deep to the transverse acetabular ligament and then is brought down inferiorly to provide inferior acetabular exposure.

The acetabular labrum is resected under direct vision and remaining islands of acetabular cartilage are removed with a large acetabular curette. The first assistant on the opposite side of the table holds the anterior and inferior retractors. The limb is allowed to lie dependent on the opposite leg. Acetabular reaming is then commenced with the largest reamer that will bottom out in the patient's socket (Figure 9.5A and B). In cases of a substantial shelf osteophyte, it is important, as in

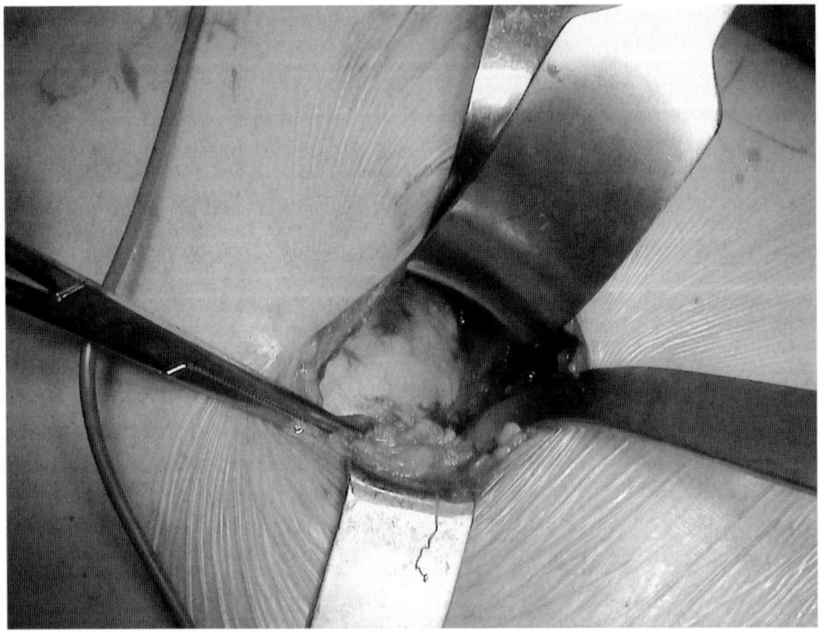

A

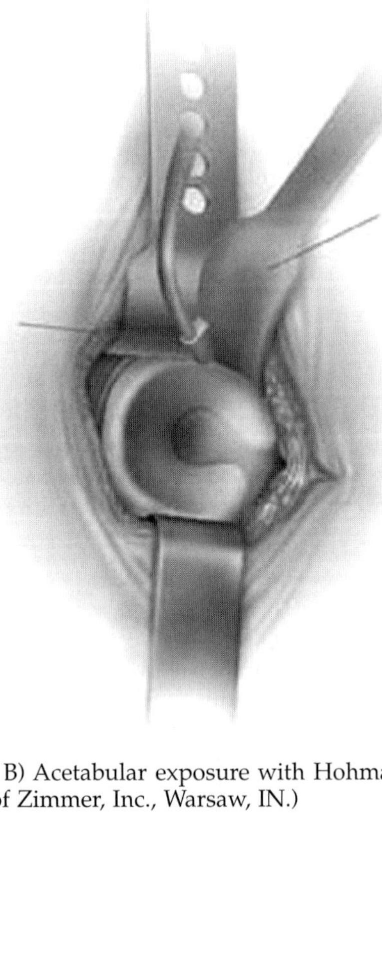

B

Figure 9.4. (A and B) Acetabular exposure with Hohmann retractor in place. (B, by permission of Zimmer, Inc., Warsaw, IN.)

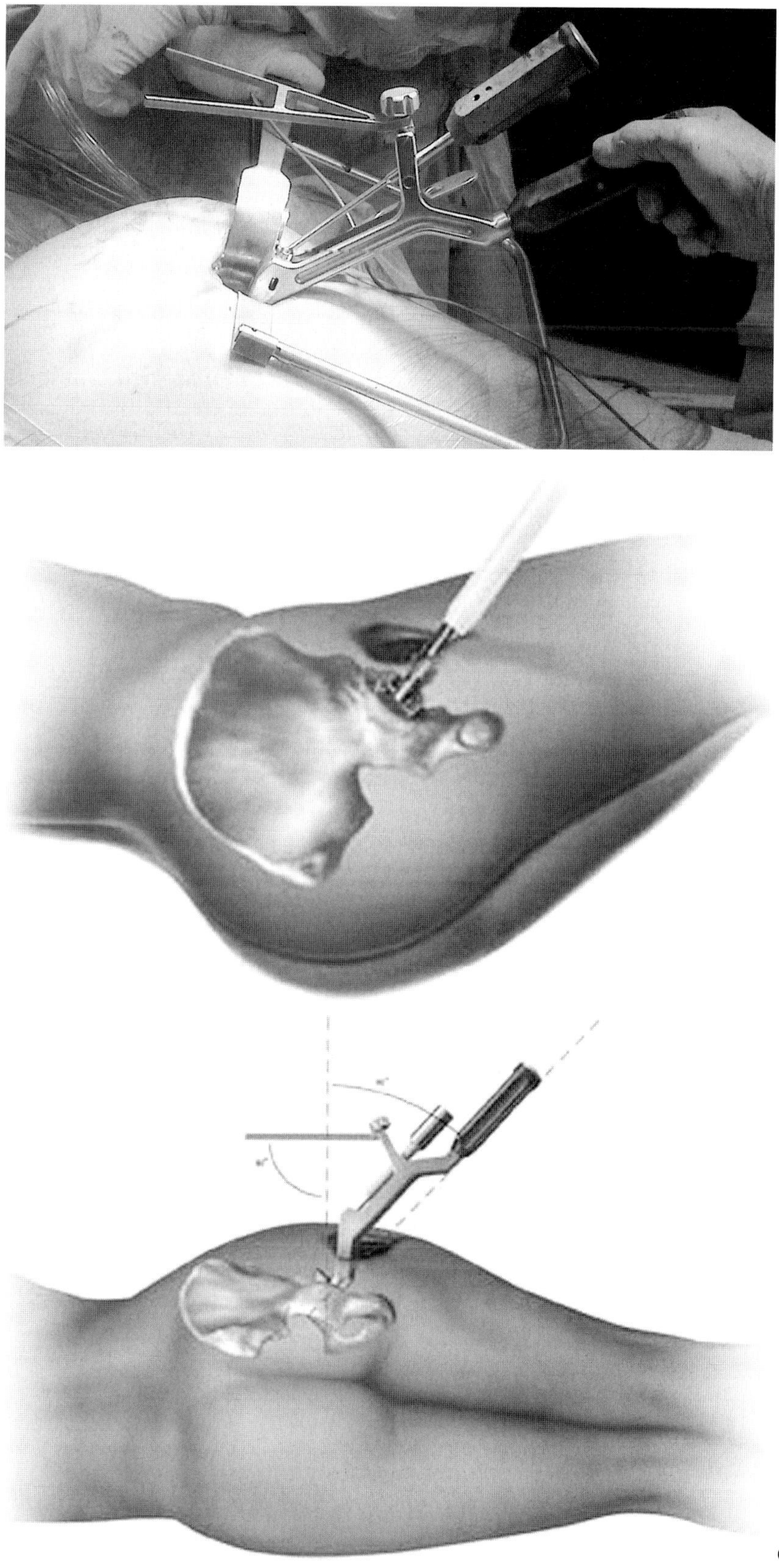

A

B

C

Figure 9.5. (A) Acetabular inserter in position. (B) Acetabular reamer in position. (C) Dogleg acetabular inserter in position. (B and C, by permission of Zimmer, Inc., Warsaw, IN.)

all approaches to total hip arthroplasty, to transversely ream the acetabulum so as to obtain appropriate acetabular component depth and return the patient's hip center to normal. The acetabular component selected is generally 2mm larger than the size of the final acetabular reamer.

If reaming is performed by the assistant on the opposite side of the table, it is crucial to avoid inadvertent levering of the reamer on the posterior border of the proximal femoral metaphysis, because this may create eccentric posterior reaming of the acetabulum and risk loss of structural integrity of the posterior wall. It is also important to ensure that the reamer sleeve protecting the soft tissue is in proper position to protect the distal pole of the skin incision.

When inserting the acetabular shell into the hip, the shell should be oriented with its internal surface directed posteriorly and its external convex surface directed anteriorly. It then is slid down along the internal radius of the anterior retractor to the level of the acetabulum and then is redirected into its appropriate position. This maneuver of utilizing the external convex geometry of the acetabular shell and orienting it to the internal concave geometry of the Charnley retractor blades is particularly important when inserting large diameter sockets in small incisions. No soft tissue should be entrapped between the outer surface of the component and the internal surface of the patient's acetabulum before impacting the shell into the acetabulum. The acetabular component is inserted with an ideal lateral opening of 40 degrees to 45 degrees and an ideal true acetabular anteversion of approximately 20 degrees. Development of a modified dogleg acetabular component inserter has greatly facilitated proper component positioning (Figure 9.5C). Its design avoids impingement on the distal corner of the skin incision and helps avoid any tendency to position the socket in an excessively vertical position.

Peripheral osteophytes are generally removed once the acetabular shell has been inserted (Figure 9.6). A 1.5-cm curved flat osteotome is used to excise anterior and anteroinferior osteophytes before insertion of the acetabular polyethylene liner. Straight osteotomes generally are used to excise posterior and posterior inferior osteophytes. Excision of posterior and posterior inferior osteophytes is made most facile if left until the trial femoral component is in place and the hip has been reduced. The posterior capsule is then under some tension and visualization will be improved.

The acetabular liner then is inserted and dialed into appropriate rotation in a free hand fashion before engagement into the outer shell (Figure 9.7). It is important to ensure that no capsule is trapped between the acetabular shell and the liner. The liner is then impacted into the shell and locking is confirmed. The anterior and inferior acetabular retractors then are removed from the wound, as is the Kocher clamp previously placed on the posterior capsule for retraction.

A combination proximal skin protector and proximal femoral elevator has been designed to elevate the proximal femur into the wound and simultaneously protect the proximal corner of the skin incision. When damage to the skin around the incision does occur, it typically

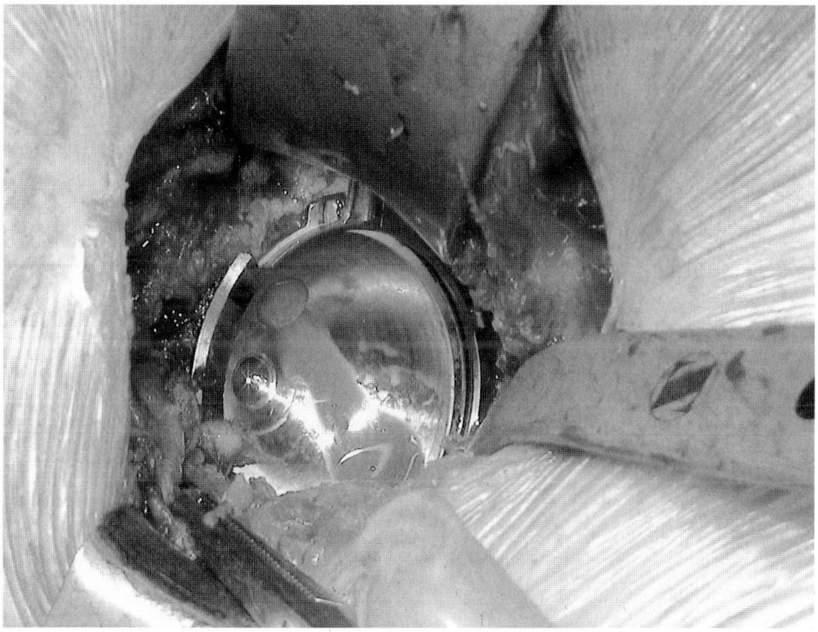

Figure 9.6. Acetabular shell in place with locking mechanism properly positioned.

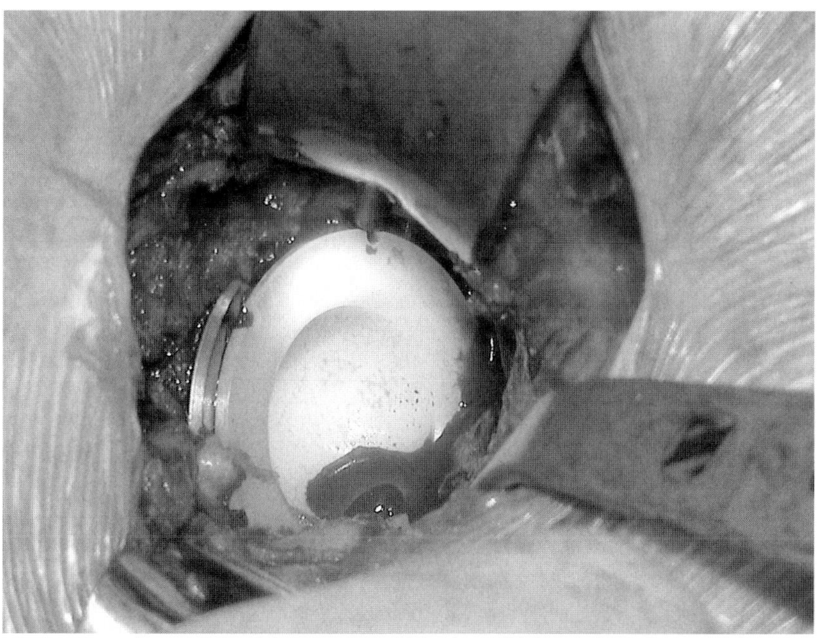

Figure 9.7. Acetabular liner inserted.

occurs at the posterior aspect of the superior pole of the wound. If this happens, the damaged skin should be trimmed prior to closure. Present skin protector/femoral elevator designs make damage to the incision edges extremely rare.

With the proximal femoral elevator held in place by the surgeon or assistant, the initial hand reamer is positioned centrally and laterally into the cancellous surface of the neck and femoral canal and directed down the femoral shaft (Figure 9.8). Care must be taken to avoid an excessively posterior starting point for this initial canal reamer, as this may tend to direct the tip of the prosthesis anteriorly and theoretically may increase the risk for impingement of the distal tip of the stem on the endosteal femur with the subsequent potential risk for femoral fracture or thigh pain. If the body habitus is such that the initial hand reamer cannot be passed in a parallel position down the femoral canal, then the proximal corner of the skin incision should be lengthened without hesitation. This is particularly critical if a fully coated, distal scratch fit type femoral component is being used.

A box chisel or lateralizing reamer then is applied laterally into the piriformis fossa (Figure 9.9). At this point, the femur, which is now held in extension, adduction and internal rotation, is slightly flexed (approximately 20 degrees) to bring the greater trochanter and piriformis fossa into a central position in the wound. A deliberate search then is made for any remaining fibrous tissue, capsule, or piriformis tendon stump in the area of the piriformis fossa, and if identified, it is excised.

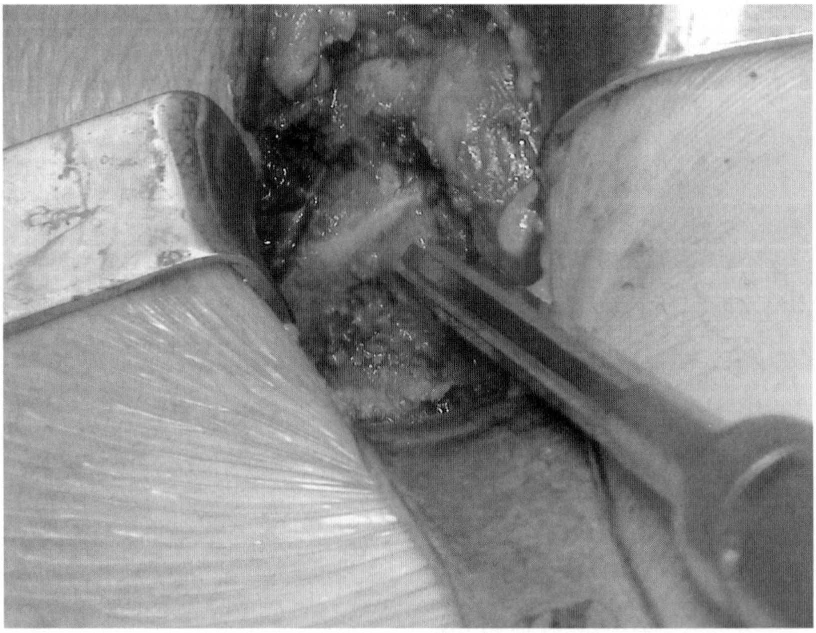

Figure 9.8. Charnley awl inserted; limb is extended, adducted and internally rotated.

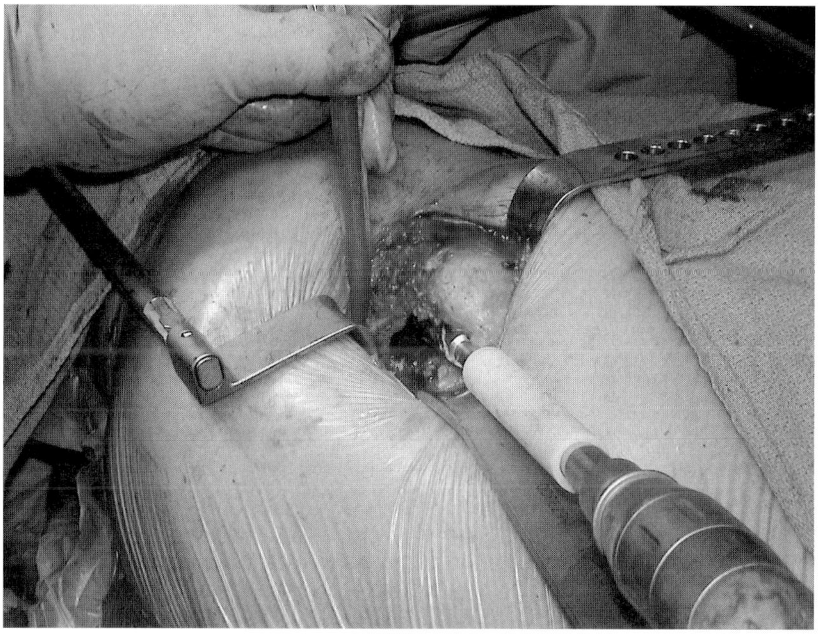

Figure 9.9. Side cutting trochanteric reamer in use.

Broaching of the femoral canal now is begun with the smallest broach. The broach handles have been modified so as to minimize impingement on the posterior superior edge of the skin incision. Despite these modifications, there remains a tendency for the proximal pole of the incision to apply a retroverting force onto the broach handle. As such, it is important to use a Tommy bar (or other means of broach handle rotational control) and to exert constant vigilance during the broaching and femoral canal preparation process so as to avoid component retroversion. The avoidance of significant flexion of the limb during femoral broaching is also important in minimizing impingement of broach handles and broaches on the posterior superior corner of the incision.

There are several ways in which the proximal pole of the skin incision is protected from broach abrasion during this portion of the procedure. One useful technique is to initially introduce the broach in retroversion. A major advantage of using a proximally coated, robustly tapered femoral component is that rotation of the rasp handle during the first 5 cm to 6 cm of its introduction has no effect on the final component interfaces. The broach is inserted in 60 degrees to 90 degrees of retroversion and as soon as its proximal teeth have moved beyond the proximal pole of the skin incision, the broach is rotated into its definitive, appropriate version. Additionally, the use of the proximal femoral elevator is critical to protection of the superior pole of the wound during this phase of femoral preparation. The elevator is applied in its normal fashion, parallel to the long axis of the shaft of the femur until the broach has seated below the proximal margin of the skin wound.

The elevator then is allowed to slide directly posteriorly and thereby protect the proximal posterior corner of the wound from any incidental broach induced abrasion (Figure 9.10).

The broaches are increased successively in 1–2-mm increments until an appropriate sense of fit and fill has been achieved and the broach has been demonstrated to be torsionally stable. Once the definitive broach has been selected, a provisional reduction is performed with the trial femoral stem in place so as to fine-tune leg length and offset. The actual prosthesis is opened, the broach is removed, and a D&C curette is lightly applied to the internal surface of the lateral femoral endosteal cortex corresponding to Gruen zone 1. In this way any fibrous tissue that may have been inadvertently introduced down the femoral canal is removed. (As a rule, irrigation is not performed at this point, as noncemented implants typically are used.) The stem then is pressed down the canal by hand and introduced initially, similar to the broach, in substantial retroversion (Figure 9.11). The stem then is dialed into appropriate anteversion as it moves down the femoral canal. This rotation of the component during insertion must be avoided when performing a hybrid arthroplasty or when utilizing a splined femoral component and, as such, the incision for these cases is translated proximally by 1 cm to 2 cm.

On occasion, particularly in cases with a small incision and a large femoral component, the hip must be hyperextended so as to facilitate reduction of the neck of the femoral component below the level of skin and fascia. Bringing the limb into neutral abduction as well as extension relaxes the skin and fascia so as to make reduction of the neck of

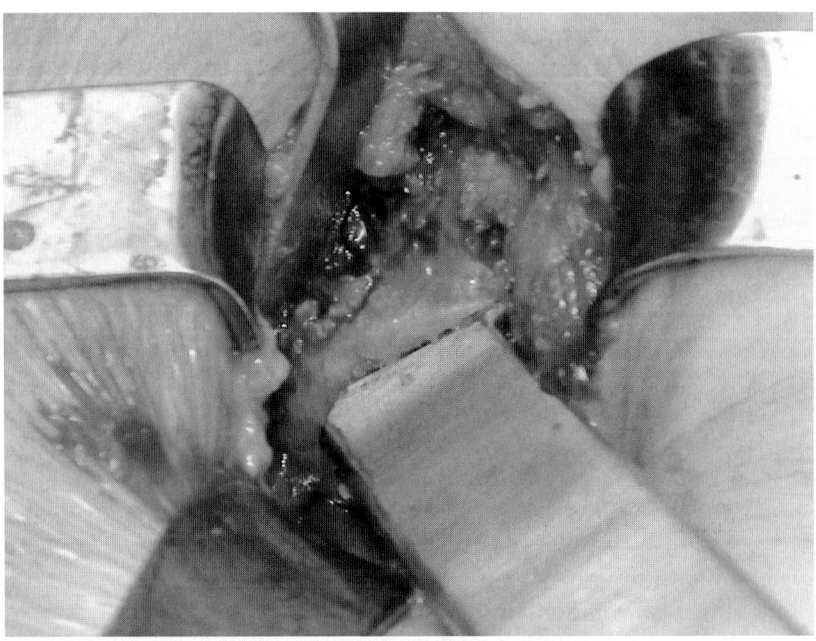

Figure 9.10. Femoral broach is seated.

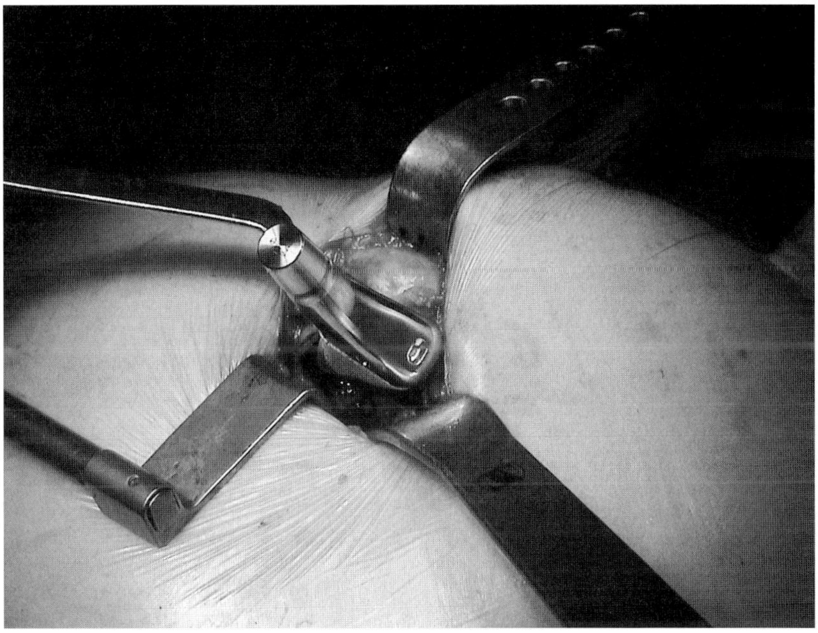

Figure 9.11. Femoral component is initially introduced in retroversion.

the femoral component under these layers easier. Correct component rotation may be confirmed with a knurled rotation control bar inserted into the extraction hole of the femoral component before the last centimeter of prosthesis seating. The bar is removed a few millimeters before final component seating.

Various femoral head trials then are applied sequentially until appropriate leg length and hip joint tension and stability have been achieved (Figure 9.12). Side mounting femoral head trials have been designed to simplify this portion of the procedure. The neck taper then is cleaned and dried. The femoral head then is placed onto the taper, twisted, and struck once with a modified, offset head impactor that greatly facilitates this portion of the procedure.

An enhanced posterior capsular closure then is performed in which a figure-of-eight suture is placed through the posterior superior corner of capsule and the priformis tendon at the point at which the radial and longitudinal portions of the capsulotomy meet. A second suture is placed approximately 1.0 cm to 1.5 cm distal to this through the posterior limb of the capsule and the conjoined tendon (Figure 9.13). Drill holes then are placed through the trochanter into the piriformis fossa, taking care that the starting point is at least 1 cm below the tip of the trochanter and 1 cm lateral to the medial-most border of the trochanter. Number 4 (22-gauge) wires are placed through the drill holes and are used as suture passers. The sutures are tied to each other with the limb in neutral rotation and 15 degrees to 20 degrees of abduction. All patients are treated with a suction drainage system that allows autotransfusion postoperatively (Figure 9.14).

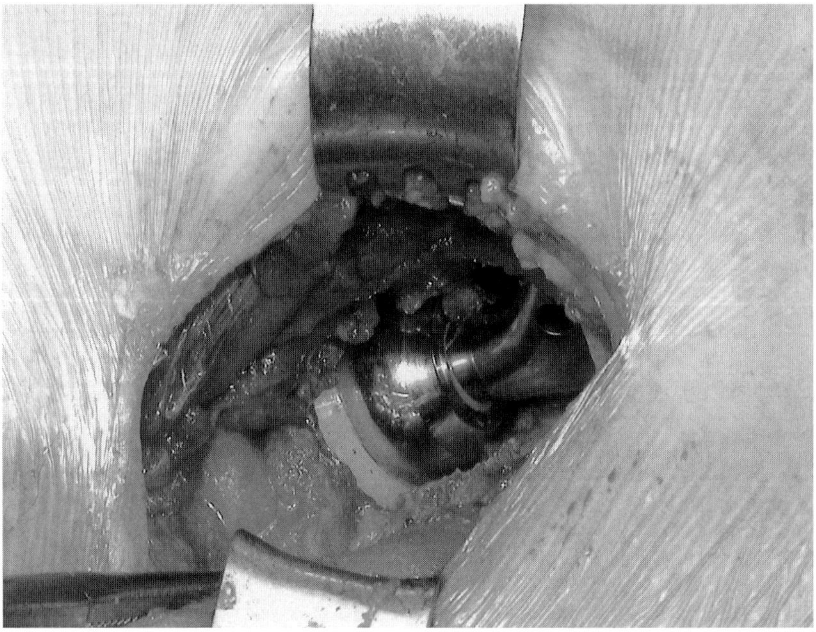

Figure 9.12. Final components in position.

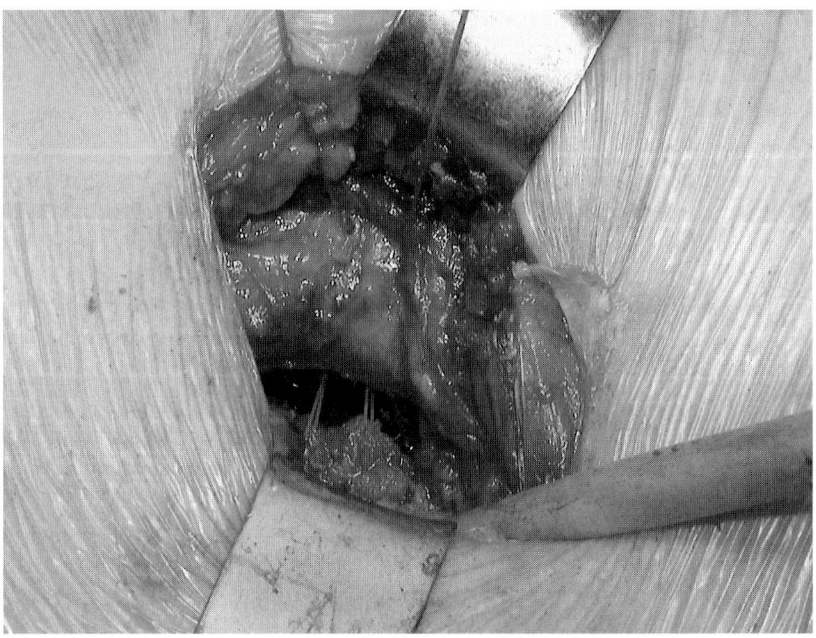

Figure 9.13. Enhanced posterior capsular closure.

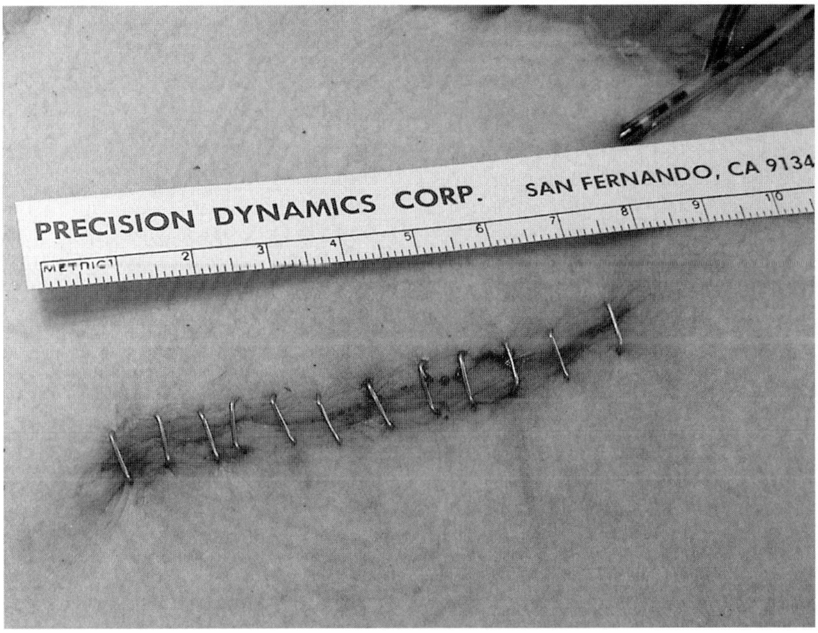

Figure 9.14. Final wound measures 7 cm in length.

Postoperative Protocol

Patients are ambulated within the first 24 hours of surgery. Hospital length of stay ranges from 48 to 72 hours. Patients are allowed to bear full weight as tolerated immediately, but are directed to use a walker or crutches for support during the first 2 postoperative weeks. They then are advanced to a single prong cane for an additional 4 weeks. Antigravity abductor strengthening is begun immediately.

Summary

There presently exists in the arthroplasty community a new and heightened level of interest in minimally invasive techniques for total joint replacement. Several investigators have published their personal experience with differing techniques,[1–3] all concluding that there are multiple advantages to this concept for total hip arthroplasty. The author's perception is that the advantages of minimally invasive posterolateral approach total hip arthroplasty are multiple. They include more rapid rehabilitation and more rapid return to activities of daily living. There is a clear impression that patients experience less postoperative pain and improved satisfaction. A concomitant decrease in hospital stay has been noted. Patients undergoing the procedure today have an average length of hospital stay of 48 hours, which represents a 30% decrease in hospital stay over the past year. Other advantages include improved cosmesis and potentially reduced blood loss.

With respect to component positioning, there may be a tendency to vertical cup placement early in one's experience. This is avoided by proper location of the skin incision and by use of a doglegged acetabular component inserter that facilitates proper positioning of the component despite the prominence of the distal angle of the skin incision. A tendency to eccentric reaming of the acetabulum may be noted if the proximal femur is not adequately retracted anteriorly. One must be aware of the potential for inadvertent levering of the acetabular reamers on the posterior aspect of the retracted femur if the operative surgeon is not performing the reaming of the acetabulum. Particularly in patients who are larger there may be a tendency toward an excessively posterior starting point in the femoral canal when broaching the femoral component. This is best avoided by careful attention at this portion of the procedure to any pressure being applied to the broach handle by the proximal corner of the skin incision. The skin incision must be lengthened at this point if the problem presents. Finally, there remains a risk for proximal skin abrasion, particularly when one is beginning to decrease the incision length in posterolateral approach to total hip arthroplasty. The evolution of proximal femoral elevators and skin protectors has decreased this risk to an extremely low level. Surgeons performing this procedure require familiarity with the local anatomy, because the technique is certainly more demanding than is traditional arthroplasty. It is perhaps a technique best applied by surgeons performing more than 50 total hip arthroplasties a year. The two keys to successful application of the technique are adequate surgical training and use of specialized instrumentation.

References

1. Berger RA. Mini-incisions: two for the price of one! Presented at: Current Concepts in Joint Replacement-Winter, 2001; December 13, 2001; Orlando, FL.
2. Waldman BS. Minimally invasive total hip replacement and perioperative management: early experience. Journal of the Southern Orthopedic Association. 2002;11(4):213–217.
3. Wenz JF, Gurkan I, Jibodh SR. Mini-incision total hip arthroplasty: A comparative assessment of perioperative outcomes. Orthopedics. 2002; 25(10):1031–1043.

10

Minimally Invasive Total Hip Arthroplasty Using the Two-Incision Approach

Richard A. Berger

Minimally invasive hip replacement has the potential for minimizing surgical trauma, pain, and recovery in total hip replacement. These minimally invasive approaches for total hip surgery include single incision and two-incision techniques.[1–3] These approaches minimize sacrificing muscle and tendon yet still allowing direct or indirect visualization for preparation and component placement.

Specifically, searching for an approach to avoid transecting any muscle or tendon, thereby minimizing morbidity and recovery, a new approach was developed; the minimally invasive two-incision total hip procedure.[4] This technique uses an anterior incision for preparation and insertion of the acetabular component and a posterior incision for preparation and insertion of the femoral component. This novel, minimally invasive, fluoroscopy assisted, two-incision total hip arthroplasty uses a number of new instruments that have been developed to facilitate exposure and component placement. Standard implants with well-established designs are used to maintain the present expectation for implant durability. The following text describes the technique of the minimally invasive two-incision, combining an anterior, Smith-Peterson and a posterior incision that is like an IM femoral nail.

Surgical Technique

The anesthesia of choice for this minimally invasive total hip arthroplasty procedure is a regional anesthesia with supplemental sedation. An epidural anesthesia with IV Propofol is the combination of choice. Propofol is a very short acting agent that is rapidly eliminated from the body and the epidural allows the medication to be titrated. This combination allows rapid recovery from the anesthesia, facilitating recovery.

The patient is placed in the supine position on a radiolucent operating room table. A special operating room table is not required; however, a pure radiolucent table is preferable. A small bolster, about 2 in., is

A

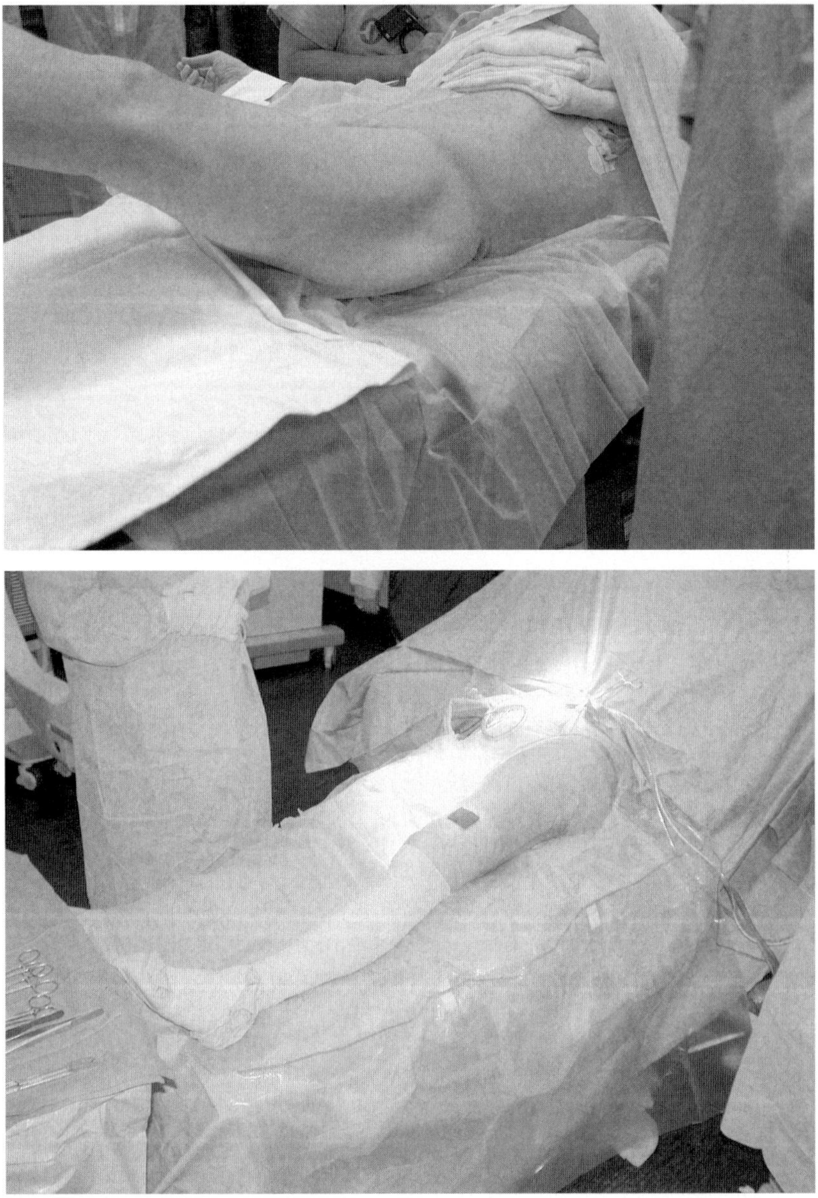

B

Figure 10.1. Preparation and drape for two-incision minimally invasive total hip. (A) Small bolster under the ischium on the affected side elevating the pelvis. (B) The entire leg prepped and draped to allow access to the anterior and posterior incision.

placed under the ischium on the affected side; this elevates the acetabulum to aid in acetabular preparation and allows the posterior buttock to be prepped and draped (Figure 10.1A). The entire leg and hip is prepped up to the chest wall including the posterior hip. After prepping, the leg is placed in an impervious sterile stockinet and is wrapped with an Ace from the foot to above the knee. The hip area is then draped superiorly from above the iliac crest, posteriorly to the posterior hip, and anteriorly to almost the midline of the patient (Figure 10.1B).

After the prepping is completed, the fluoroscope is used to define the femoral neck. The femoral neck lies approximately two finger-widths distally from the anterior superior iliac spine. A metal marker is used to mark the midline of the femoral neck from the junction of the head distally 1.5 in. to 2.0 in. (Figure 10.2). This incision is then made through the skin and the subcutaneous fat, directly over the femoral neck from the base of the femoral head distally. Care must be taken, as the subcutaneous fat in this area is very thin. The fascia is exposed. The sartorius muscle is present in the proximal medial incision while the tensor fascia lata lies at the distal lateral tip of the incision. The sartorius muscle and tensor fascia lata can be seen beneath the fascia. The fascia at the medial border of tensor fascia lata is incised longitudinally parallel to the tensor fascia lata. The lateral femoral cutaneous nerve is located over the sartorius muscle; therefore, an incision made lateral to the sartorius, at the medial border of tensor fascia lata avoids the lateral femoral cutaneous nerve. The nerve should not be dissected out, as postoperative scarring may cause a lateral thigh hypoesthesia. After the fascia is incised, a retractor is used to retract the sartorius medially. A second retractor is used to retract the tensor fascia lata laterally. This exposes the lateral border of the rectus femoris (Figure 10.3A). The

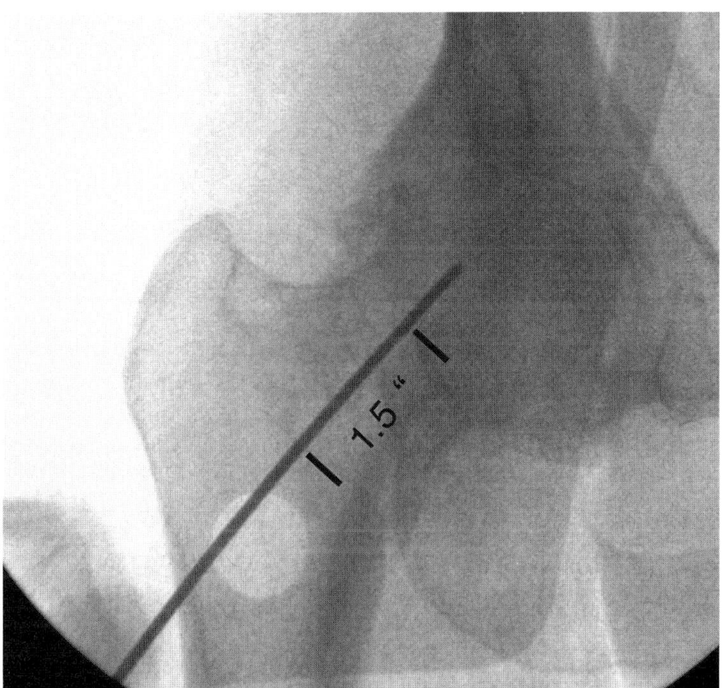

Figure 10.2. Fluoroscope picture of incision site over femoral neck. The incision is made from the head/neck junction distally to the intertrochanteric line, approximately 1.5 in.

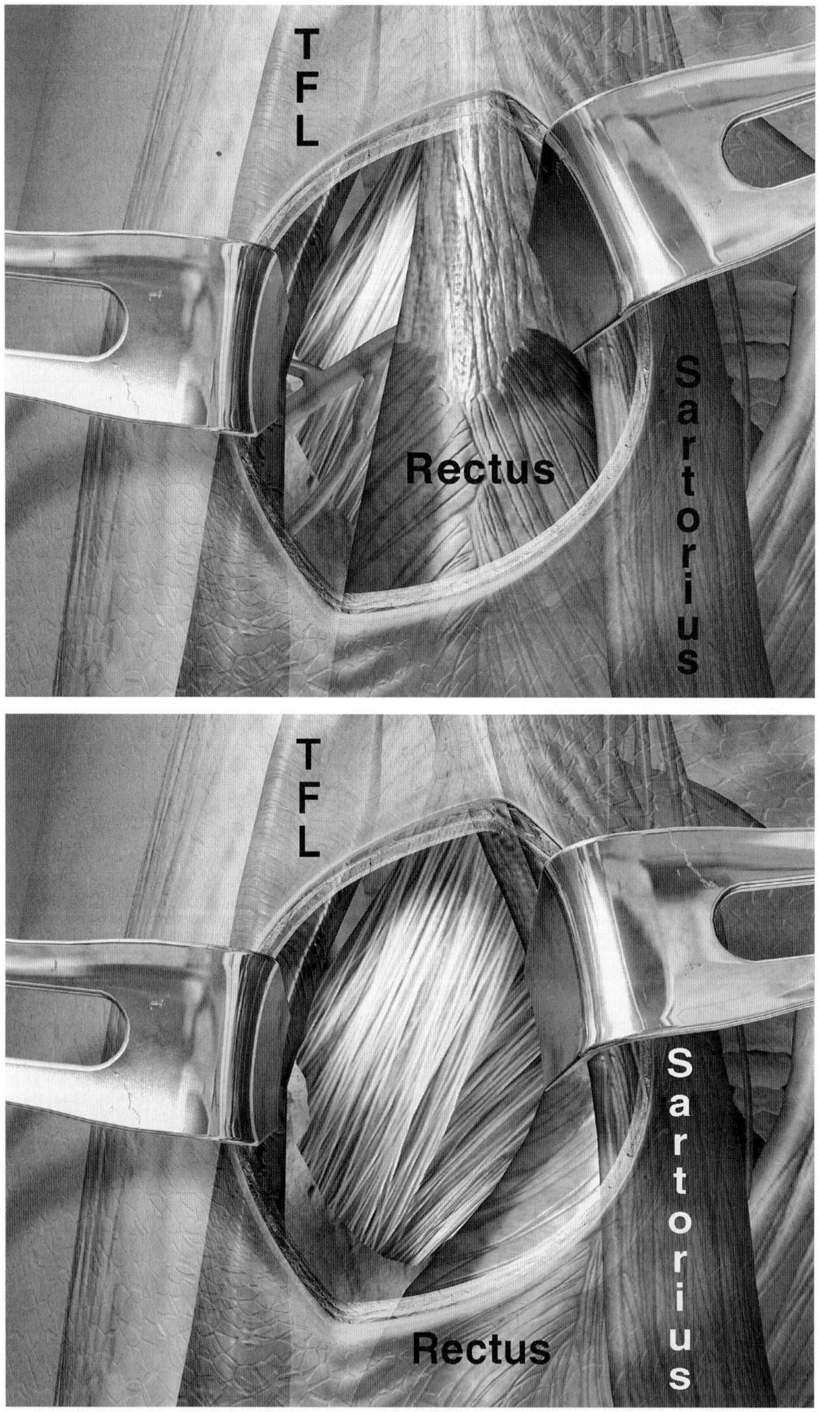

Figure 10.3. The anterior dissection. (A) The sartorius and tensor fascia latae after being retracted. Note rectus femoris. (B) The rectus femoris is retracted, exposing the capsule.

medial retractor is repositioned to retract the rectus muscle medially (Figure 10.3B). This exposes the fascia overlying the lateral circumflex vessels and the femoral capsule. This thin fascia lying over the lateral circumflex vessels is incised carefully as the lateral circumflex vessels are adherent to the undersurface. The lateral circumflex vessels are then carefully found within the small fat pad over the capsule of the femoral neck. The lateral femoral vessels are carefully coagulated with an electrocautery. The fat pad is then incised in the line of the femoral neck and gently moved medially and laterally off the femoral neck exposing the capsule over the femoral neck.

Two curved lit Hohmann retractors, part of the minimally invasive instrument set (Zimmer), are then placed extracapsularly around the femoral neck perpendicular to the femoral neck. These lit retractors afford an excellent view of the capsule (Figure 10.4A). The capsule, having been identified, is incised in line with the femoral neck just lateral to the middle of the femoral neck. This incision is made from the edge of the acetabulum distally to the intertrochanteric line (Figure 10.4B). If necessary for enhanced exposure, the capsule can be elevated about 1 cm medially and laterally along the intertrochanteric line. The femoral neck and femoral head are now visible.

The two curved lit Hohmann retractors, which were extracapsular, are now placed intracapsular along the femoral neck, one medially and one laterally. The lit retractors in place afford excellent visualization of the femoral neck (Figure 10.5). The femoral neck should now be visualized from the acetabulum distally to the intertrochanteric line. With the two curved lit Hohmann retractors still in place, a high neck cut is made at the equator of the femoral head with an oscillating saw. This is made perpendicular to the axis of the femoral neck. A second cut is then made 1 cm distal to the first cut in the femoral head (Figure 10.6). First, the small 1-cm wafer of bone is removed using a threaded Steinmann pin; gentle traction placed on the leg will facilitate removing this piece of bone (Figure 10.7). Next, a threaded Steinmann pin or corkscrew is then placed into the femoral head and is used to slightly dislocate the femoral head. A curved Cobb elevator osteotome is used to transect the ligamentum teres. Again, gentle traction placed on the leg usually allows the femoral head to be removed completely (Figure 10.7). If the femoral head cannot be completely removed due to osteophytes or soft tissue attachments, the head may be morseled in situ, but this is unusual.

The fluoroscope is used to assess the angle and length of the femoral neck resection based upon the lesser trochanter. Based upon preoperative templating, the final neck resection is then made. The resection length is checking with fluoroscopy. Alternatively, flexing and externally rotating the hip in a figure of four can directly visualize the lesser trochanter. In this position, the lesser trochanter is easily seen and is used as a landmark to measure the neck resection. Alternatively, the fluoroscope can be used to check the angle of resection as well as the

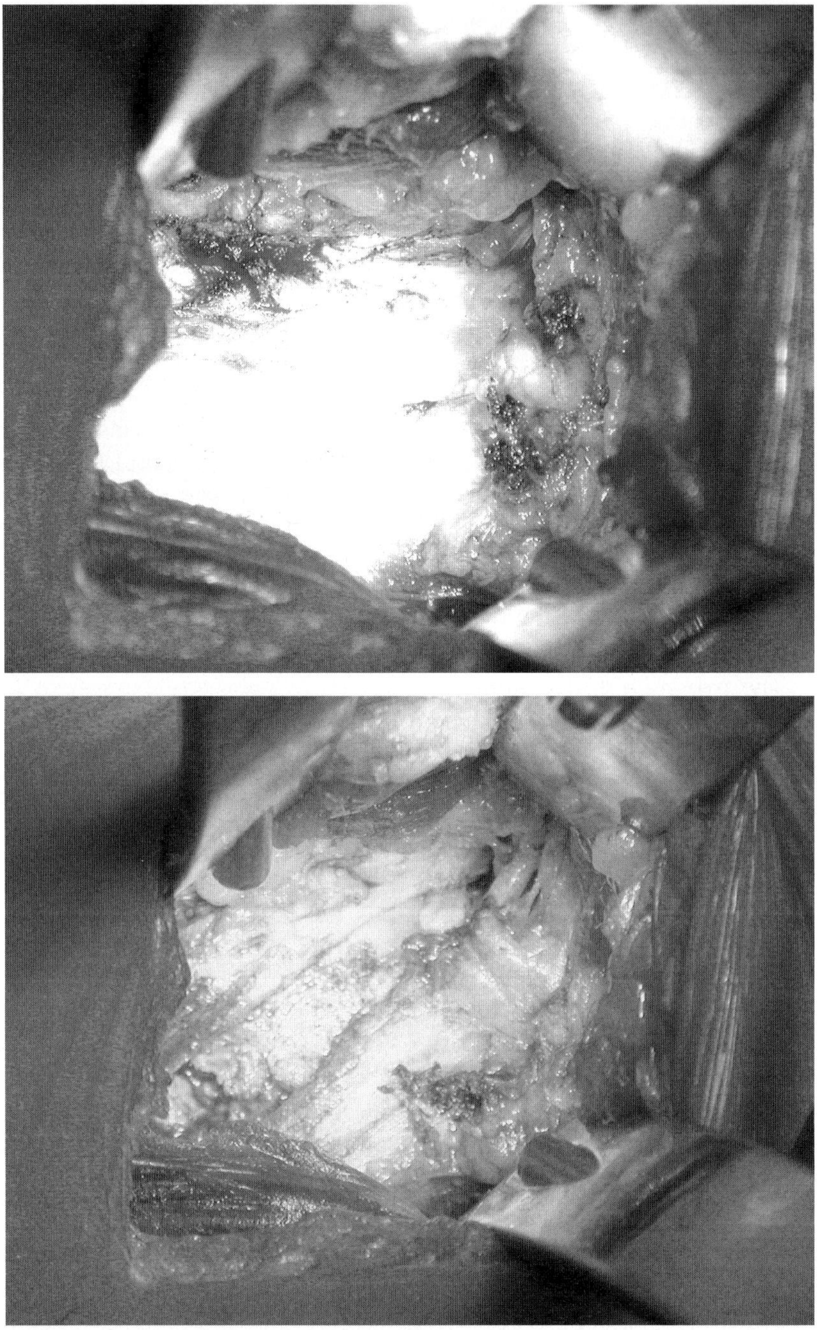

Figure 10.4. (A) The lit Hohmann retractors positioned around the capsule and exposing the hip capsule. (B) The hip capsule is incised in line with the femoral neck, exposing the femoral head and neck.

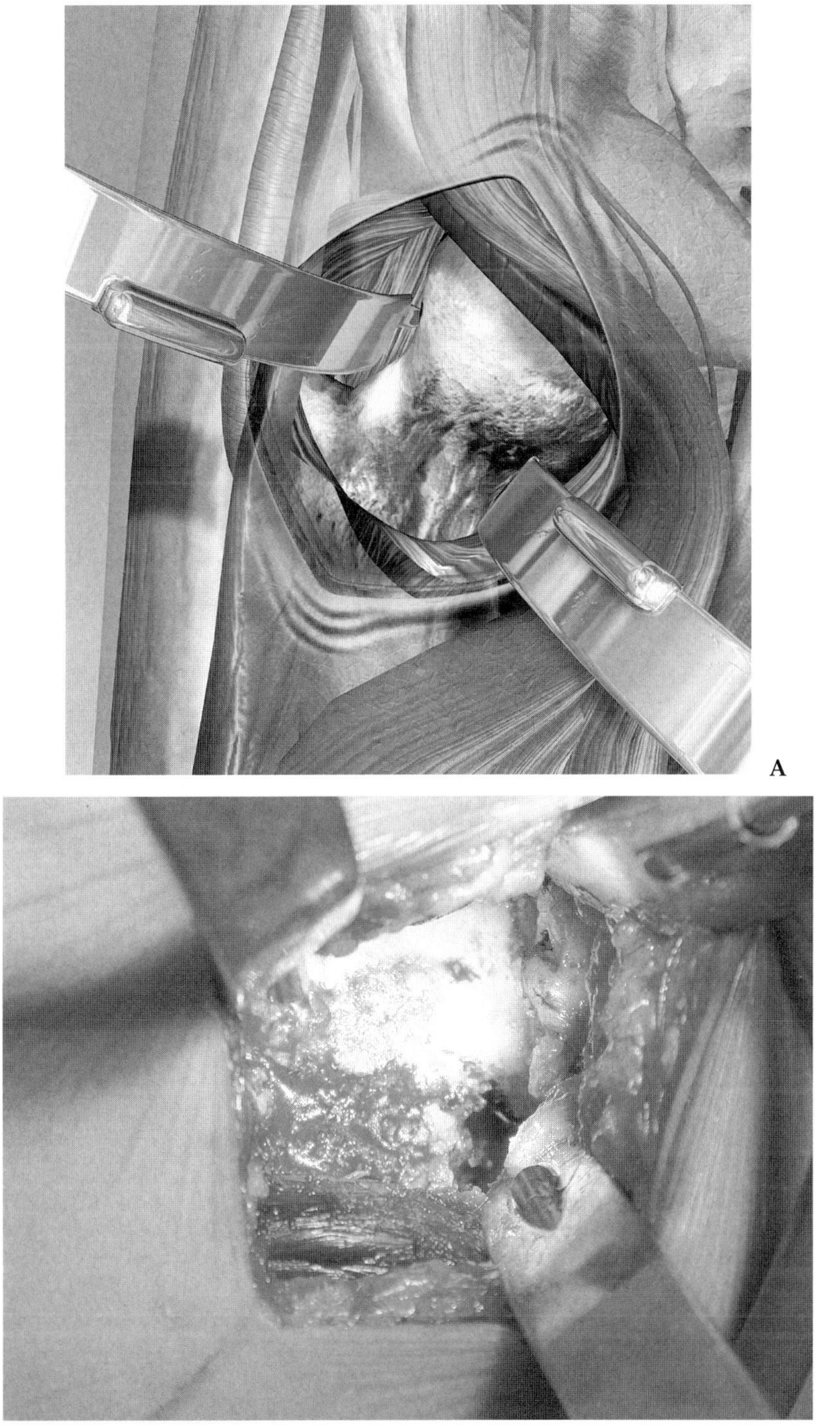

A

B

Figure 10.5. (A) The Hohmann retractors intracapsular around the femoral neck, exposing the femoral head and neck. (B) Picture of the femoral head and neck. The hip capsule is incised in line with the femoral neck and the Hohmann retractors are placed intracapsular around the femoral neck, exposing the femoral head and neck.

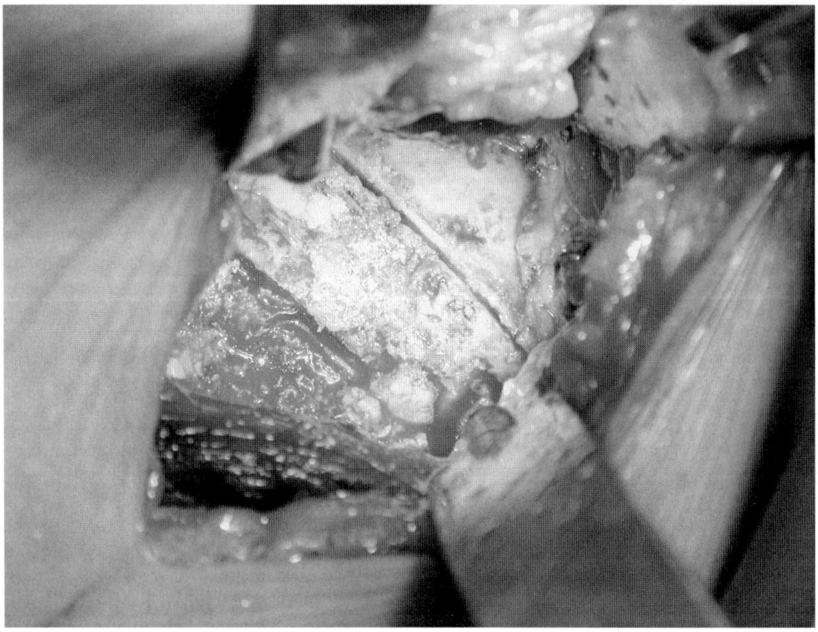

Figure 10.6. The Hohmann retractors intracapsular around the femoral neck, exposing the femoral head and neck. Two lines show the placement of the initial two cuts in the femoral head and neck.

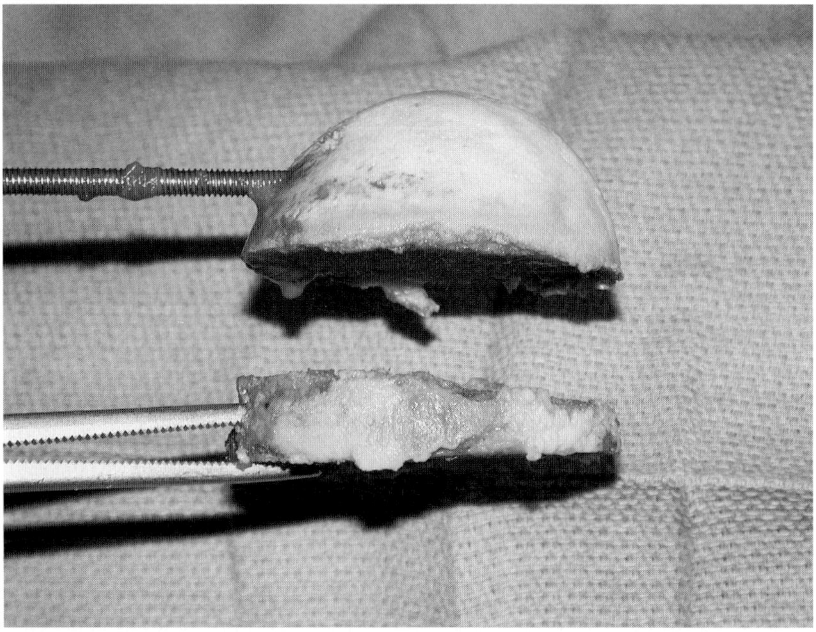

Figure 10.7. The removed femoral head and upper neck in two pieces to facilitate removal.

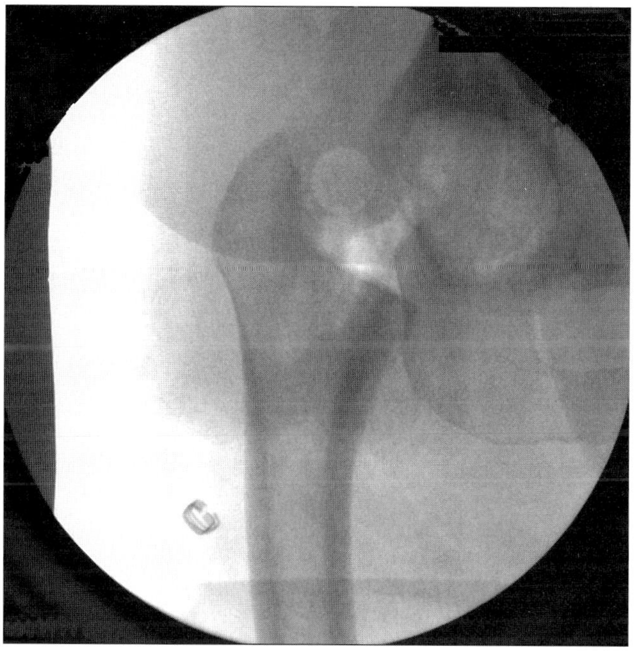

Figure 10.8. Fluoroscopy of the final femoral neck cut.

length of resection based upon the lesser trochanter (Figure 10.8). If an additional neck cut is needed, the oscillating saw is used to make the final neck resection and a sagittal saw was then used to make a longitudinal neck cut as to not disrupt the trochanteric bed. This final thin wafer of bone is then removed. Again, the resection length is checked with fluoroscopy or by rotating the hip in a figure-of-four position, exposing the lesser trochanter.

With the final neck resection made, attention is turned to acetabular preparation. Having the pelvis elevated (with the bolster) allows the femur to fall posteriorly, facilitating access to the acetabulum. Three curved lit Hohmann retractors were placed around the acetabulum, one directly superiorly in the line of the incision that was placed over the brim of the acetabulum, a second is placed anteriorly at the anterior margin of the transverse acetabular ligament, and a third is placed posteriorly around the acetabulum. This allows excellent retraction of the entire capsule. The lit retractors in these positions allow excellent visualization of the acetabulum. However, unlike conventional exposure, where the entire acetabulum can be seen in one view, with this exposure, only about three-quarters of the acetabulum can be seen at one time. To visualize the entire acetabulum, the retractors can be shifted slightly anteriorly or posteriorly to see anteriorly or posterior as needed. With this technique, the acetabulum is assessed (Figure 10.9). Of note, pulling hard on opposing retractors paradoxically limits visualization by shortening the incision. Gentle retraction of one retractor should be associated with a release of the opposite retractor.

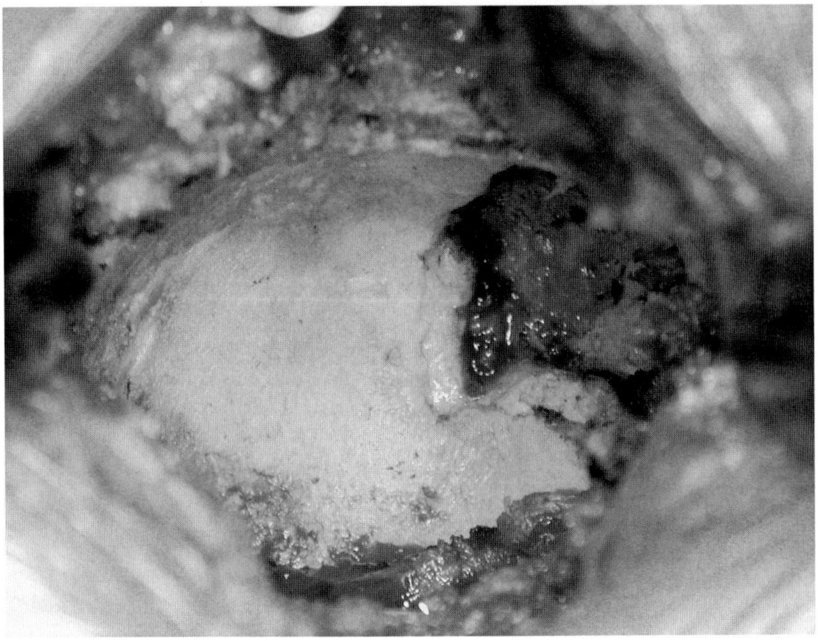

Figure 10.9. A lit Hohmann retractor placement and superior view of the acetabulum.

The labrum and redundant synovium is then excised around the entire periphery of the acetabulum. After the superior acetabulum is excised the superior retractor can be removed and is repositioned more inferiorly, allowing better visualization of the inferior acetabulum. The remaining labrum and redundant synovium is then removed exposing the entire periphery of the acetabulum (Figure 10.9). The acetabulum, now clear of invaginating soft tissue, is prepared for reaming.

At this point acetabular reaming is begun. The anterior and posterior retractors are left in place and the superior retractor is removed. Specially designed, low profile reamers, which are cut out on the sides, are used to ream the acetabulum (Figure 10.10A). These reamers are especially aggressive with square cutting teeth; therefore, it is useful to start with a reamer that is very close in size to the intended final reamer. It is useful to ream with as few reamers as necessary to avoid inserting and extracting reamers. In addition, the open design of these reamers allows good visualization of the acetabulum during reaming. The reamer is inserted in line with the femoral neck, with the cutouts of the reamer aligned with the two retractors. This position allows the reamer to be easily inserted. Gentle traction on the leg facilitates the reamer into the acetabulum (Figure 10.10B).

With the reamer at 45 degrees of abduction and 20 degrees of anteversion, the acetabulum is reamed. The fluoroscope is used to visualize as the acetabular as bone is gradually removed (Figure 10.10C). The acetabulum is appropriately reamed and the reamer is then removed. The lit retractors, which remain in place around the acetabulum, afford good visualization. Any redundant tissue, which had been invaginated due to reaming, can be removed at this time. The acetabulum is sequentially reamed until good bleeding bone is present throughout the entire acetabulum. Any remaining pulvinar is cut away from the fossa with an electric cautery. Again, the entire acetabulum rim is fully evaluated and care is taken to remove any excess labrum.

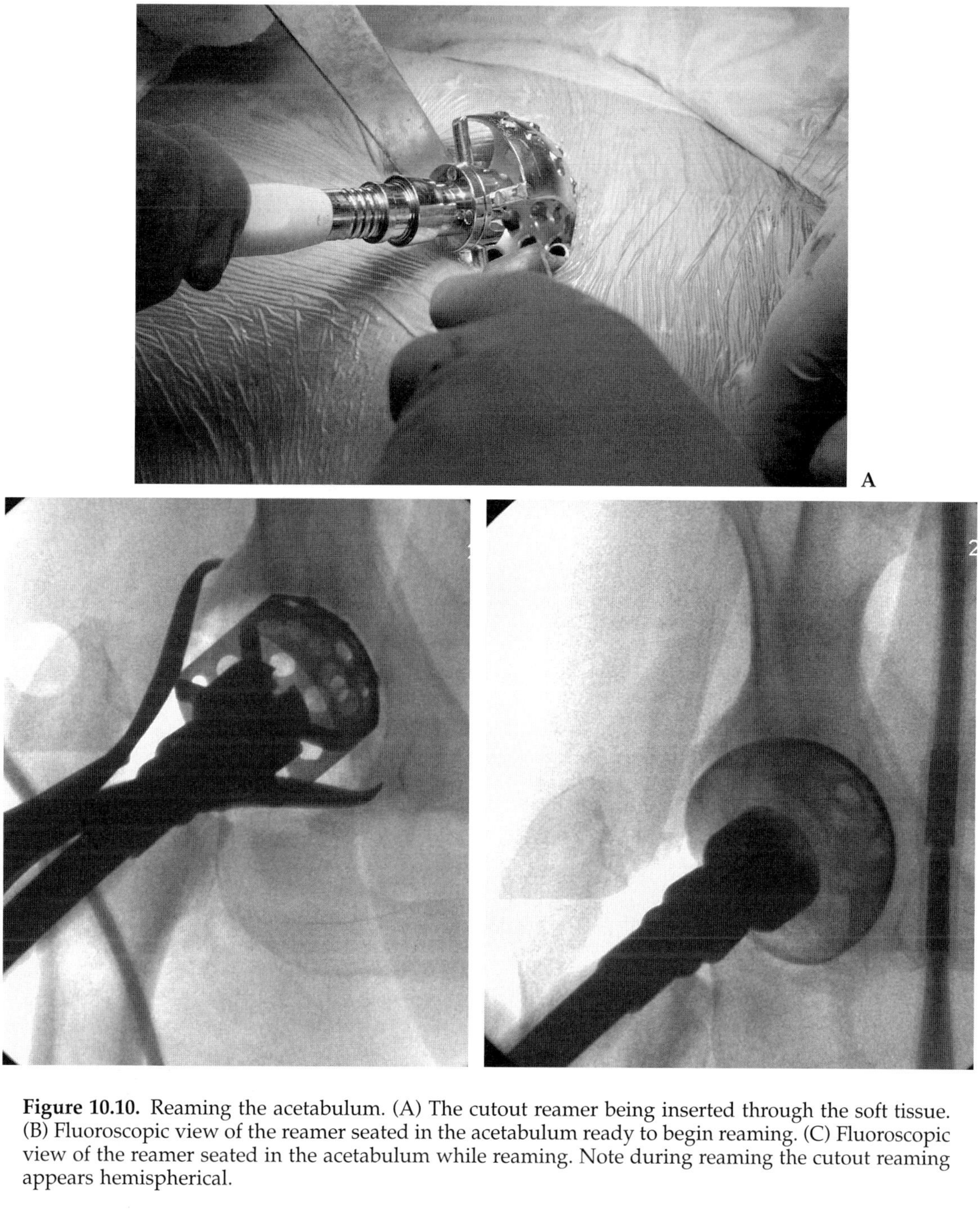

Figure 10.10. Reaming the acetabulum. (A) The cutout reamer being inserted through the soft tissue. (B) Fluoroscopic view of the reamer seated in the acetabulum ready to begin reaming. (C) Fluoroscopic view of the reamer seated in the acetabulum while reaming. Note during reaming the cutout reaming appears hemispherical.

A specialized dogleg acetabular inserter with the supine positioner is used to place an acetabulum shell that is 2 mm larger than the last reamer used. This will give a 2 mm press-fit. The two acetabular retractors, one anterior and one posterior, are left in place as gentle traction is placed on the leg. The acetabular component is then inserted into the acetabulum (Figure 10.11A). The bolster beneath the pelvis is then removed and the patient is now directly supine on the operating room table. Fluoroscopy is again used to check to make sure that the pelvis is flat and does not have any obliquity. The fluoroscope should also be

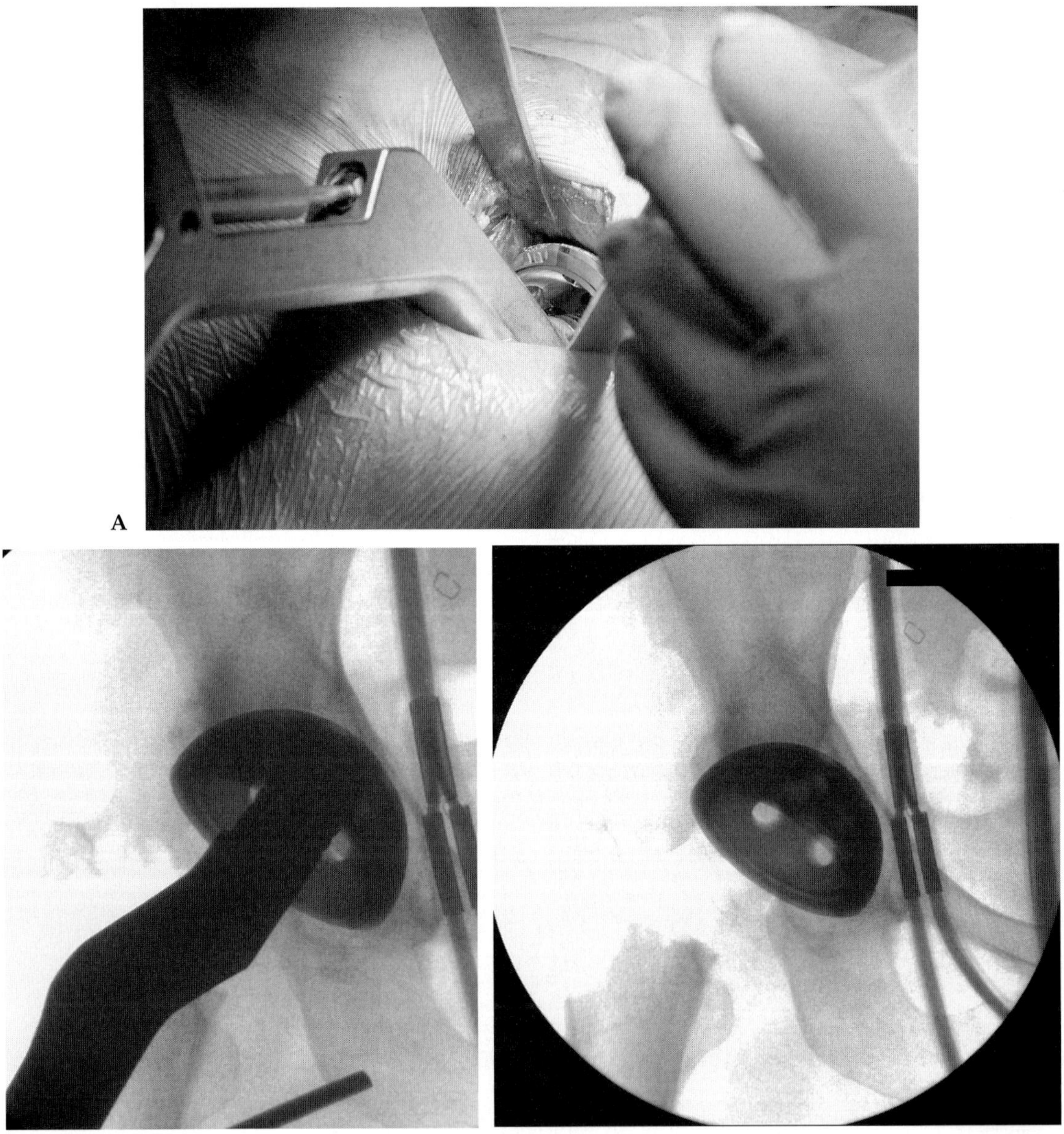

A B C

Figure 10.11. Inserting the acetabulum. (A) The acetabulum being inserted through the soft tissue. (B) Fluoroscopic view of the acetabular component with the inserter seated in the acetabulum. (C) Fluoroscopic view of the final acetabular component placement.

rotated so that the pelvis is directly horizontal. This allows proper assessment of the abduction angle of the acetabular component.

The acetabular shell is then manipulated in place; the retractors keep the capsule from invaginating. The retractors are then removed. The acetabulum is viewed with the fluoroscope as the cup is positioned in 45 degrees of abduction and 20 degrees of anteversion. The cup is impacted in place, keeping the cup in 45 degrees of abduction and 20 degrees of anteversion (Figure 10.11B). When the cup is fully seated, the dogleg acetabulum inserter is removed (Figure 10.11C).

The curved lit acetabular retractors are replaced around the acetabulum. The lit retractor allows excellent visualization of the acetabular shell. Stability of the shell can then be assessed. Two screws are used. Two screws may be placed using the posterior superior quadrant of the shell; these were placed up the wing of the ileum and slightly posteriorly over the sciatic notch. These screws usually measure 30 mm and 35 mm. Finally, a small curved osteotome is used to remove any osteophytes around the rim of the acetabulum and the liner is then impacted in place. With the acetabulum complete, all retractors are removed from the acetabulum and attention is turned to the femur.

The femur is placed back in a figure of four and a burr is used to mark the medial apex of the calcar. This mark is then used for palpation and visualization for femoral component rotation. The leg is then fully adducted and placed in neutral rotation. A finger is placed into the piriformis fossa to allow assessment of where to make the starting point on the skin on the posterior lateral buttocks. This point is colinear with the piriformis fossa to allow access to the femoral canal. A small stab wound is made in the posterior lateral buttock corresponding to the location of the piriformis fossa to allow access to the femoral canal. A Charnley awl is then used as a finger is left in the piriformis fossa. The Charnley awl is guided posteriorly, posterior to the abductors, anterior to the piriformis under direct palpation. The Charnley awl is then manipulated down the femur with the aid of fluoroscopy.

The initial insertion point into the femur is usually slightly medially to the desired starting point. Specially designed side-cutting reamers are used to enlarge this starting hole and position the starting point lateral against the trochanteric bed. The reamers are used sequentially starting with the smallest, 9 mm reamer. This reamer is placed in the canal from posteriorly within the same track as the Charnley awl has made. The reamers are used with visualization from the fluoroscope to allowed lateralization of the starting hole to the lateral edge of the femoral canal (Figure 10.12). The initial stab wound is opened in line with the femur neck extending approximately 1.25 in. A self-retaining retractor is used to spread the fat and the fat is cauterized. The lateralization reamers are then used sequentially from 9 mm up to the intended size stem. Fluoroscopy is used to assure that the starting point is lined up with the lateral cortex of the femur. This corresponds to the tip of the trochanter in most patients but should be based upon the preoperative templating. Care is taken with periodic fluoroscopy views of the leg in a frog position lateral to make sure this is well centralized anteriorly and posteriorly. In addition, palpation from posterior

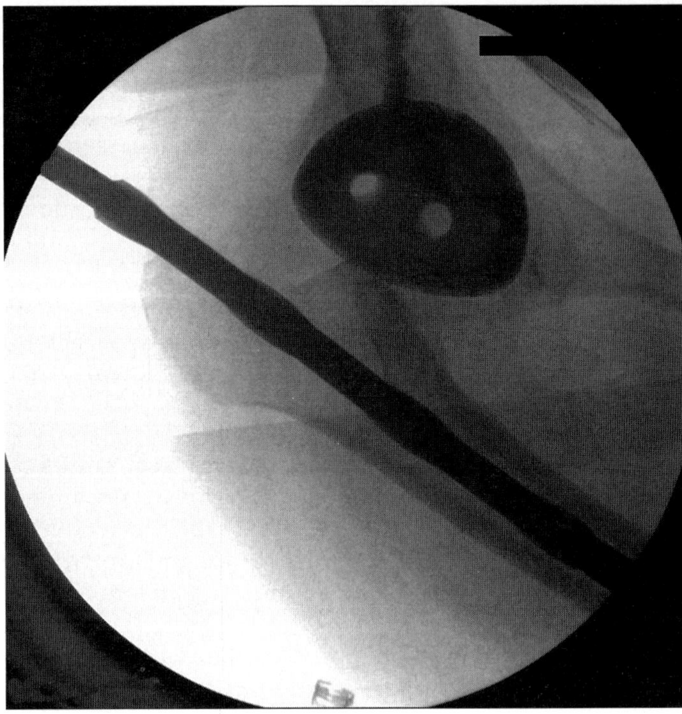

Figure 10.12. Fluoroscopic view of the lateralization reamer clearing the trochanteric bed, getting to a neutral alignment.

straight down the canal can be used to palpate the anterior and the posterior wall of the trochanter to make sure that this is well centralized anteriorly and posteriorly.

With the starting point being fully lateralized, flexible reamers are used to gently ream the canal, starting until cortical chatter is obtained. Straight reamers with a tissue-protecting sleeve are then used to ream down the femoral shaft until good cortical chatter is obtained. Fluoroscopy is used to assure the reamers were well centralized both on the anterior fluoroscopy view as well as the lateral radiograph fluoroscopy view (Figure 10.13). A full-coated stem is used; therefore the cortex is reamed 0.5 mm less than the stem that is chosen. Good cortical chatter must be obtained before reaming is discontinued.

After reaming is completed, broaching is performed. The leg remains adducted and in neutral rotation while rasps are placed down the canal. The rasps have a medial groove cut in them that can be palpated as the rasp is introduced. The rasp is aligned, by palpation or visualization through the anterior incision, to the mark that had been made in the calcar. The rasp is fully seated and checked with fluoroscopy. Rasps are then sequentially introduced and seated ending with the size stem that was reamed (Figure 10.14). When the final rasp is seated, the rotation of the rasp should be viewed through the anterior incision to ensure that it is aligned with the apex of the calcar.

At this point the rasp handle is removed and a trial reduction can be performed. Traction is placed on the leg to pull the rasp completely

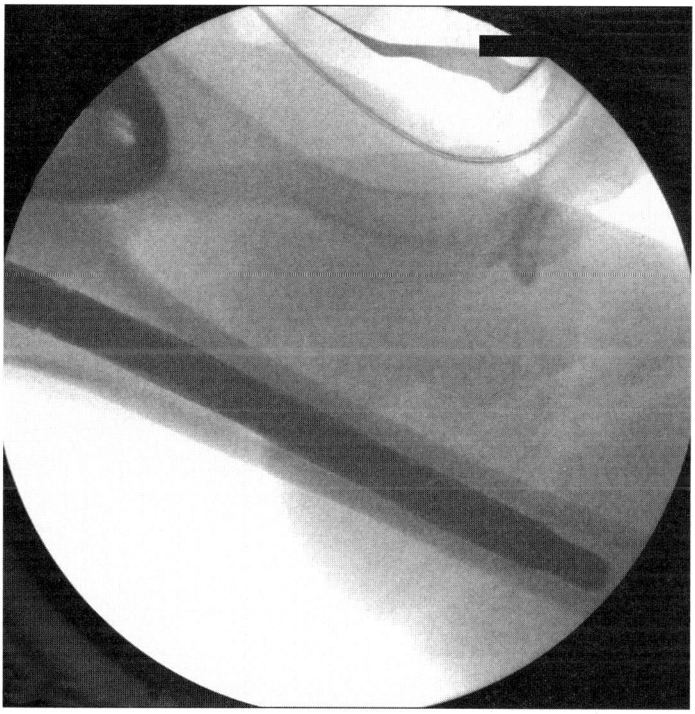

Figure 10.13. Fluoroscopic view of distal femoral diaphysis showing fill and alignment of stem.

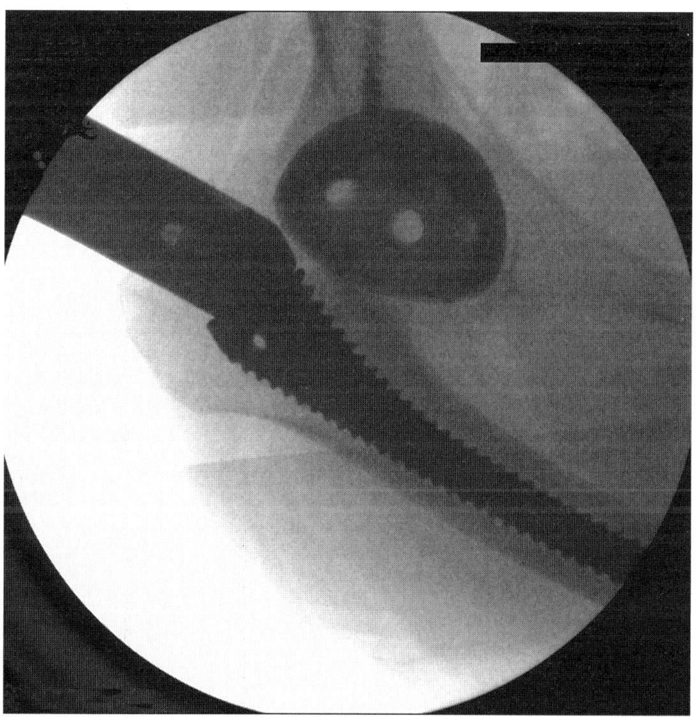

Figure 10.14. Fluoroscopic view of final femoral rasp being seated.

within the capsule of the hip. The trial neck and head are placed on the neck from the anterior wound. Externally rotating the hip and a bone hook around the neck gently pulls the neck anteriorly through the wound. Traction on the leg at this point can make placing the head more difficult. The head is placed on the neck and then the leg is pulled with gentle traction as internal rotation is placed on the leg; this locates the hip. If the calcar requires trimming, this is done from the anterior incision with a sagittal saw. The calcar is easily accessed from the anterior incision with the leg in external rotation. The hip is then put through a range of motion to assess stability. The hip should be stable in full extension with 90 degrees of external rotation as well as 90 degrees of flexion and 20 degrees of adduction with at least 50 degrees of internal rotation. The fluoroscope can be used to assess leg lengths by comparing the level of the lesser trochanters to the obturator foramen. In addition, with the patient in the supine position, the medial malleoli may be checked to assess leg length. When the trial reduction is complete, the head and neck are removed though the anterior incision and the rasp is removed through the posterior incision.

Hohmann retractors are placed into the posterior wound, and placed anterior around the femoral neck. This will keep the anterior soft tissue clear from the stem as it is placed into the femoral canal. Gravity keeps the posterior soft tissue clear from the stem as it is placed into the femoral canal. The stem is then introduced into the femoral canal from the posterior incision (Figure 10.15). The stem is rotationally aligned as

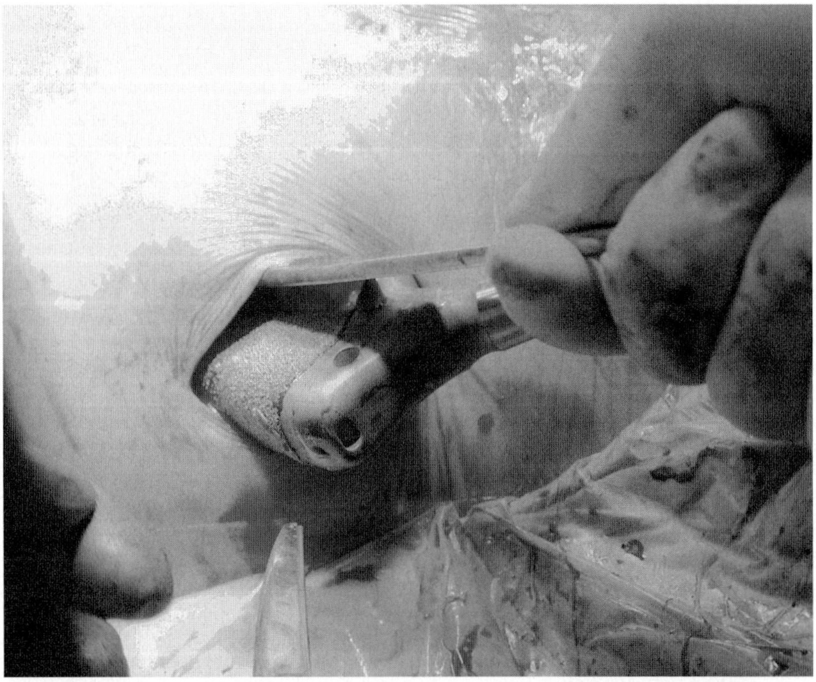

Figure 10.15. Inserting the femoral component through the skin in the posterior incision.

the rasp is placed, this should be in line with the mark that was made on the tip of the calcar. The stem is impacted in place until about a centimeter from being seated. Gentle traction is then placed on the leg with the leg in neutral abduction. This allows the soft tissue to come around the neck of the prosthesis. In addition this pulls the entire femoral component though the capsule to lie within the hip. In this position the version of the femoral component can be easily assessed through the anterior incision (Figure 10.16A). The leg is then put back into abduction and care is taken to make sure all soft tissue is cleared from around the collar and around the neck. The stem is then impacted into place and seated (Figure 10.16B).

If the neck is not fully through the capsule, traction is again placed on the leg, which brings the neck through the capsule lying into the acetabulum (Figure 10.17). Care is taken again to look in the anterior incision to assure that no soft tissue is caught between the calcar and the collar as well as making sure the rotation of the stem is correct, being aligned with the apex of the calcar and the mark that was placed.

A trial reduction is performed, placing the heads from the anterior incision. The hip should be stable in full extension with 90 degrees of external rotation as well as 90 degrees of flexion and 20 degrees of adduction with at least 50 degrees of internal rotation. The fluoroscope can be used to assess leg lengths by comparing the level of the lesser trochanters to the obturator foramen. In addition, with the patient still in the supine position, the medial malleoli may be checked to assess leg length. When the trial reduction is complete, the head is removed though the anterior incision.

Prior to placing the final head, two stitches are put in the capsule, one on the medial and one on the lateral side. This is done prior to reducing the head, as the capsule can become invaginated posteriorly once the hip is located. With the hip in external rotation and the bone hook around the neck, the neck is gently pulled anteriorly through the anterior incision and the final head is then placed on the neck and gently impacted in place. Then the leg is pulled with gentle traction as internal rotation is placed on the leg and the hip is located. During the location process, the two stitches, which were put on the medial and lateral capsule, are kept taut so the capsule does not invaginate posteriorly. With the hip located, it is again put through a full range of motion and stability and leg length are assessed.

Both anteriorly and posteriorly, a total of 40 mm to 60 mm of 0.25% Marcaine with epinephrine is infiltrated into the capsule, the surrounding tissue, and skin. Care is taken not to infiltrate the femoral nerve. The two sutures in the capsule are tied and one or two additional stitches are used to fully close the capsule anatomically. The fascia is closed between the sartorius and tensor fascia lata. Care is taken not to entrap the lateral femoral cutaneous nerve. A few 2-0 Vicryl stitches are placed into the fat layer and then the skin is closed anteriorly with 2-0 Vicryl and staples. Posteriorly the small rent in the maximus fascia is closed with 2-0 Vicryl and a few deep sutures are put in with 2-0 Vicryl in the subcutaneous fat. The skin is then closed with 2-0 Vicryl and staples. Two 2 in. × 2 in. bandages with

A

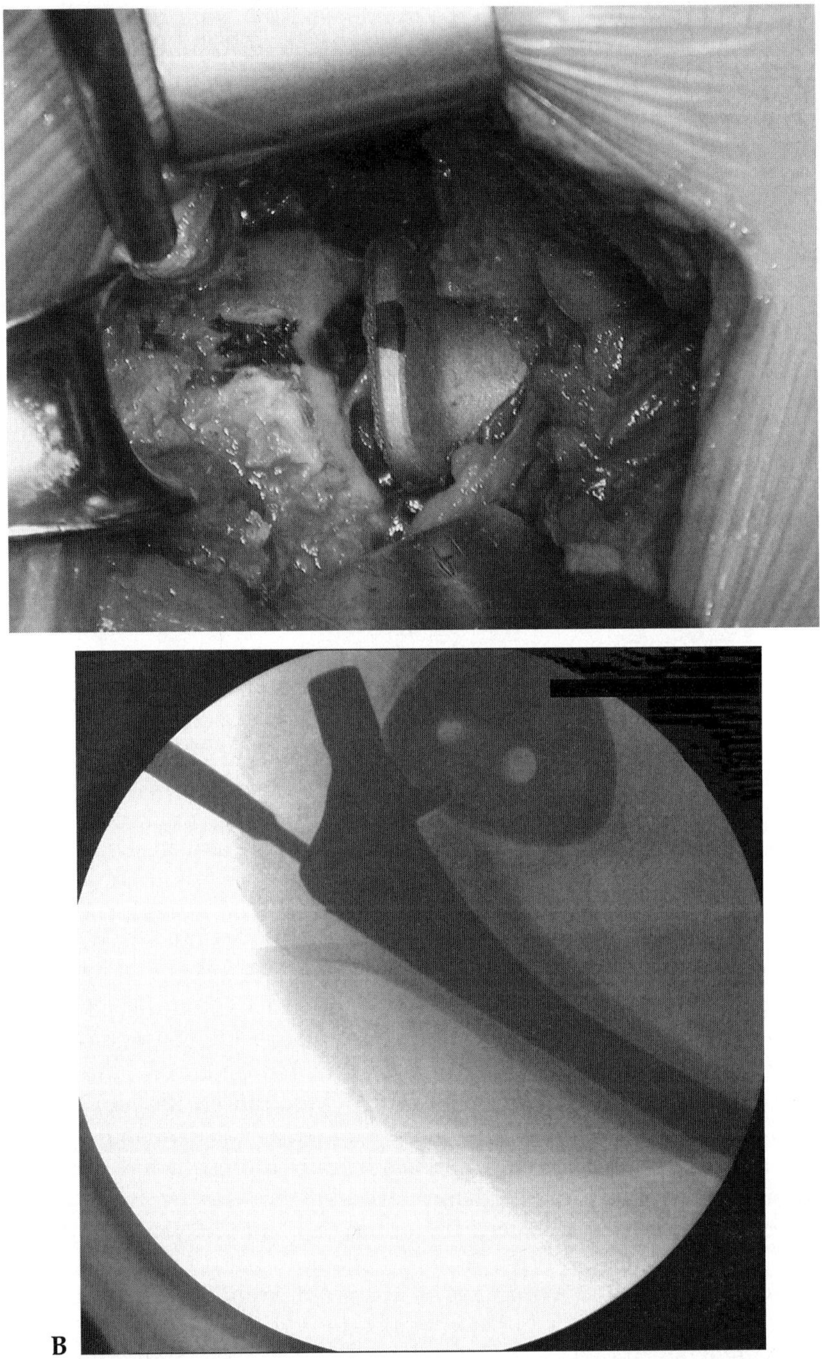

B

Figure 10.16. Inserting the femoral component. (A) The femoral rotation as seen through the anterior incision, aligning the stem with the apex of the calcar. (B) Fluoroscopic view of the femoral component during insertion. The component is seated to the final position.

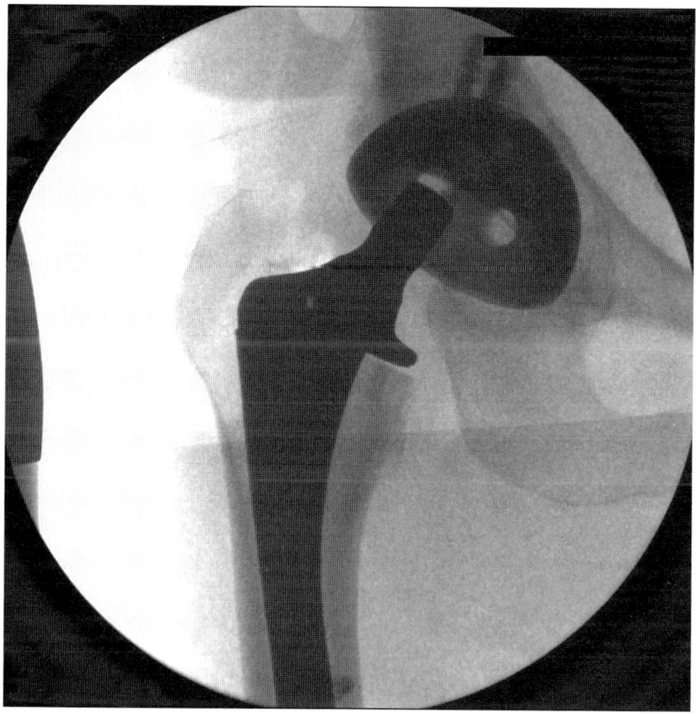

Figure 10.17. Fluoroscopic view of the femoral component with the neck reduced into the acetabulum.

Tegaderm are used to cover the incisions (Figure 10.18). Figure 10.19 shows the preoperative and postoperative radiographs of a patient who received a total hip with this minimally invasive two-incision approach.

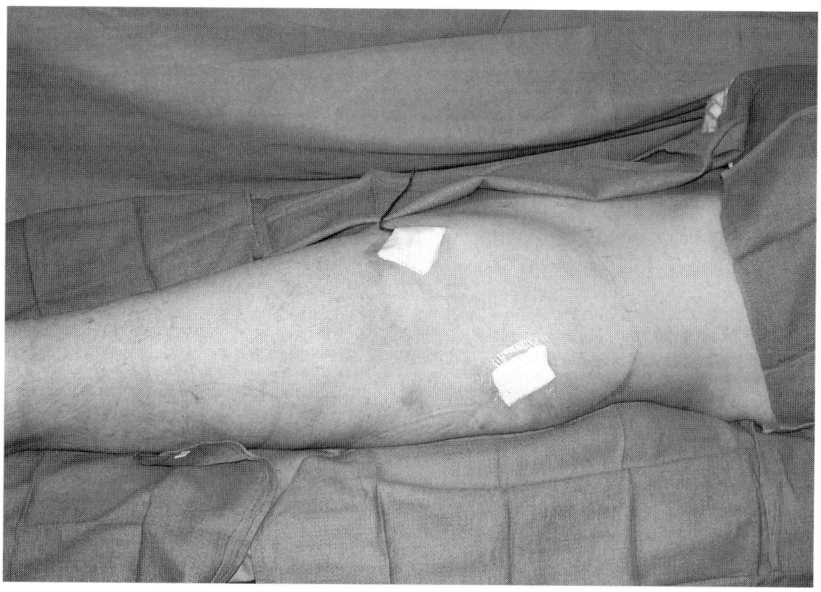

Figure 10.18. Final dressing on minimally invasive two-incision total hip with two 2 in. × 2 in. bandages with Tegaderm covering the incisions.

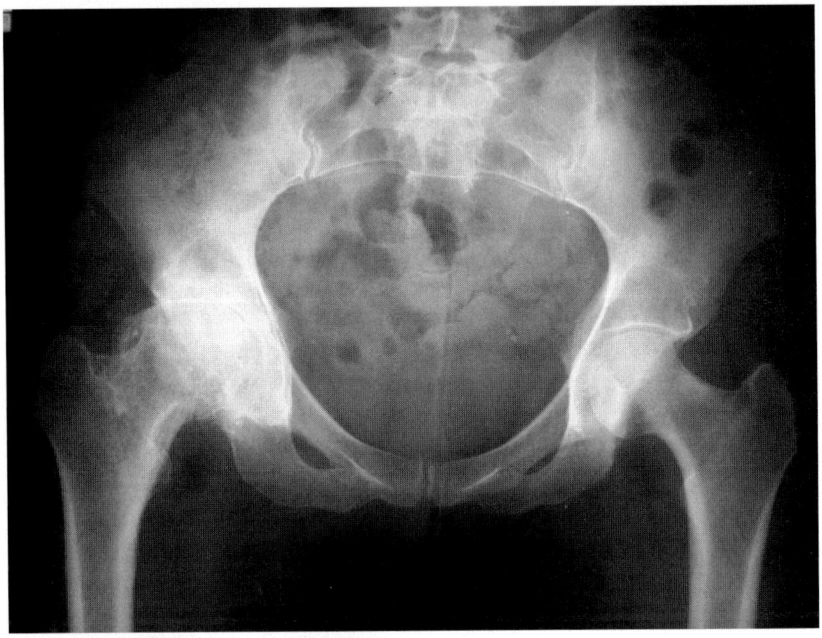

A

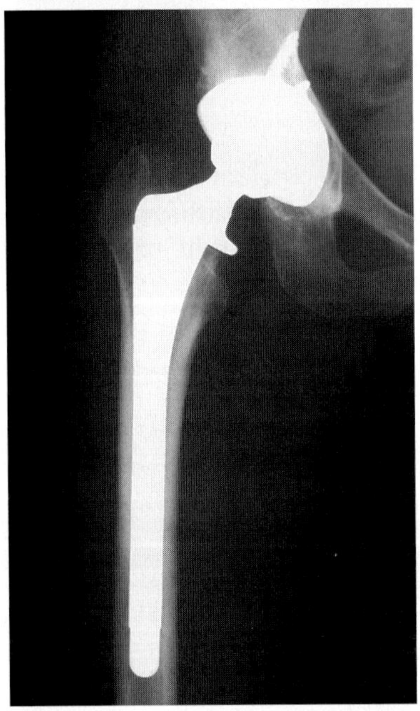

B

Figure 10.19. Radiographs of a patient who received a total hip with this minimally invasive two-incision approach. (A) Preoperative radiograph shows a patient with an arthritic right hip. (B) Postoperative radiograph shows the minimally invasive two-incision THA reconstruction.

Summary

Minimally invasive surgery has the potential for minimizing surgical trauma, pain, and recovery in total hip arthroplasty. This two-incision minimally invasive total hip procedure was found to be safe and facilitated a rapid patient recovery. In the first 100 minimally invasive two-incision total hip arthroplasty preformed at Rush Presbyterian St.

Luke's hospital, the 1% complication rate was acceptable, a single femoral fracture.[5] There have been no dislocations, no failure of ingrowth, and no re-operations. Since initiating an accelerated hospital pathway to allow a shorter length of stay, 85% of patients have chosen to go home the same day with no patient staying more than a 23-hour admission. Furthermore, there have been no readmissions for any reason and no post-discharge complications. Last, radiographically, since fluoroscopy is used during insertion, the overall alignment and ingrowth of the components have been excellent.

In conclusion, this two-incision minimally invasive total hip technique has demonstrated great results; however, this technique is technically extremely challenging and is very different from a standard total hip. When performed in the hands of a trained surgeon, the minimally invasive two-incision procedure achieves excellent success; nevertheless, the minimally invasive two-incision procedure employs novel techniques that must be learned. Optimizing patient outcomes using the minimally invasive two-incision approach requires meticulous surgical technique, specialized instrumentation, and special instruction. As such, active participation in the pretraining exercises, anatomy labs, cadaver training, and proctoring program are essential to minimize complications and ensure success of this procedure.

References

1. Berger RA. Mini-incisions: two for the price of one. Orthopedics. 2002;25: 472–498.
2. Digioia AM III, Plakseychuk AY, Levison TJ, Jaramaz B. Mini-incision technique for total hip arthroplasty with navigation. J Arthroplasty. 2003; 18:123–128.
3. Wenz JF, Gurkan I, Jibodh SR. Mini-incision total hip arthroplasty: a comparative assessment of perioperative outcomes. Orthopedics. 2002;25: 1031–1043.
4. Berry DJ, Berger RA, Callaghan JJ, et al. Minimally invasive total hip arthroplasty. Development, early results, and a critical analysis. J Bone Joint Surg. 2003;85A:2235–2246.
5. Berger RA. Total hip arthroplasty using the minimally invasive two-incision approach. Clin Orthop. 2003;417:232–241.

11

Minimally Invasive Metal-on-Metal Resurfacing Arthroplasty of the Hip

Hari P. Bezwada, Phillip S. Ragland, Craig M. Thomas, and Michael A. Mont

Resurfacing arthroplasty is not a new concept as this type of prosthesis actually predated the use of stemmed femoral components.[1] Resurfacing is bone conserving on the proximal femur, which involves preparing the femoral head with special tools that allows for capping the remaining femoral head and neck. There has been a recent resurgence in interest in resurfacing because of the advent of new metallurgical manufacturing techniques, which have produced precise metal-on-metal articulations. Currently, the resurfaced femoral head articulates with a mated acetabular component and forms a metal-on-metal couple. There have been several reports of excellent mid-term results with a number of these particular devices.[2–4] This chapter focuses on our technique for a minimally invasive approach to hip resurfacing with the Conserve Plus (Wright Medical, Arlington, TN) device. However, most resurfacing devices are similar in design, and the techniques that are described in this chapter can be applied to most of the available implants.

Indications

The indications for resurfacing hip arthroplasty are essentially similar to those used for conventional hip arthroplasty for nearly any arthritic condition, and this device may be especially attractive for the young patient with hip pathology. The indications include all forms of primary osteoarthritis, as well as developmental hip dysplasia, posttraumatic arthritis, osteonecrosis, and inflammatory arthritis as long as there is adequate bone stock. Preoperative bone mineral density of the proximal femur may also be used to assess bone stock. Specific indications for hip resurfacing might include patients who have retained hardware of the proximal femur that would be difficult to remove for a conventional hip arthroplasty, patients with certain diagnoses that may have a high risk for failure or dislocation in standard total hip replacements, and patients with a proximal femoral deformity that might make a conventional hip prosthesis difficult or impossible to place (Figure 11.1).

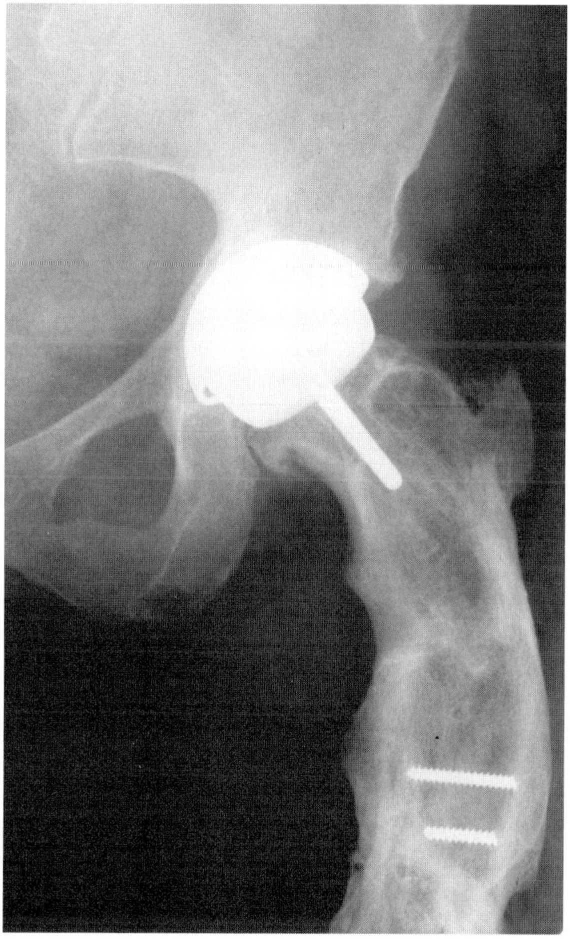

Figure 11.1. Metal-on-metal resurfacing in a patient with an extra-articular deformity of the proximal femur.

The obvious contraindications for resurfacing include patients who lack adequate femoral head or neck bone stock to support a resurfacing femoral component. Patients who are tall, of female gender, and who have femoral head cysts greater than 1 cm, may be at increased risk for component failure.[2] In addition, patients with bone-deficient acetabulae may not be candidates as most resurfacing acetabular components lack additional screw holes necessary for ancillary screw fixation. As future second-generation devices are developed with ancillary fixation aids for the acetabulum, additional patients with severe dysplasia or acetabular bone deficiency might become candidates for this procedure.

Surgical Technique: Anterolateral Approach

Placement of Incision

The appropriate placement of the initial skin incision is essential to the minimally invasive resurfacing hip arthroplasty approach, as inade-

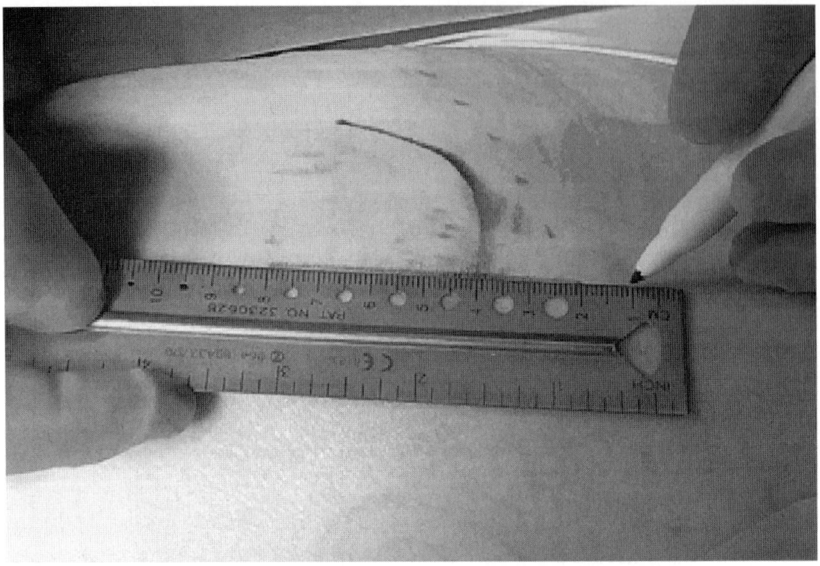

Figure 11.2. Figure showing the landmarks used for placement of the initial skin incision.

quate exposure may compromise component placement. First, the greater trochanter is outlined and the location of the center of the femoral head is grossly determined from the preoperative radiographs since many young patients may also have proximal femoral deformity, with variable neck-shaft angles. As a result, the landmarks for the incision may vary from patient to patient. From the approximate center of the femoral head, mark a direct lateral line 3 cm proximal and distal (Figure 11.2). This serves as a mark for the initial base incision. Additionally, the surgeon can extend the mark 2 cm, on either end, if extension is required during surgery. The overall incision length ranges from 6 cm to 8 cm for most patients. The next step is to deepen the skin incision through the subcutaneous tissue to the level of the tensor fascia lata. A single self-retaining retractor is usually sufficient for tissue retraction and also provides tamponade of subcutaneous bleeding vessels. Ideally, the use of electrocautery should be limited at this superficial level so as to minimize the extent of fat necrosis created. A less destructive type of hemostatic device such as Tissue Link (Dover, NH) may be helpful.

Deep Exposure

The tensor fascia lata is identified and a Cobb elevator is used to establish a plane of exposure of approximately 5 cm in every direction. This step allows for mobilization of the skin incision and essentially converts a 6-cm skin incision into an 8-cm to 10-cm working incision (Figure 11.3). The leg is held in slight abduction to relax the tensor fascia lata and the fascia is sharply incised both proximally and distally, with care not to extend the tensor fascia lata incision much beyond the boundaries of the mobile skin window. The abductor mass should be identified and any overlying bursal tissue is excised. Next, the anterior 30% of the gluteus medius muscle is detached from its insertion on the greater trochanter with electrocautery. It is important to leave an adequate soft tissue sleeve on the trochanter for subsequent repair. The dissection should be continued along the femoral neck, until the plane between the gluteus minimus and the anterior capsule is identified. At this point, Hohmann retractors are placed around the superior and inferior margins of the femoral neck. A Cobb elevator may be used to additionally develop the plane between the gluteus minimus and anterior capsule. The tip of the Cobb is placed on the anterior-superior rim of the acetabulum and used to elevate the abductor mass and free the reflected head of the rectus femoris from the anterior capsule. The anterior capsule is dissected free of any gluteus minimus fibers with dissecting scissors. Once the entire anterior capsule is completely exposed, a standard anterior capsulectomy is performed. Any of the remaining capsular insertion can be released from the neck with a Smillie meniscal knife. The Smillie knife is carefully placed along the femoral neck and the capsule is then incised in both a superior and inferior direction. Next, the hip is dislocated anteriorly. A bone hook should be avoided in resurfacing as the point of the hook can penetrate the femoral neck, leading to a stress riser. The posterior limb of the tensor fascia lata may impede dislocation unless an angled greater trochanteric retractor or a blunt Hohmann retractor is placed directly along the posterior aspect of the greater trochanter to keep this limb of the tensor fascia lata posterior. Once the femoral head is dislocated, any remaining capsule is excised from the femoral neck and a direct measurement of the femoral neck is obtained. This is an important step as the neck measurement determines the appropriate femoral component size and its corre-

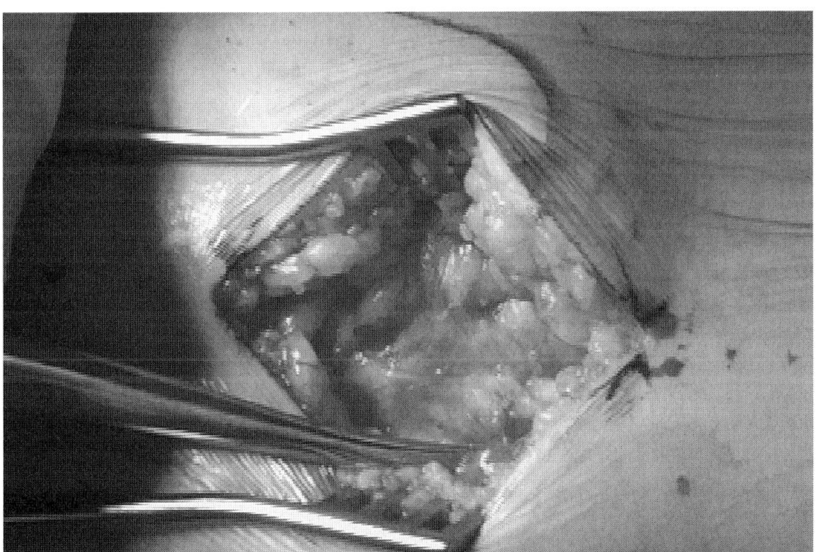

Figure 11.3. The development of a plane at the tensor fascia lata allows mobilization of the incision proximally and distally.

sponding acetabular shell size. This turns out to be a critical step as femoral component undersizing may lead to notching of the femoral neck and a potential stress riser. For example, the approximate neck diameter measurement will be the minimum diameter cylindrical reamer that can be used for femoral preparation to avoid notching the femoral neck. This minimum diameter will then direct the minimum acetabular cup size that must be obtained to avoid a corresponding femoral component size that notches the femoral neck. Any femoral neck osteophytes must also be considered during femoral neck sizing. The leg is then brought back into extension, and the acetabulum is exposed and prepared for placement of the acetabular component. When the head is dislocated through a small incision, it may be tempting to lengthen the incision at this time. However, the surgeon should resist this tendency as the incision may often stretch an additional 1 cm to 2 cm as a result of soft tissue retraction during acetabular preparation.

Exposing the Acetabulum

This may be the most challenging part of a resurfacing arthroplasty to master. The hip is placed in varying degrees of flexion to obtain adequate acetabular exposure. Usually, 30 degrees to 40 degrees of hip flexion is sufficient to allow the femoral head to be posteriorly retracted. First, an angled anterior retractor is placed in an anterior-inferior direction (approximately 4:30 position). Next, an angled Hohmann retractor is positioned along the posterior-inferior acetabular rim (approximately 7:30 position). Many patients have deficient anterior and/or posterior walls; therefore, it is important to avoid levering the retractors on the acetabular walls thus creating a fracture. At this point, only 20% of the acetabulum may be visualized (Figure 11.4).

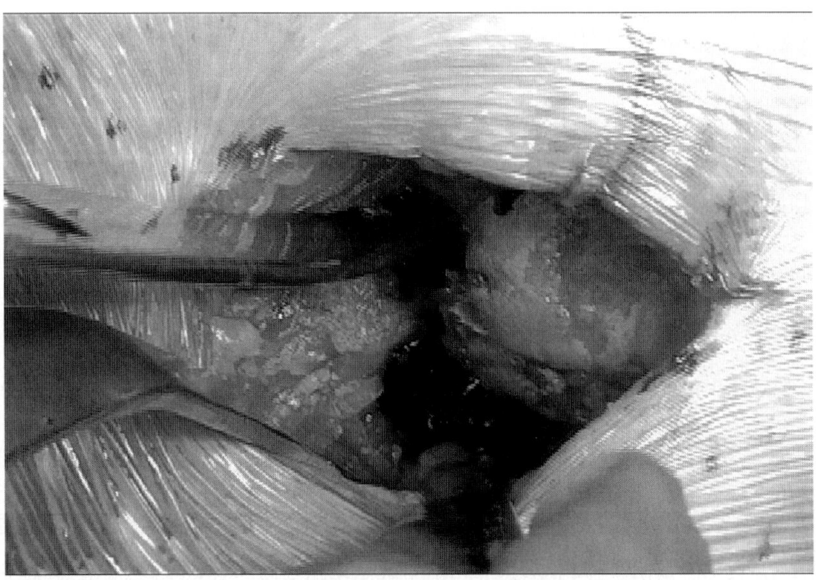

Figure 11.4. An angled anterior retractor, angled Hohmann, and a spiked Mueller permit adequate visualization of the acetabulum.

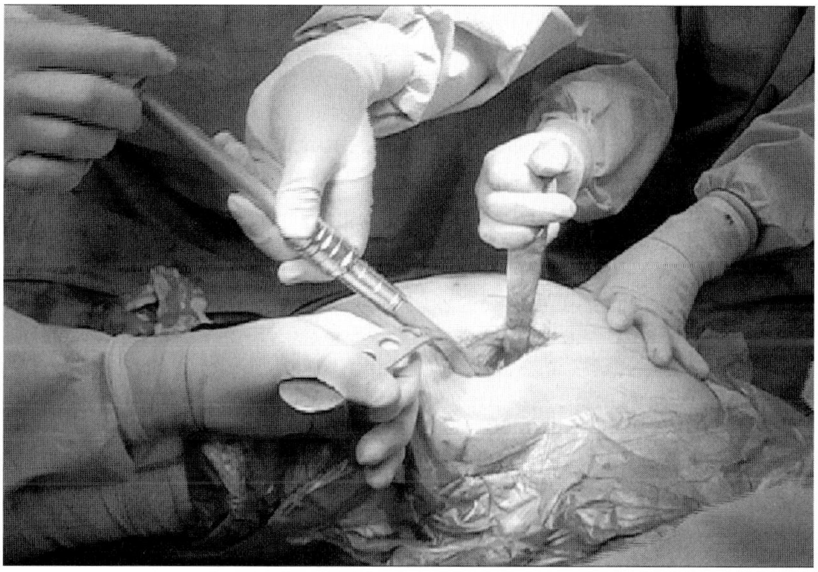

Figure 11.5. Impaction of acetabular component with retractors in position.

A spiked Mueller or Taylor retractor is then placed above the superior rim of the acetabulum between the labrum and superior capsule. Inferiorly, the medial capsule is excised in an elliptical fashion and the psoas tendon is identified to avoid cutting it. This medial capsular release allows additional posterior translation of the femur for additional acetabular exposure. In the majority of patients, these steps will be sufficient to provide adequate exposure for acetabular preparation. There may be specific situations in which the femoral head deformity, as in the case of a previous slipped capital femoral epiphysis, will not allow adequate exposure. In these particular patients a superficial osteotomy of the femoral head in line with the femoral neck may be performed to obtain additional exposure. Again, it is important to avoid notching the femoral neck, as this may increase the risk of subsequent femoral neck fracture. Once adequate exposure and visualization are obtained, reaming of the acetabulum is initiated. As there are few acetabular components made for resurfacing with screw fixation available, concentric reaming is a must, and an intraoperative radiograph may be necessary to confirm appropriate acetabular component position and impaction. After acetabular component placement (Figure 11.5), any overhanging anterior or posterior osteophytes should be carefully removed with either an osteotome or a burr. Osteophyte excision is an important step in achieving maximal range of motion and avoiding femoral component or femoral neck impingement.

Femoral Resurfacing

The hip is now externally rotated into view and delivered through the incision with the leg held in a figure-of-four position. The skin margins should be protected with a variety of smooth retractors. The authors prefer to use a combination of smooth Bennett retractors and

Richardson retractors to protect the soft tissues. A smooth 3.2-mm guide pin is placed in the femoral head in line with the femoral neck at an angle between 135 degrees and 140 degrees, with the aid of a goniometer. Appropriate pin placement in the center of the femoral neck is confirmed with the spin-around guide to make sure there is no eccentric pin placement (Figure 11.6). After the guide pin is inserted, the trans-epicondylar axis of the knee is placed parallel to the plane of the floor and the pin-femoral shaft angle is measured to confirm an angle between 135 degrees and 140 degrees. A cutout drape is then placed around the femoral neck to capture any bony reaming. Next, the femoral head is initially reamed with a cylindrical reamer 6 mm larger than the final size, as determined by the inner diameter of the acetabular component (Figure 11.7). The spin-around guide is again used to confirm central placement in the femoral neck and that notching will be avoided. If the potential for notching exists, the pin is translated 1 cm or 2 mm, using a pin translating device, in the appropriate direction, with care not to change the pin-femoral shaft angle. If there is any doubt, the pin-femoral shaft angle should be rechecked with the goniometer. With confirmation of the appropriate pin position, the final femoral head cylindrical reaming is performed. The initial smooth 3.2-mm guide pin is removed and the doughnut guide is placed around the cylindrically reamed femoral head and positioned to resect approximately 5 mm to 10 mm of the proximal femoral head depending on the amount of wear or shape of the remaining arthritic head. The central hole is then drilled through the *doughnut tower* guide to the appropriate depth to provide for the short central stem. A short central guide pin is placed in the central drill hole for the chamfer cutting reamer.

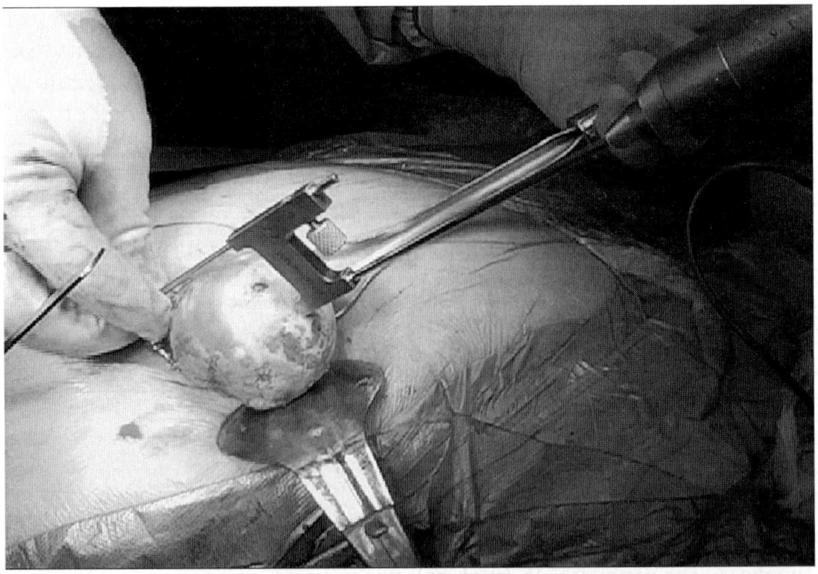

Figure 11.6. The circumferential guide ensures centralization of the guide pin.

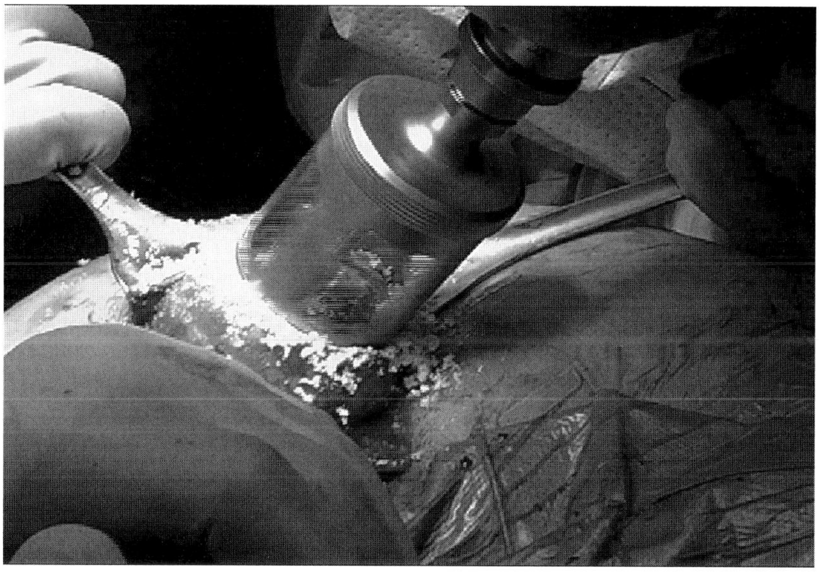

Figure 11.7. The initial cylindrical reaming is oversized by 6 mm and incrementally decreased to avoid notching cortical bone.

The chamfer cuts are made with special care not to torque on the femoral neck. The chamfer reamer must be started off the bone and then gradually advanced onto the femoral head. A trial head component is placed on the cut surface to ensure that the central hole is deep and large enough to allow the trial head to seat flush with the proximal femoral head cut. If this is not the case, then the central hole should be enlarged.

The real femoral component is cemented into place after the femoral head is irrigated, dried, and cleared of any soft tissue or debris (Figure 11.8). Excess cement should be removed once the cement has cured. The hip is taken through a full range of motion to establish that there is no femoral neck-acetabular impingement. Although patients may have a shock with distraction, this is usually of no clinical significance, due to the large diameter femoral component. Heavy nonabsorbable sutures are placed in the gluteus minimus with a locking stitch and it is repaired back to the greater trochanter through drill holes. A drain can be placed and the gluteus medius is repaired back to the remaining tissue sleeve on the greater trochanter with interrupted heavy absorbable suture. The fascia lata and wound are closed in a routine manner.

Postoperative Care

Patients undergo a regimen of protected weight bearing following surgery. Typically, this is 20% weight-bearing on the operated extremity for 6 weeks, followed by advancement to 50% weight-bearing from weeks 6 through 12. If bilateral procedures were performed then patients typically ambulate with a four-point gait with crutches or a

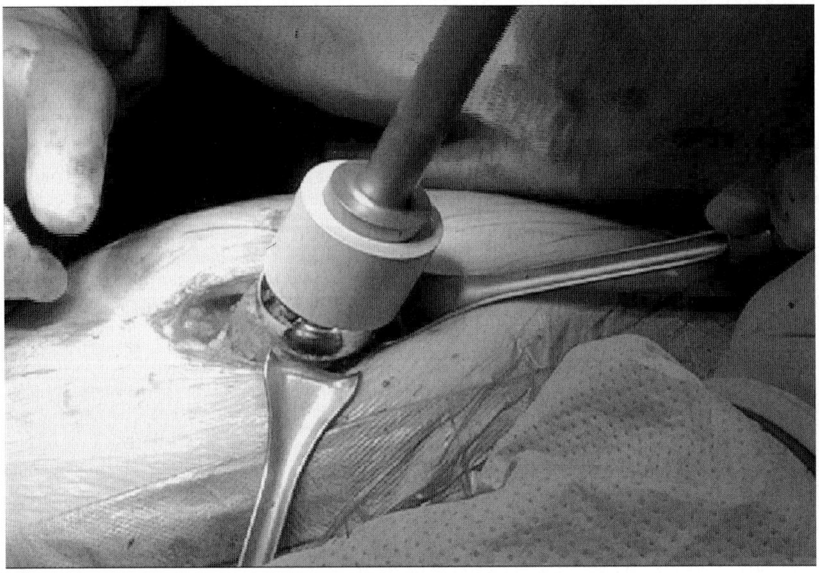

Figure 11.8. Impaction of the femoral component.

walker for the first 6 weeks, followed by full weight-bearing. In addition, patients are encouraged to follow hip precautions during this period of 12 weeks as well. There are no restrictions after 12 weeks.

Discussion

Although resurfacing the worn joint surfaces of a hip has uncommonly been used as a method for total hip replacement, this procedure offers a number of theoretical advantages. It is directly bone conserving on the proximal femur and avoids the use of an intramedullary femoral device that is typical in standard total hip arthroplasties. In addition, a truly conservative procedure should sacrifice little acetabular bone stock. Until recent design modifications of the available acetabular components, this was not necessarily the case as more acetabular bone stock was sacrificed in the past. Resurfacing may provide better stress transfer to the proximal femur and because of the large diameter femoral head (typically, sizes range from 36 mm to 54 mm), there is tremendous range of motion with an extremely low dislocation rate. In a recent report, the gait mechanics appear to more closely resemble that of a normal hip than conventional hip arthroplasties.[2–4] A final advantage may be that, when necessary, the revision of a resurfacing femoral component is less complicated than revising a standard intramedullary femoral component in a conventional total hip arthroplasty. The contemporary resurfacing implants have an acetabular component that removes very little acetabular bone stock and in the event of a revision, there is less osteolysis from the metal-on-metal bearing couple. In the event of a femoral-sided failure, the acetabular component can be retained and be mated to a conventional femoral component with a large diameter femoral head.[5]

Many of the techniques used in this minimally invasive approach have evolved from our standard anterolateral approach to the hip. Although this chapter has specifically focused on the anterolateral approach, many of these same concepts can be applied to the posterior approach. In general, surgeons should initially start with a larger incision (more than 10 cm long) and progressively downsize the incision. This should certainly be an evolutionary process, as an important feature of performing hip resurfacing is to be able to develop adequate acetabular exposure while keeping the femoral head in place.

In the authors' experience, patients with this minimally invasive approach have had improved short-term results when compared with patients with a standard approach. These patients have reported less pain, required less narcotic analgesics, and are discharged from the hospital almost a full day earlier than patients with a more conventional approach. In addition, the patients appear to be pleased with the overall cosmesis of the minimal incision. The authors are also presently evaluating other outcome measures, such as gait analyses, to more objectively evaluate the potential benefits of this minimally invasive approach and determine if these apparent short-term gains materialize into improved long-term outcomes.

In summary, this minimally invasive approach to hip resurfacing appears to have distinct advantages over standard or conventional approaches to hip resurfacing. It should be an evolutionary process that most surgeons, familiar with the techniques of hip resurfacing, should be able to perform. Further refinements to this technique will allow its general use.

References

1. Amstutz HC, Grigoris P, Dorey FJ. Evolution and future of surface replacement of the hip. J Orthop Sci. 1998;3:169–186.
2. Amstutz HC, Beaule PE, Dorey FJ, LeDuff MJ, Campbell PA, Gruen T. Metal-on-metal hybrid surface arthroplasty: Two to six-year follow-up study. J Bone Joint Surg Am. 2004;86:28–39.
3. Mont MA, Bhave A, Etienne G, Ragland PS, Starr R, Erhart J. Gait analysis of resurfacing hip arthroplasty compared to hip osteoarthritis and standard total hip arthroplasty. Presented at: Hip Society Interim Meeting; 2003. Clin Orthop. 2004 (in press).
4. Mont MA, Etienne G, Schmalzried TP. Hip resurfacing arthroplasty: Past, present, and future. J Am Acad Orthop Surg. 2004 (in press).
5. Etienne GE, Ragland PS, Mont MA. Use of modular large femoral heads without liners in hip arthroplasty: A case report. Am J Orthop. 2004 (in press).

Section III

The Knee: Unicondylar Knee Arthroplasty

12

Minimally Invasive Surgery for Unicondylar Knee Arthroplasty: The Bone-Sparing Technique

John A. Repicci and Jodi F. Hartman

When considering treatment options for osteoarthritis of the knee, the pathology and progression of the disease must be considered. Past studies examining osteoarthritis of the knee have demonstrated that the disease is slow, progressive, and typically limited to the medial tibiofemoral compartment.[1–4] Moreover, the erosion of cartilage in the medial compartment is almost always limited to the anterior half of the medial tibial plateau and the corresponding contact area on the distal portion of the medial femoral condylar.[4] Anteromedial osteoarthritis was coined by White et al. to describe this distinct clinicopathological condition.[4] The ensuing anatomic defect, namely, loss of articular cartilage in the extension gap with no corresponding loss of articular cartilage in the flexion gap, results in a 6-mm to 8-mm disparity between the extension and flexion gaps. For this reason, medial osteoarthritis also may be considered an extension gap disease (Figure 12.1). The joint surface asymmetry also accounts for the varus alignment and lateral tibial thrust commonly associated with medial unicompartmental osteoarthritis. At this stage in the disease process, the medial meniscus is either partially torn or completely compromised and tension is compromised in the anterior cruciate (ACL) and medial collateral (MCL) ligaments.[5] To compensate for the varus deformity, a sclerotic layer of bone, or medial tibial buttress is formed. As varus angulation increases, the medial tibial buttress hypertrophies to resist the increasing varus stresses. Although this may appear to be a rather inefficient solution, this layer of sclerotic bone allows the medial compartment to withstand joint loading and to support weight, permitting continued ambulation for 10 to 19 years after initiation of the disease.[3] Eventually, however, patients experience weight-bearing pain as a result of the plastic deformation of bone at the articular surface, instability because of ligamentous laxity, and mechanical symptoms due to meniscal damage.[5]

The clinical presentation of this early, unicompartmental form of osteoarthritis must be differentiated from that of patients with more advanced forms of the disease. The pain associated with the tricompartmental form of the disease often is so debilitating that activities of daily living are severely restricted, independence is lost, and ambula-

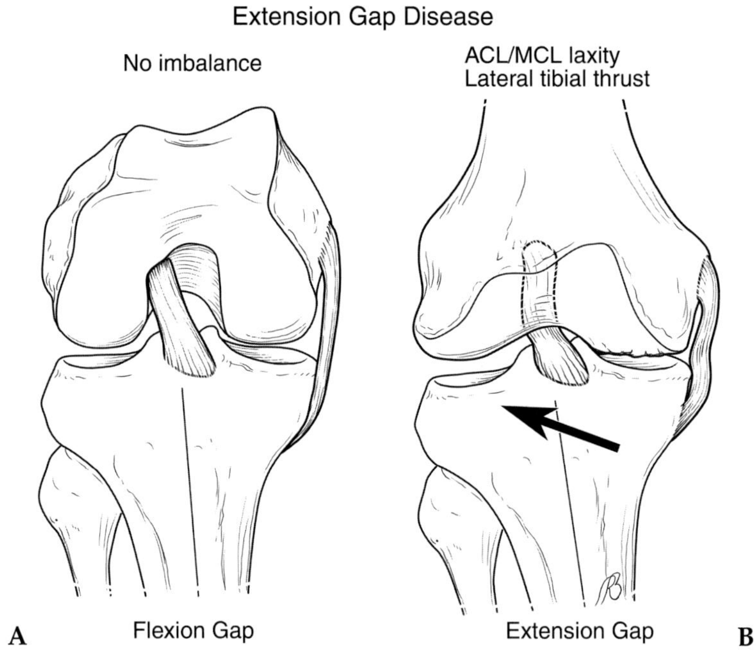

Figure 12.1. Medial unicompartmental osteoarthritis is an extension gap disease. (A) There is no articular surface loss in the flexion gap. (B) In contrast, a loss of approximately 5 mm is present in the extension gap. This narrowing of the medial compartment joint space is evident on radiographic evaluation and is responsible for ACL and MCL laxity, the lateral tibial thrust, or varus deformity, present in the extension gap, and the absence of deformity in the flexion gap, which are all clinical observations characteristic of medial unicompartmental osteoarthritis.

tory aids, such as crutches, a walker, or wheelchair, are required. For these patients, total knee arthroplasty (TKA) is the most appropriate surgical option to relieve pain and to restore some degree of independence. Fortunately, however, unicompartmental osteoarthritis is far more prevalent than the tricompartmental form of the disease[1,3] and the associated pain usually is not as disabling. In general, patients exhibiting unicompartmental osteoarthritis are more active than those with the tricompartmental variant and, therefore, are not satisfied with simple pain relief. These patients typically are inconvenienced by their pain and are seeking restoration of function and a return to activities of daily living. Unicompartmental knee arthroplasty (UKA) is a viable surgical option for many of these patients, as it addresses articular surface pathology, restores anatomic alignment, and reinstates appropriate tension to the ACL and MCL. Utilization of a resurfacing UKA design preserves the medial tibial buttress, which provides peripheral support for the inlay tibial component. Combining a minimally invasive surgical technique with UKA avoids soft tissue trauma, which greatly reduces rehabilitation time and the need for formal postoperative physical therapy,[6–8] making the procedure an even more appealing option to many patients.

Patient Selection

One of the most significant factors contributing to UKA success, whether minimally invasive or traditional techniques are employed, is proper patient selection. According to the senior author's selection criteria, all patients between 50 and 90 years of age who are diagnosed with osteoarthritis and have failed nonoperative treatment are candidates for UKA if presenting with weight-bearing pain that significantly impairs quality of life. Radiographic assessment identifies pathological changes and establishes the extent of osteoarthritis, whereas the preoperative physical examination determines the degree of pain, function, and deformity. In addition, patient discussion identifies restrictions in the activities of daily living, as well as occupational and recreational demands, which are of particular significance in electing UKA.[9,10] Although this preoperative evaluation assists in selecting potential UKA candidates, the decision to perform UKA may only be finalized at the time of surgery, at which point the status of the contralateral compartment and meniscus may be evaluated.

Weight-bearing anteroposterior, lateral, and patellofemoral radiographs, in addition to Ahlback classification to grade the progression of medial compartment disease,[1,11] are critical components of the patient selection process. The anatomic tibiofemoral alignment averages 6 degrees varus for medial disease.[5] Osteoarthritis must be confined to a single tibiofemoral compartment on weight-bearing radiograph. Studies have suggested that some degenerative changes in the contralateral compartment are permissible and do not adversely affect the results of UKA, provided that the articular cartilage on weight-bearing surface of the contralateral compartment appears adequate.[12–16] Large osteophytes on the femoral condyle of the uninvolved compartment, however, may be indicative of bi- or tricompartmental disease, so, if present, the surgeon should be prepared to perform a TKA.[15,17,18] During the course of medial osteoarthritis, the joint line becomes elevated by several millimeters in the weight-bearing position, which consequently affects the patellofemoral compartment. As a result, most patients with medial osteoarthritis also exhibit an altered patellofemoral compartment, which is not a contraindication for UKA.[12,15,16] If, however, the Merchant's view demonstrates sclerosis with loss of lateral patellofemoral joint space, UKA should not be considered.[5] Most patients selected for UKA demonstrate Ahlback stage 2 (absence of joint line) or stage 3 (minor bone attrition), but the procedure may be considered in select cases with Ahlback stage 4 (moderate bone attrition).[5] Patients with Ahlback stage 1 disease are too early in the disease process to be considered for UKA; patients with Ahlback stage 5 have advanced osteoarthritis with gross bone attrition and, therefore, are better treated with TKA.[5]

All patients with Ahlback stage 2, 3, or 4 osteoarthritis are candidates if range of motion is at least 10 to 90 degrees.[19] Instability, including a compromised anterior cruciate ligament (ACL), is a relative contraindication to medial UKA,[14,18–23] but an absolute contraindication to lateral UKA.[19] Absolute contraindications include rheumatoid arthritis, extensive avascular necrosis, and active or recent infection.[19] As long as absolute indications are met, certain relative contraindications, including obesity and high activity, do not appear critical in determining UKA survivorship.[23–25] According to Sisto et al. the key to UKA success is to be absolutely certain that the osteoarthritic process is confined only to the involved compartment that is to be replaced.[26] In this context, a surgeon may elect to perform UKA in spite of relative contraindication(s), as long as the surgeon and patient are aware that the survivorship of the prosthesis may be affected.

Although other surgeons may recommend adherence to strict selection criteria,[27–30] concentrating on absolute indications and contraindications, the senior author follows a broad approach,[8,19] focusing on patient choice rather than on definitive criteria. According to this serial prosthetic replacement concept, UKA is used to treat patients with unicompartmental osteoarthritis who wish to avoid or postpone UKA. The objective is to delay the need for TKA, either indefinitely or for as long as possible, so that if TKA use is required, the UKA may be converted to a primary TKA, which may survive the duration of the patient's life. The use of UKA in this context is minimally invasive in that it is less aggressive than TKA. After other conservative treatment modalities have failed, UKA is inserted in a segmental fashion into the middle of a disease process and, consequently, is considered as the last reconstructive procedure. TKA, on the other hand, is a salvage procedure, signifying the end of the disease process and marking the beginning of a new predictable construct.

In the senior author's twenty years of implementing UKA, patients readily accept the concept of a temporizing arthritic bypass to delay or prevent TKA. When patients exhibiting unicompartmental osteoarthritis are given a choice between UKA and TKA, they tend to choose the less invasive procedure.[8,19] In addition, based on the preoperative discussion, most patients understand that, when used under broad indications, UKA may require conversion to TKA. Because most patients with unicompartmental osteoarthritis are inconvenienced by pain, but remain involved in leisure or professional pursuits, many are interested in UKA as a means of reducing their symptoms, while avoiding or postponing UKA.

Surgical Technique

The surgical technique for performing minimally invasive UKA with medial inlay preparation has been described previously[31] and is summarized, focusing on medial implantation, the most common indication for UKA. The goal of the procedure is to replace one tibiofemoral compartment and to subsequently balance the forces so that the opposite compartment and replaced compartment equally share the weight. General, spinal, or regional anesthesia may be implemented. The anesthesia team must, however, be cognizant of the goal for out-patient or short-stay rehabilitation, which requires the patient to begin physical therapy and walking within 2 to 4 hours postsurgery. Patient preparation and closure are performed per standard protocols. The patient is placed in a supine position and a thigh holder with an arterial tourniquet set at 300 mm Hg is used to secure the leg. A standard operating table is used, with the foot end of the table in a flexed position. In order to accomplish the minimally invasive surgical approach, continuous repositioning of the knee will be required throughout the surgical procedure to optimize visualization, as certain structures are better visualized at low or high degrees of flexion. Because the knee must be positioned from 0 degrees to 120 degrees of flexion, the lower leg and knee are drape free.

Diagnostic Arthroscopy

Before beginning the UKA procedure, arthroscopy is used to corroborate the preoperative diagnosis of unicompartmental osteoarthritis by verifying that the contralateral compartment is unaffected. The status of the contralateral meniscus also must be assessed at this time, because it cannot be visualized through the flexion gap during the open procedure. In addition, the extent of medial compartment damage and the status of the ACL should be observed. The arthroscope is introduced through a medial portal. The UKA procedure should proceed only if the osteoarthritis is limited to one tibiofemoral compartment and the contralateral meniscus is functional. If the disease is more progressive, the surgeon must be prepared to perform a TKA, the potential of which should be preoperatively discussed and consented to by the patient.

Exposure with Posterior Femoral Condyle Resection

To proceed with the UKA, a limited 7-cm to 10-cm skin incision is made from the superomedial edge of the patella to the proximal tibial region, incorporating the arthroscopic portal (Figure 12.2). A subcutaneous dissection, producing a 2-cm to 5-cm skip flap surrounding the entire incision improves skin mobility and visualization. A medial parapatellar capsular arthrotomy, from the superior pole of the patella to the tibia, is produced. A 2-cm transverse release of the vastus medialis further enhances visualization. If additional exposure of the femoral condyle is required, 2-cm to 3-cm of medial patellar osteophyte may be resected with a sagittal saw.

The medial parapatellar capsular arthrotomy does not violate the extensor mechanism and does not dislocate the patella, which is fundamental to the minimally invasive surgical technique. By avoiding patellar dislocation, the suprapatellar pouch remains intact and able to unfold the required four times in length when the knee is flexed 90 degrees.[5,32] The patellar eversion that occurs during traditional open TKA and UKA procedures damages the suprapatellar pouch, thereby necessitating extensive physical therapy to reverse the iatrogenic damage.

Because medial compartmental osteoarthritis is an extension gap disease (see Figure 12.1), there is no defect in the flexion gap, which necessitates the creation of approximately 10 mm of space in the flexion gap to accommodate the prosthesis. A 5-mm to 8-mm resection of the posterior femoral condyle is the first step in generating space for insertion of the prosthesis. The articular defect is located at the distal femur

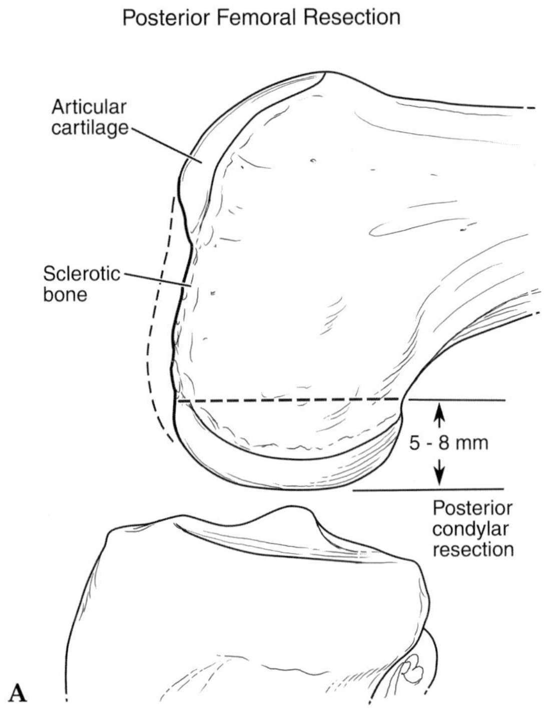

B
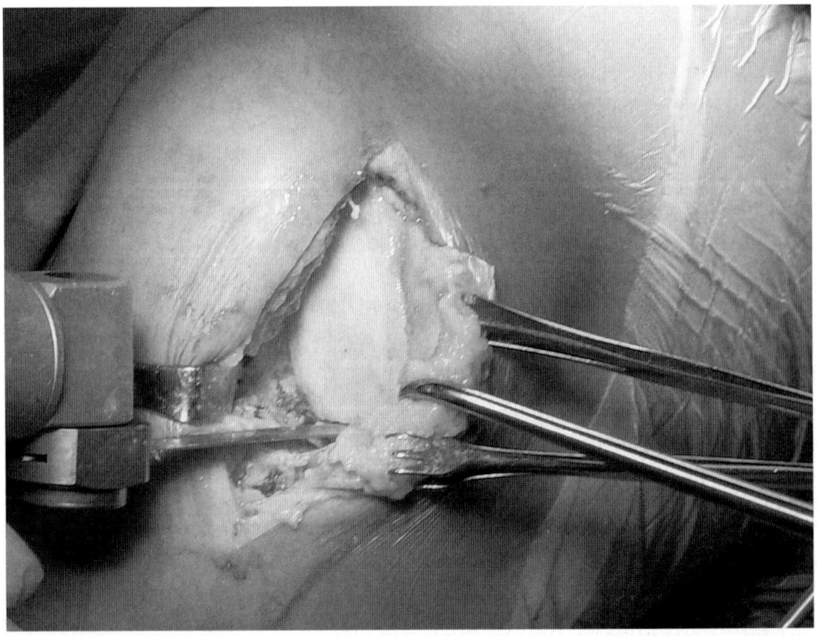

Figure 12.2. (A and B) Exposure with posterior femoral condyle resection.

and the anterior tibia. When the knee is flexed 90 degrees, the femur rolls back onto the tibia, exposing an area of preserved articular cartilage. This area of retained cartilage is an excellent reference point for reconstruction.

Distraction with Tibial Inlay Preparation and Resection

To improve visualization of the tibial plateau, curved distractor pins are placed at the femoral and tibial levels to allow placement of a joint distractor (Figure 12.3). Tibial bone adjacent to the posterior tibial rim is resected with a high-speed burr to create the additional 4-mm to

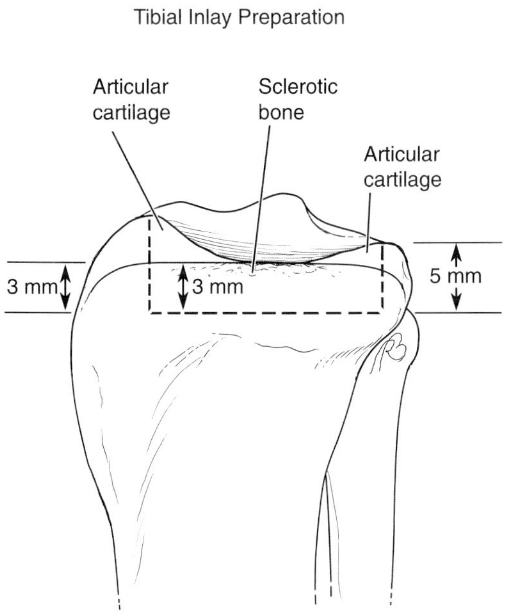

A

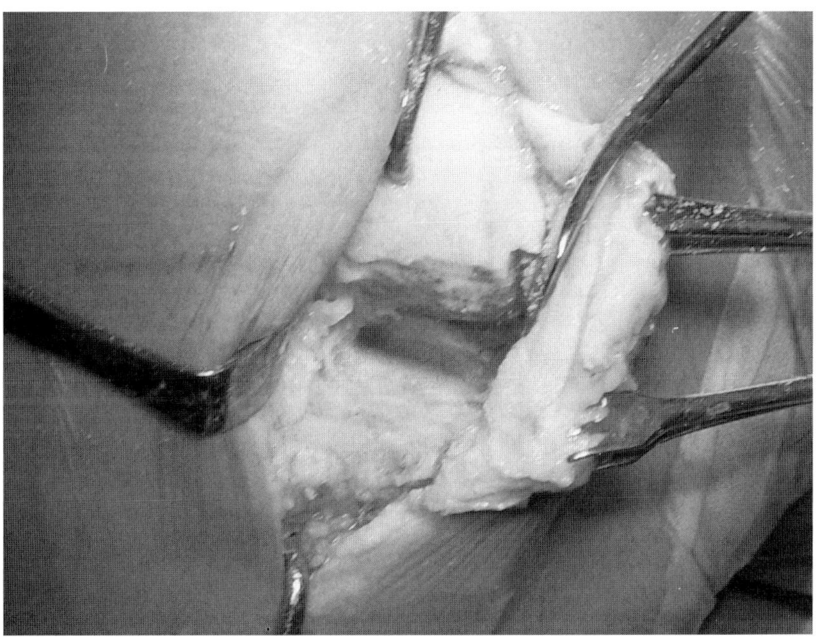

B

Figure 12.3. (A and B) Distraction with tibial inlay preparation and resection.

5-mm of space in the flexion gap necessary for prosthetic insertion. To preserve the medial tibial buttress, the burr only is buried at a half-depth (3 mm) at the anterior tibial region, which corresponds to the area of articular cartilage loss and sclerotic bone formation. In addition, a 2-mm to 3-mm circumferential rim of tibial bone is preserved to aid in stabilizing the component. This careful resection process creates a bed for the all-polyethylene tibial inlay component. A crosshatch is created at the anterior tibial level, which is the natural location of femoral-weight transfer. The tibial inlay component may be fitted and adjusted as necessary.

By preserving the layer of sclerotic bone, a stable platform for the tibial component is created and medial tibial bone loss is minimized, which is a major cause of UKA revision.[33,34] The importance of protecting this medial tibial buttress may be likened to the preservation of the posterior acetabular rim in total hip arthroplasty in that, if lost, future reconstruction is severely compromised. Therefore, the use of a resurfacing UKA design that implements a tibial inlay component and preserves the medial tibial buttress is advantageous compared to the use of a UKA design that requires saw-cut resections and sacrifices the valuable layer of sclerotic bone (Figure 12.4).

A

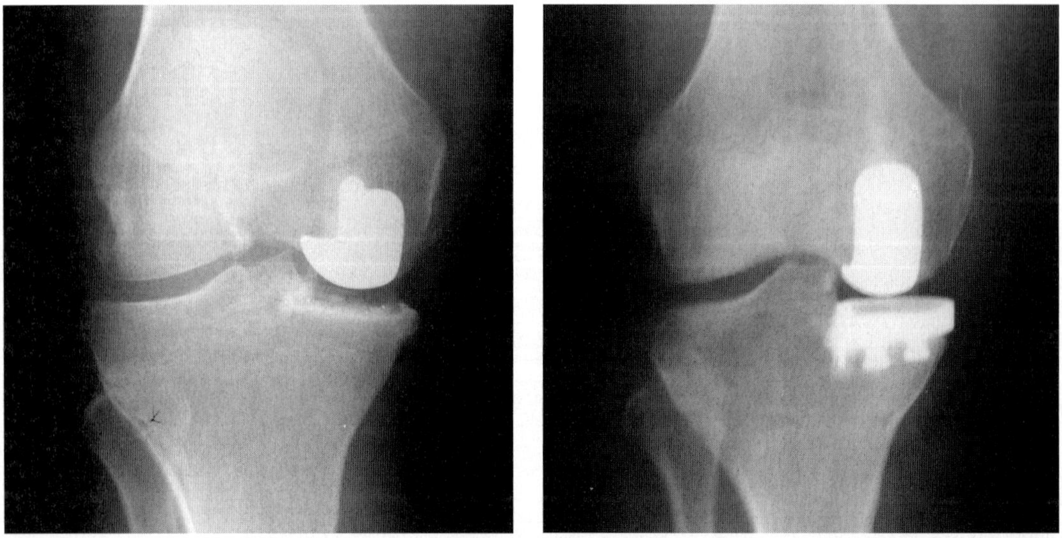

B

Figure 12.4. Inlay all-polyethylene versus saw-cut tibial component. AP weight-bearing postoperative radiographs of knee joints exhibiting Ahlback 3 osteoarthritis with complete loss of medial joint space. (A) Limited bone resection and preservation of the medial tibial buttress associated with the use of the inlay all-polyethylene tibial component. (B) More aggressive bone resection and corresponding medial tibial buttress sacrifice required with the use of saw-cut polyethylene designs.

Femoral Preparation and Resection

To prepare for femoral component insertion, the 5.5-mm round burr is used to drill to a half-depth of 3 mm into the femoral extension gap surface, which will serve as a depth gauge (Figure 12.5). Next, an additional full-depth of 5 mm is created at the junction with the previous saw cut and the distal femoral surface, which will allow the curved portion of the femoral component to set midway between the

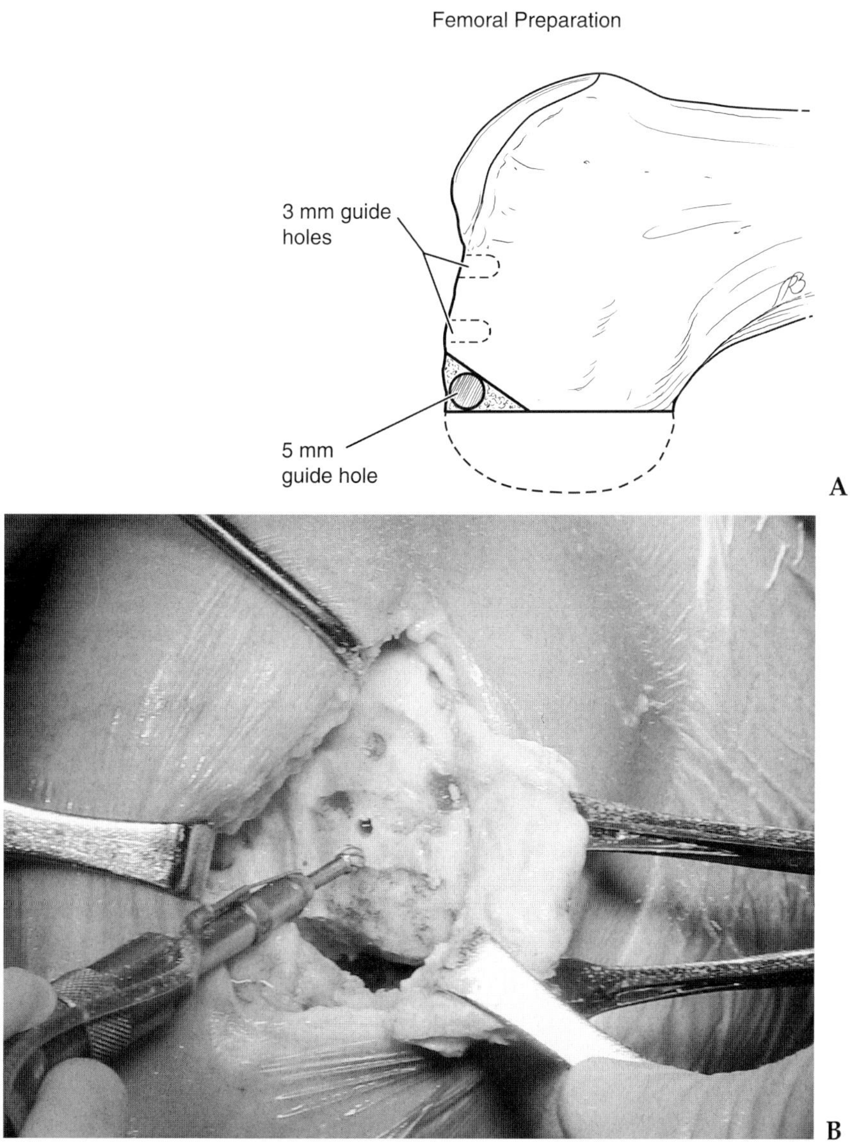

Figure 12.5. (A and B) Femoral preparation and resection.

flexion and extension gaps (45-degree flexion position). Bulk bone is removed with the burr. By performing the femoral resection in this manner, adequate space for the component is created, while preventing settling.

Femoral-Tibial Alignment

Methylene blue marks on the sclerotic tibial bone and on the corresponding area of the femoral condyle are created with the knee in full extension and flexion to indicate the desired center of rotation, or contact point, of the femoral component in relation to the tibial component and to indicate the desired center point of the femoral component (Figure 12.6). A femoral drill guide, manufactured with a large central slot to visualize component alignment, is inserted to assist in this alignment process. A sagittal saw or side-cutting burr may be used to create a keel-slot for the fin of the femoral component referencing the methylene blue markings. The trial femoral component is placed using the femoral inserter.

Trial Reduction and Local Anesthetic Injection

Trial reduction is performed to evaluate range of motion through 115 degrees of flexion and to assess soft-tissue balance (Figure 12.7). Lack of complete extension or flexion indicates inadequate tibial or femoral preparations. Insertion and proper alignment of appropriately sized implants should result in ligament balancing. If, however, the ligaments are tight only in the extension gap, tension may be adjusted by further bone removal at the distal femoral level. Tension in both the flexion and extension gaps requires additional tibial bone resection, as previously described, in 1 mm increments until proper tension is achieved.

When satisfactory range of motion and proper soft tissue balancing is achieved, the trial components are removed, the joint is irrigated thoroughly, and a dry field is established. At this stage, the femoral and tibial preparations will be visible. Prior to component insertion, all incised tissues are infiltrated with anesthesia (0.25% bupivacaine and 0.5% epinephrine solution) for postoperative pain relief and hemostasis.

Component Insertion and Final Preparation

Methylmethacrylate cement is used to insert all components into gauze-dried bone after irrigation with pulse lavage and antibiotic solution (Figure 12.8). Sponge packs are placed in the suprapatellar pouch, posterior to the femoral condyle, and on the femoral and tibial surfaces to dry the field and to aid in cement removal. Excess cement should be removed from the posterior recess and perimeter of the tibial component after insertion, but before femoral component placement, using a narrow nerve hook. Following femoral component insertion, excess cement should be removed from the perimeter using a dental pick. Following final prosthetic implantation, range of motion should be performed to evaluate the flexion-extension gaps. The cement is cured with the knee in full extension. Once the cement mantle has hardened,

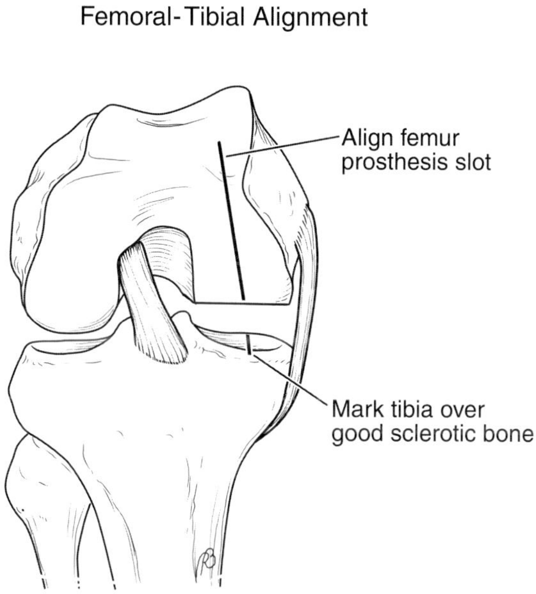

A

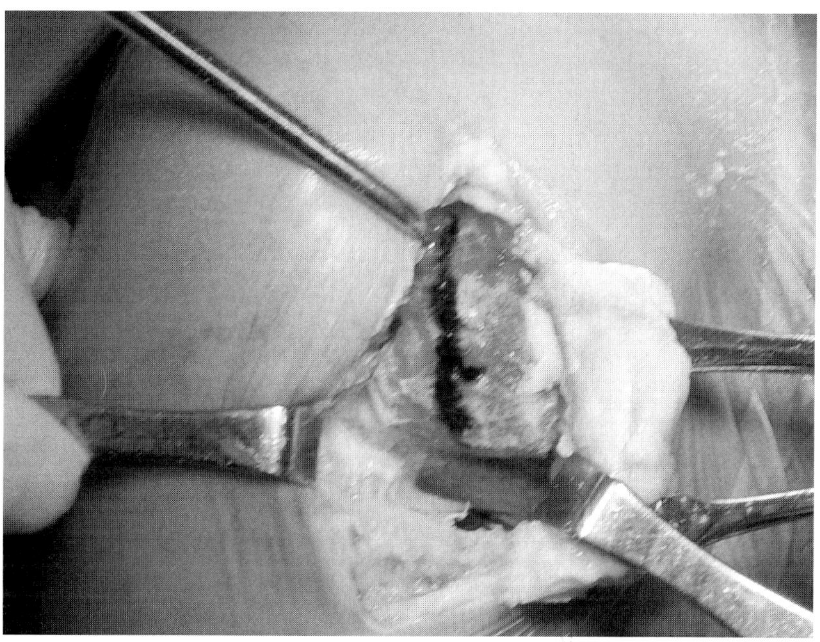

B

Figure 12.6. (A and B) Femoral-tibial alignment.

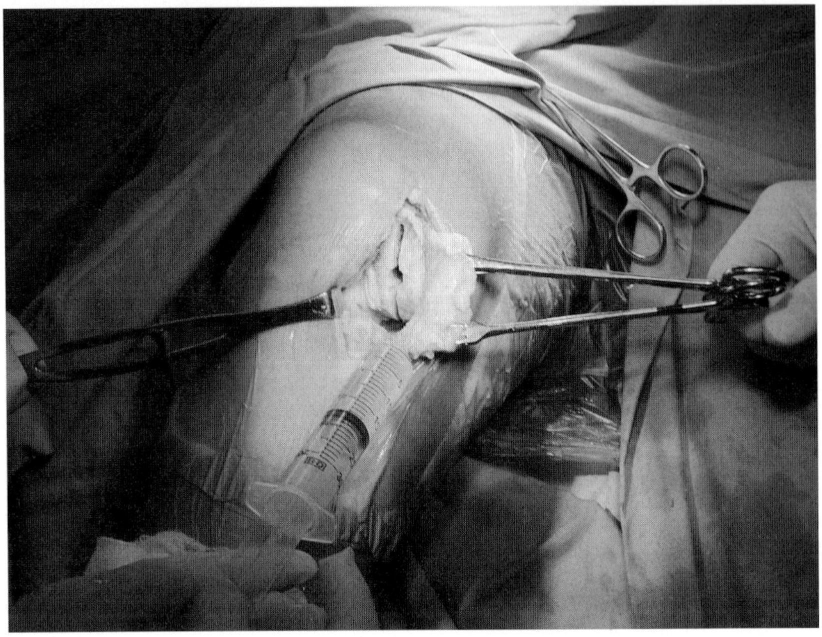

Figure 12.7. Local anesthetic injection.

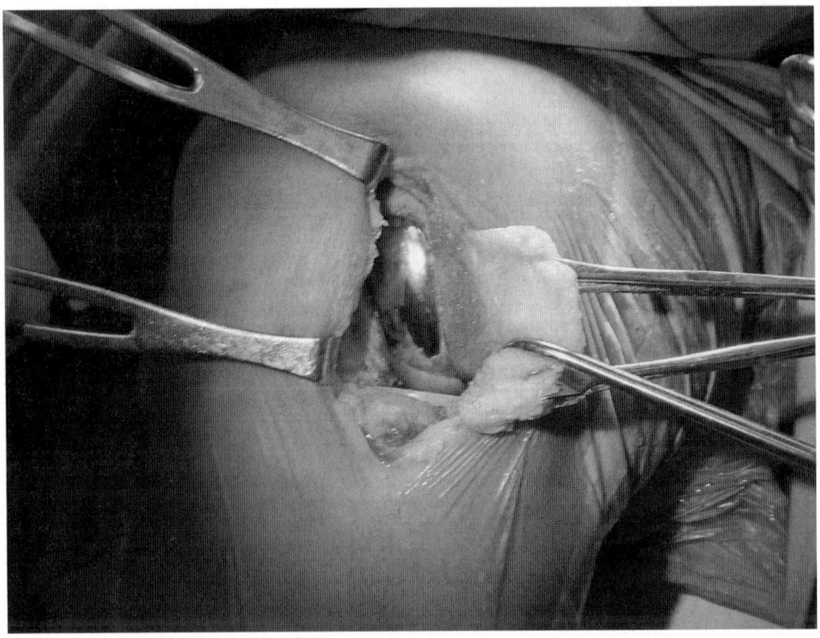

Figure 12.8. Implantation of UKA resurfacing prosthesis.

any remaining osteophytes should be removed. If necessary, patella contouring or notchplasty may be performed. As a final step, the joint should be thoroughly irrigated with sterile saline. The tourniquet then is deflated and hemostasis is achieved with electrocautery. A tube drain is inserted into the contralateral compartment via a stab wound. Capsular closure is performed with 0-Vicryl suture (Ethicon Company; Somerville, NJ). The skin is closed with subcuticular 0-prolene suture and sterile dressing. Before exiting the operating room, final knee preparation involves applying a circumferential ice cuff, a pneumatic compression device, and an immobilizer.

Avoiding Complications

The minimally invasive surgical technique described previously provides adequate visualization to effectively perform UKA. If, however, visualization or technique is compromised at any point, the technique should be converted from the minimally invasive approach to an open procedure, with full dislocation of the patella.

Many of the surgical errors associated with early UKA failures are avoidable. The most common error associated with resurfacing UKA is overly aggressive resection of the tibial surface.[5] Maintaining the medial tibial buttress is crucial, which may require slight varus positioning of the tibial component. If the sclerotic layer of bone is broached, the all-polyethylene tibial inlay component will subside into the proximal tibia. Another frequent error in resurfacing UKA is using an undersized tibial component, which will cause the femoral component to roll off the posterior margin of the tibial component in flexion, resulting in early failure.[5] A careful medial meniscectomy and a well-defined posterior edge of the tibia prior to bone preparation will ensure that adequate tibial coverage is achieved, while maintaining the posterior rim of the tibia. The 2-mm to 3-mm circumferential rim of tibial bone is necessary to counteract sheer forces and increase the surface area for interdigitation of the cement mantle.

Aggressive initial resection of the posterior femoral condyle, which results in a loose flexion gap and predisposes the femoral component to patellar impingement, is another common error that should be avoided.[5] Instead, erring towards underresection is recommended initially, as modification of the transition from extension surface to flexion surface with the round burr during selection of the femoral jig size allows a more precise fit of the femoral component and better flexion-extension gap balance.

Perhaps the largest obstacle in performing UKA, regardless of using a traditional open or minimally invasive approach, is overcoming the learning curve, which is a well-established phenomenon associated with UKA.[10,16,17,35–39] While the main causes of UKA failures, including improper patient selection and technical errors, are not unique to UKA, but to any arthroplasty procedure, UKA is particularly affected by these failure modes because the device is implanted in the middle of a progressing disease process. Patient selection decisions alone greatly influence survivorship. In addition, overcorrection may lead to aseptic loosening, subsidence, and secondary degeneration of the contralateral compartment. Furthermore, a minimally invasive surgical technique adds a significant variable to the procedure. These challenges stress the importance of obtaining UKA-specific training, the significance of strong surgical technique, and the advantage of surgeon experience, all of which enhance UKA survivorship. Robertsson et al. emphasized that surgeon skill, judgment regarding patient selection, and operative routine are assumed to be influenced by the volume of procedures performed.[40] Christensen acknowledged the need for UKA-specific training by contending that TKA systems with good instrumentation may be implanted referring to written instructions, but stressing that UKA technique is best learned in the operating room.[21] Centers performing UKA on a regular basis do, indeed, demonstrate better results compared to those centers where the procedure is performed on an occasional basis.[38,41]

Results

Author's Experience

A retrospective study conducted by the senior author of 136 patients (Ahlback stages 2, 3, and 4) involving minimally invasive UKA with medial inlay preparation and using broad selection criteria demonstrated an overall 7% revision rate requiring TKA at 8 years.[8] The revision rate at 8 years among the 20 Ahlback 4 cases was 25%.[8] The Repicci II unicondylar knee system (Biomet, Inc., Warsaw, IN) was used in all cases. All patients ambulated with a walker within 4 hours after surgery and most (98%) were discharged from the hospital within 23 hours.[8] Hospitalization for 48 hours was required for refractory nausea in one case and for telemetry observation for new onset atrial fibrillation in another case.[8] Primary TKA designs were utilized in the 8 cases requiring revision, with good (25%) or excellent (75%) Knee Society clinical ratings at follow-up.[8] The results from this study support the safety and efficacy of the minimally invasive surgical technique, highlight the decreased recovery and rehabilitation time associated with the technique, and substantiate the relative ease of conversion to TKA, if required, of this particular resurfacing UKA design.

Minimum 10-Year Results of Other Resurfacing UKA Designs

Nondesigning surgeons have reported survivorship of 90% or greater at a minimum follow-up of 10 years for other resurfacing UKA designs.[20,24] Squire et al. reported a 22-year survivorship of 93%, defined by revision due to aseptic loosening, at a minimum follow-up of 15 years.[24]

Minimally Invasive UKA Program

A successful minimally invasive program, regardless of its application, must meet the following goals:

- Minimal physiologic disruption;
- Minimal interference in patient lifestyle; and
- Minimal obtrusion to future treatment options.

In 1992, the senior author implemented a minimally invasive UKA program[31] that is significantly different from simply the use of a small incision or implementation of only a minimally invasive surgical approach. The following concepts, which are all minimally invasive in nature, were combined into a single program to meet the previously mentioned goals:

- Minimally invasive surgical approach avoiding patellar dislocation;
- Adjunct use of arthroscopy;
- Resurfacing UKA design with an inlay tibial component; and
- Pain management with local anesthetic and without the use of narcotics.

The purpose of arthroscopic evaluation prior to arthroplasty allows assessment of articular cartilage in the contralateral compartment and permits the evaluation of the contralateral meniscus, which cannot be visualized through traditional surgical exposure alone. If advanced osteoarthritic involvement of the contralateral compartment is observed or if the contralateral meniscus is not intact, the pre-planned UKA procedure may be abandoned in favor of TKA, the preferred procedure for more advanced cases of osteoarthritis. Verification of a fully functioning, intact contralateral meniscus is critical before proceeding with UKA, as the surface area of load bearing and the stability of the knee joint are enhanced by intact menisci.[42–48] The average tibiofemoral surface contact area when the menisci are intact is 765 mm to 1150 mm^2, but is reduced to approximately 520 mm^2 if the menisci are removed.[49–51] Based on these findings, Kuster et al. concluded that a contact area of approximately 400 mm^2 is necessary to avoid polyethylene stress and to prevent cold flow in knee prostheses.[51] Although a certain degree of cold flow is acceptable in UKA designs, due to the lower tibiofemoral contact area compared to TKA designs, an absent contralateral meniscus will result in an inadequate amount of tibiofemoral contact. This lack of tibiofemoral contact, combined with continued osteoarthritic progression, may hasten the rate of degeneration of the untreated contralateral side and may lead to early failure of the UKA device.[52] Therefore, although eliminating overcorrection has reduced the incidence of UKA failures in recent years,[10,13,15,16,18,22,24,25,30,35,43,52–56] contralateral compartment degeneration and early UKA failure remain a concern if the status of the contralateral meniscus is not assessed.

A minimally invasive surgical approach is considerably different from a "mini incision," which is merely a small hole and may result in significant distortion of soft tissue. A minimally invasive surgical approach preserves soft tissue, while maintaining the function of the suprapatellar synovial pouch, the quadriceps tendon, and the patella. The advantages of a minimally invasive surgical approach in combination with UKA include a reduction in postoperative morbidity; a reduction in postoperative pain; decreased rehabilitation time without the need for formal physical therapy; and the ability to perform the procedure on a same-day or short-day basis.[7,8,31,57–60] Several studies have demonstrated a faster rate of recovery and earlier discharge in minimally invasive UKA compared with traditional open UKA or TKA.[6,7,60] UKA also may be performed as reliably with a minimally invasive approach as through a wide incision, without compromising proper component placement or long-term results.[7,57,60] The preservation of the quadriceps tendon, opposed to the short skin incision itself, is most likely responsible for the diminished postoperative pain and decreased rehabilitation time associated with the minimally invasive surgical technique.[7]

A major problem in converting UKA to TKA is medial tibial bone loss.[33,34] The use of an inlay all-polyethylene component, which requires minimal bone resection and preserves the medial tibial buttress, therefore, is advantageous compared with use of their modular, saw-cut tibial counterparts, which are thicker and require significantly more bone resection (Figure 12.9). The full exposure that often is required for jig instrumentation requires additional bone resection. Because such saw-cut tibial designs frequently use peg or fin fixation, tibial bone will be compromised on implant removal and may necessitate the use of bone grafts, special custom devices, or metal wedge tibial trays to sta-

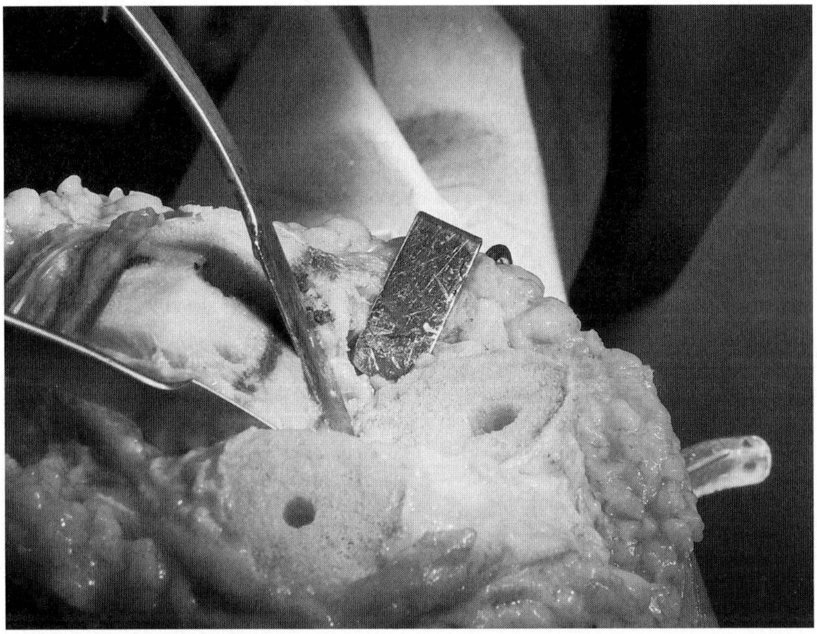

Figure 12.9. Intraoperative photograph depicting the conversion of a bone sparing, resurfacing medial UKA to TKA. After 10 years, revision to a primary TKA was required due to advanced disease of the lateral compartment. With the use of an inlay tibial component, the medial tibial buttress is preserved and the amount of tibial bone loss at revision is minimal, allowing a relatively easy conversion to TKA.

bilize the tibia if conversion to TKA is required, further complicating the revision surgery.[33,34,61–63]

Outpatient status requires a structured pain management program. Spinal or general anesthesia is used in all cases. Patient education, avoidance of cerebral-depressing injectable narcotics, infiltration of all incised tissues with long-acting local anesthetics, and the preemptive use of scheduled oral 400 mg ibuprofen every 4 hours and oral 500 mg acetaminophen/5 mg hydrocodone bitartrate every 4 hours for the first 3 days postoperatively, all aid in controlling pain. In addition, 30 mg ketoroloc tromethamine (15 mg for patients over 65 years of age) is administered either intramuscularly or intravenously during surgery and is repeated after 5 hours in patients with normal renal function. This pain management program results in fully alert patients in the recovery room with no local knee pain. When pain is absent, patients are able to perform straight leg raises and to actively participate in their postoperative rehabilitation process. In addition to the minimally invasive surgical approach, the use of the local anesthetic and avoidance of narcotics are credited for shortening the recovery and rehabilitation time, permitting the procedure to be performed on an outpatient basis.

Conclusion

The senior author's multipronged minimally invasive UKA program is a highly desirable treatment option for patients suffering from unicompartmental osteoarthritis of the knee, as it results in minimal interference in physiology, lifestyle, and future treatment options. In summary, by thorough preoperative clinical and radiographic evaluation, corroborated by diagnostic arthroscopy, patients with more advanced stages of osteoarthritis are excluded from UKA and, instead, may receive the more appropriate TKA, reducing morbidity and increasing survivorship. By avoiding patellar dislocation and nonessential tissue dissection, interference in physiology is avoided, resulting in lower morbidity and rapid rehabilitation. The minimally invasive surgical approach, combined with the specific pain management program, allows UKA to be performed on an outpatient basis, with full independence achieved by 4 hours postoperatively. This rapid rehabilitation and return to activities of daily living addresses patient satisfaction regarding minimizing lifestyle interference. The use of a resurfacing UKA design diminishes bone resection compared to other UKA designs. Consequently, future treatment options are not interfered with and UKA use is permitted in a broader range of patients, including younger, heavier or active patients.

Because UKA is an extension of conservative management, osteoarthritis will continue to progress following prosthetic implantation. Therefore, long-term survivorship of UKA is variable and is affected by many factors, including the stage of osteoarthritis at insertion, limited tibial bone support, and material constraints, such as polyethylene deformity and wear. Although the surgeon does not directly control these aforementioned variables, the single factor affecting UKA survivorship, regardless of design or use of a minimally invasive approach, is proper surgical technique. Therefore, for those surgeons choosing to perform UKA, receiving proper instructional training is critical to ensure the surgical expertise required to successfully perform UKA. Combining a minimally invasive surgical approach with UKA is appealing due to lower morbidity and decreased rehabilitation; however, it adds a significant variable to an already demanding surgical procedure. Proper component positioning and accurate cement removal in spite of decreased visualization must be achieved. In this context, UKA is feasible as a minimally invasive, bone-sparing outpatient procedure with low morbidity.

References

1. Ahlback S. Osteoarthrosis of the knee. A radiographic investigation. Acta Radiol Diagn. 1968;277(suppl):7–72.
2. Brocklehurst R, Bayliss MT, Maroudas A, et al. The composition of normal and osteoarthritic articular cartilage from human knee joints. With special reference to unicompartmental replacement and osteotomy of the knee. J Bone Joint Surg Am. 1984;66(1):95–106.
3. Hernborg JS, Nilsson BE. The natural course of untreated osteoarthritis of the knee. Clin Orthop. 1977;123:130–137.
4. White SH, Ludkowski PF, Goodfellow JW. Anteromedial osteoarthritis of the knee. J Bone Joint Surg Br. 1991;73(4):582–586.
5. Romanowski MR, Repicci JA. Unicondylar knee surgery: development of the minimally invasive surgical approach. In: Scuderi GR, Tria AJ Jr, eds. MIS of the hip and the knee: a clinical prospective. New York: Springer-Verlag; 2004:123–151.
6. Price A, Webb J, Topf H, Dodd C, Goodfellow J, Murray D. Oxford unicompartmental knee replacement with a minimally invasive technique. J Bone Joint Surg Br. 2000;82(suppl 1):24.
7. Price AJ, Webb J, Topf H, Dodd CA, Goodfellow JW, Murray DW. Rapid recovery after Oxford unicompartmental arthroplasty through a short incision. J Arthroplasty 2001;16(8):970–976.
8. Romanowski MR, Repicci JA. Minimally invasive unicondylar arthroplasty. Eight-year follow-up. Am J Knee Surg. 2002;15(1):17–22.
9. Kozinn SC, Scott RD. Surgical treatment of unicompartmental degenerative arthritis of the knee. Rheum Dis Clin North Am. 1988;14(3):545–564.
10. Kozinn SC, Scott R. Unicondylar knee arthroplasty. J Bone Joint Surg Am. 1989;71(1):145–150.
11. Bauer GC, Knutson K, Lindstrand A. Knee surgery for arthrosis. Scientific Exhibit, 54th Annual AAOS Meeting;1987; San Francisco.
12. Carr A, Keyes G, Miller R, O'Connor J, Goodfellow J. Medial unicompartmental arthroplasty. A survival study of the Oxford meniscal knee. Clin Orthop. 1993;295:205–213.
13. Goodfellow JW, Tibrewal SB, Sherman KP, O'Connor JJ. Unicompartmental Oxford meniscal knee arthroplasty. J Arthroplasty. 1987;2(1):1–9.
14. Jackson RW. Surgical treatment. Osteotomy and unicompartmental arthroplasty. Am J Knee Surg. 1998;11(1):55–57.
15. Marmor L. Unicompartmental knee arthroplasty. Ten- to 13-year follow-up study. Clin Orthop. 1988;226:14–20.
16. Murray DW, Goodfellow JW, O'Connor JJ. The Oxford medial unicompartmental arthroplasty: a ten-year survival study. J Bone Joint Surg Br. 1998;80(6):983–989.

17. Marmor L. Unicompartmental knee arthroplasty of the knee with a minimum ten-year follow-up period. Clin Orthop. 1988;228:171–177.
18. Thornhill TS, Scott RD. Unicompartmental total knee arthroplasty. Orthop Clin North Am. 1989;20(2):245–256.
19. Repicci JA, Hartman JF. Unicondylar knee replacement: the American experience. In: Fu FH, Browner BD, eds. Management of osteoarthritis of the knee: an international consensus, 1st ed. Rosemont, Illinois: American Academy of Orthopaedic Surgeons; 2003:67–79.
20. Cartier P, Sanouiller JL, Grelsamer RP. Unicompartmental knee arthroplasty surgery. 10-year minimum follow-up period. J Arthroplasty. 1996; 11(7):782–788.
21. Christensen NO. Unicompartmental prosthesis for gonarthrosis. A nine-year series of 575 knees from a Swedish hospital. Clin Orthop. 1991;273: 165–169.
22. Stockelman RE, Pohl KP. The long-term efficacy of unicompartmental arthroplasty of the knee. Clin Orthop. 1991;271:88–95.
23. Voss F, Sheinkop MB, Galante JO, Barden RM, Rosenberg AG. Miller-Galante unicompartmental knee arthroplasty at 2- to 5-year follow-up evaluations. J Arthroplasty 1995;10(6):764–771.
24. Squire MW, Callaghan JJ, Goetz DD, Sullivan PM, Johnston RC. Unicompartmental knee replacement. A minimum 15 year follow-up study. Clin Orthop. 1999;367:61–72.
25. Tabor OB Jr, Tabor OB. Unicompartmental arthroplasty: a long-term follow-up study. J Arthroplasty 1998;13(4):373–379.
26. Sisto DJ, Blazina ME, Heskiaoff D, Hirsh LC. Unicompartmental arthroplasty for osteoarthrosis of the knee. Clin Orthop. 1993;286:149–153.
27. Berger RA, Nedeff DD, Barden RM, et al. Unicompartmental knee arthroplasty. Clinical experience at 6- to 10-year follow-up. Clin Orthop. 1999; 367:50–60.
28. Bert JM. 10-year survivorship of metal-backed, unicompartmental arthroplasty. J Arthroplasty 1998;13(8):901–905.
29. Capra SW Jr, Fehring TK. Unicondylar arthroplasty. A survivorship analysis. J Arthroplasty. 1992;7(3):247–251.
30. Laskin RS. Unicompartmental tibiofemoral resurfacing arthroplasty. J Bone Joint Surg Am. 1978;60(2):182–185.
31. Repicci JA, Eberle RW. Minimally invasive surgical technique for unicondylar knee arthroplasty. J Southern Orthop Assoc. 1999;8(1):20–27.
32. Kapandji IA. The physiology of the joints. 5th ed. Vol 2. New York: Churchill Livingstone; 1987.
33. Barrett WP, Scott RD. Revision of failed unicondylar unicompartmental knee arthroplasty. J Bone Joint Surg Am. 1987;69(9):1328–1335.
34. Padgett DE, Stern SH, Insall JN. Revision total knee arthroplasty for failed unicompartmental replacement. J Bone Joint Surg Am. 1991;73(2):186–190.
35. Bohm I, Landsiedl F. Revision surgery after failed unicompartmental knee arthroplasty. A study of 35 cases. J Arthroplasty. 2000;15(8):982–989.
36. Bourne RB. Reevaluating the unicondylar knee arthroplasty. Orthopedics. 2001;24(9):885–886.
37. Lewold S, Knutson K, Lidgren L. Reduced failure rate in knee prosthetic surgery with improved implantation technique. Clin Orthop. 1993;287: 94–97.
38. Lindstrand A, Stenstrom A, Lewold S. Multicenter study of unicompartmental knee revision. PCA, Marmor, and St. Georg compared in 3,777 cases of arthrosis. Acta Orthop Scand. 1992;63(3):256–259.
39. Weale AE, Halabi OA, Jones PW, White SH. Perceptions of outcomes after unicompartmental and total knee replacements. Clin Orthop. 2001;382: 143–153.

40. Robertsson O, Knutson K, Lewold S, Lidgren L. The routine of surgical management reduces failure after unicompartmental knee arthroplasty. J Bone Joint Surg Br. 2001;83(1):45–49.
41. Robertsson O, Borgquist L, Knutson K, Lewold S, Lidgren L. Use of unicompartmental instead of tricompartmental prostheses for unicompartmental arthrosis in the knee is a cost-effective alternative. 5,437 primary tricompartmental prostheses were compared with 10,624 primary medial or lateral unicompartmental prostheses. Acta Orthop Scand. 1999;70(2):170–175.
42. Fithian DC, Kelly MA, Mow VC. Material properties and structure-function relationships in the menisci. Clin Orthop. 1990;252:19–31.
43. Grelsamer RP. Current concepts review. Unicompartmental osteoarthrosis of the knee. J Bone Joint Surg Am. 1995;77(2):278–292.
44. Ihn JC, Kim SJ, Park IH. In vitro study of contact area and pressure distribution in the human knee after partial and total meniscectomy. Int Orthop. 1993;17(4):214–218.
45. Johnson RJ, Kettelkamp DB, Clark W, Leaverton P. Factors affecting late results after meniscectomy. J Bone Joint Surg Am. 1974;56(4):719–729.
46. Kurosawa H, Fukubayashi T, Nakajima H. Load-bearing mode of the knee joint: physical behavior of the knee joint with or without menisci. Clin Orthop. 1980;149:283–290.
47. Shrive NG, O'Connor JJ, Goodfellow JW. Load-bearing in the knee joint. Clin Orthop. 1978;131:279–287.
48. Walker PS, Erkman MJ. The role of the menisci in force transmission across the knee. Clin Orthop. 1975;109:184–192.
49. Fukubayashi T, Kurosawa H. The contact area and pressure distribution pattern of the knee. A study of normal and osteoarthritic knee joints. Acta Orthop Scand. 1980;51(6):871–879.
50. Kettelkamp DB, Jacobs AW. Tibiofemoral contact area—determination and implications. Bone Joint Surg Am. 1972;54(2):349–356.
51. Kuster MA, Wood GA, Stachowiak GW, Gachter A. Joint load considerations in total knee replacement. J Bone Joint Surg Br. 1997;79(1):109–113.
52. Marmor L. Results of single compartment arthroplasty with acrylic cement fixation. A minimum follow-up of two years. Clin Orthop. 1977;122:181–188.
53. Goodfellow JW, Kershaw CJ, Benson MK, O'Connor JJ. The Oxford knee for unicompartmental osteoarthritis. The first 103 cases. J Bone Joint Surg Br. 1988;70(5):692–701.
54. Kennedy WR, White RP. Unicompartmental arthroplasty of the knee. Postoperative alignment and its influence on overall results. Clin Orthop. 1987;221:278–285.
55. Marmor L. Marmor modular knee in unicompartmental disease. Minimum four year follow-up. J Bone Joint Surg Am. 1979;61(3):347–353.
56. Swank M, Stulberg SD, Jiganti J, Machairas S. The natural history of unicompartmental arthroplasty. An eight-year follow-up study with survival analysis. Clin Orthop. 1993;286:130–142.
57. Brown A. The Oxford unicompartmental knee replacement for osteoarthritis. Issues Emerg Health Technol. 2001;23:1–4.
58. Deshmukh RV, Scott RD. Unicompartmental knee arthroplasty: long-term results. Clin Orthop. 2001;392:272–278.
59. Keys GW. Reduced invasive approach for Oxford II medial unicompartmental knee replacement—a preliminary study. The Knee. 1999;6(3):193–196.
60. Murray DW. Unicompartmental knee replacement: now or never? Orthopedics. 2000;23(9):979–980.

61. Insall J, Dethmers DA. Revision of total knee arthroplasty. Clin Orthop. 1982;170:123–130.
62. Lai CH, Rand JA. Revision of failed unicompartmental total knee arthroplasty. Clin Orthop. 1993;287:193–201.
63. Rand JA, Bryan RS. Results of revision total knee arthroplasties using condylar prostheses. A review of fifty knees. J Bone Joint Surg Am. 1988; 70(5):738–745.

13

Minimally Invasive Surgery for Unicondylar Knee Arthroplasty: The Intramedullary Technique

Richard A. Berger and Alfred J. Tria, Jr.

Minimally invasive surgery (MIS) for unicondylar knee arthroplasty (UKA) was instituted in the early 1990s by John Repicci.[1,2] While there had been a long history of UKA dating back to the early 1970s,[3–6] the techniques and surgical approaches were modeled after total knee arthroplasty (TKA). The results were not equal to TKA and many surgeons abandoned the procedure. The MIS approach introduced a new method to perform the surgery and helped to improve the results by emphasizing the differences between TKA and UKA. MIS forced the surgeon to consider UKA as a separate operation with its own techniques and its own principles.

Preoperative Planning

The preoperative evaluation of the patient should include the history, physical examination, and radiography. It is critical to choose the correct patient for the operation and to observe the limitations that it imposes. The patient should identify a single compartment of the knee as the primary source of the pain. The physical examination should correlate with the history. Tenderness should be isolated to one tibiofemoral compartment and the patellofemoral exam should be negative. The posterior cruciate and collateral ligaments should be intact with distinct endpoints. The literature suggests that the anterior cruciate ligament (ACL) should be intact[7]; however, the authors will accept some ACL laxity when implanting a fixed bearing UKA. The varus or valgus deformity does not have to be completely correctable to neutral; but, the procedure is more difficult to perform with fixed deformity. The range of motion in flexion should be greater than 105 degrees.

The standing x-ray is the primary imaging study (Figure 13.1). While it is ideal to have a full view of the hip, knee, and ankle, it is not absolutely necessary. The 14 in. × 17 in. standard cassette allows measurement of the anatomic axes of the femur and the tibia which will

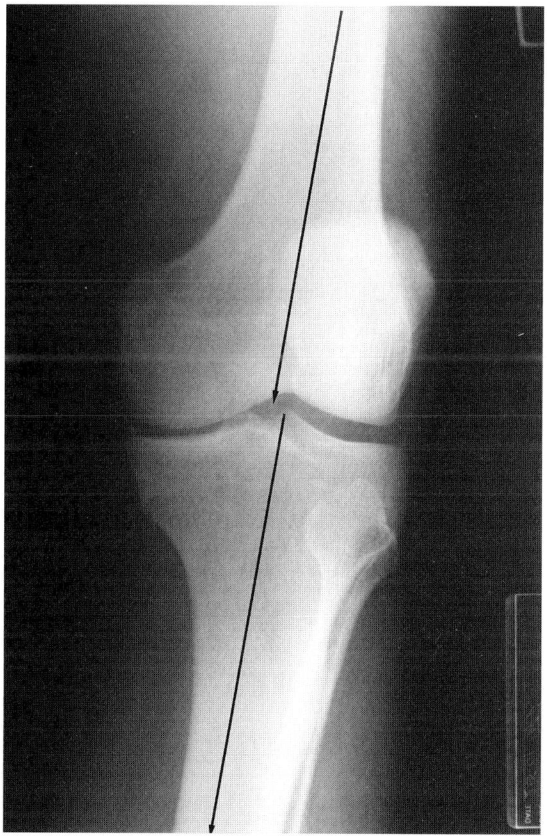

Figure 13.1. The anteroposterior standing x-ray of a left knee. (By permission of Choi YJ, Tanavalee A, Chan A, et al. Unicondylar knee arthroplasty: surgical approach and early results of the minimally invasive surgical approach. In Scuderi GR, Tria, Jr., AJ [eds]: MIS of the Hip and the Knee: A Clinical Perspective. New York: Springer, 2004.)

permit adequate preoperative planning for the surgical procedure. An anteroposterior flexed knee view (notch view) is helpful to rule out any involvement of the opposite condyle. The patellar view, such as a Merchant, will allow evaluation of that area of the knee and will confirm that there is no significant malalignment. The lateral x-ray is used to further judge the patellofemoral joint and to measure the slope of the tibial plateau (Figure 13.2). The tibial slope can vary from 0 degrees to 15 degrees and can be changed during the surgery to adjust the flexion extension gap balancing.

The x-rays are important guidelines for the surgery. The varus deformity should not exceed 10 degrees; the valgus should not exceed 15 degrees; and the flexion contracture should not exceed 10 degrees. Deformities outside these limits will require soft tissue releases and corrections that are not compatible with UKA. There should be minimal translocation of the tibia beneath the femur (Figure 13.3) and the opposite tibiofemoral compartment and the patellofemoral compartment should show minimal involvement. Translocation indicates

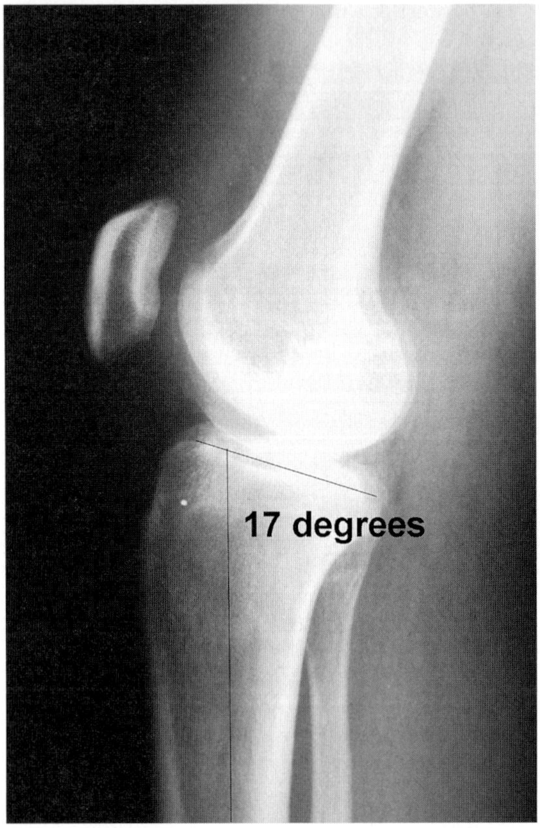

Figure 13.2. The lateral x-ray of the knee showing a 17-degree tibial slope. (By permission of Choi YJ, Tanavalee A, Chan A, et al. Unicondylar knee arthroplasty: surgical approach and early results of the minimally invasive surgical approach. In Scuderi GR, Tria, Jr., AJ [eds]: MIS of the Hip and the Knee: A Clinical Perspective. New York: Springer, 2004.)

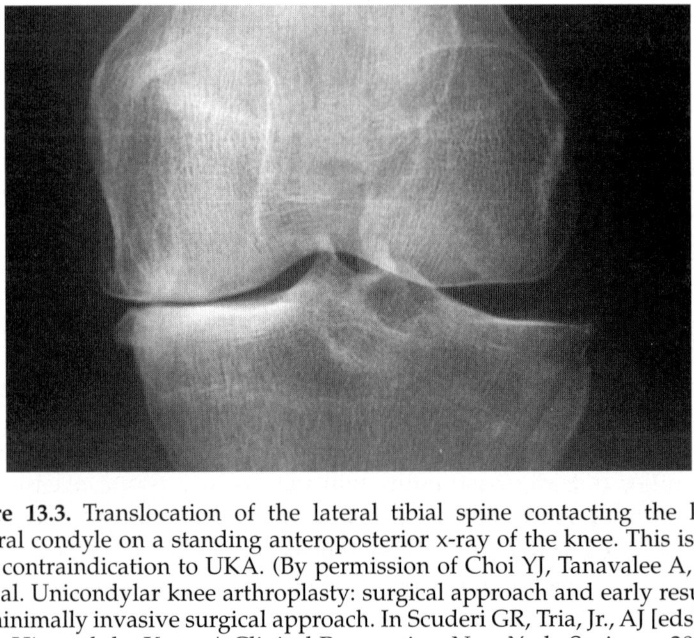

Figure 13.3. Translocation of the lateral tibial spine contacting the lateral femoral condyle on a standing anteroposterior x-ray of the knee. This is a relative contraindication to UKA. (By permission of Choi YJ, Tanavalee A, Chan A, et al. Unicondylar knee arthroplasty: surgical approach and early results of the minimally invasive surgical approach. In Scuderi GR, Tria, Jr., AJ [eds]: MIS of the Hip and the Knee: A Clinical Perspective. New York: Springer, 2004.)

that the opposite femoral condyle has degenerative changes and this will certainly compromise the clinical result. While Stern and Insall indicated only 6 percent of all patients satisfy the requirements for the UKA,[8] the authors found the incidence to be about 10 to 15 percent. However, it is important to avoid broadening the indications outside the limitations noted in order to preserve a high success rate with good longevity.

Magnetic resonance imaging (MRI) is sometimes helpful for evaluation of an avascular necrosis of the femoral condyle or to confirm the integrity of the meniscus in the opposite compartment when the patient complains of an element of instability. However, MRI is not necessary on a routine basis.

Scintigraphic studies are sometimes helpful to identify the extent of involvement of one compartment versus the other. But, once again, this is not a routine diagnostic test.

Surgical Technique (Intramedullary Approach)

The operation can be performed with epidural, spinal, or general anesthesia. Femoral nerve blocks have become very popular but the authors do have some hesitation concerning the technique because of the occasional associated motor block that inhibits the patient's ability to move the knee through active range of motion immediately after the surgical procedure. It is important that the anesthesia team understand that the patients will be required to walk and begin physical therapy within two to four hours of the completion of the operation and the anesthesia must be in harmony with this approach.

The surgery is usually performed with an arterial tourniquet; however, this is not mandatory. The limited MIS incision necessitates continuous repositioning of the knee. The surgeon should be prepared for this and the authors have found that a leg holding device facilitates the exposure (Figure 13.4).

The incision is made on either the medial or lateral side of the patella (depending on the compartment to be replaced) at the superior aspect and is carried distally to the tibial joint line. It is typically 7 cm to 10 cm long. The incision should not be centered on the joint line because this will limit the exposure to the femoral condyle. In the varus knee the arthrotomy is performed in a vertical fashion and the authors initially included a short, transverse cut in the capsule approximately 1 cm to 2 cm beneath the vastus medialis (Figure 13.5). The capsular extension is helpful when the surgeon's experience is limited and when exposure is difficult in the tight knee. With greater experience, the extension is not necessary. It is important to emphasize that this transverse cut is not a subvastus approach but merely an incision in the capsule of the knee midway between the vastus medialis and the tibial joint line. The deep MCL is released on the tibial side to improve the exposure of the joint. The release is not performed for the purposes of alignment correction. This is the beginning of the divergence of UKA from the TKA surgery. It is important to remember that the surgery is only

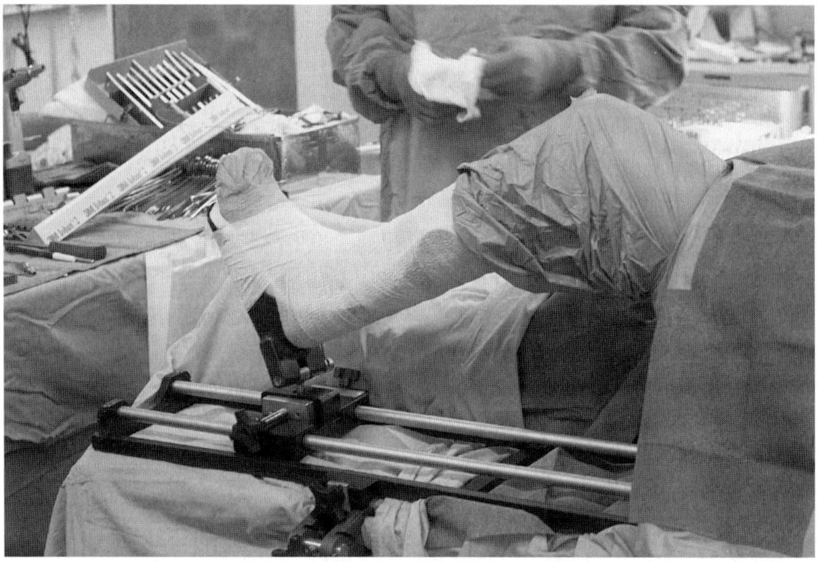

Figure 13.4. The leg holder (Innovative Medical Products, Inc., Plainville, CT) allows flexion and extension of the knee along with internal and external rotation. (By permission of Choi YJ, Tanavalee A, Chan A, et al. Unicondylar knee arthroplasty: surgical approach and early results of the minimally invasive surgical approach. In Scuderi GR, Tria, Jr., AJ [eds]: MIS of the Hip and the Knee: A Clinical Perspective. New York: Springer, 2004.)

performed on one side of the joint. The goal of the surgery is to replace one side and to balance the forces so that the arthroplasty and the opposite compartment share the weight bearing equally. If the medial ligamentous complex is released, there is the potential for overloading the opposite side with resultant pain and failure.

In the lateral UKA, the T extension is not necessary. The vertical incision is taken down to the tibial plateau and the iliotibial band (ITB) is sharply released from Gerdy's tubercle and elevated posteriorly (Figure 13.6). The arthrotomy is closed in a vertical fashion and the ITB is left to scar down to the tibial metaphysis.

The patella is not everted in the procedure and the vastus medialis is not violated either by a dividing incision or a subvastus approach. The sparing of the surrounding soft tissue structures and the preservation of the extensor mechanism in its entirety makes the procedure minimally invasive.

With the completion of the arthrotomy, the peripheral osteophytes should be removed from the femoral condyle and the tibial plateau. All compartments of the joint should be inspected. It is not unusual to see some limited arthritic involvement in the other compartments of the knee. The preoperative evaluation should be thorough enough to preclude a conversion to a TKA. Diagnostic arthroscopy is not necessary but can sometimes be included to confirm the anatomy of the opposite side in an unusual case. The addition of this procedure should be undertaken with care to avoid the possibility of increasing the associated infection rate.

The intramedullary technique requires an entrance hole centered just above the roof of the intercondylar notch (Figure 13.7). The intramedullary canal is suctioned free of its contents to discourage fat embolization and the instrument is positioned. The depth of the distal femoral cut affects the extension gap and also the anatomic valgus of

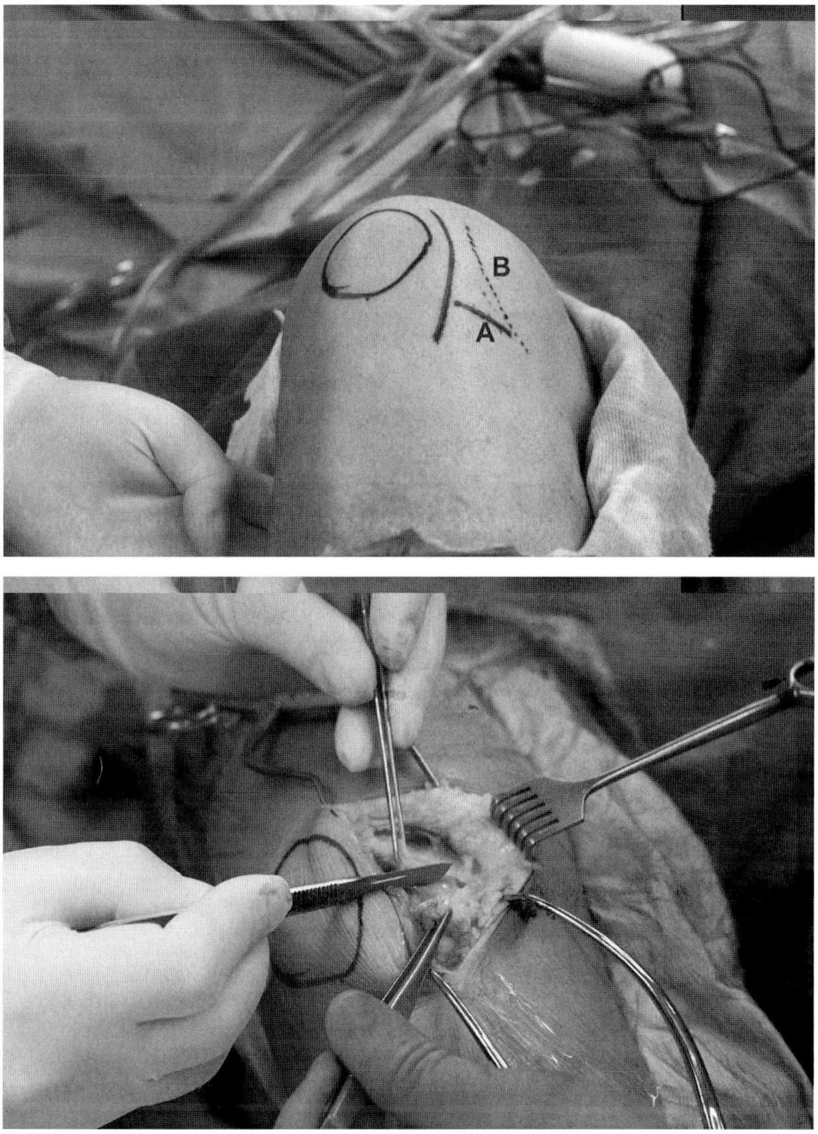

A

B

Figure 13.5. (A) The medial incision extends from the top of the patella to just below the tibial joint line (A). B is the outline of the margin of the medial femoral condyle. (B) The medial arthrotomy can include a T in the capsule (made with the tip of the knife blade). (B, by permission of Choi YJ, Tanavalee A, Chan A, et al. Unicondylar knee arthroplasty: surgical approach and early results of the minimally invasive surgical approach. In Scuderi GR, Tria, Jr., AJ [eds]: MIS of the Hip and the Knee: A Clinical Perspective. New York: Springer, 2004.)

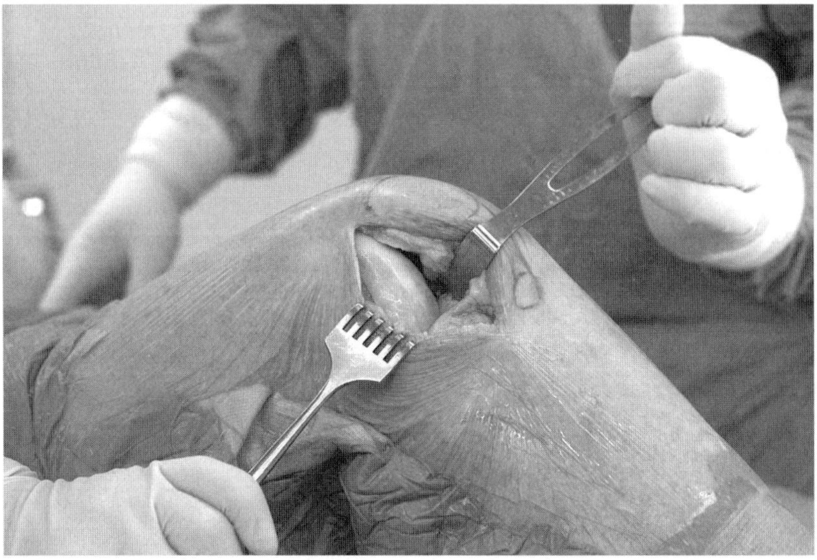

Figure 13.6. The lateral view of a right knee shows the anterior tibial joint line after the iliotibial band has been released and retracted posteriorly. (By permission of Choi YJ, Tanavalee A, Chan A, et al. Unicondylar knee arthroplasty: surgical approach and early results of the minimally invasive surgical approach. In Scuderi GR, Tria, Jr., AJ [eds]: MIS of the Hip and the Knee: A Clinical Perspective. New York: Springer, 2004.)

the distal femur (Figure 13.8). The angle (or tilt) of the cut determines the perpendicularity of the component to the tibial plateau surface in full extension (Figure 13.9). This angle can be precisely determined by measuring the difference between the anatomic and mechanical axis of the knee on long-standing x-ray films. In the clinical setting the authors arbitrarily choose a 4-degree angle for the varus knee and a 6-degree angle for the valgus knee.

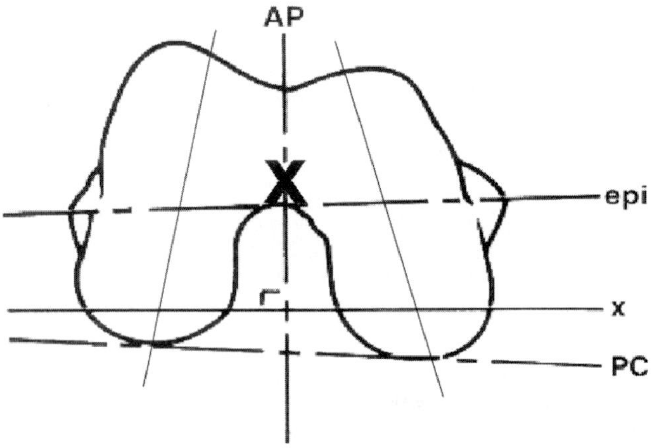

Figure 13.7. The intramedullary hole is located just above the roof of the intercondylar notch (marked with the letter "X").

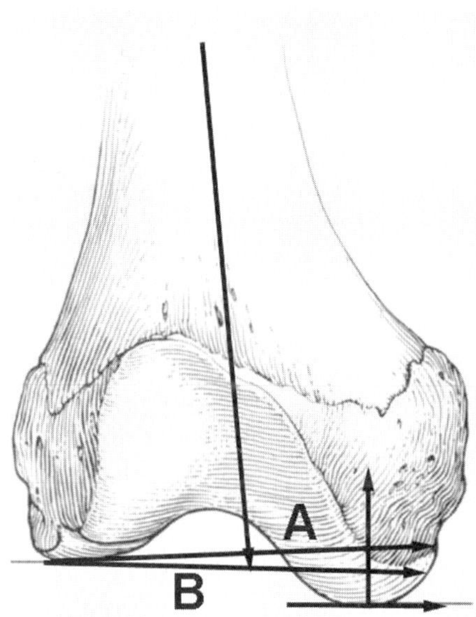

Figure 13.8. The two cuts on the medial femoral condyle show that the deeper resection (line A) results in less valgus than line B (3 degrees versus 5 degrees). This also allows for more space in full extension. (From Tria AJ, Jr., Klein KS. An illustrated Guide to the Knee. New York: Churchill Livingstone, 1992 with permission from Elsevier.)

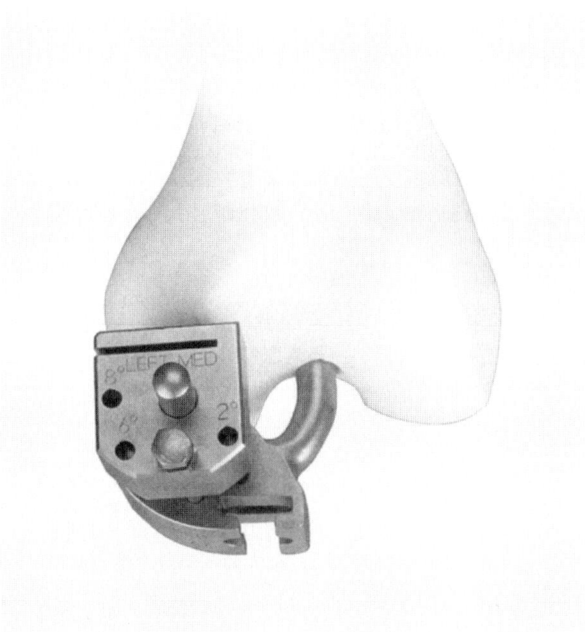

A

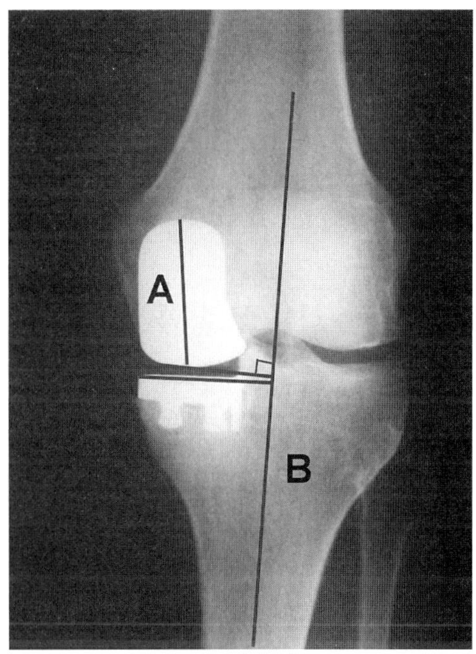

B

Figure 13.9. (A) The intramedullary guide allows for a distal cut of 2, 4, 6, or 8 degrees. This setting adjusts the angle of the femoral component with relation to the tibial plateau cut surface. It does not adjust the overall varus or valgus of the knee because it is only cutting one condyle. (B) The femoral component "tilt" is defined as the angle between the long axis of the component (line A) referenced to the axis of the tibial shaft (line B). (B, by permission of Choi YJ, Tanavalee A, Chan A, et al. Unicondylar knee arthroplasty: surgical approach and early results of the minimally invasive surgical approach. In Scuderi GR, Tria, Jr., AJ [eds]: MIS of the Hip and the Knee: A Clinical Perspective. New York: Springer, 2004.)

Flexion contractures of the knee can be corrected with the medial UKA but not with the lateral replacement. If there is a flexion contracture and the distal anatomic femoral valgus is 5 degrees or less in the varus knee, the standard amount of bone is removed to replace millimeter for millimeter with the prosthesis. If the distal femoral valgus is 6 degrees or more in the varus knee, 2 mm of additional bone are removed from the distal femur to decrease the excess valgus and to increase the space in full extension. Increasing the space in full extension helps to correct the flexion contracture and enables the surgeon to decrease the associated depth of the tibial cut. The deeper femoral cut saves 2 mm of bone on the tibial side and results in a total distal femoral resection of 8 mm. The resection does not elevate the femoral joint line as it would in a TKA. Most TKA femoral components remove a minimum of 9 mm for the prosthesis so that this change does not adversely affect revision to a TKA.

In the valgus knee, the maximum acceptable deformity is 15 degrees and the distal femur is cut millimeter for millimeter for replacement. The deformity will be slightly decreased with a standard resurfacing because the prosthesis and the cement mantle are slightly thicker than the bone that is removed. Because the lateral femoral condyle is less prominent than the medial condyle in full extension, flexion contractures cannot be corrected as easily on the lateral side. A deeper cut on the lateral femoral condyle will only increase the distal femoral valgus without changing the extension gap significantly.

After completing the distal femoral cut, it is easier to proceed to the tibial preparation because this in turn opens up the space in 90 degrees of flexion and makes the femoral finishing cuts much easier. The tibial cut is made with an extramedullary instrument (Figure 13.10). In the MIS setting, intramedullary instrumentation is difficult on the tibial

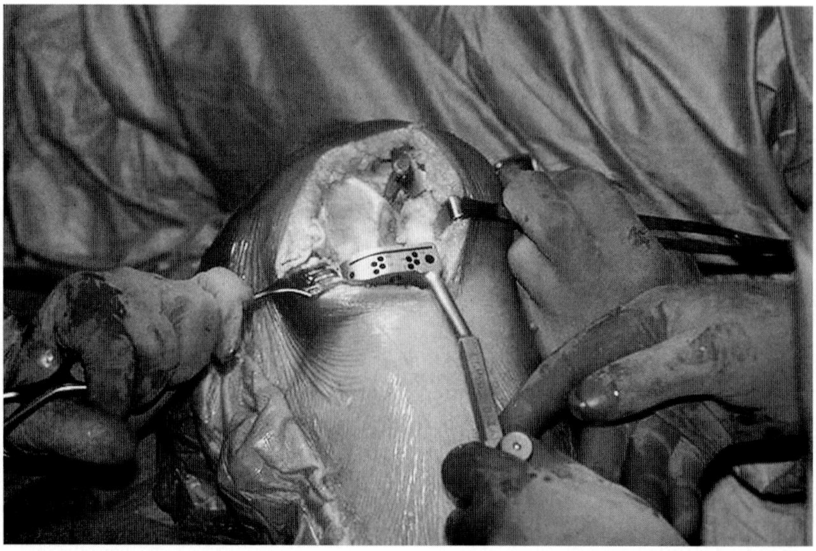

Figure 13.10. The tibial cut is complete with an extramedullary guide.

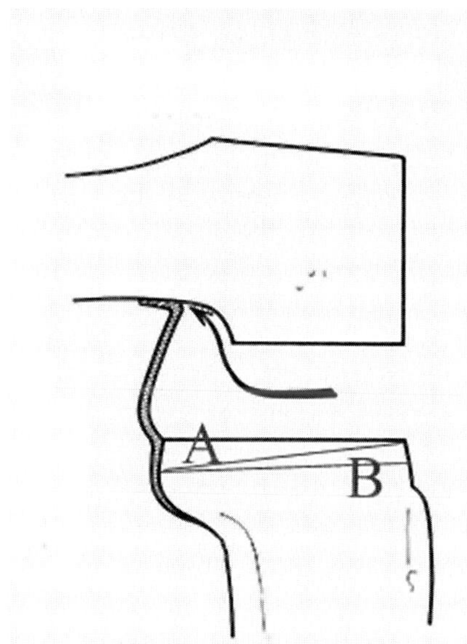

Figure 13.11. The slope of the tibial cut can be changed to correct flexion extension imbalance. The flexion gap is often larger than the extension gap. The cut A can be lowered anteriorly and the slope decreased to line B, which will equalize the gaps.

side without everting the patella. The tibial cut can be angled from anterior to posterior. Most systems favor a 5 degree to 7 degree posterior slope for roll back. The slope of the cut also affects the flexion-extension balancing. The balancing is not the same as the techniques for TKA. In the UKA surgery, the flexion gap is usually larger than the extension gap because of the flexion contracture that is present in almost all arthritic knees. As the flexion contracture increases to 10 degrees, the extension gap becomes tighter. If the slope of the tibial cut is decreased from the anatomic slope of the preoperative tibial x-ray, the cut can be made deeper anteriorly to give greater space in extension while maintaining the same flexion gap posteriorly (Figure 13.11). This is the alternate technique for flexion contracture correction if the distal femoral valgus is normal at 5 degrees or less.

With the completion of the tibial cut, the remainder of the femoral cuts can be completed with the appropriate blocks for guidance of the saws. An intramedullary retractor can be used to retract the patella (Figure 13.12). The femoral runner should be a slight bit smaller than the original femoral condyle surface and should be perpendicular to the tibial plateau at 90 degrees of flexion and centered medial to lateral on the condyle. If the femoral condyle divergence is extreme in 90 degrees of flexion, the femoral component should be positioned perpendicular to the tibial cut surface (parallel to the long axis of the tibia). This positioning may result in some overhang of the femoral runner into the intercondylar notch (Figure 13.13).

The tibial tray should cover the entire cut surface out to the cortical rim without overhang on the medial or lateral side of the tibia. The component is not in/aid and any degree of varus positioning should be avoided. The inlay technique depends on the subchondral bone surface for support and if this is violated during the tibial preparation, sinkage of the component will certainly follow. Varus inclination can lead to early component loosening and should be avoided.

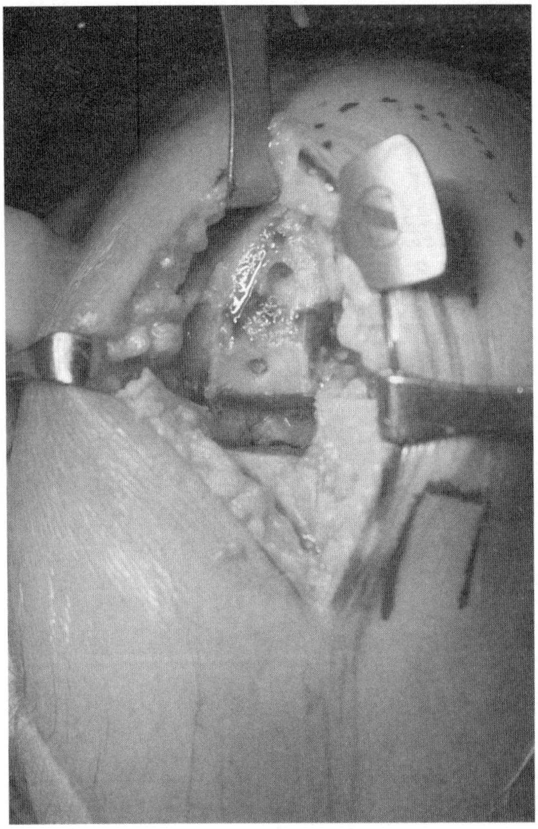

Figure 13.12. The intramedullary retractor is useful to visualize the joint (labeled Z).

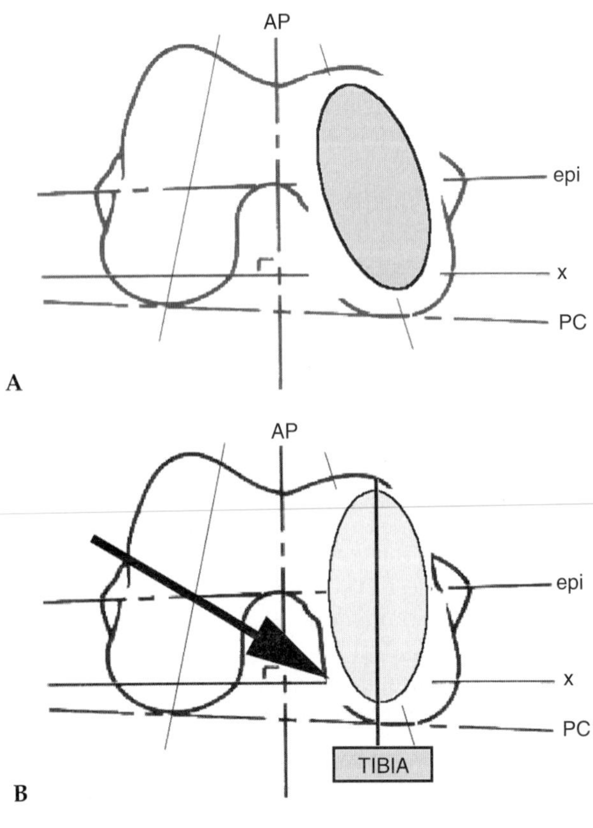

Figure 13.13. (A) If the femoral component is aligned with the cut articular surface of the femur, the divergence of the condyles may be too great and the subsequent position may lead to edge loading on the polyethylene tibial insert. (B) The femoral component should be perpendicular to the tibial insert even if this leads to a nonanatomic position on the femoral surface and slight overhang of the component into the intercondylar notch.

Once the cuts are completed, the flexion-extension gap should be tested with the trial components in position. In the ideal case there should be 2 mm of laxity in both positions (Figure 13.14). It is best not to overtighten the joint and to accept greater rather than less laxity. Excess tightness may lead to early polyethylene failure and also contributes to increased pressure transmission to the opposite side. Three

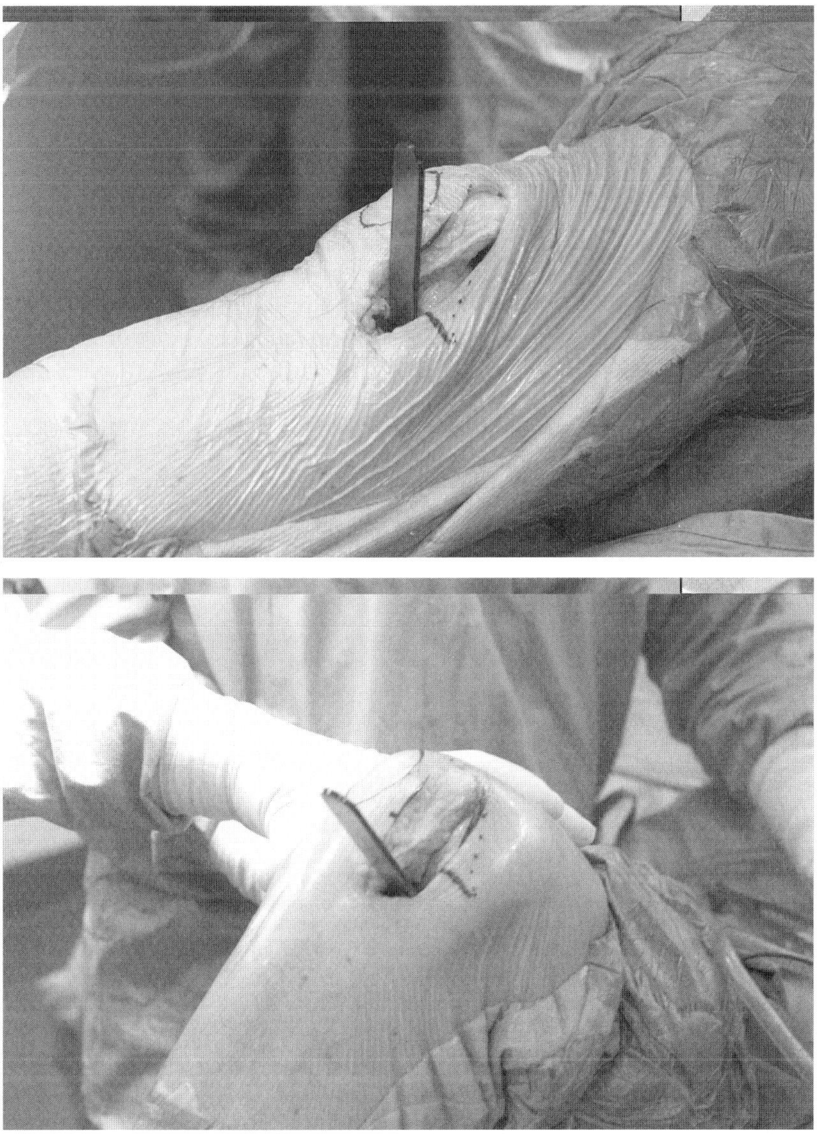

A

B

Figure 13.14. (A) The tongue depressor is 2 mm thick and demonstrates the proper laxity in full extension of the knee. (B) The tongue depressor demonstrates the matching proper laxity in 90 degrees of flexion. (By permission of Choi YJ, Tanavalee A, Chan A, et al. Unicondylar knee arthroplasty: surgical approach and early results of the minimally invasive surgical approach. In Scuderi GR, Tria, Jr., AJ [eds]: MIS of the Hip and the Knee: A Clinical Perspective. New York: Springer, 2004.)

separate items determine the overall varus or valgus of the knee: the depth of the tibial cut, the tibial polyethylene thickness, and the depth of the femoral cut. The tibia can be cut exactly perpendicular and the distal femoral cut can be set in 4 degrees of valgus; but with the insertion of an excessively thick polyethylene, the knee can be shifted into 6 or more degrees of valgus and overcorrected despite properly aligned bone cuts. In the setting of the TKA, changing the thickness of the tibial insert affects spacing in full extension and 90 degrees of flexion but it does not affect the varus of valgus of the knee which remains the same.

If the UKA spacing is not symmetric, the tibial cut should be altered. Typically, the extension space will be smaller than the flexion space. This can be corrected by starting the tibial cut slightly deeper on the anterior surface and decreasing the slope angle. Once again, in TKA the extension space is easily increased by removing more bone from the distal femur. In UKA deepening the femoral cut will change the distal femoral valgus and will also increase the size of the component because the anteroposterior surface will be widened. This may lead to poor bone contact with the new femoral component and possible early loosening. Thus, it is best to modify the spacing with changes on the tibial side. If the space in extension is larger than the flexion space, this usually means that the slope of the tibial cut was made too shallow and the slope should just be increased. Figure 13.15 outlines the corrections that can be made if the spacing is not ideal.

After testing the components for stability, range of motion, and flexion-extension balance, the final components are cemented in place. Cementless fixation for UKA has not been very successful and the

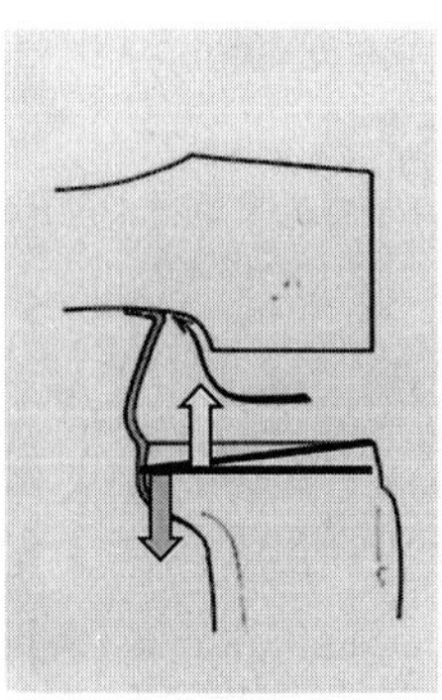

S = Slope

FLEX/EXT → / ↓	0	1	2
0	RECUT 2mm	⇩S	⇩S
1	⇧S	RECUT 1mm	⇩S
2	⇧S	⇧S	PERFECT!

AJT

Figure 13.15. UKA spacing. Measurements of laxity of the knee in full extension and in 90 degrees of flexion with the appropriate changes that should be made in the slope of the tibial cut to equalize the gaps. (By permission of Choi YJ, Tanavalee A, Chan A, et al. Unicondylar knee arthroplasty: surgical approach and early results of the minimally invasive surgical approach. In Scuderi GR, Tria, Jr., AJ [eds]: MIS of the Hip and the Knee: A Clinical Perspective. New York: Springer, 2004.)

authors do not recommend that approach. When the tibial component is a modular design, the metal tray can be cemented in place first and this allows excellent visualization of the posterior aspect of the joint and also allows more space for the femoral component cementing. The all polyethylene insert does give more thickness to the prosthesis. However, the thicker polyethylene blocks visualization for the cementing; and, if full thickness polyethylene failure occurs, the exchange will require invasion of the underlying tibial bone. The modular tibial tray allows polyethylene exchange without bone invasion and backside wear is not a problem in UKA surgery. The femoral runner is cemented after the tibial tray, and the polyethylene is inserted last.

The tourniquet is released before the closure and adequate hemostasis is established. The closure of the arthrotomy is performed with nonabsorbable sutures in an interrupted fashion over a single drain. The medial closure should be clinically checked to be sure that it is neither too loose nor too tight. The patellar tracking should be checked before closing the subcutaneous tissues.

At the time of closure, some surgeons prefer to inject the surrounding tissues with a local anesthetic to permit more comfortable activity immediately after the surgery. The authors have not found this to be particularly helpful but it is certainly not contraindicated.

Results

At present there are few reports using the MIS surgical approach. Berger's report[9] included a 10 year follow-up with 98% longevity using standard open arthrotomy techniques. The average age of the patients was 68 and the indications for the procedure were quite strict. Price reported early follow-up of an abbreviated incision for UKA with good results.[10] He compared 40 Oxford UKAs using an MIS type incision with 20 Oxford UKAs performed with a standard incision. The average rate of recovery of the MIS UKAs was twice as fast. The accuracy of the implantation was evaluated using 11 variables on fluoroscopically centered postoperative x-rays and was found to be the same as the open UKAs. Price concluded that more rapid recovery was possible with less morbidity. The technique did not compromise the final result of the UKA. Repicci reported on 136 knees with eight years of follow-up using the MIS technique.[2] There were ten revisions (7%): three for technical errors, one for poor pain relief, five for advancing disease, and one for fracture. The revisions for technical errors occurred from 6 to 25 months after surgery. The revisions for advancing disease occurred from 37 to 90 months after surgery. Repicci concluded that MIS UKA is "... an initial arthroplasty procedure (that) relieves pain, restores limb alignment, and improves function with minimal morbidity without interfering with future TKA."

The senior author has performed 320 UKAs using the Miller-Galante Unicondylar Knee Arthroplasty (Zimmer, Warsaw, IN). Fifty-seven patients underwent UKA in the first year (2000); 41 (72%) patients have 2 or more years of follow up.[11] There are 24 women and 17 men including 6 bilateral surgeries, 4 simultaneous, and 2 staged 6 to 8 weeks apart. There are 47 knees, 45 varus and 2 valgus. Average age is 68 with a range from 42 to 93; 10 patients (30%) are under age 60 and 8 patients (20%) are over age 75. Average weight is 189 pounds. The range of motion went from 120 degrees before the operation to 132 degrees after the surgery. One knee has been converted to a TKA because of patellar subluxation occurring 9 months after the surgery. The revision was performed at 14 months after the original TKA. One patient sustained an undisplaced tibial plateau fracture two weeks after surgery and healed this without intervention. All patients have obtained their full range of motion within three weeks and no components have shown any signs of loosening, thus far. While these are very early results, most of the series with poor results started to see failures within the first two years following the procedure.

Conclusions

The results of UKA have improved steadily through the late 1990s into 2000. The MIS technique has fostered better results and has helped to set UKA apart from TKA in the minds of the operating surgeons. The intramedullary instrumentation has been well adapted to the MIS technique. As the prosthetic designs and surgical techniques continue to improve, MIS UKA should have results similar to those of TKA in the first 10 to 15 years and give patients a choice before TKA that will permit greater activity and improved quality of life without compromising the result of a later TKA.

References

1. Repicci JA, Eberle RW. Minimally invasive surgical technique for unicondylar knee arthroplasty. Journal of the Southern Orthopaedic Association. 1999;8(1):20–27.
2. Romanowski MR, Repicci JA. Minimally invasive unicondylar arthroplasty, eight year follow-up. Journal Knee Surgery. 2002;15(1):17–22.
3. Marmor L. Marmor modular knee in unicompartmental disease. Minimum four-year follow-up. JBJS. 1979;61A:347–353.
4. Insall J, Walker P. Unicondylar knee replacement. Clinical Orthopaedics. 1976;120:83–85.
5. Laskin RS. Unicompartment tibiofemoral resurfacing arthroplasty. JBJS. 1978;60A:182–185.
6. Goodfellow J, O'Connor J. The mechanics of the knee and prosthesis design. JBJS. 1978;60B:358–369.
7. Goodfellow JW, Kershaw CJ, Benson MK, O'Connor JJ. The Oxford knee for unicompartmental osteoarthritis. The first 103 cases. J Bone Joint Surg Br. 1988;70:692–701.
8. Stern SH, Becker MW, Insall J. Unicompartmental knee arthroplasty. An evaluation of selection criteria. CORR. 1993;286:143–148.
9. Berger RA, Nedeff DD, Barden RN, et al. Unicompartmental knee arthroplasty. CORR. 1999;367:50–60.

10. Price AJ, Webb J, Topf H, Dodd CAF, Goodfellow JW, Murray DW and the Oxford Hip and Knee Group. Rapid recovery after Oxford Unicompartmental Arthroplasty through a short incision. J Arthroplasty. 2001;16: 970–976.
11. Gesell MW, Tria AJ Jr. MIS Unicondylar Knee Arthroplasty: Surgical approach and early results. Clin Orthop Relat Res. 2004;428:53–60.

14

Minimally Invasive Surgery for Unicondylar Knee Arthroplasty: The Extramedullary Tensor Technique

Paul L. Saenger

The extramedullary (EM) tensor tools and surgical technique were developed to orient cutting guides for the implantation of the MG uni prosthesis with greater ease and accuracy and to reduce the surgical morbidity of this limited reconstruction. Unicompartmental knee replacement attempts to reduce pain and improve function by restoring the extremity's alignment and the joint's soft tissue balance with the positioning of an implant limited to that compartment. All uni implants, be they monoblock wafers, mobile bearing devices, or fixed articular prostheses, must effect this restoration to enjoy whatever success they may provide.

Various surgical techniques for their implantation are available. Instrument systems without direct linkage of the femoral and tibial cuts require intuitive estimates. With such a technique the implant must, in effect, be retrofitted. The cuts are made and then a device of a given volume and width is chosen that best fits the flexion and extension gaps created. Those cuts were not predetermined for a given implant and thus are approximations. Approximations can work well should there be unlimited prosthetic sizes from which to choose.

The relationship between the bone cuts and the subsequent insertion of an implant with its particular geometry filling the created extension and flexion gaps, it should be remembered, is the key to the angular and soft tissue balance one is attempting to achieve. Instruments now exist that allow the anticipated cuts to be positioned relative to a knee's corrected posture. There is a direct relationship such that the cuts made are specific for a given implant's dimensions. The EM tensor technique herein described uses patented instrumentation with direct linkage, referencing off the femur and tibia simultaneously. Knowing the dimensions of the intended implant in both extension and flexion then allows the use of cutting guides that create spatial dimensions, that is,

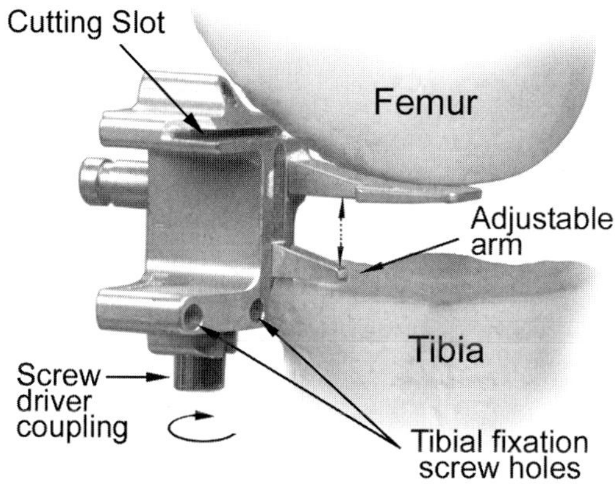

Figure 14.1. The tensor device.

extension and flexion gaps, to accommodate a particular composite implant.

The Tensor

The tensor device is an adjustable interposed spacer with incorporated tibial and femoral cutting surfaces that is positioned in extension between the femur and tibia while their articular surfaces are held in a corrected position. The space to be created for a given implant can then be made with a specific width and slope oriented at will prior to setting the surface cutting guides. The relationship of the two cut surfaces is set with respect to a preachieved correction of the soft tissue tension and overall limb alignment (Figure 14.1).

Predetermined flexion and extension gaps lessen the need to modify or compensate for an imbalance potentially created by guesswork. The need for subsequent *eye ball* revisions is reduced. Alignment instruments that measure first and cut second attempt to eliminate the inaccuracies and secondary complexities of the bone preparation.

Minimally Invasive Surgery

Central to developing the EM tensor system was the desire to lessen the morbidity associated with this limited reconstruction. The invasiveness of any surgical procedure is certainly more than the length of the incision. In the case of knee reconstruction, the extent of the quadriceps division, the intrusion of the intramedullary canal,[1,2] or the use of a tourniquet add to the morbidity of the effort. To avoid or limit such compromising elements is the goal of MIS. The tensor technique requires a small skin incision, usually 4 cm to 7 cm, a modest division of the vastus medialis oblique (VMO), no intrusion of the intramedullary canal and no need for a tourniquet.

The instruments and implants detailed in this chapter will likely be soon replaced with new versions. However, the concept and use of artificial implants that adhere to the host bone so as to anatomically reconstruct articular surfaces will likely endure. Their surgical implantation will require an ever more accurate and less morbid technique. Understanding the nature of this implant, the Zimmer MG uni, and its attendant EM tensioning instrumentation and technique is apropos to the consideration of future developments.

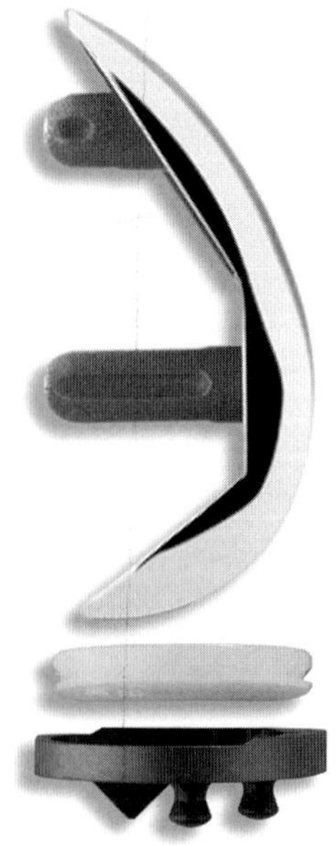

Figure 14.2. The MG uni prosthesis.

The Implant

Unicompartmental knee reconstruction using femoral and tibial implants that mimic the original geometry of the host articular surfaces and that are secured to cut bone with cement has been shown to offer reliably good to excellent results.[3–8] Several series have demonstrated the MG uni (Zimmer, Inc., Warsaw, IN) prosthesis to offer success for at least 10 years equal to or better than TKA in middle aged or older populations.[9–11] The prosthesis consists of a biconvex chrome cobalt femoral component with three precoated backside facets. It is cemented to three matching cut femoral bone surfaces; planed cuts that determined the implant's position and orientation. The tibial implant, either monoblock or modular, is available in incremental widths of 8 mm, 10 mm, 12 mm, and 14 mm. It, too, is cemented to a cut, planed surface (Figure 14.2).

Measure First, Cut Second

Regardless of future navigational aids for yet to be designed implants, it will likely require orienting the bone preparation for a given implant relative to a specifically corrected and thereafter maintained joint and limb posture.

The tensor technique uses a space filling tensioner that serves as an adjustable expansive unit between the femur and tibia that maintains the corrected alignment and tissue balance in extension. With that done, the femoral and tibial cutting blocks, using shared fixation screws, are set so as to create a space equal to the intended implant's composite width. The orientation of the surfaces to be cut can be accurately established. As presently configured, those surfaces are parallel to one another in the coronal plane. In the sagittal plane, the slope on the tibia is adjustable to 3 degrees, 5 degrees, or 7 degrees. These cut surface relationships could be readily altered if it is determined to be otherwise optimal (Figure 14.3A and B).

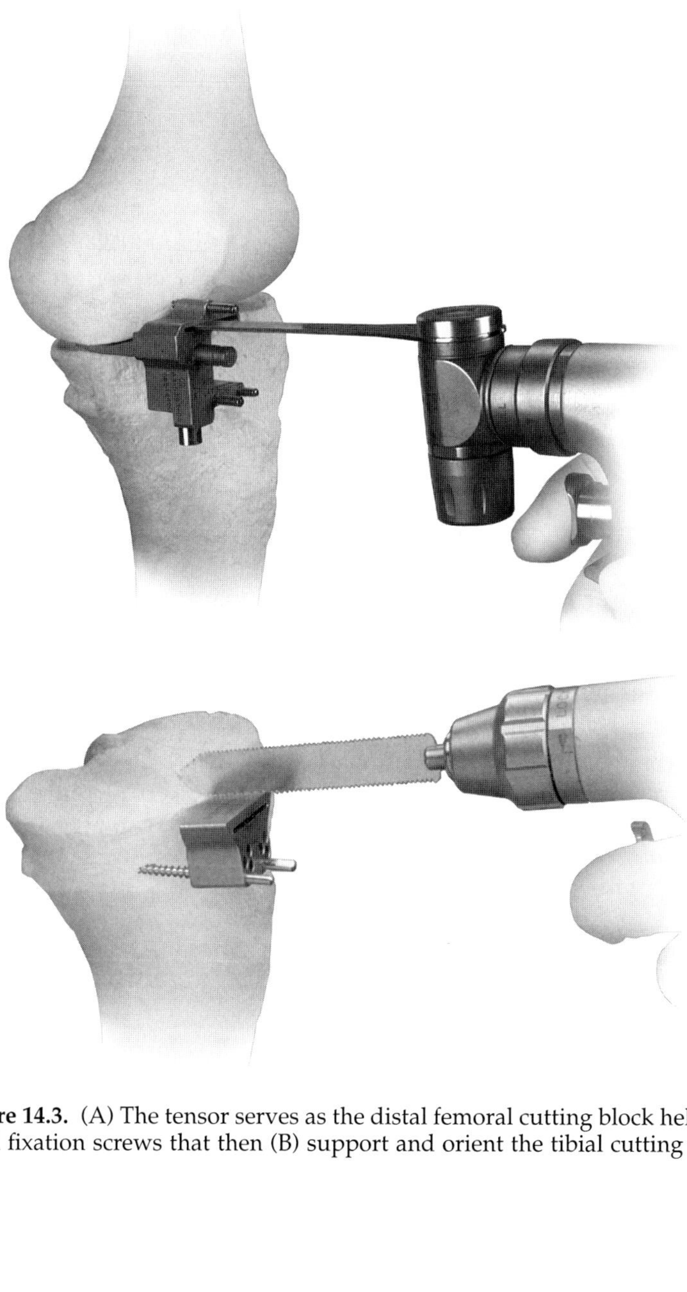

A

B

Figure 14.3. (A) The tensor serves as the distal femoral cutting block held with tibial fixation screws that then (B) support and orient the tibial cutting block.

How Much Correction?

Occasionally, unicompartmental pathology does not involve significant deformity of the joint space and thus the alignment and tissue balance are intact. In that case, maintaining the existing dynamic geometric relationships is a fundamental goal of the procedure. More often, with the eccentric loss of articular and meniscal cartilage seen in unicompartmental disease, the knee falls into varus or valgus. This intraarticular loss secondarily affects the ligamentous stability. By restoring the intraarticular spacing, the ligaments are again tensioned. Assuming there is no soft tissue contracture, replacing the lost cartilage and bone with an implant of equal dimensions should restore both the joint's soft tissue tension and overall alignment relative to the mechanical and anatomical axes.

Alignment and soft tissue balance are critical to the success of total knee arthroplasties, too. However, it must be understood that the alignment of the extremity as a whole in TKA is a function of the angle of the cuts. That is not true for a uni. For instance, in TKA, a 6-degree femoral cut combined with a standard 0 degree cut on the tibia can be expected to result in a femoral-tibial angle of 6 degrees. Varying the thickness of the plastic insert will affect the soft tissue tension but not the angle of the extremity's alignment.

Varying the thickness of the insert in a uni directly affects the soft tissue tension as well. But unlike the TKA, in a uni it is an eccentric variation and changes the alignment, too. In that sense it is similar to the angular alteration seen with wedge resection or insertion used in high tibial osteotomies. However, unlike HTO, a uni insert is intraarticular and thus the addition of a thicker implant will, once the soft tissues are already snug, overstuff the joint. Too wide a prosthesis creates intraarticular compressive forces detrimental to not only the implant, but to the uninvolved compartment as well and can be expected to be deleterious to both.[12] It is very important to avoid overstuffing the joint throughout its arc of movement from extension to flexion.

The mechanical axis of the lower extremity is that line that passes through the center of the hip, knee and ankle. This system assumes that a mechanical axis of 0 degrees is a reference point, not a target. It is thought that knees that fall into varus for want of medial cartilage were likely in some varus relative to a 0 degree mechanical axis even before the pathology notably altered the alignment. Thus, to force that knee to 0 degrees would presumably go beyond what was once normal and in so doing would tighten the medial ligaments beyond their norm. Therefore, when using the mechanical axis as a guide, the correction will typically fall slightly short of full correction to 0 degrees.[13]

While the two, alignment and soft tissue tension, are directly related and can each be used to help assess the correction, it is the latter, the soft tissue tension, that is thought to be most critical. Until such time as a more sophisticated method of measuring intracompartmental pressure is used, the present system relies on the manual and visual perceptions of the surgeon such that a valgus stress (or varus in the

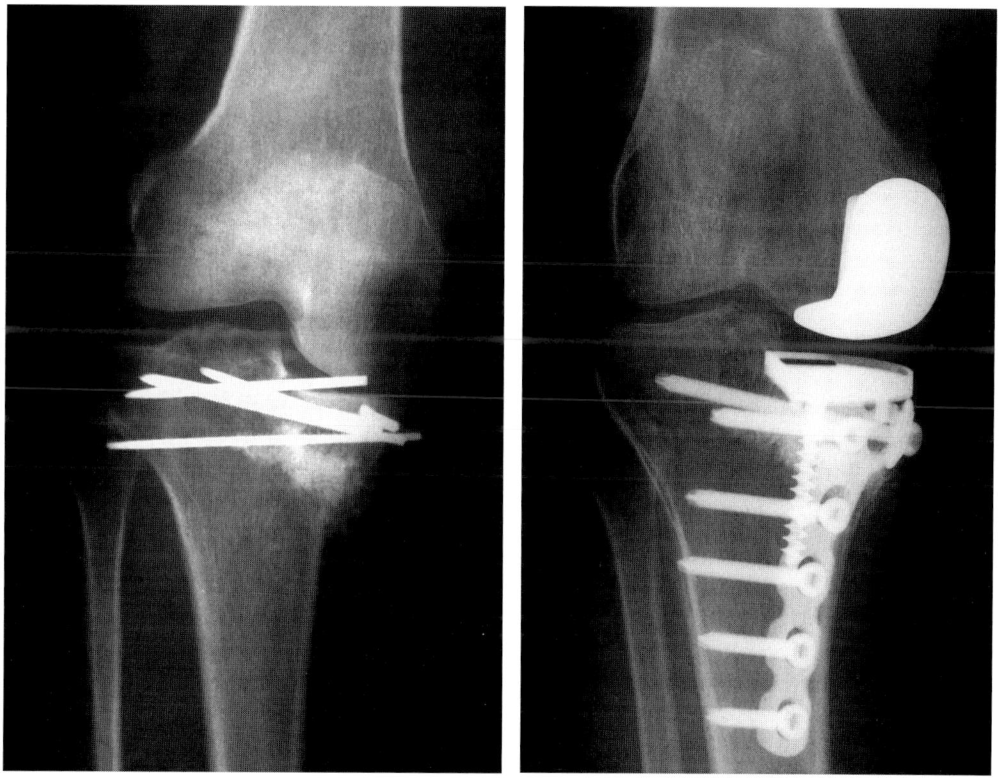

A B

Figure 14.4. (A) Nonunion with varus nine months status post inadequate fixation of medial tibial plateau fracture in a 51-year-old woman. (B) Four year postoperative x-ray of uni reconstruction with soft-tissue release for a contracture using Sulzer Natural Knee Uni. Pre-op ROM, 5–65 degrees; postoperative, 3–122 degrees.

case of lateral reconstruction) should allow approximately 2 mm of opening. Regardless of the alignment, if the ligaments are too tight and the knee overstuffed, the long-term success of the procedure is likely to be compromised.

In the author's experience, most knees felt to be appropriate for this procedure can be adequately corrected without soft tissue release. Indeed, for many knees, there may be little or no angular or ligamentous deformity. However, in selected cases, a correction towards an improved alignment and appropriate soft tissue tension requires the release of the soft tissue contracture (Figure 14.4A and B).

Surgical Technique

Medial unicompartmental degenerative joint disease can be seen as a disease of extension.[14] Cartilage loss on the femur, for instance, is often minimal on the posterior condyle where it articulates with the tibia in flexion. Rather, the more profound compromise occurs on the distal end of the condyle in the area that articulates with the tibia as the knee

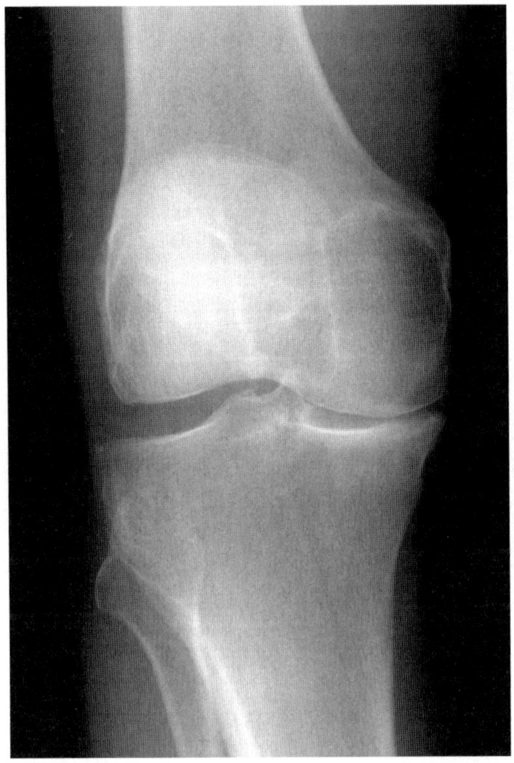

Figure 14.5. X-ray of medial DJD with varus deformity.

extends. Genu varum is an extension deformity. The correction to be made is in extension (Figure 14.5).

Keying off the distal femur with a cutting guide that allows the reestablishment of the appropriate joint line, the EM tensor, a variable spacing block inserted into the involved compartment, is adjusted to maintain a corrected extension alignment. Secured to both femur and tibia by shared fixation posts, coordinated cutting blocks serve to allow the distal femoral and then the tibial cuts to be made in a directly linked fashion that will prepare this predetermined space to be filled by an anticipated implant (Figure 14.6A–E).

With the extension pathology restructured, it is time to balance the flexion gap. It is important that the knee not be compromised in flexion by over- or undertensioning the flexion gap with inappropriate bone preparation or inaccurate femoral sizing. To avoid that complication, a gauge is used to predict the ensuing flexion gap. This ensures that the subsequent cut on the posterior femur combined with the cut already made on the tibia creates a flexion space whose soft tissue tension is consistent with that established for extension.

The EM tensor technique is intended to follow sequential steps. Altering the sequence may compromise the end result. With experience, the procedure can be regularly accomplished with a 4-cm

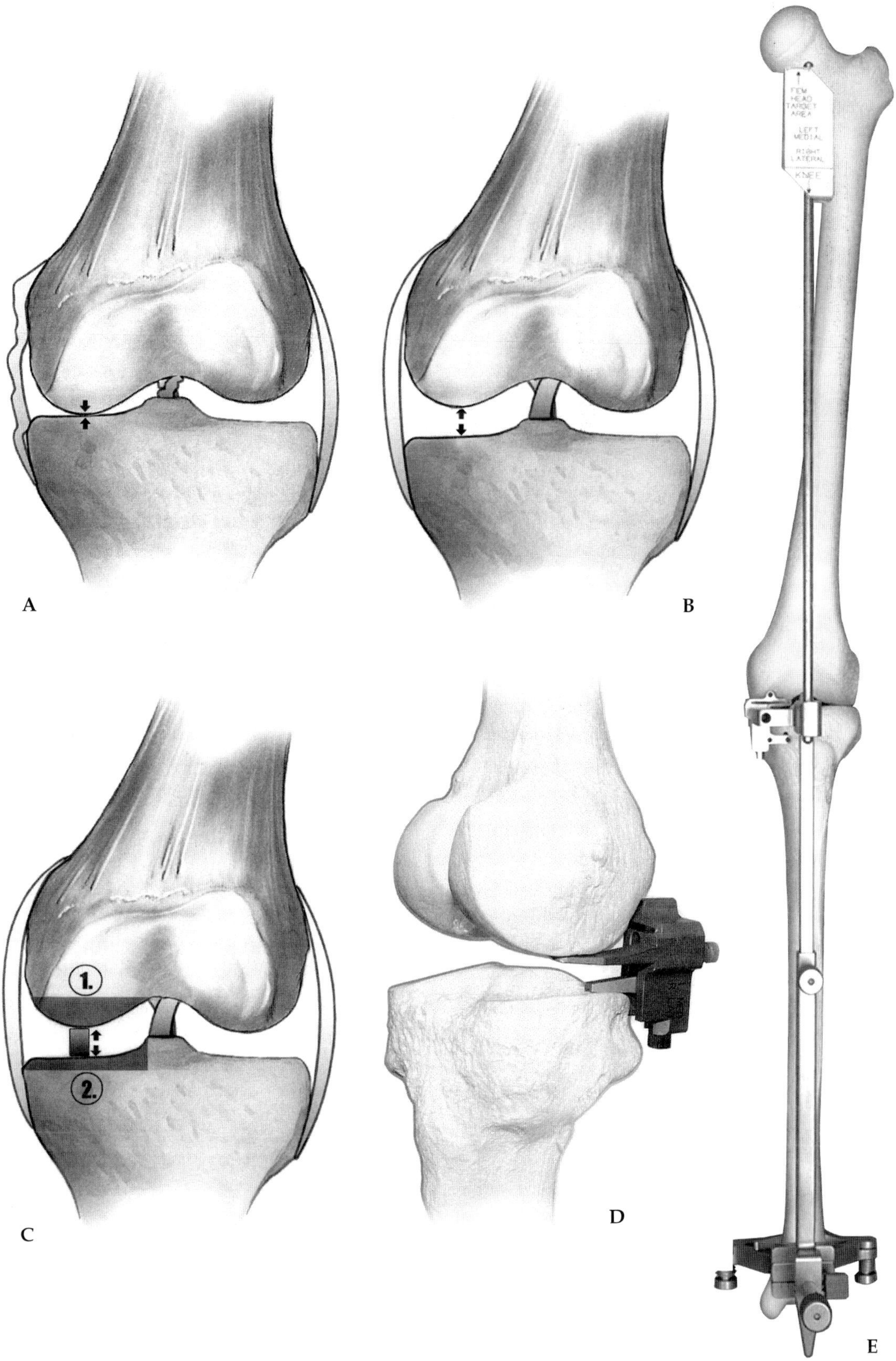

Figure 14.6. (A) The narrowed medial compartment is opened until (B) the medial ligaments are tensioned. (C) The space is filled with the tensor, (D) setting parallel cuts (1 and 2) for the intended implant. (E) Attached alignment rods confirm orientation.

to 7-cm skin incision, the extent of which has the potential to shrink further with future innovation.

Given the restricted space, the intact ligaments and the modest incision, adequate exposure requires that the limb be postured and manipulated in specific ways to facilitate the various steps. For instance, knee extension relaxes the quad mechanism and allows displacement of the patella not possible with even slight flexion with the VMO intact. Thus, certain steps are best done in full extension, whereas other steps require flexion to as much as 120 degrees. In that case, maintaining a valgus stress while holding the leg externally rotated for a medial reconstruction will, along with the wise use of retractors, enhance greatly the exposure.

The following description of the surgical technique reflects one surgeon's way of doing things. It represents a considered effort to minimize the morbidity and ensure proper implant positioning. It involves obtaining a preoperative AP hip x-ray with markers over the hip joint in an effort to determine accurately the mechanical axis as a reference point for limb alignment. Also, the use of a tourniquet is thought to be unnecessary. That uni procedures are routinely done successfully without x-rays and with tourniquets is recognized. It is also known that large numbers of prosthetic devices of this and similar design have been implanted with reported good results using indirectly linked cutting or measuring guides. That is a credit to the skill and understanding of those surgeons implanting the prosthesis. It also suggests the potential and adaptability of these secured implants. The EM tensor technique was developed to lessen the guesswork by providing accurate, reproducible cuts with minimally invasive instruments that can diminish many of the complexities inherent to this procedure.

The great majority of uni reconstructions are done medially and of those, most are in middle-aged to older men and women with a narrowed medial compartment secondary to osteoarthritis as seen on physical examination and standing x-rays. The procedure is thus described for that compartment with that pathology in mind and assumes some varus misalignment with associated medial ligament laxity that allows correction without soft tissue release. The steps of the procedure are the same whether this deformity is a little or a lot. Lateral reconstruction is essentially the same other than the incision is made lateral to the patella.

Surgical Steps

Incision

The length and position of the incision is dependent on the exposure required for certain surgical steps done in flexion (Table 14.1). In extension, the arthrotomy is a window that can be moved about for better viewing. In flexion, however, the quad is tight and the patella locked

Table 14.1. Surgical steps for extramedullary tensor technique for unicondylar knee arthroplasty

1. Incision
2. Removal of the anterior boss of the tibia
3. Alignment correction
4. Distal femoral cut
5. Tibial cuts
6. Flexion and extension gaps
7. Anterior femoral marking
8. Femoral finishing guide sizing and positioning
9. Tibial sizing and finishing
10. Trial and cementing

into the trochlea. Knowing what must be seen in flexion, that is, the anterior aspect of the distal femur down to the tibial joint line just medial to the patellar tendon, can then serve to guide the proximal and distal extent of the skin and retinaculum incision.

Therefore, with the knee flexed, an incision is made slightly medial to the midline from near the superior pole of the patella to just a few millimeters below the joint line. Likewise, divide the medial retinaculum and fat pad. Excise a portion of the fat pad in the area along with the anterior third of the meniscus. Use electrocautery for hemostasis. Excise osteophytes found on the femur, tibia and patella. For exposure now and whenever the knee is flexed, use a 90 degree bent sharp Hohmann's retractor positioned in the notch and a similar retractor or two along the medial tibia. Importantly, this also protects the cruciates and MCL while using saw blades (Figures 14.7 and 14.8).

Removal of the Anterior Boss of the Tibia

Positioning and manipulating the tensor is made easier by removing the anterior tibial boss normally encountered. With the reciprocating saw, make a 2 cm or 3 mm deep cut along the medial edge of the tibial spine parallel to the tibial axis. Then, with the oscillating saw, remove the tibial boss perpendicular to the tibial axis to a depth of about 3 mm. This additional space makes easier the insertion of the spacer arms and also improves the interface between the active (it moves) tibial arm and the surface of the anterior tibial plateau (Figure 14.9).

Alignment Correction

The tensor and alignment rods are positioned with the knee in extension. To ease their assembly, put the tensor into the joint with the

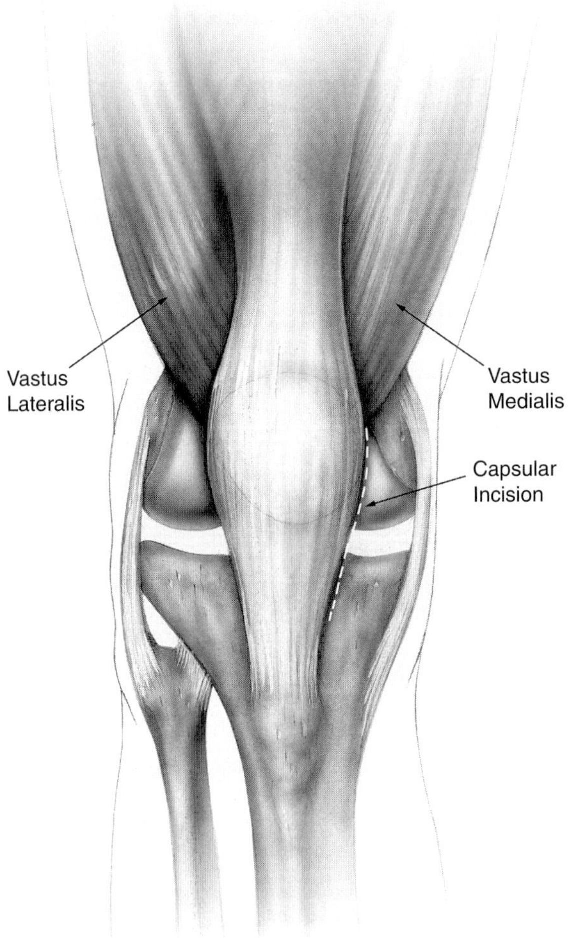

Figure 14.7. The incision.

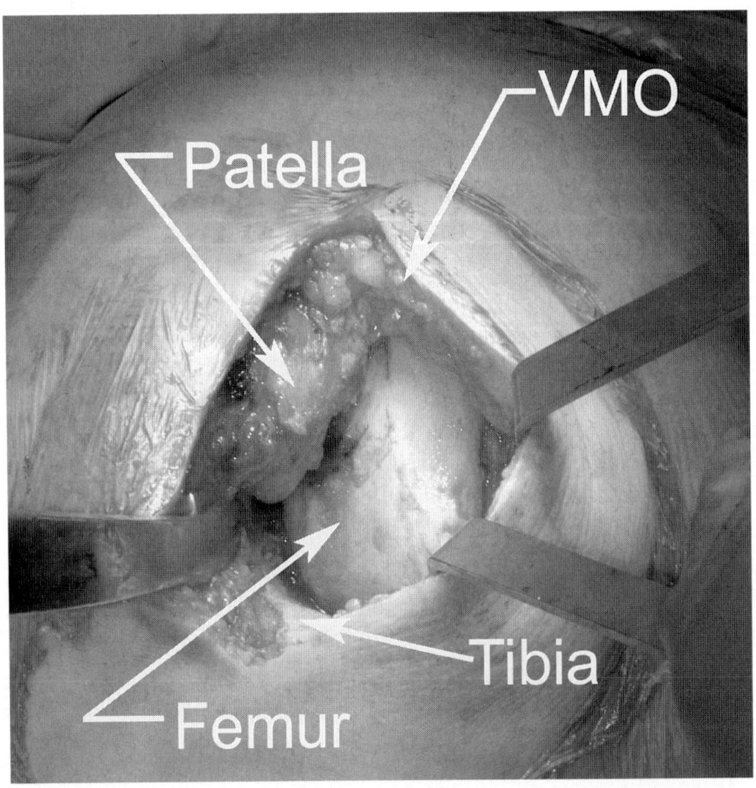

Figure 14.8. The exposure in flexion. VMO, vastus medialis oblique.

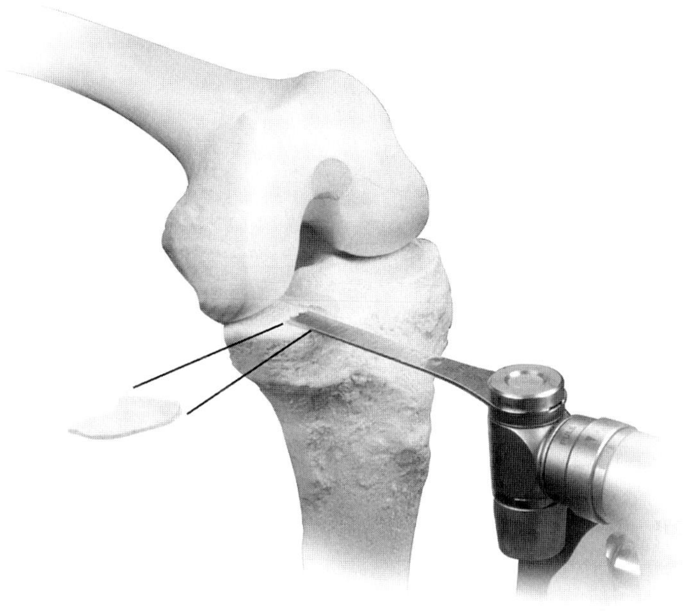

Figure 14.9. Excise the anterior tibial boss.

connecting tower attached. Clamp the tibial alignment rod to the distal leg with the locking screws loose so as to allow multidirectional adjustments. Now, insert the tibia's square alignment rod into the square hole in the tower by manipulating the tensor and tower with the round femoral rod held proximally (Figure 14.10).

With that done, align the tibial rod parallel to the tibia in both the AP and lateral planes and tighten the locking screws (Figure 14.11). So doing determines the orientation but not yet the depth of the tibial cut. The femoral rod should now, in the uncorrected varus knee, project lateral to the marked femoral head. Manually correct the varus with a valgus stress until the soft tissue tension feels snug. Do not force the knee beyond this point. The femoral rod typically still projects lateral to the femoral head, but only slightly (Figure 14.12).

While maintaining this manual correction in extension, have an assistant turn the tensor screw to expand the spacer until contact is felt, implying that the space within the joint created with the manipulation is now filled with the spacing device. Release the manual stress to see that the correction is maintained and that the soft tissue tension is not excessive. If satisfied, position a collared screw in the proximal femoral hole and then two uncollared screws (posts) into the tibia.

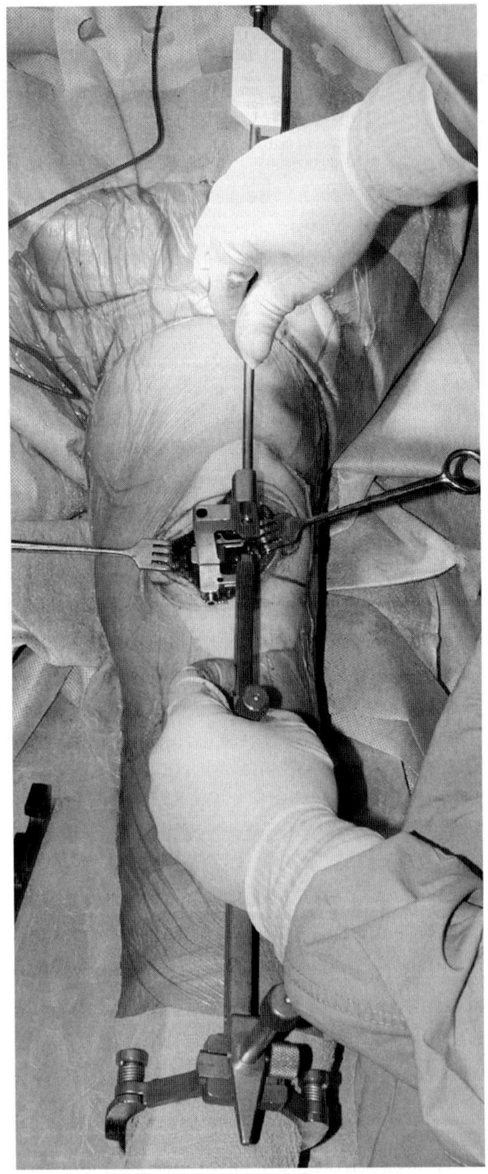

Figure 14.10. Assemble the tensor device, connecting tower, and rods.

Distal Femoral Cut

Remove the tower and rods leaving the spacer and distal femoral cutting guide in place. Using an angled retractor medially and a skin retractor along the patella, resect the distal femur with the oscillating saw. The knee is in extension so be wary of soft tissue injury as the posterior extent of the cut is approached. Remove the femoral collared

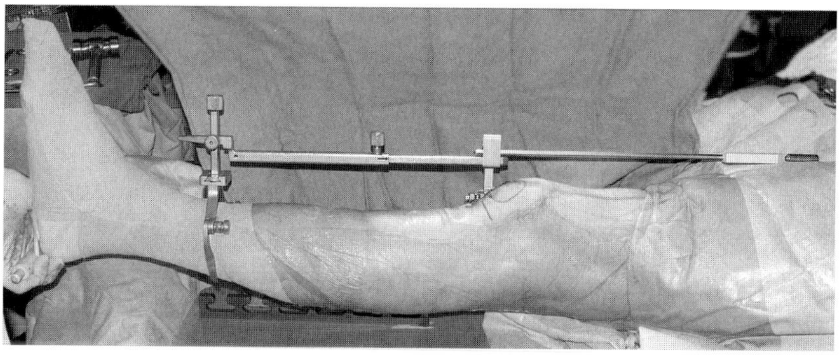

A

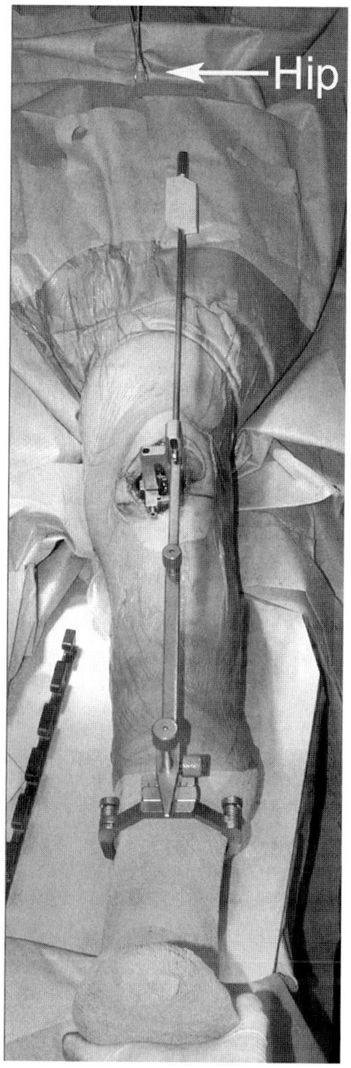

B

Figure 14.11. (A) The tibial rod is aligned parallel to the tibia in the AP and (B) ML planes.

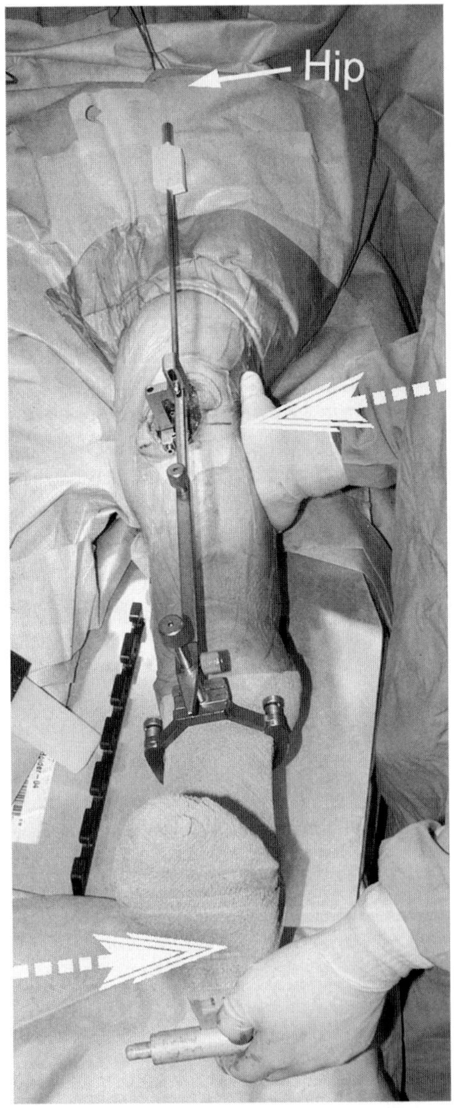

Figure 14.12. Manually correct the alignment.

screw, retract the tensor and slide it off the retained tibial screws (posts) (Figure 14.13).

Tibial Cuts

While still in extension so as to accommodate a small incision, position the tibial cutting block of choice (3-degree, 5-degree, or 7-degree slope) at the desired level (8 mm, 10 mm, 12 mm, or 14 mm) and secure it with a Kocher clamp to each uncollared screw (post). Now flex the knee to 90 degrees so as to relax and protect the posterior soft tissues. Manipulate the leg into valgus and external rotation and then position the retractors.

First, with the reciprocating saw blade just inside the notch in the sagittal plane, cut down to the cutting block. Leave the blade in place to serve as a visual and physical guide for the lateral extent of the ensuing cut. Now, with the oscillating saw, make the sloped cut of the tibial plateau between the protected cruciates and MCL (Figure 14.14A and B).

Flexion and Extension Gaps

The femoral component's sizing and placement keys off the posterior condyle. Therefore, it is important to confirm that the yet to be created flexion gap corresponds to the established extension gap before sizing the femoral component. This is done with the paired extension/flexion gap gauges. If at this time the space is found to be tight, before committing to the posterior condylar cut and its concomitant prosthetic width, open up the flexion gap by shaving off the necessary cartilage and bone from the posterior condyle. Now size the femur. It is easy to adjust the flexion gap before sizing and finishing the femoral cuts. It is difficult to do so afterward (Figure 14.15A and B).

First check the extension gap with an extension gap gauge. It is the thicker end that is equal to the composite width of a given femoral and tibial implant. Determine the one that is optimal in establishing the

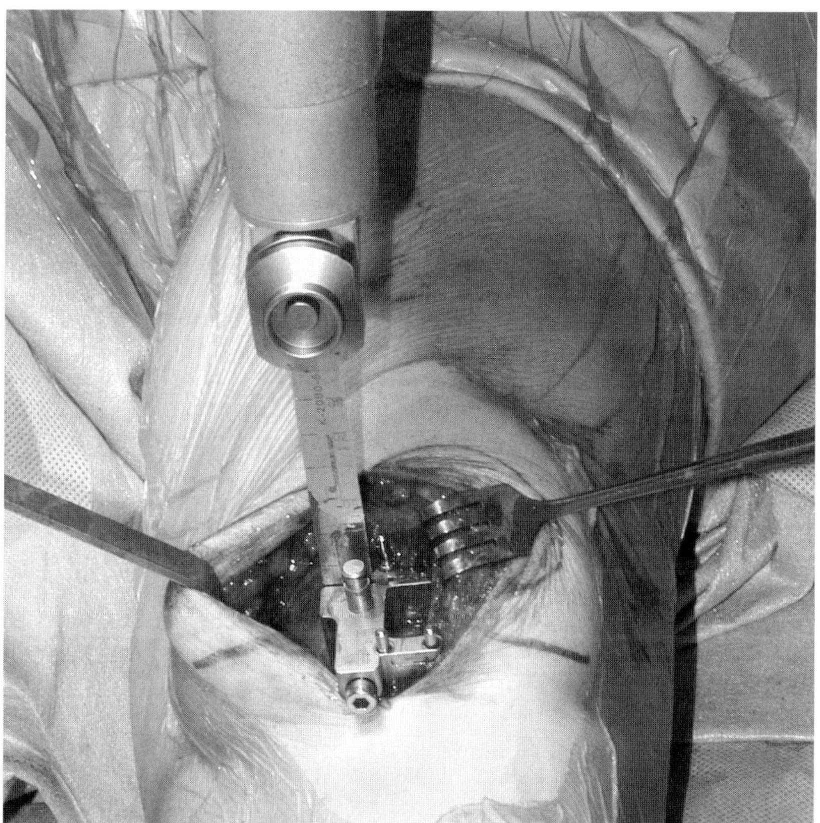

Figure 14.13. Cut the distal femur.

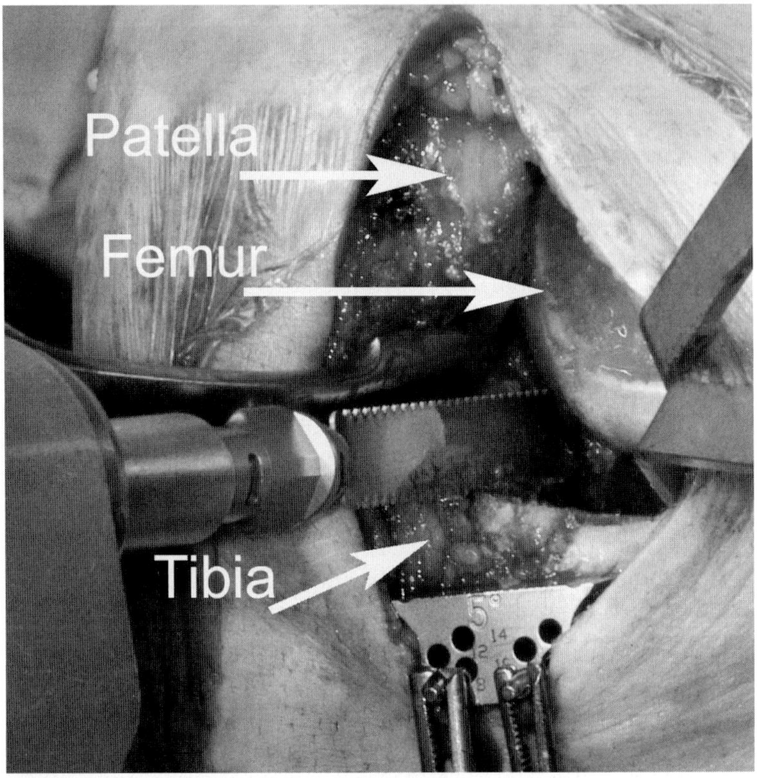

A

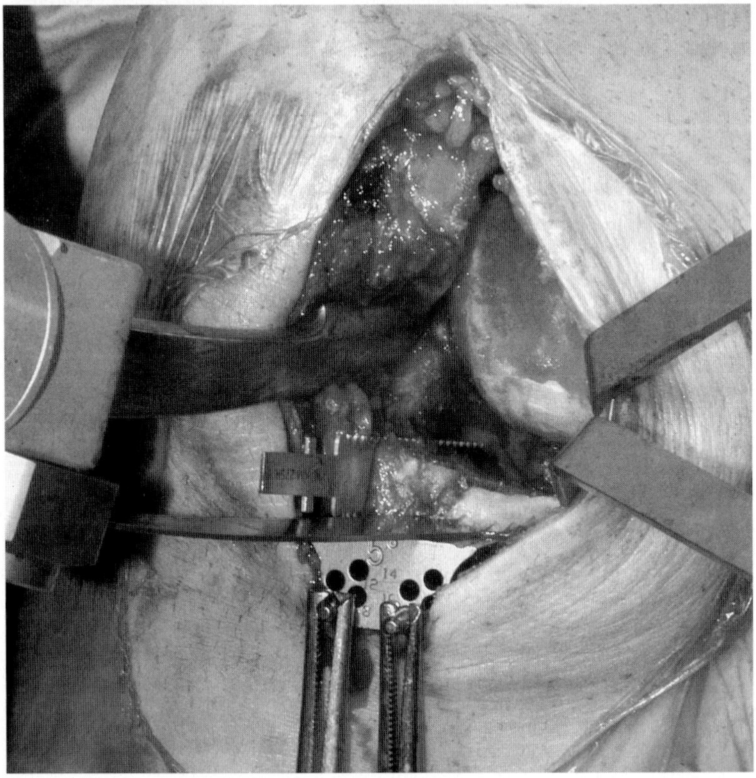

B

Figure 14.14. (A) With the reciprocating saw just lateral to the medial condyle, cut down to the tibial cutting block. (B) Leave the blade in place and protect the MCL with retractors for the oscillating saw cut.

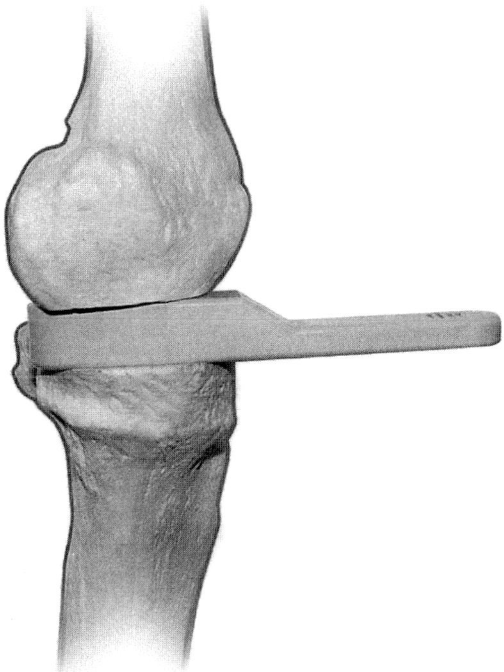
A

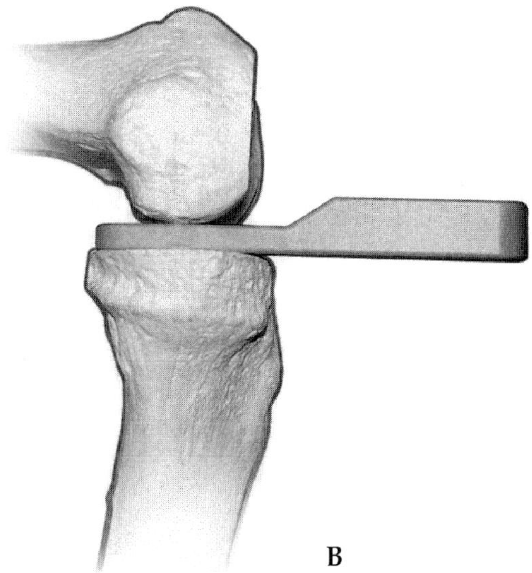
B

Figure 14.15. (A) Extension and (B) flexion gauges.

desired alignment and soft tissue balance. Presumably and usually this corresponds to the cut chosen for the tibia, that is, 8 mm or 10 mm as a rule. Whatever composite width is chosen, 8, 10, 12, or 14, be sure the flexion gap then accommodates those projected components by inserting the thinner end of the gauge, the width of which corresponds to the intended tibial component only. If the flexion gap is tight, unless the posterior reference point for the femoral guide is moved anteriorly, the implant when implanted recreates the tight space. Thus, if tight, resect the cartilage and, occasionally, bone necessary to adequately open up the flexion space.

Anterior Femoral Marking

It is time now for sizing and positioning the femoral component. For that to be done accurately requires clear visualization of the entire cut distal surface of the femur. Doing so in flexion is compromised anteriorly by the tight quad and patella. However, while in extension and with the quad relaxed, the entire cut surface is readily seen. Taking advantage of this clear view in extension, a mark can be made anteriorly on that cut distal surface that corresponds to where the femoral finishing guide should go. Then, when the knee is next brought into flexion, only this mark need be seen, not the entire distal femoral cut surface. This reduces the need for a more extended division of the quad mechanism or the displacement of the patella (Figure 14.16A and B).

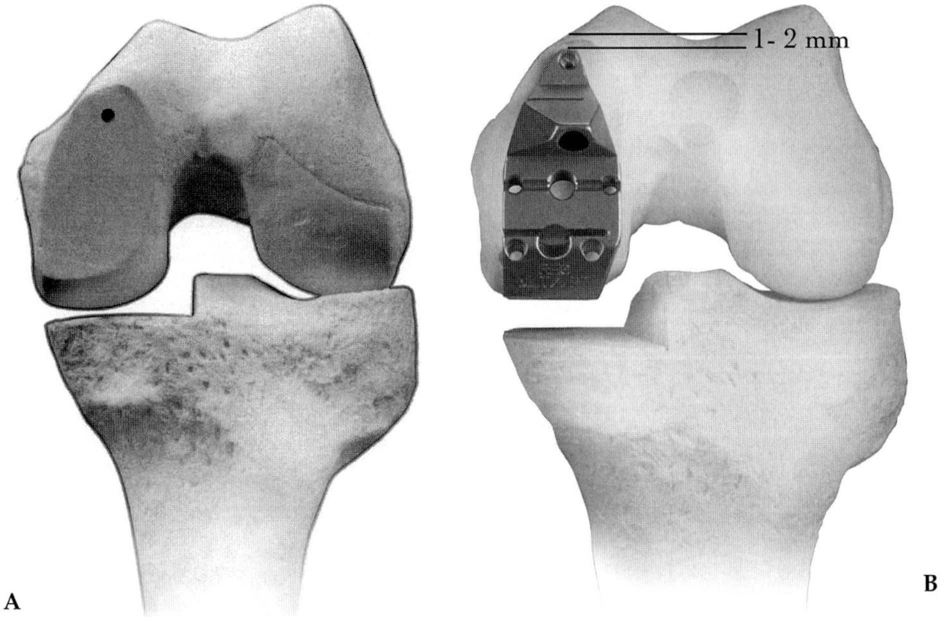

Figure 14.16. (A) Mark the anterior femur at the (B) intended screw fixation site.

Also, an advantage of marking the femur in extension for subsequent positioning of the finishing guide is the ability to center the anterior femoral component relative to the cut tibial surface. If the cuts and post holes for the femoral component are centered in extension and then next in flexion relative to the tibial cut surface, the components will be presumably centered upon one another throughout the arc of motion to, thus, avoid edge loading of the tibial plastic.

Femoral Finishing Guide Sizing and Positioning

Having marked the anterior femur with a bovie or pen in extension, flex the knee to 90 degrees and position the retractors. Choose the femoral finishing guide that when keyed off the posterior condyle has an anterior screw hole that corresponds to the mark. If in doubt as to which size fits best, choose the smaller size to avoid having the femoral implant extend beyond the cut femoral surface anteriorly where it might impinge on the patella.

Secure the guide anteriorly with a collared screw through the hole overlying the mark. With the knee still flexed, rotate the posterior aspect of the guide to a position that again centers it over the cut tibial surface. This typically is accomplished by lining up the notch side of the guide to the very edge of the notch side of the femoral cut surface, that is, rotate the guide to the extreme lateral edge of the femoral cut surface. With the guide secured posteriorly with one or two screws, the post holes are drilled, the chamfer cut is made, and then last, the posterior condyle. Remove the anterior screw and then the guide with its attached posterior condylar fragment (Figure 14.17A–D).

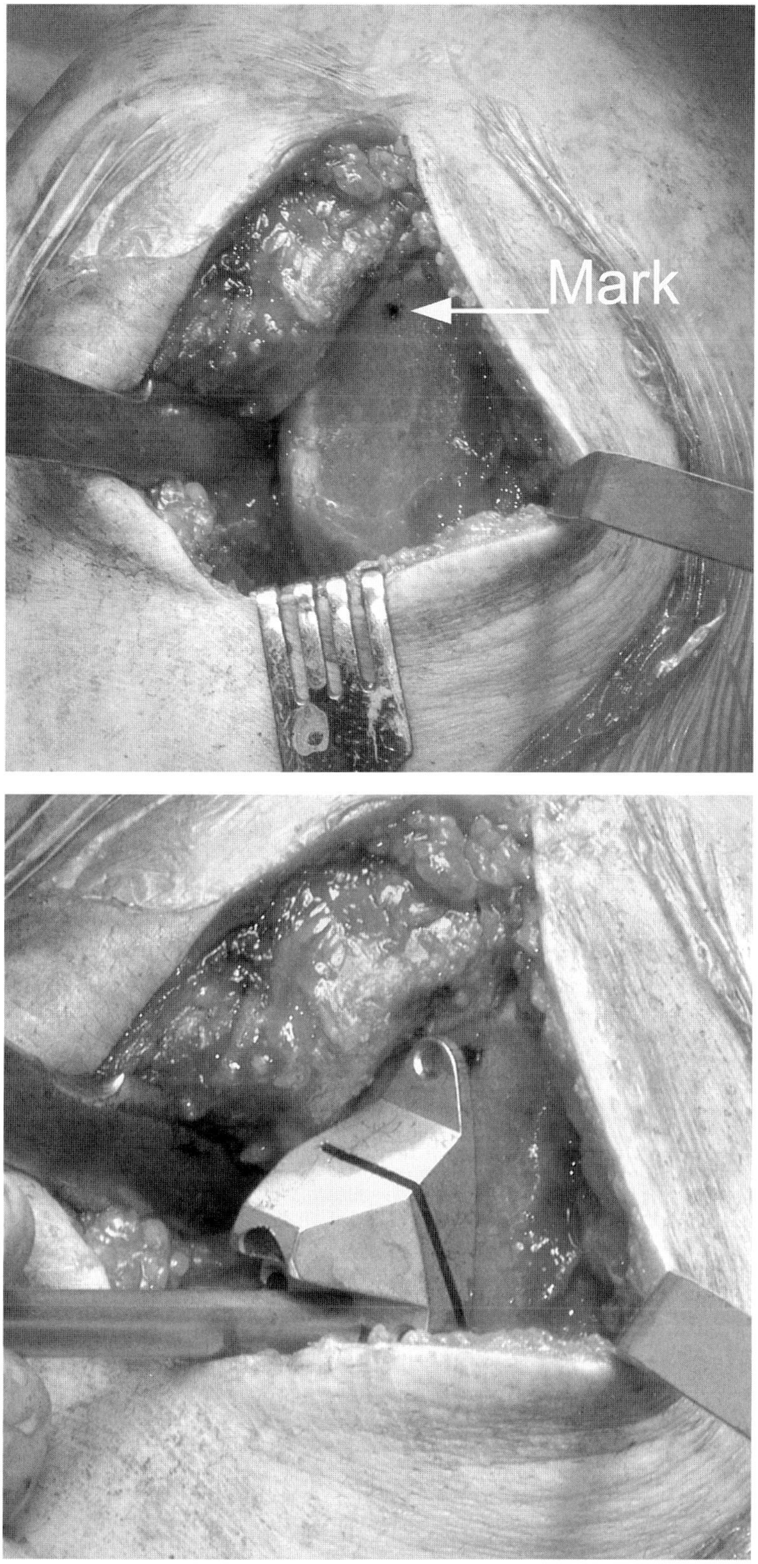

Figure 14.17. (A) The mark is used as (B) a target for securing the femoral cutting guide anteriorly before (C) pivoting it into position posteriorly and (D) securing it with screws.

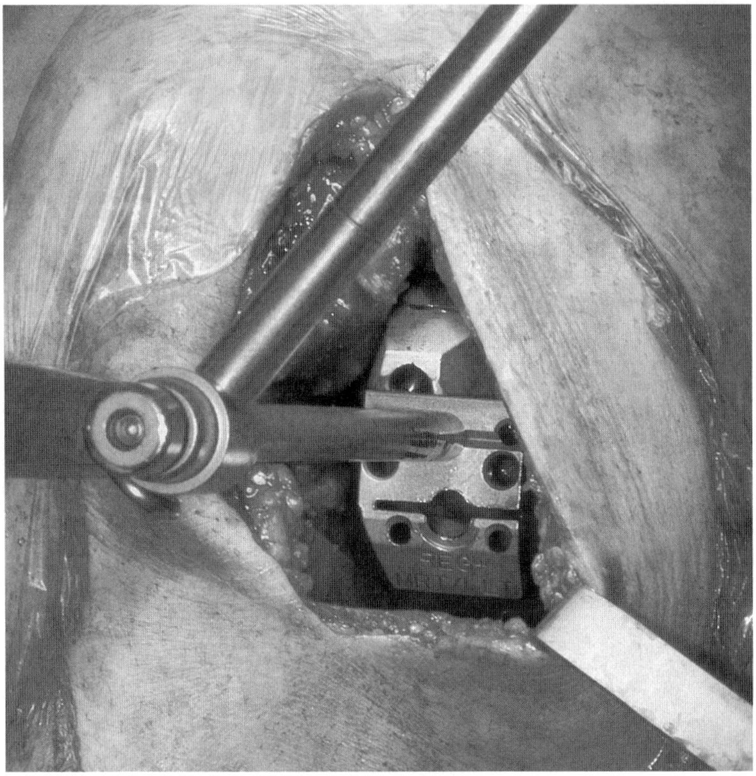

C

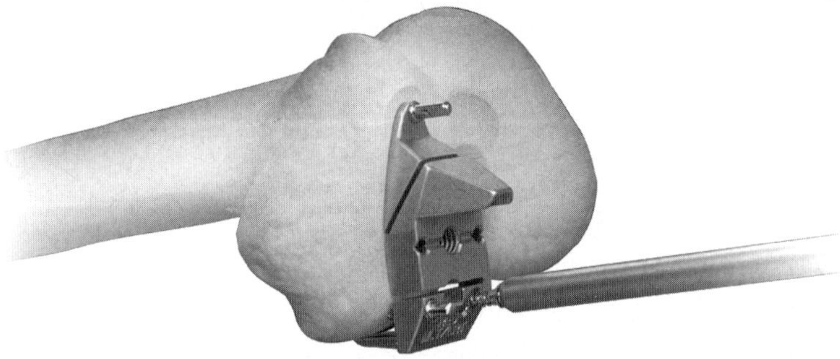

D

Figure 14.17. *Continued*

With all cuts now made, visualization of the posterior aspect of the compartment is maximized. First, remove the remaining medial meniscus and then debride the posterior condyle with a curved osteotome to assure an unrestricting flexion recess.

Tibial Sizing and Finishing

Determine optimal coverage of the tibial cut surface with the sizing paddles. If in between sizes, cut away from the tibial spine the small amount necessary to accommodate the larger size. Impact that provisional plate into place and drill the holes. Impacting the plate will tend to push it posterior. Stabilizing the plate first with a short screw anteriorly can prevent this displacement (Figure 14.18A and B).

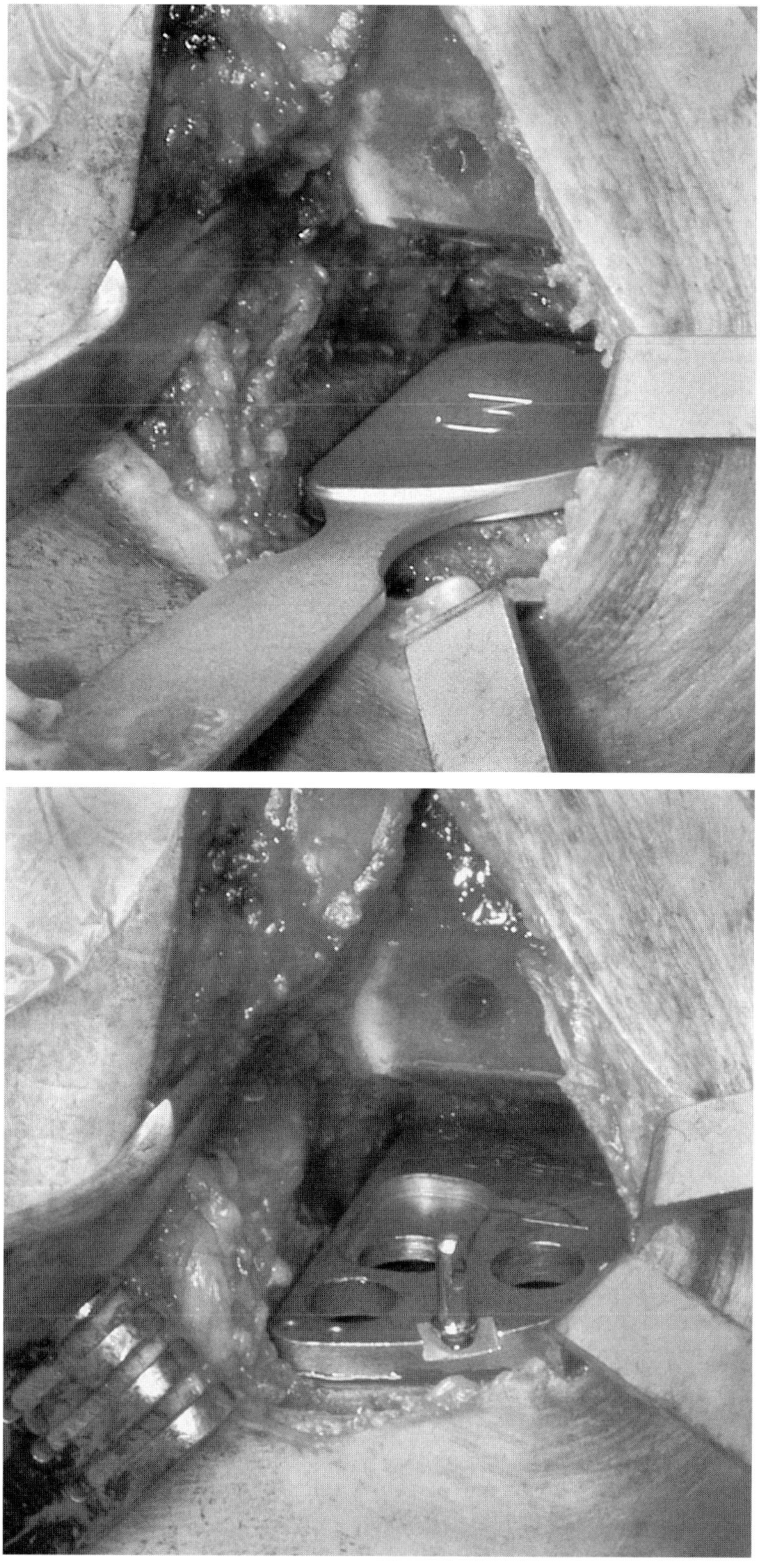

A

B

Figure 14.18. (A) Size and (B) secure the provisional tibial plate.

Trial and Cementing

The knee is flexed with the tibial plate in place. With a small incision and a patella that is not displaced, positioning of the trial femoral component, and later the prosthesis, is challenging. It is made easier by flexing the knee to 120 degrees while maintaining a valgus and external rotational stress. With the femoral trial rotated away from the patella, place the longer posterior post into its hole in the femur and impact it slightly. Then slowly extend the knee until the patella is lax enough to allow the trial to be rotated into place beneath it. With the shorter anterior post aligned with its hole, impact the trial fully.

Flexing and stressing the knee once again, slip the plastic trial into place. In extension, the limb alignment should be noted. Of particular importance is to again check that the tissue balance is proper. For a given set of implants it is thought that in both flexion and extension a valgus stress should produce about 2 mm of opening. A 2-mm wide tension gauge is available. Do not accept a tight space. If all cuts were made in the sequence described, that should not at this point be a problem. Nonetheless, check the tension carefully. Also, check to see that the femoral component tracks centrally over the tibial implant through its arc of motion and confirm that there is no trochlear impingement (Figure 14.19A–D).

Having checked for debris, cleanse the cut bone surfaces with pulsatile lavage, dry and then impact over cement the tibial implant with the knee in flexion. A valgus and external rotation stress to the leg improves viewing the extraction of excess cement using a small curved spatula.

For the femoral component, again flex the knee to 120 degrees and position the femoral implant as previously described. With the posterior post positioned first, extend the knee until the shorter post can be rotated into place and then impacted fully. Remove all excess cement. Now insert the chosen plastic and prop the foot so as to maintain the knee in extension while the cement hardens. Insertion of a drain and closure of the wound can commence at this time (Figure 14.20).

Conclusion

Implants such as the MG uni prosthesis are known to work well for an intermediate time, at least. With improved materials and optimal designs it is assumed that longer term success can be achieved. Meanwhile, the challenge is to develop surgical techniques that will further diminish the morbidity of the implantation while enhancing the surgeon's ability to better align and balance the knee. The EM Tensor technique using linked femoral and tibial cuts oriented after the alignment and soft tissue correction has been achieved with modestly sized extramedullary instruments is consistent with those goals.

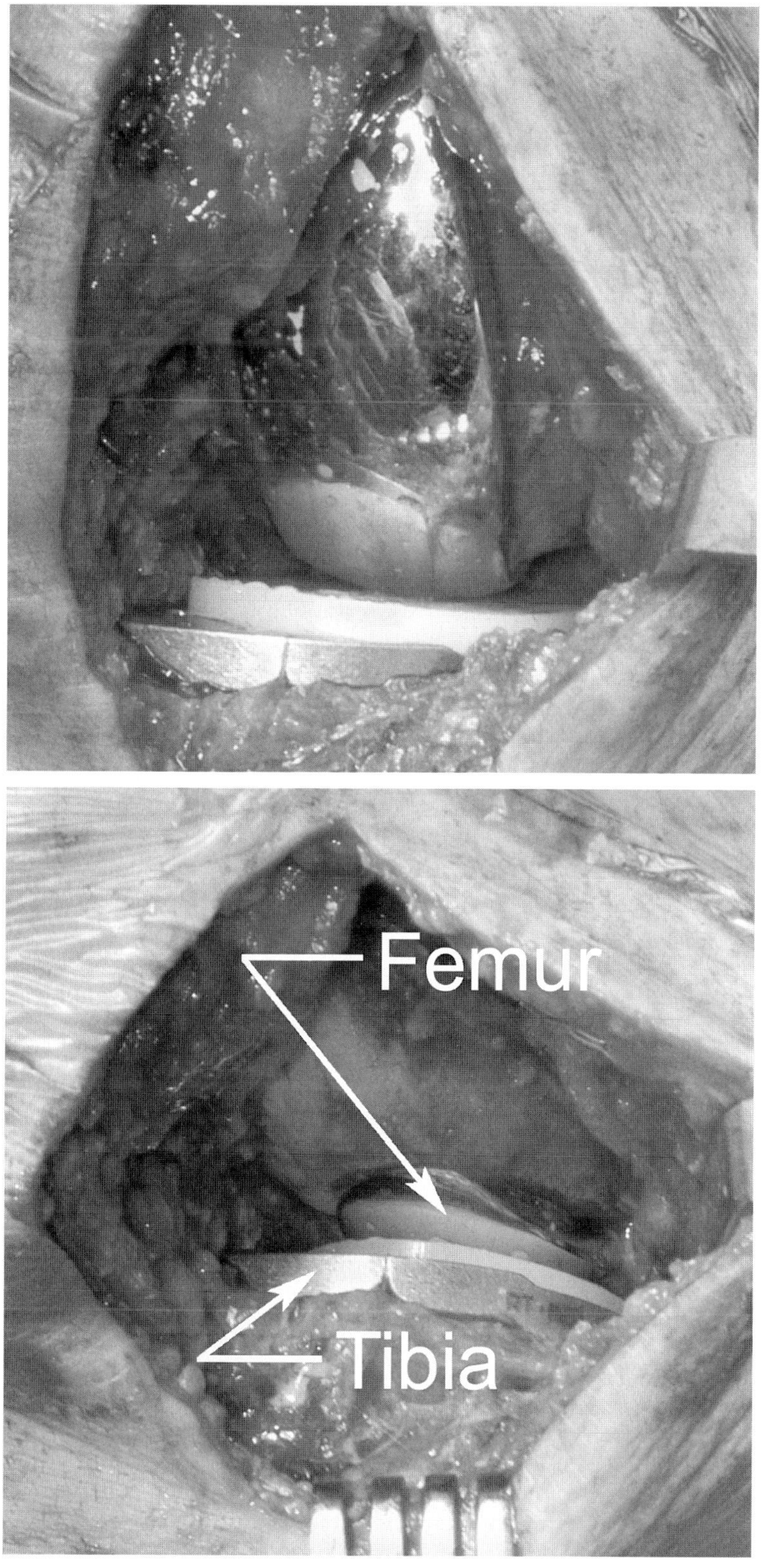

A

B

Figure 14.19. (A) The femoral component should be centered over the tibia in both flexion and (B) extension. (C) Check the tissue tension and (D) the limb alignment.

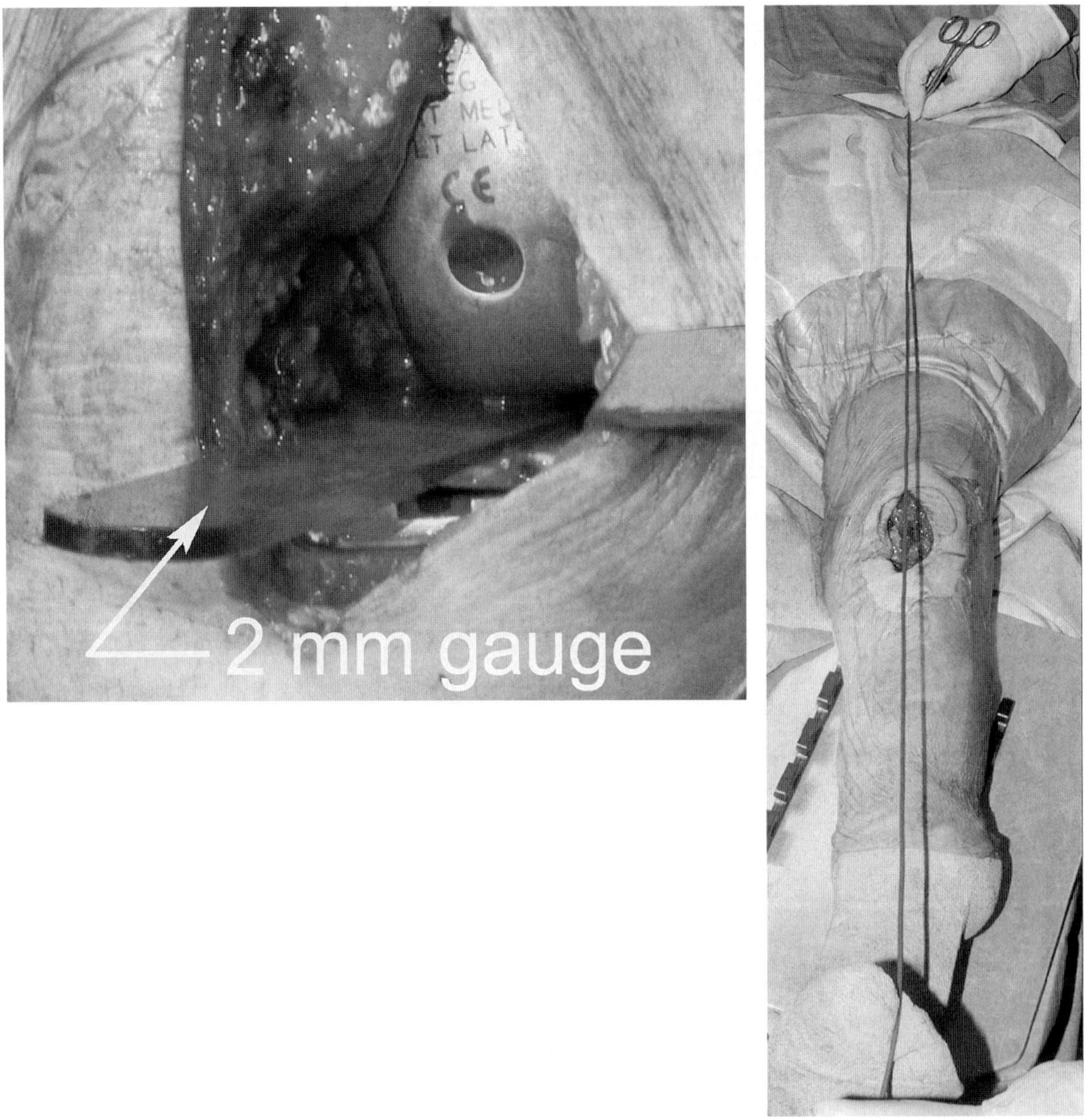

C

D

Figure 14.19. *Continued*

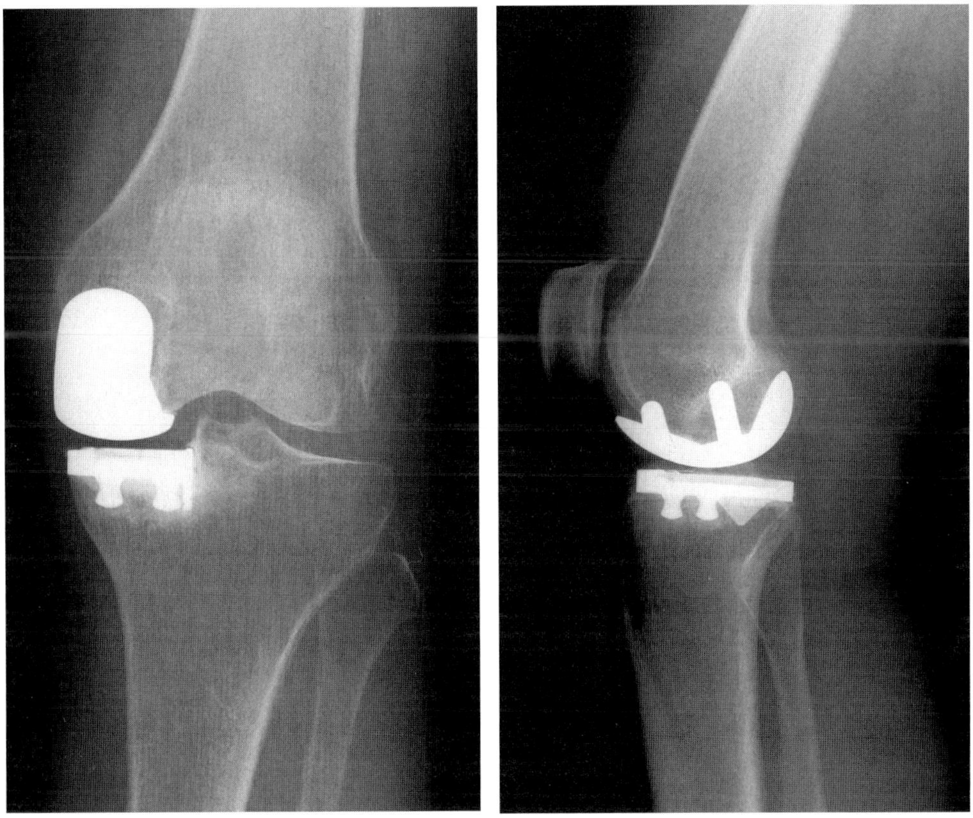

A B

Figure 14.20. (A) Postoperative AP and (B) lateral x-ray of an MG unicompartmental knee.

References

1. Caillouette JT. Fat embolism syndrome following the intramedullary alignment guide in total knee arthroplasty. Clin Orthop. 1990;251:198–199.
2. Kolettis GT. Safety of one-stage bilateral total knee arthroplasty. Clin Orthop. 309:102–109.
3. Hasegawa Y, Opishi Y, Shimizu T. Unicompartmental knee arthroplasty for medial gonarthrosis. Arch Orthop Trauma Surg (Germany). 117(4–5):183–187.
4. Murray DW, Goodfellow JW, O'Connor JJ. The Oxford medial unicompartmental arthroplasty: a ten-year survival study. JBJS Br. November 1998;80(6):983–999.
5. Newman JW, Ackroyd DE, Shah NA: Unicompartmental or total knee replacement? Five-year results of a prospective, randomized trial of 102 osteoarthritic knees with unicompartmental arthritis. JBJS Br. September 1998;80(5):862–865.
6. Tabor OB Jr, Tabor OB. Unicompartmental arthroplasty; a long-term follow-up study. J Arthroplasty. June 1998;13(4):373–379.
7. Marmor L. Unicompartmental knee arthroplasty: Ten to thirteen year follow-up study. Clin Orthop. 1988;226:14.
8. Scott RD. Unicompartmental knee arthroplasty. Clin Orthop. 1991;271: 96–100.

9. Berger RA, Nedeff DD, Barden RM, et al. Unicompartmental knee arthroplasty: Clinical experience at 6- to 10-year follow up. Clin Orthop. 1999; 367:50–60.
10. Argenson JN, Chevrol-Benkeddache Y, Aubniac JM. Modern cemented metal-backed unicompartmental knee arthroplasty: a 3 to 10 year follow-up study. 68th annual Meeting of the American Academy of Orthopaedic Surgeons; 2001.
11. Pennington DW, Swienckowski JJ, Lutes WB. Unicompartmental knee arthroplasty in patients sixty years of age or younger. JBJS. 2003;85-A: 1968–73.
12. Laskin RS. Unicompartmental tibiofemoral resurfacing arthroplasty. JBJS. 1978;60:182–185.
13. Cartier P, Sanouiller JL, Dreisamer RP. Unicompartmental knee arthroplasty: 10-year minimum follow-up period. J Arthroplasty. 1996;11970: 782–788.
14. Romanowski MR, Repicci JA. Technical aspects of medial versus lateral minimally invasive unicondylar arthroplasty. Orthopedics. 2003;26:289–293.

15

Minimally Invasive Surgery for Unicondylar Knee Arthroplasty: The Extramedullary Technique

Giles R. Scuderi

MIS unicondylar knee arthroplasty was introduced in the mid-1990s by Repicci and Eberle.[1] The procedure was essentially a freehand technique that used limited instrumentation. Over the years there have been modifications in the surgical instruments in order to perform the procedure accurately and reproducibly through a limited incision. The Miller Galante Unicondylar prosthesis (Zimmer, Warsaw, IN) introduced intramedullary instrumentation and most recently extramedullary instrumentation.[2] The smaller modified instruments clearly help in bone preparation and component position. Reliable instrumentation and surgical technique produce clinical results that are comparable with a conventional procedure.[3] Reproducible and predictable placement of the components is based on sound surgical principles.[4] Improved instrumentation allows the surgeon to operate through a minimally invasive arthrotomy, without everting the patella, and permits more accurate bone resection. It is the refinements in instrumentation that have contributed to successful clinical results.

General Principles

Alignment in unicondylar knee arthroplasty is determined by femoral and tibial bone resection, and not soft tissue release. Since soft tissue releases to correct deformity are not performed, if the varus or valgus deformity exceeds 15 degrees or if there is a flexion contracture greater than 10 degrees, a total knee arthroplasty should be considered. In unicondylar knee arthroplasty, overcorrection of the knee should be avoided, because this overloads the contralateral compartment and increases the potential for progression of the degenerative arthritis. Reports have shown that slight undercorrection of the knee alignment is correlated with long-term survivorship.[5,6]

The advantage of extramedullary instrumentation in MIS is that it eliminates the need for violation of the femoral intramedullary canal. Extramedullary instruments are designed to provide a means of achieving precision in limb alignment. With the limb aligned in extension, the deformity may be passively corrected. By coupling an extramedullary femoral and tibial guide, the angle of resection for the distal femur and the proximal tibia can be determined. This should create a parallel resection of the femur and tibia in extension. The linked cuts are perpendicular to the mechanical axis of the femur and tibia, respectively.

Approach

The skin incision is made with the knee in flexion and begins from the superior pole of the patella to 2cm distal to the joint line. This straight incision is placed along the medial border of the patella for a medial unicondylar replacement. A limited medial parapatellar arthrotomy is performed, extending from the lower border of the vastus medialis to a point just distal to the joint line along the proximal tibia. To aid visualization, the fat pad is excised along with the anterior horn of the medial meniscus. Subperiosteal dissection is then carried out along the proximal medial tibia, releasing the meniscal tibial attachment, but not releasing the medial collateral ligament. A retractor is then placed to protect the collateral ligament. Medial tibial and femoral osteophytes are removed along with any osteophytes along the femoral intercondylar notch. With the spacer block technique the tibia is prepared first.[2]

Tibial Preparation

The tibia is resected with an extramedullary tibial cutting guide. The shaft of the resection guide is set parallel to the tibial shaft. The proximal cutting head is secured to the tibia and the depth and slope of resection is determined. A depth gauge is used so that 2mm to 4mm of bone is removed from the lowest point on the tibial plateau. Once the desired depth of resection is determined, a retractor is placed medially to protect the medial collateral ligament. With the knee flexed, the proximal tibia is resected (Figure 15.1). Caution must be taken not to undercut the attachment of the anterior cruciate ligament and the lateral tibial plateau. With a reciprocating saw, the sagittal tibial cut is made in line with the medial wall of the intercondylar notch down to the level of the transverse cut. The resected tibial bone is then removed. The gap is checked with a spacer block to ensure that the appropriate

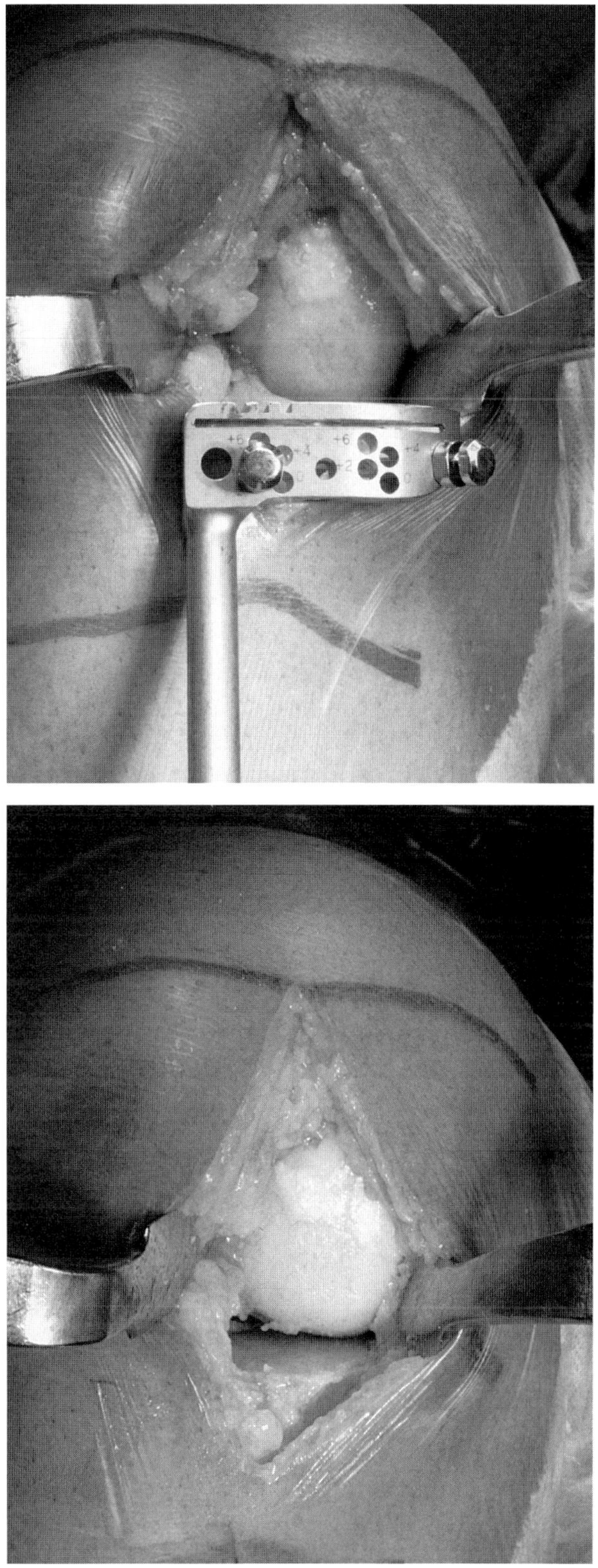

A

B

Figure 15.1. (A and B) Resection of the proximal tibia with the extramedullary guide (A) following resection the bone is removed (B).

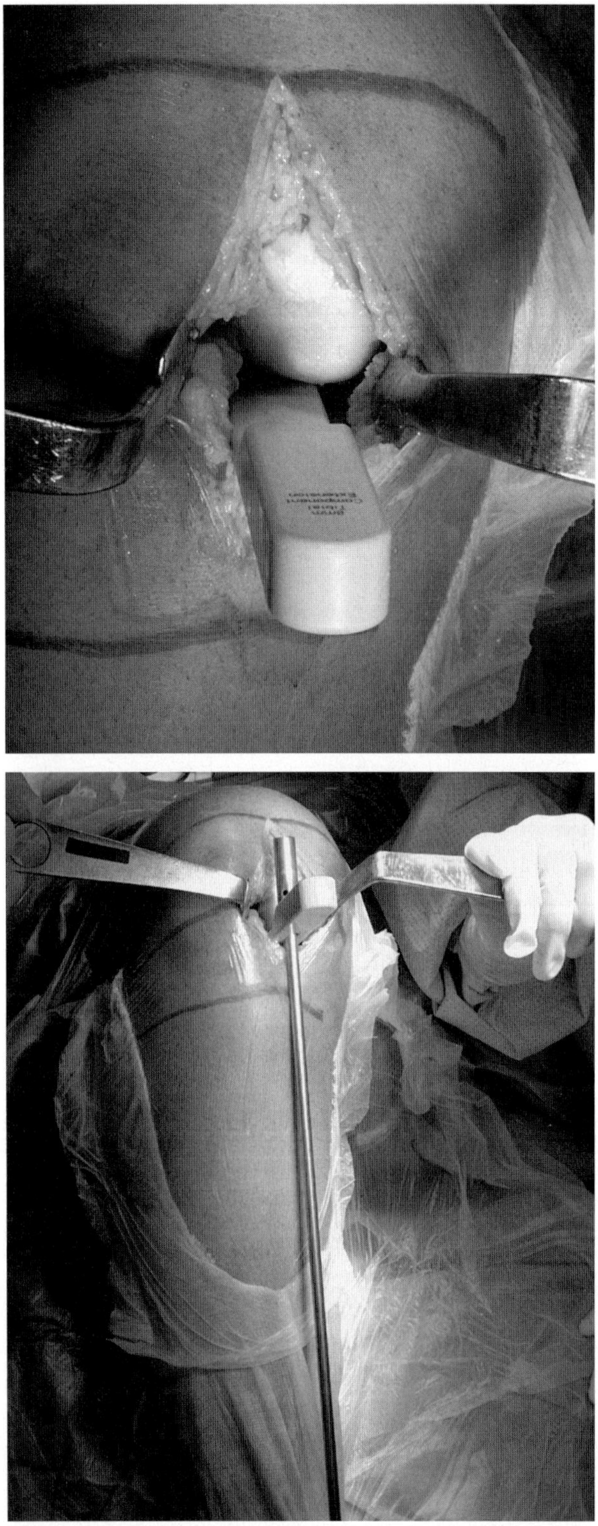

A

B

Figure 15.2. (A and B) Following the tibial resection, the gap is checked in extension (A) and flexion (B).

amount of bone has been resected and that the axial alignment is correct (Figure 15.2). If the gap is too tight, additional bone should be resected from the proximal tibia. If the gap is too loose, a thicker spacer block, which correlates to a thicker tibial component, should be inserted.

Femoral Preparation

Following resection of the proximal tibia, the knee is brought into full extension and the 8-mm spacer block is inserted into the joint space. It should be fully inserted and sit flat on the resected tibia to ensure that the proper amount of distal femur will be resected (Figure 15.3). If there is any difficulty inserting the 8-mm spacer block, then additional bone needs to be resected from the proximal tibia. In contrast, if the 8 mm spacer block is too loose then a thicker spacer block should be inserted.

With the appropriate spacer block in place and the knee in extension, the alignment tower is attached so that the position of the guide can be checked relative to the femoral head (Figure 15.4). The alignment tower is then removed and the distal femoral resection guide is attached to the spacer block (Figure 15.5). The distal femoral resection guide is secured to the distal femur and the distal femur is resected. The cut can be completed in full extension, but caution must be taken not to overcut the distal femur and have the saw blade extend into the popliteal area. If desired, the femoral cut can be started in extension and finished in flexion. Once the distal femur is resected, the extension gap is checked with a spacer block and alignment rod (Figure 15.6).

Finishing the Femur

The appropriate sized MG femoral finishing guide is selected (Figure 15.7). This guide rests on the flat surface of the distal femur and the posterior extension lies against the posterior condyles. There should be 1 mm to 2 mm of exposed bone along the anterior edge of the guide. If the guide appears to be in between sizes, it would be preferable to pick the smaller size. This guide should also be rotationally set so that the posterior surface is parallel to the resected tibia. With the guide secured to the femur the final cuts and lug holes are made. This completes the femoral preparation.

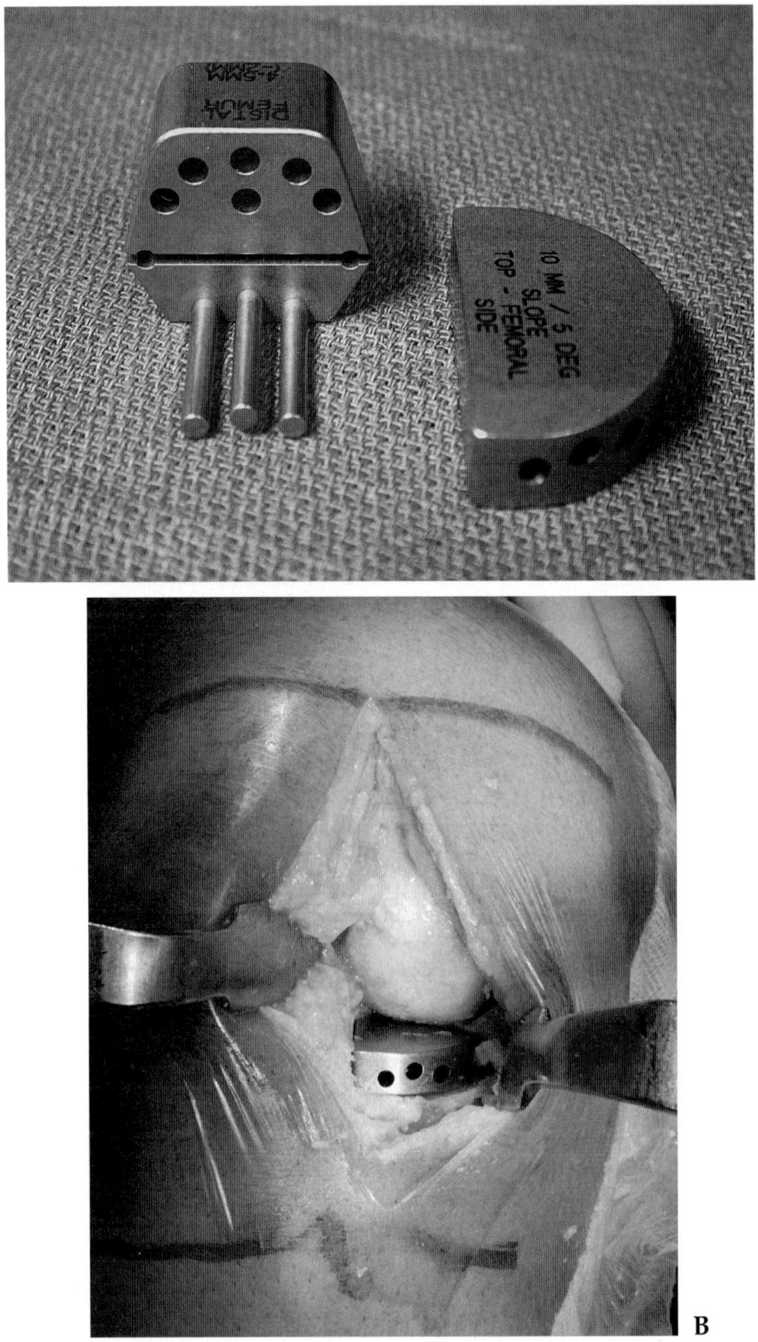

A

B

Figure 15.3. (A and B) The spacer block (A) is inserted into the joint on the resected tibia (B).

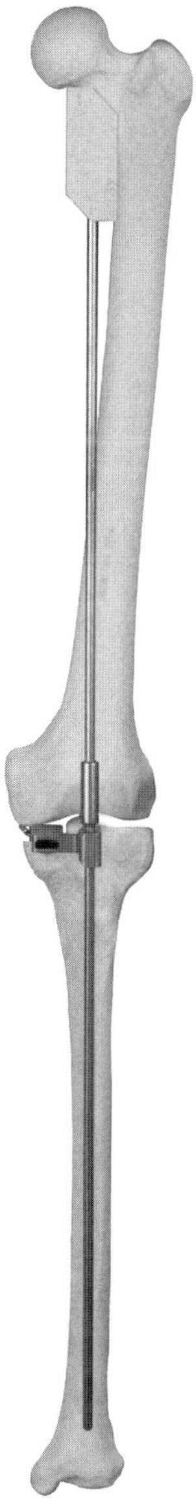

Figure 15.4. The Alignment Tower is attached to the spacer block.

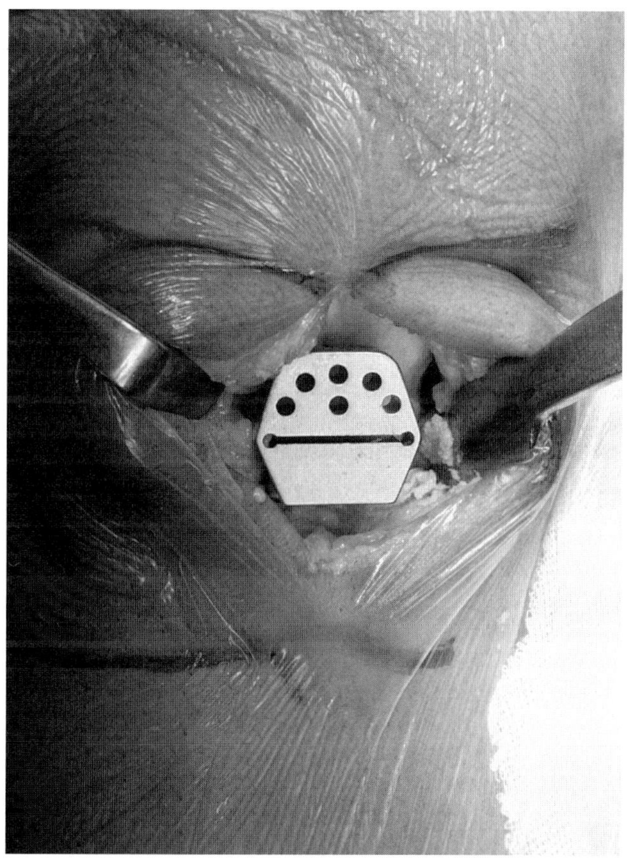

Figure 15.5. The distal femoral resection guide is attached to the spacer block.

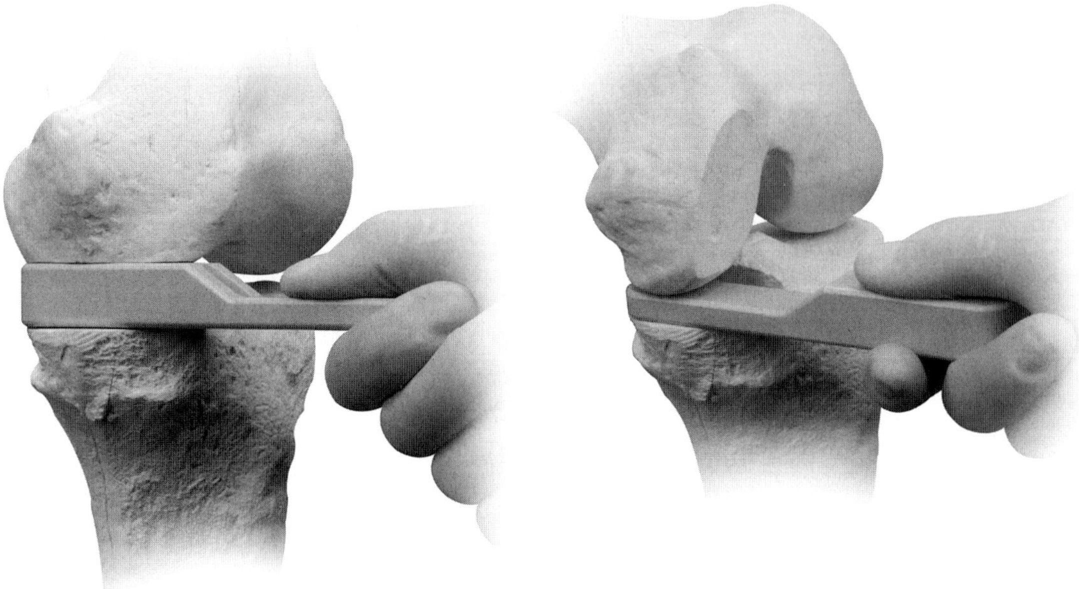

A

B

Figure 15.6. (A and B) The gaps are checked, in extension (A) and flexion (B).

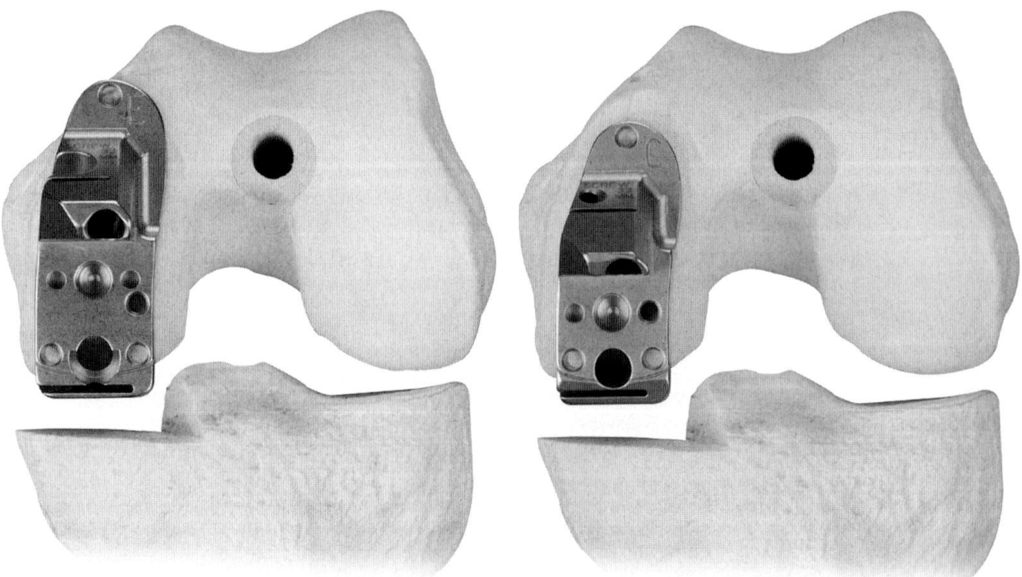

A

B

Figure 15.7. (A-C) The correct femoral finishing guide is selected. (A) too big (B) too small (C) correct size.

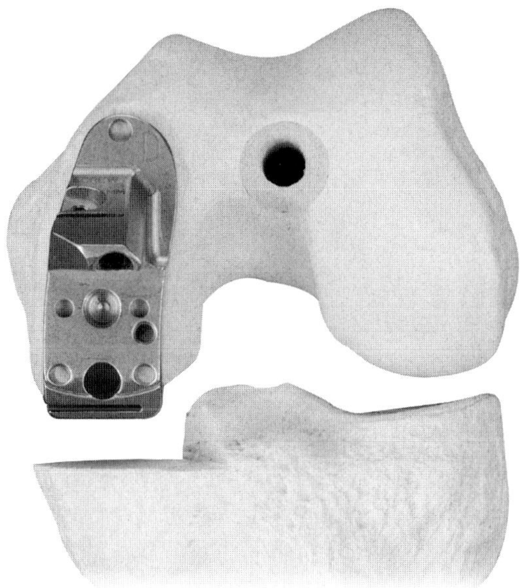

C

Figure 15.7. *Contined*

Finishing the Tibia

At this point the remaining meniscus and osteophytes are removed. The appropriate sized MG tibial template, which covers the entire surface without overhang, is selected (Figure 15.8). The template is secured to the proximal tibia and the lug holes are drilled. The tibial template is left in place for the trial reduction.

Trial Reduction

With the knee in 90 degrees of flexion and a retractor in the intercondylar notch to pull back the patella, the provisional femoral component is seated on the distal femur. A trial tibial articular surface is then placed on the tibial template. With all the components in place, the knee is checked for range of motion and stability. Appropriate soft tissue tension is checked with the 2 mm tension gauge that should fit snugly, but not overly tight, between the femur and the tibial articular surface in both flexion and extension (Figure 15.9). In general the correct thickness of the prosthesis should allow for approximately 2 mm of joint laxity when a valgus stress is applied to the knee in full extension.

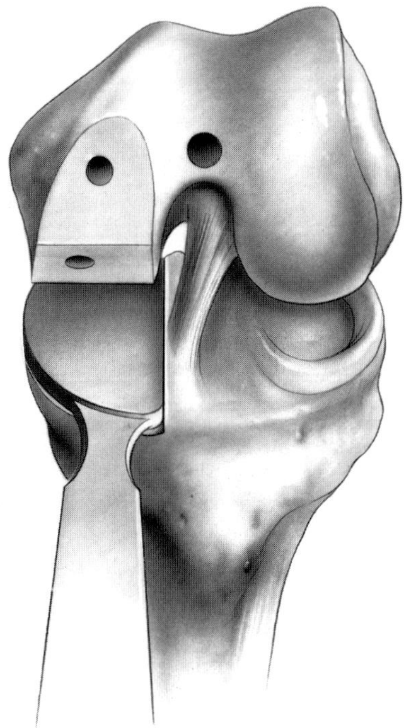

Figure 15.8. The tibial template is placed on the resected tibia.

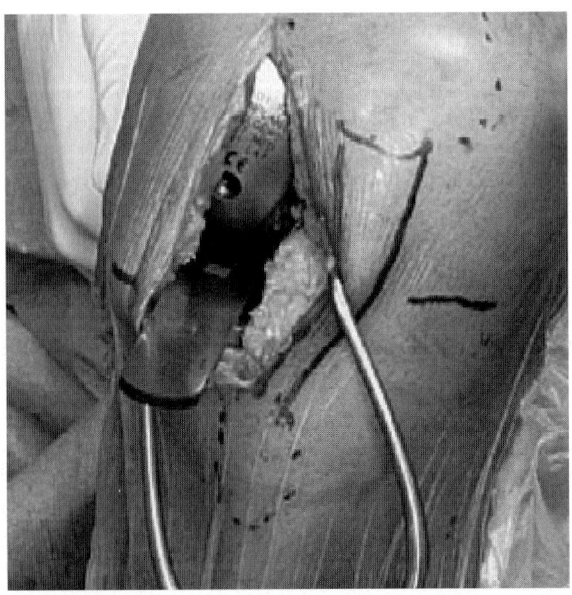

Figure 15.9. With the provisional components in place, the 2 mm tension gauge is inserted in the joint.

Final Components

The trial components are removed and the bone surfaces are cleansed with water pick lavage in an effort to remove blood and debris from the surfaces. In preparation for cementing, the bone is dried. The modular tibial component is cemented in place first. With the knee hyperflexed and externally rotated, a small amount of cement is placed on the exposed surface of the tibia. An additional amount of cement is placed on the undersurface of the tibial component. The final tibial component is then pressed into place and the excess cement is removed. To fully seat the tibial component it is impacted into place and any extruded cement is removed.

With the knee in 90 degrees of flexion, a retractor is placed in the intercondylar notch to hold the patella back so that the femur is exposed. A small amount of cement is placed on the distal femur and along the backside of the femoral component. The MG femoral component is impacted in place and all excess cement is removed. The modular tibial polyethylene articular surface is then inserted and a final check of motion and stability is performed.

With the final components in place (Figure 15.10), the knee is irrigated with an antibiotic solution. The arthrotomy, subcutaneous layer and skin are closed in a routine fashion.

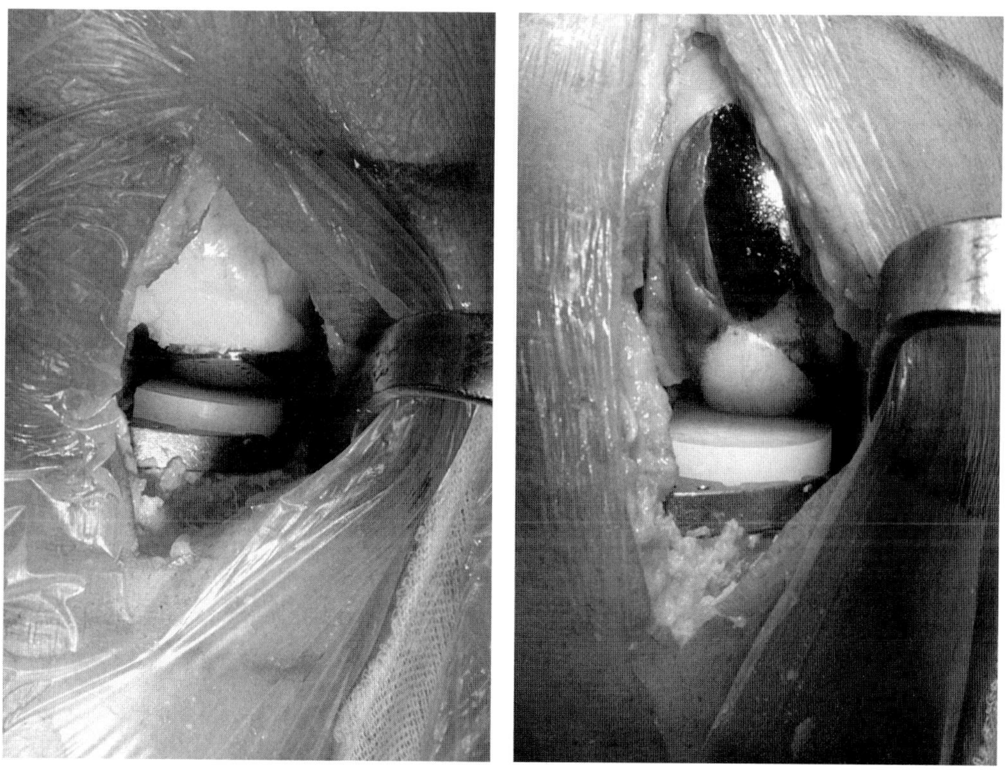

A B

Figure 15.10. (A and B) The final components are in place, (C) with the resultant radiograph.

C 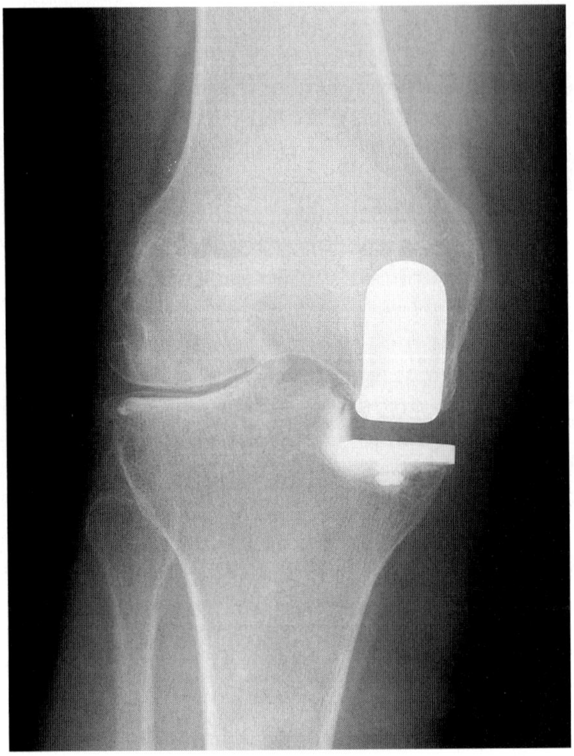

Figure 15.10. *Continued*

Summary

Minimally invasive unicondylar knee arthroplasty implanted with extramedullary instrumentation minimizes soft tissue dissection, does not violate the femoral intramedullary canal, and ensures accurate component positioning. Since the proximal tibial resection and the distal femoral resection are linked in extension, this coupled resection and desired soft tissue tension set limb alignment. The cuts are parallel and result in a preset gap that is calculated to match the thickness of the implants. Gap balancing reduces the need for recutting, helps preserve bone stock, and ensures accurate component positioning. Final postoperative alignment is determined by the composite thickness of the components. Reliable instrumentation results in accurate bone resection and component position, which are necessary for a successful clinical outcome.

References

1. Repicci JA, Eberle RW. Minimally invasive surgical technique for unicondylar knee replacement. J South Orthop Assoc. 1999;8:20–27.
2. Zimmer monograph. The Zimmer Unicompartmental High Flex Knee: Intramedullary, Spacer Block Option and Extramedullary Minimally Invasive Surgical Techniques; 2004.

3. Scuderi GR. Instrumentation for Unicondylar Knee Replacement. In: Scuderi GR, Tria AJ, eds. MIS of the Hip and the Knee: A Clinical Perspective. New York: Springer; 2004:87–104.
4. Barnes CL, Scott RD. Unicondylar Replacement. In: Scuderi GR, Tria AJ, eds. Surgical Techniques in Total Knee Arthroplasty. New York: Springer-Verlag; 2002:106–111.
5. Berger RA, Nedeff DD, Barden RM, et al. Unicompartmental knee arthroplasty: Clinical Experience at 6- to 10-year follow-up. Clin Orthop. 1999; 367:50–60.
6. Cartier P, Sanouiller JL, Grelsamer RP. Unicompartmental knee arthroplasty: 10-year minimum follow-up period. J Arthroplasty. 1996;11:782–788.

16

Minimally Invasive Surgery for Arthroplasty with the UniSpacer

Richard H. Hallock

MIS Arthroplasty with the UniSpacer

Middle-age osteoarthritis of the knee remains a problem with many treatment options. It can be treated in its earlier stages with a combination of oral medication, intra-articular injection with cortisone or viscosupplementation, physical therapy, and arthroscopic debridement. Once the patient has reached a level of disability which is not responding to these less invasive treatment modalities, the patient and physician are both faced with the decision to choose a more invasive surgical option. The selection of the best surgical alternative will depend on many nonsurgical issues including the patient's age, weight, sex, activity level, and occupation. This decision will also be based on the extent of cartilage degeneration, as well as bony deformity. These options include high tibial osteotomy, unicompartmental knee arthroplasty, total knee arthroplasty, and the UniSpacer. The final decision on which of these techniques is ultimately used will come down to patient and surgeon preference based on the individual set of circumstances.

The UniSpacer was designed on both very traditional orthopedic principles as well as some nontraditional orthopedic concepts.[1–5] It is a cobalt chrome metallic device that is inserted into the medial compartment of the knee. The bearing surfaces of the device have a metal on cartilage/bone interface on both the femoral and tibial surfaces. Metal on biologic interfaces have been used traditionally in orthopedics in hemiarthroplasty of the shoulder, hemiarthroplasty of the hip, and nonresurfaced patellae in total knee replacement. It serves as a self-centering shim, which replaces the missing articular and meniscal cartilage of the medial compartment.

As such, the thickness of the shim is determined by the amount of missing articular and meniscal cartilage within the constraints of the collateral and cruciate ligaments. The varus deformity will thus only be corrected back to the patient's premorbid knee alignment. This realignment will off-load the medial compartment of the knee without overcorrecting the alignment and accelerating lateral compartment degeneration. What is different about this device from traditional arthroplasty is that it is neither fixed to the bony surfaces of the tibia or the femur, nor requires bone cuts or bone removal for implantation. The geometry of the device with its concave femoral surface and convex tibial surface allows it to function as a self-centering shim between the biological femoral and tibial surfaces of the patient. These nontraditional concepts avoid the traditional modes of arthroplasty failure including loosening, polyethylene wear, and malpositioning of components. As such, it can function either as a final arthroplasty or as a safe bridge procedure in younger patients, which does not alter the bony and ligamentous anatomy for a next step procedure.

Preoperative Evaluation

The preoperative evaluation for the UniSpacer requires the same type of evaluation that would be necessary to perform a high tibial osteotomy, unicompartmental knee replacement, or total knee replacement. Routine x-ray evaluation should include AP erect views of the knee, which allows evaluation of the loss of joint space as well as the femoral tibial axis (Figure 16.1). The surgeon should pay particular attention to medial subluxation of the femur relative to the tibia and deformity of the tibial plateau (Figure 16.2).

Either of these two conditions would preclude the use of the UniSpacer. The lateral x-ray of the knee is necessary to view the relative

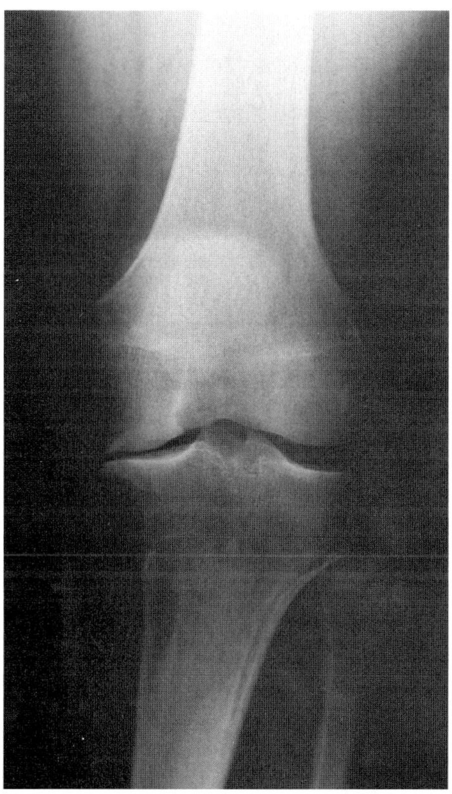

Figure 16.1. Loss of medial joint space without deformation of the tibia.

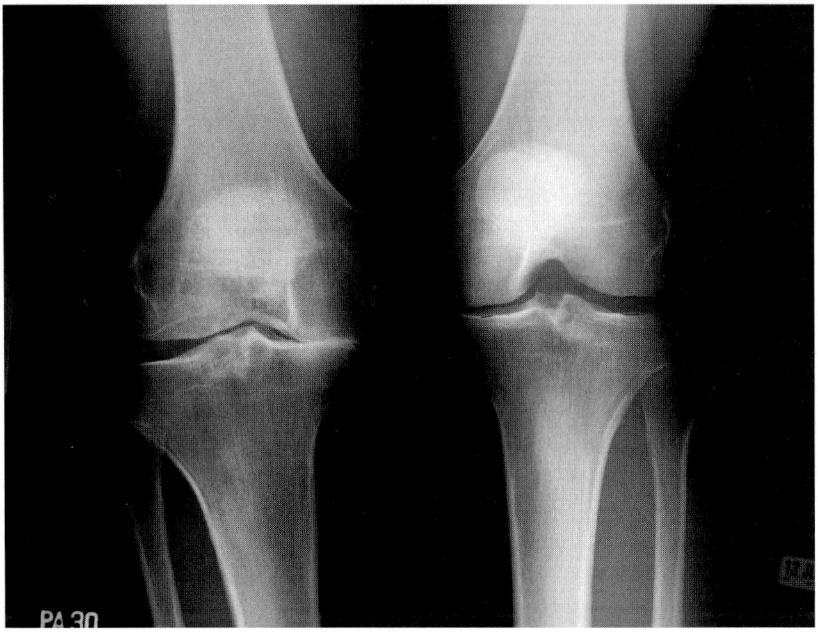

Figure 16.2. Deformity of the tibia and medial subluxation of the femur.

position of the femoral condyle with respect to the tibia. Anterior translation of the tibia relative to the femur may indicate chronic anterior cruciate ligament insufficiency, which may also be a contraindication for the use of the UniSpacer (Figure 16.3). The lateral view also demonstrates

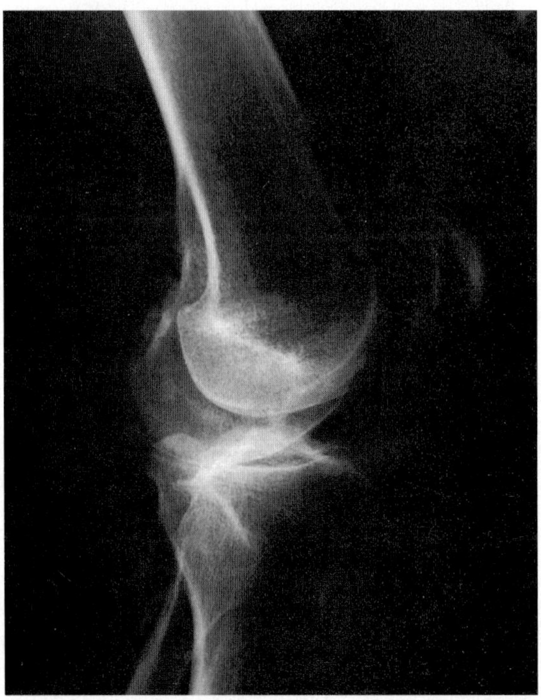

Figure 16.3. A anterior subluxation of the tibia suggestive of chronic ACL deficiency.

posterior femoral osteophytes. Large posterior femoral osteophytes can produce a flexion contracture greater than five degrees, which is also a contraindication for the use of the UniSpacer. The skyline view is necessary to evaluate the patellofemoral joint. Any significant loss of joint space or osteophyte formation may also contraindicate the use of the UniSpacer especially if the patient has symptoms, which can be confused with medial joint pain. An MRI scan can also be useful in evaluating the status of the knee. Questions concerning the integrity of the anterior cruciate ligament as well as the status of the patella femoral joint can also be answered with an MRI scan.

Surgical Technique

Since the UniSpacer requires no bone cuts and has no fixation, the surgical technique is decidedly different from traditional arthroplasty. The surgical technique focuses on restoring the knee alignment through thorough joint debridement and implantation of an intra-articular shim. This will be broken down into steps including arthrotomy, osteophyte resection and anterior medial meniscectomy, chondroplasty, tweenplasty, sizing, insertion technique, fluoroscopy and final implantation and closure.

Surgical Preparation

Preoperative antibiotic prophylaxis is utilized on all patients. The use of a thigh tourniquet is optional and left to surgeon preference. The arthroscopy portals and incision line can be infiltrated with local anesthetic with epinephrine, to decrease intraoperative bleeding especially if the patient does not have a tourniquet. The patient is placed in the supine position with the knee prepped and draped in routine fashion.

Rigid leg holders should be avoided since they will inhibit the surgeon from placing the knee through a range of motion, and they will interfere with use of the fluoroscopy equipment later in the case.

Arthroplasty

Every patient who is considered for the UniSpacer should have an arthroscopy performed either at the time of surgery or during the previous 12 months. Inappropriate candidates can be deselected based on the extent of degeneration present at the time of the arthroscopy. The arthroscopy is also useful with some of the initial debridement necessary to proceed with insertion of the UniSpacer. An initial evaluation of the patellofemoral joint, lateral compartment including the lateral meniscus, as well as the cruciate ligament complex should be performed. Any significant degeneration in the patellofemoral compartment or the lateral compartment should result in deselection of the current UniSpacer candidate. Mild Grade I to Grade II chondromalacia of the patellofemoral joint and lateral compartment is acceptable. Any grade of chondromalacia worse than that degree of degeneration should lead to deselection of that patient for a UniSpacer. Since an intact lateral compartment, including an intact lateral meniscus, is critical when weight bearing is going to be shifted to that compartment, every patient should have an intact lateral meniscus as well as only mild chondromalacic changes involving the lateral femoral condyle and lateral tibial plateau. It is very difficult to distinguish anteromedial knee pain originating from the medial compartment versus the patellofemoral joint. Any patient with significant degeneration involving the patella or femoral sulcus also should be deselected. The cruciate ligament complex also needs to be thoroughly examined.

Many of these patients have had previous arthrotomies for medial meniscectomy as a result of old injuries. When that occurs the cruciate ligament complex should be examined for complete integrity of both the anterior and the posterior cruciate ligaments. Any patient with deficiency of either the anterior or posterior cruciate ligament will require either reconstruction of these ligaments or consideration of other treatment options. The most common reason for deselection of any UniSpacer candidate is evaluation of the medial compartment. Most UniSpacer candidates have bipolar degenerative disease involving both the femoral condyle and tibial plateau. If the patient has deformity of the tibial plateau subchondral bone plate resulting in remodeling of the medial edge of the tibial plateau, that patient should also be deselected. When this occurs the tibial plateau has essentially a convex surface instead of the normal shallow, concave surface for the UniSpacer to translate on (Figure 16.4). Any convex surface of the tibial plateau will

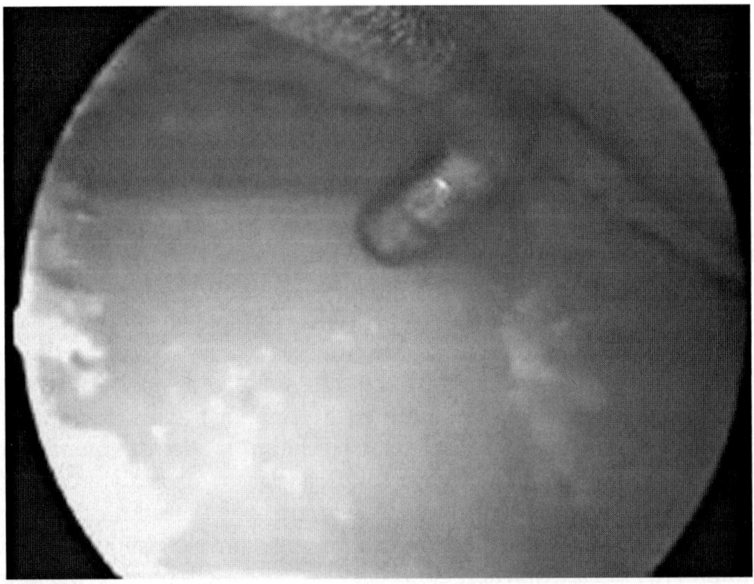

Figure 16.4. Medial tibial bone loss, which cannot be contoured to create normal UniSpacer kinematics. The subchondral bone has been remodeled to create a convex surface.

inhibit normal translational and rotatory motion that is required for restoration of normal knee kinematics. If, after initial arthroscopic evaluation, the patient is considered to be a satisfactory candidate for utilization of the UniSpacer, several of the initial debridement steps can be performed arthroscopically. This includes resection of the posterior horn of the medial meniscus. The medial meniscus is usually degenerated in these patients, and completion of the posterior meniscectomy can be performed arthroscopically back to the junction of the red and white zones. Any residual leading edge of the meniscus should be resected as this can result in translation of the UniSpacer over the leading edge of the meniscus. The residual boundary of the meniscus will act as a partial physical constraint. Once posterior meniscectomy has been completed, the evaluation of the intercondylar osteophytes can proceed. It is not unusual for osteophytes to form in the intercondylar regions in these patients.

Osteophytes abrading the anterior cruciate ligament can cause degeneration of an intact anterior cruciate ligament and eventually result in incompetency. These osteophytes adjacent to the anterior cruciate ligament should be resected if visualized arthroscopically. The osteophytes on the lateral/posterior aspect of the medial femoral condyle can also be difficult to visualize after the arthroscopy has been performed. If that is the case, it is often easier to resect these osteophytes using the aid of the arthroscope. Again, the goal of osteophyte resection adjacent to the intercondylar notch is to restore normal cruciate ligament excursion, in addition to removing any abnormal femoral anatomy that may cause aberrant UniSpacer motion.

Arthrotomy

The arthrotomy for insertion of the UniSpacer is very similar to the arthrotomy performed for insertion of a traditional unicompartmental arthroplasty. The incision usually extends from the mid-patella down to the tibial joint line (Figure 16.5). The subcutaneous tissue is undermined to allow a mobile view of the medial compartment. The medial retinaculum is incised from the superior pole of the patella down to the proximal tibia. The anteromedial corner of the knee is released including transection of the anterolateral horn of the medial meniscus. Subperiosteal release of the proximal 2 cm of the tibia should be performed when it is necessary to resect osteophytes off the medial aspect of the tibia (Figure 16.6). This release is not necessary when there is only minimal medial tibial osteophyte formation present. The arthrotomy should allow visualization of the medial facet of the patella, intercondylar notch, medial femoral condyle, and medial tibial plateau when necessary. A small portion of the infrapatellar fat pad can be resected when visualization of the intercondylar notch or medial compartment is impaired with just the medial arthrotomy.

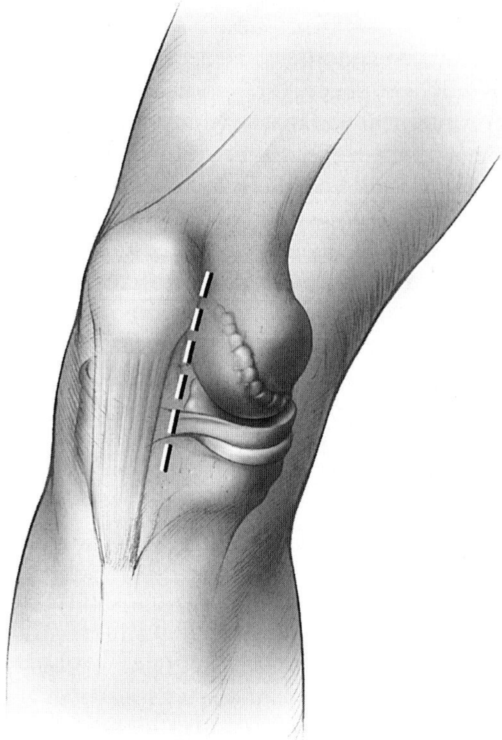

Figure 16.5. A medial parapatellar incision from mid-patella to the tibial joint line.

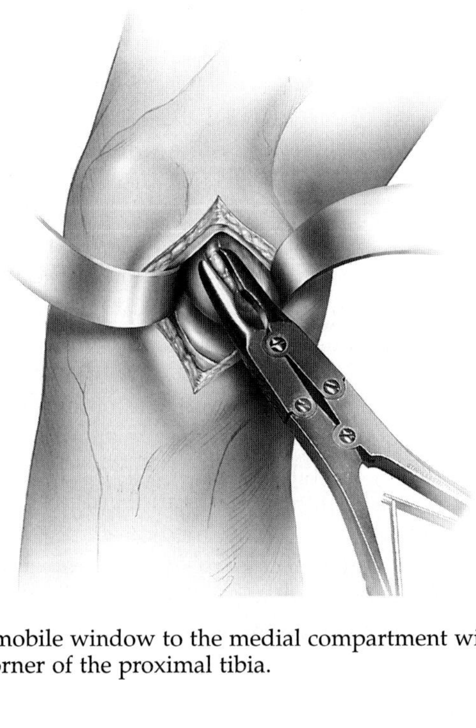

Figure 16.6. A mobile window to the medial compartment with release of the anteromedial corner of the proximal tibia.

Osteophyte Resection and Anteromedial Meniscectomy

Following the arthrotomy a complete debridement of medial compartment osteophytes is necessary to allow full excursion of the medial collateral and cruciate ligament complex. Initially, any overhanging osteophytes adjacent to the medial aspect of the patella should be resected. Osteophytes are frequently present along the medial border of the patella. When the femoral tibial axis is corrected from varus to valgus alignment, these osteophytes can impinge on the medial aspect of the femoral sulcus. It is imperative to debride these osteophytes to avoid residual medial patellofemoral pain. Osteophytes are then resected completely from the anterior aspect of the femoral condyle to the posterior aspect of the femoral condyle. This can be performed usually using a rongeur. The osteophytes need to be resected down to the original borders of the femur.

A retractor is supplied with the instrumentation to allow resection of the posterior osteophyte formation on the femoral condyle (Figure 16.7). This is most easily accomplished by placing the knee in the figure-of-four position with the knee flexed. An osteotome can be utilized to shear off the posterior osteophytes to restore the original bony contours. It is also imperative to resect any significant osteophyte formation along the medial border of the tibial plateau. When this occurs, it is necessary to release the deep fibers of the medial collateral ligament and meniscal tibial ligament along the proximal 2-cm region of the tibial plateau. Once this is released, osteophytes can easily be resected that overhang the medial border of the original tibial plateau.

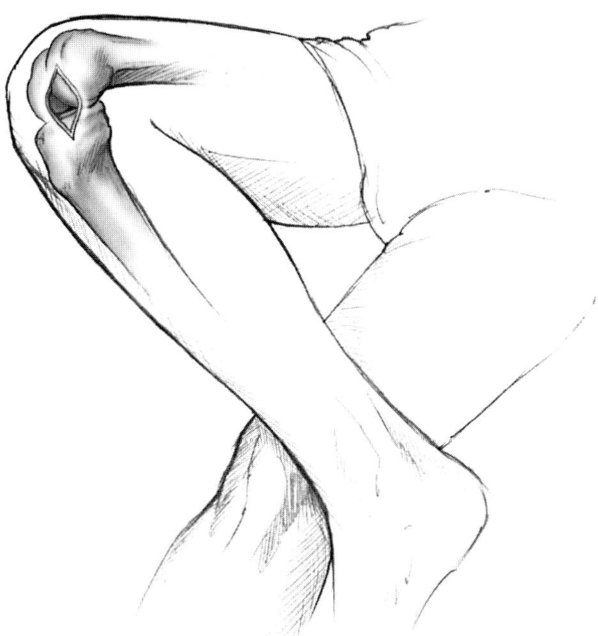

Figure 16.7. The figure-of-four position necessary to resect osteophytes from the posterior region of the medial femoral condyle.

It is not unusual for the anterior and middle thirds of the medial meniscus to remain relatively intact in these patients. When this occurs, an open anteromedial meniscectomy should be performed at the level of the junction of the red and white zones to avoid any impingement of the UniSpacer on a residual leading edge of the meniscus. Leaving the red zone of the meniscus intact will create a stable border for the UniSpacer. The surgeon should be careful not to violate the superficial fibers of the medial collateral ligament during this procedure.

Chondroplasty

The degenerative surfaces of the femoral condyle and tibial plateau typically have irregular shapes created by variations in thickness of the remaining articular cartilage. The tibial surface of the UniSpacer has a uniform, shallow convexity despite the size of the device. In an effort to create the most conformal surface that articulates against the UniSpacer, it is necessary to contour the patient's femoral condyle and tibial plateau. This femoral and tibial "sculpting" will ultimately create the best fit and sizing for the UniSpacer. The surgeon must, therefore, attempt to recreate the anatomic J-curve of the femoral condyle in addition to recreating the shallow dish curvature of the tibial plateau. Despite the fact that the UniSpacer will span cartilage defects on either of these surfaces, it is best to restore the most uniform surfaces, which, ultimately, distributes the load over a greater surface area during loading. Convex and concave rasps are provided with the instrumentation that can be utilized to restore a "best fit" contour to the patient's biological surfaces. The rasps are utilized to smooth out divoted regions of the patient's articular surfaces in addition to restoring more uniform thickness to the remaining articular cartilage (Figure 16.8). This process is necessary to create more stable kinematics for the UniSpacer during its normal translational/rotational motion. This often requires smoothing out ridges of articular cartilage that create an

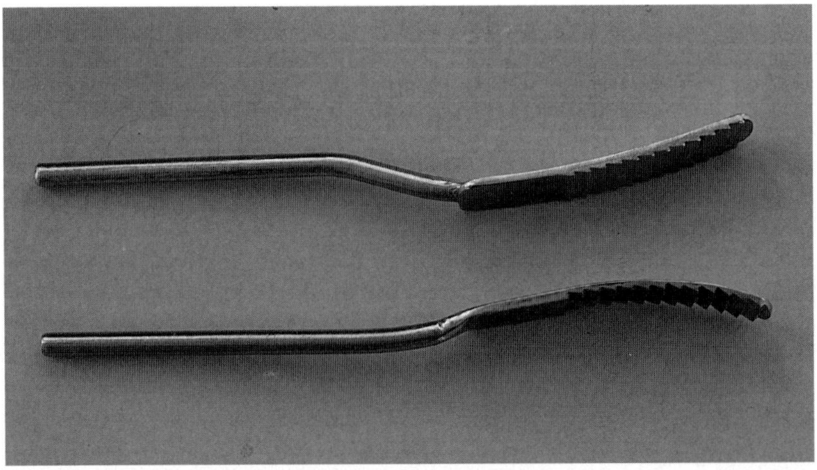

Figure 16.8. The rasps are shown, which are available to contour the femoral and tibial surfaces to restore a smooth articular surface.

impediment to normal motion. Areas of full thickness articular cartilage may tend to exaggerate normal motion of the UniSpacer. This is most often seen on the posterior aspect of the femoral condyle where full thickness cartilage often remains. The concave rasp can be used to thin this remaining articular cartilage to avoid an exaggerated posterior translation of the device during flexion.

Although it is not necessary for the surgeon to create a fully conformal surface to the UniSpacer in extension, any attempt to do so will decrease the patient's recovery time. Increased conformity ultimately leads to distribution of medial compartment load over a greater surface area. This is confirmed when evaluating the clinical results that show improvement occurs not only during the first postoperative year, but also improvement continues to occur during the second postoperative year.

Tweenplasty

There is one special area that needs to be addressed during the contouring procedure to allow normal anterior rotation of the UniSpacer in full extension. This area, the junction of Whitesides line and the superior aspect of the intercondylar notch, is critical in allowing normal anterior rotation of the UniSpacer in full extension. Since the UniSpacer is driven by the femoral condyle toward the femoral sulcus in full extension, this area needs to be recessed to allow normal rotational motion.

Full thickness cartilage just above the intercondylar notch must be removed to allow the anterior flange of the device to "screw home" in full extension. If this cartilage is not removed, the UniSpacer will be driven out into an anteromedial position causing impingement and pain during full extension (Figure 16.9). The degree of articular degen-

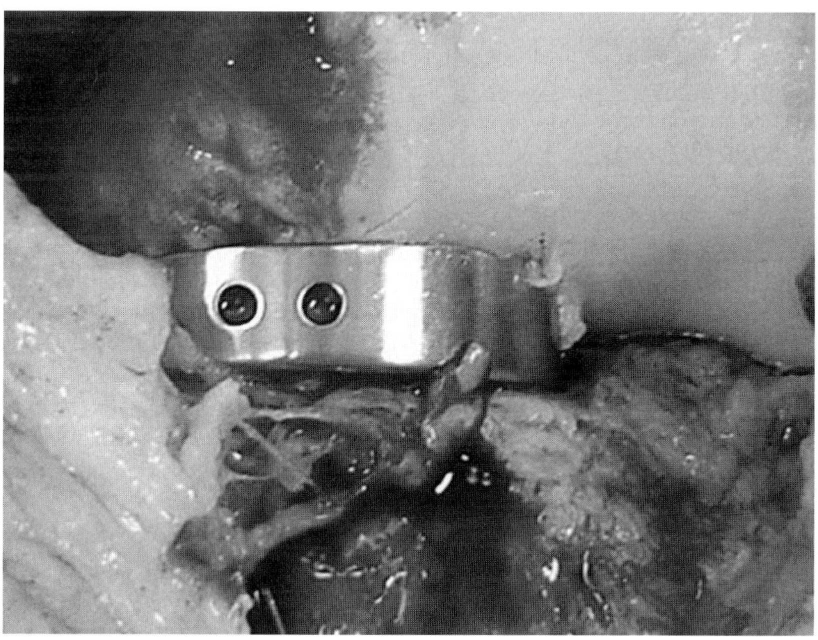

Figure 16.9. A UniSpacer in position without a proper tweenplasty. Note the impingement on the femoral condyle.

eration on the femoral surface of the patient will dictate how deep this recess needs to be. Most patients require removal of full thickness articular cartilage in this zone.

Sizing

The UniSpacer comes in six different sizes with respect to length/width and four different thicknesses for each knee. Thus, both the left and right knee each have 24 different sized implants. The AP length of the device remains proportional to the medial/lateral width of the device as the size increases and decreases. Thus the dimensions of the device increase and decrease proportionally relative to the size. Standard sets range in size between 38 mm in length to 58 mm in length. The device also comes in four varying thicknesses from 2 mm to 5 mm. Initially, the size of the device is estimated by measuring the AP length of the tibia.

The ultimate sizing, however, is determined by the remaining contour of the femoral condyle. The femoral surface of the UniSpacer must have a radius that is greater than or equal to the surface remaining on the contoured femoral condyle. In other words, the femoral condyle must fit the femoral surface of the UniSpacer without producing any edge loading anteriorly or posteriorly as this creates impingement and eventually may lead to pain or dislocation.

Sizing the Implant

The size of the implant that is ultimately chosen is based on length and thickness. The implant must restore the joint space of the medial compartment that corrects the axial alignment. There is a thickness gauge with the instrument set that can be used to help determine the appropriate thickness. The thickness gauge comes in four different thicknesses ranging from 2 mm to 5 mm, in 1-mm increments. This gauge is placed between the medial femoral condyle and tibial plateau in both flexion and extension. The correct thickness implant will retension the medial collateral ligament and anterior cruciate ligament while allowing full extension and maximum flexion. The thickness gauge gives the surgeon an initial trial size that may have to be modified after the initial implant trial. The implant must ultimately be sized to fit the contour of the femoral condyle, however, the initial length measurement is taken from the AP dimension of the tibia. An arthroscopy probe is used to hook the posterior aspect of the tibial plateau and then mark the anterior aspect of the tibia using a hemostat (Figure 16.10). There is a ruler with the instruments that can then be used to check the AP dimension off the arthroscopy hook. This gives the surgeon an initial trial size with respect to length.

Once the initial measurements have been taken with respect to length and thickness, an implant trial is selected out of the set. The trial is placed on the insertion handle, and then implanted into the medial compartment. The final sizing is actually confirmed by evaluation of the conformity of the femoral surface of the UniSpacer to the femoral

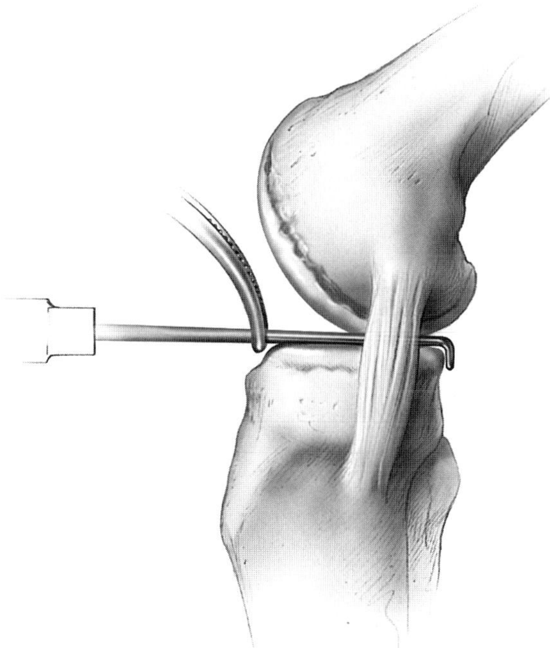

Figure 16.10. The length initial measurement for the UniSpacer taken off the AP dimension of the tibial plateau.

condyle. Once the implant is in place, the knee should be placed through a vigorous range of motion to ensure that the UniSpacer has both uniform translation and rotation during flexion and extension cycles. In extension the UniSpacer should always translate and rotate toward the intercondylar notch, and demonstrate a small amount of anterior overhand off the tibia. In flexion, the UniSpacer should rotate around the tibial spine, translate posteriorly, and frequently show posterior translation off the tibia.

Insertion Technique

The insertion of both the UniSpacer trials as well as the final implant is often the most intimidating portion of the procedure to learn. Once this technique is mastered, however, it is relatively simple and reproducible. The handle of the trial device allows 360 degrees of rotation, which allows the surgeon to choose the most optimal position of the handle to avoid impingement on the soft tissues during insertion. During the insertion, the trial is tucked into the medial compartment underneath the medial edge of the patella. With the knee flexed to approximately 45 degrees to 60 degrees, a valgus stress is applied to the knee and the UniSpacer is held against the femoral condyle with the trial handle. Using some posterior pressure on the handle in addition to a small wiggle, the knee is pulled into full extension and the

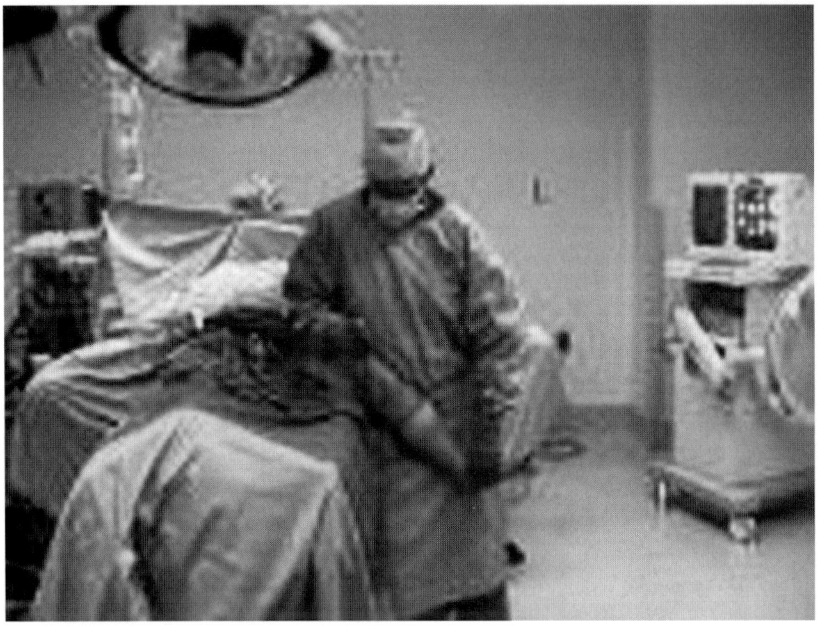

Figure 16.11. Proper surgeon positioning for UniSpacer insertion.

UniSpacer will drop into the medial compartment. The surgeon must be careful to exert pressure, which is directly posterior on the tibial plateau to allow the device to slide into position (Figure 6.11). The most common error during this technique is improper insertion angle, which results in driving the UniSpacer into the tibial spine instead of into a posterior position on the tibial plateau. Once in position, the implant should center itself under the femoral condyle. To remove the trial implant from the knee, the reverse of this technique is performed. The knee is held in extension with a valgus stress applied to the knee. With the UniSpacer held against the femoral condyle, the knee is flexed. With that maneuver the UniSpacer can easily be removed from the medial compartment.

Fluoroscopy

It is necessary to confirm correct implant sizing and motion using fluoroscopic guidance. Fluoroscopy allows the surgeon to check the size of the implant relative to the femoral condyle, again ensuring that the UniSpacer has the most anatomic fit to the femoral condyle without undersizing the implant. Fluoroscopy also allows the surgeon to view the motion of the device through normal range of motion. In the fully extended position, the UniSpacer should translate several millimeters anterior to the tibial plateau on the lateral view (Figure 16.12). In flexion the UniSpacer should translate to the posterior aspect of the tibia or extend several millimeters past the posterior aspect of the tibial plateau (Figure 16.13). On the AP view in full extension, the UniSpacer should

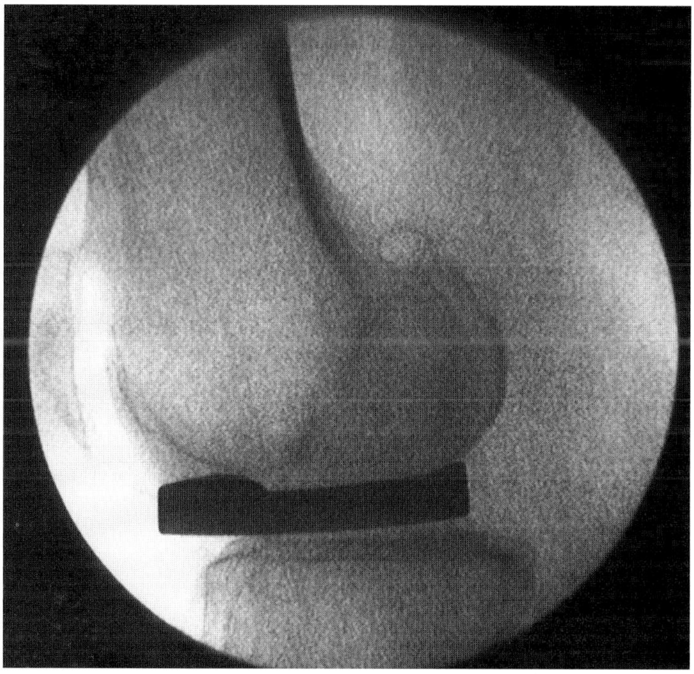

Figure 16.12. Lateral fluoroscopy view with the knee extended. Note the anterior position of the UniSpacer on the tibial plateau.

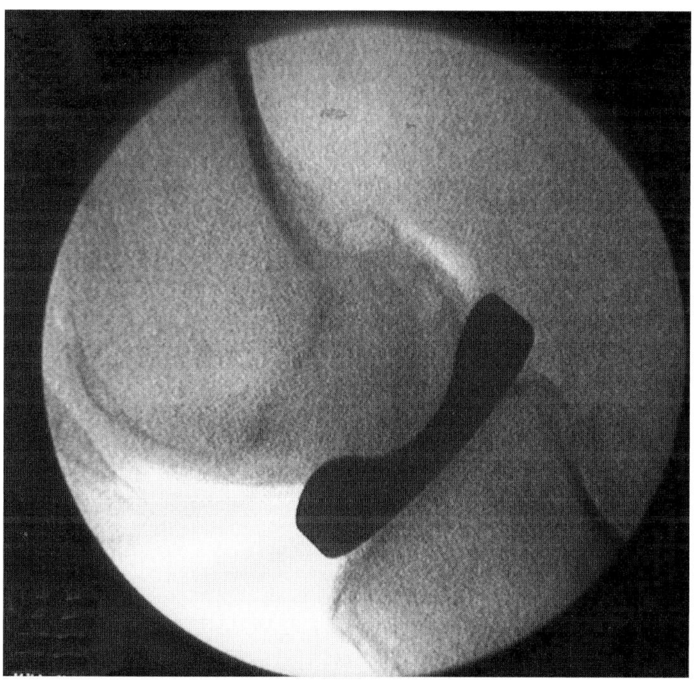

Figure 16.13. A lateral fluoroscopy view with the knee flexed. Note the posterior translation of the UniSpacer on the tibial plateau. The UniSpacer follows the femoral condyle during femoral roll back.

appear rotated with the anterior horn of the UniSpacer rotated centrally toward the tibial spine. As the surgeon becomes more comfortable with the technique, the fluoroscopy can be kept to a minimum.

Final Implantation and Closure

Once the optimum implant size has been selected, and fluoroscopy is completed, the final implant is inserted into the medial compartment. The handle of the insertion tool is slightly different from the trial tool. The implant is connected to the insertion handle using converging pins. These pins are more fragile than the large pin on the anterior aspect of the trial implants. The insertion technique, however, is basically the same. Once the final implant is in position, the surgeon should place the knee through a range of motion to confirm proper kinematics. The wound is closed in a standard fashion using heavier suture material in the deeper retinacular layer and the routine subcutaneous and skin closure preferred by the surgeon. Patients do not require immobilization unless the surgeon feels the patient would have improved initial ambulation with the extra support.

References

1. Hallock RH, Fell BM. Unicompartmental tibial hemiarthroplasty: early results of the UniSpacer knee. Clin Orthop. November 2003;(416):154–163.
2. Hallock RH. The UniSpacer Knee System: have we been there before? Orthopedics. September 2003;26(9):953–954.
3. Geier KA. UniSpacer for knee osteoarthritis. Orthop Nurs. September–October 2003;22(5):369–370.
4. Friedman MJ. UniSpacer. Arthroscopy. December 2003;19(suppl 1):120–121.
5. Dressler K, Ellermann A. UNISPACER—a new minimally-invasive therapeutic concept for the isolated medial knee joint disease. Z Orthop Ihre Grenzgeb. March–April 2004;142(2):131–133.

17

Minimally Invasive Technique for Insertion of a Unicompartmental Knee Arthroplasty

A.J. Price and D.W. Murray

Prosthesis Design

The Oxford meniscal unicompartmental knee arthroplasty has been used to treat anteromedial arthritis of the knee since 1982.[1] The design of the prosthesis employs a spherical femoral component with a flat tibial base-plate, between which a fully congruent unconstrained mobile bearing is inserted (Figure 17.1). This provides a large contact area for articulation in all angles of flexion, reducing contact stress, and the design has been shown to provide low wear rates in clinical practice.[2,3] The bearing is held in place by the shapes of the components together with the tension in the ligaments of the knee. It is free to move and allows near normal sliding and rolling movements of the femoral condyle in the medial compartment.[4]

Indications

The prosthesis has achieved 10-year survival results of 95% to 98% in the hands of surgeons experienced in its use.[5,6] Appropriate patient selection is vital to the success of the device and the indications for its use are now well established. The device is most commonly used to treat anteromedial osteoarthritis of the knee, but can be employed in cases of focal medial compartment osteonecrosis.[7,8] In all cases the anterior cruciate ligament should be functionally intact.[9] Full thickness cartilage must be retained in the lateral compartment and any varus deformity must be correctable, as demonstrated by preoperative stress radiographs. Contraindications include inflammatory arthropathy and previous high tibial osteotomy.[5,10] Age, weight, chondrocalcinosis and the state of the patellofemoral joint are not considered contraindications.[1]

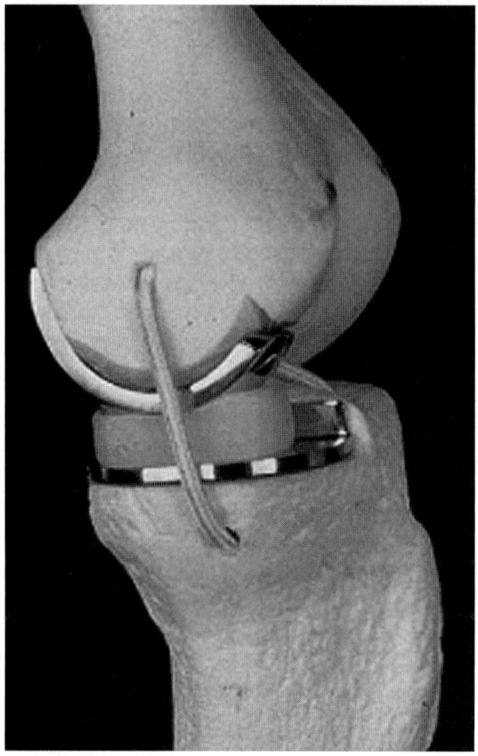

Figure 17.1. The Phase 3 Oxford unicompartmental knee arthroplasty inserted into a saw-bone model.

Introduction of the Phase 3 Oxford Unicompartmental Knee Arthroplasty

Phase 1 and 2 Oxford unicompartmental knee arthroplasty were both inserted through a standard approach used for total knee procedures, where the patella was dislocated. In 1998, in an attempt to reduce perioperative morbidity, Phase 3 was introduced. This allowed the device to be inserted through a much smaller incision, where the suprapatellar pouch was not violated and the patella not dislocated (Figure 17.2). The bone-resecting mill, a key feature of the Phase 2 instrumentation, could be used through such a small incision. With the mill, bone can be removed in 1-mm increments from the distal femur until ligament balance and tension are restored to normal. In addition, new instrumentation was designed to facilitate accurate component insertion through a small wound.

The early results of Phase 3 prostheses implanted in Oxford, show that small incision patients mobilize approximately twice as fast as those where the more extensive approach was used, while there was no reduction in the accuracy of component insertion.[11]

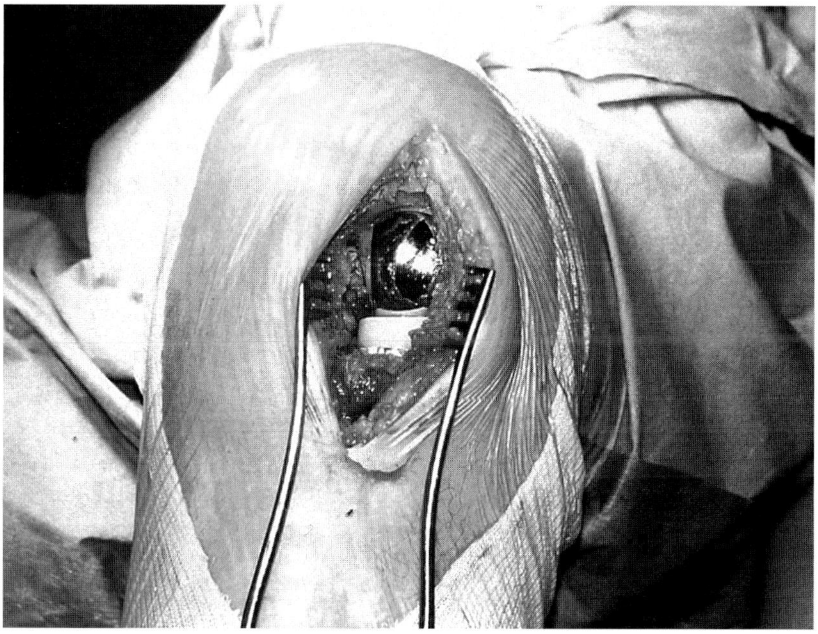

Figure 17.2. Intraoperative picture of Phase 3 prosthesis following final reduction prior to skin closure.

Operative Technique

Templating the Preoperative Radiographs

Prior to starting a case, the lateral knee radiograph should be templated to establish the size of femoral component to be used: small, medium, large or extra large. Templates with 105% magnification are available, corresponding to the magnification that occurs if the radiographic source is about 100 cm from the knee and the x-ray cassette rests against the knee.

Positioning the Patient

The patient is placed supine at the edge of the operating table and the hip is abducted and flexed to 30 degrees, to allow the thigh to sit in a trough support attached to the side of the table (Figure 17.3). The support must not impinge on the popliteal fossa. A tourniquet is placed at the same level as the support and the knee is free to flex fully. The knee is draped in standard fashion. An experienced assistant is required, who despite having a poor view of the operation, can retract and hold the knee in appropriate positions giving the surgeon an excellent view and good access.

Incision and Debridement of Osteophytes

With the knee flexed at 90 degrees, a skin incision is made from the medial margin of the patella to the medial border of the tibial tuberosity,

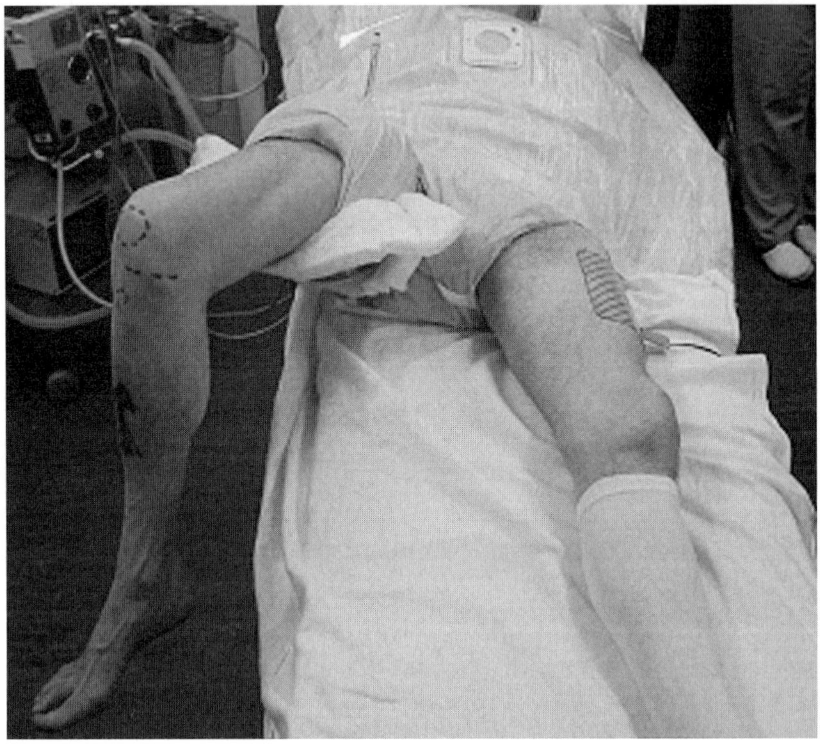

A

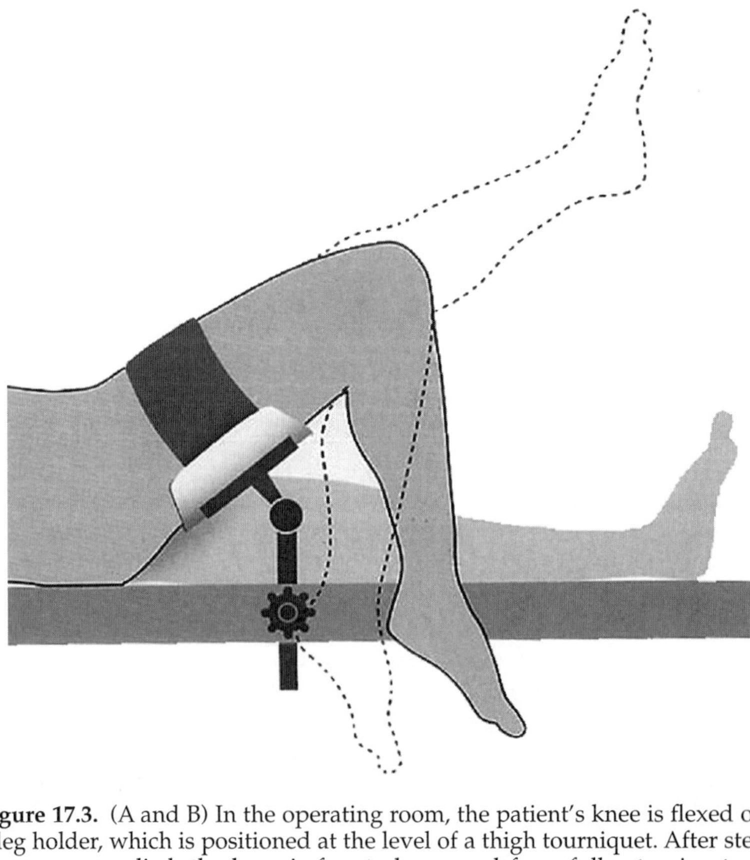

B

Figure 17.3. (A and B) In the operating room, the patient's knee is flexed over a leg holder, which is positioned at the level of a thigh tourniquet. After sterile drapes are applied, the knee is free to be moved from full extension to 120 degrees of flexion.

approximately 3 cm below the joint line (Figure 17.4). Beginning from the upper pole of the patella a medial capsulotomy is made in the same line as the skin incision and the joint is entered. The upper end of the capsular incision can be extended by 1 cm to 2 cm into the vastus medialis. Part of the fat pad and medial meniscus is excised to expose the articular surfaces and a self-retaining retractor is placed in the wound. All instruments for the procedure are passed through the incision in the anteroposterior plane.

The anterior cruciate ligament is examined and assessed with a hook to determine whether it is intact. The lateral compartment is inspected to ensure that articular surfaces are intact. Commonly a full thickness ulcer is seen on the medial side of the lateral condyle, caused by impingement on the tibial spine. This is ignored. If the anterior cruciate ligament is deficient or if there is significant articular damage centrally on the lateral condyle, then the procedure is abandoned and a total knee replacement is implanted.

Using a chisel, osteophytes are removed from the margins of the medial femoral condyle and the intercondylar notch. Particular care must be taken to remove the osteophytes that are found on the posterolateral aspect of the medial condyle. Additional osteophytes around the anterior margin of the tibia, the intercondylar notch and the patella are removed. Flexion and extension of the knee, controlled by an assistant allows adequate exposure. The knee is washed out with saline.

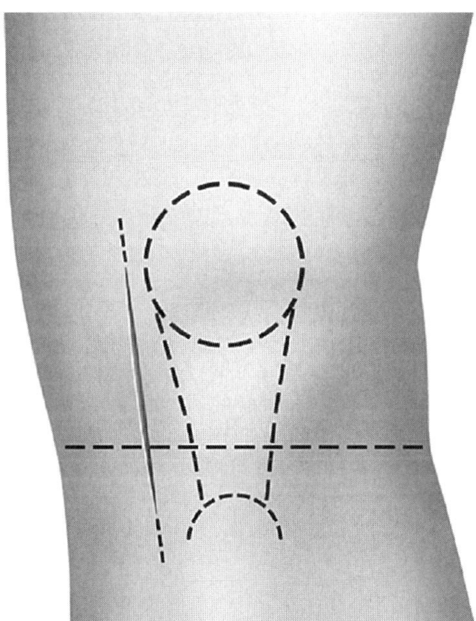

Figure 17.4. The incision is made from the medial margin of the patella to the medial border of the tibial tuberosity, approximately 3 cm below the joint line.

Making the Tibial Plateau Bone Cuts

The anterior aspect of the tibia is exposed, without releasing any fibers of the medial collateral ligament. An extramedullary jig is employed and is placed against the front of the tibia, with the recessed shape of the cutting block accommodating the patellar tendon. The rod is positioned in line with the tibial crest in the coronal plane and parallel to it in the saggital plane. In this orientation the tibial cut will have 7 degrees of posterior slope.

The level of resection should normally pass 2 mm to 3 mm below the deepest part of the tibial erosion. Once the level of resection has been selected the tibial jig is pinned to the tibia. The vertical saw cut is made with a reciprocating saw. The saw blade is passed alongside the lateral side of the medial condyle and is directed toward the femoral head, which is identified by an assistant (Figure 17.5). The cut is made down to the level of the cutting block, taking care to ensure the posterior cortex is included.

A retractor is inserted to protect the medial collateral ligament and the horizontal cut is made with an oscillating saw (Figure 17.6). Care should be taken not to damage the medial collateral ligament. The cut

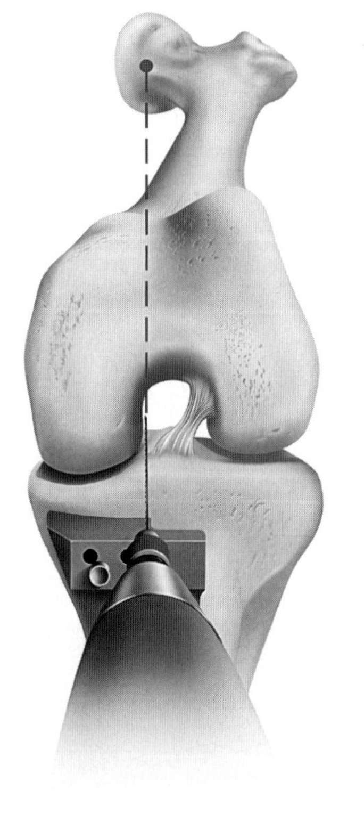

Figure 17.5. The reciprocating saw blade is passed through the intercondylar notch, resting against the lateral wall of the medial condyle. With the blade pointing toward the femoral head, the vertical cut can then be made. The anteriorly placed tibial saw guide acts as a stop.

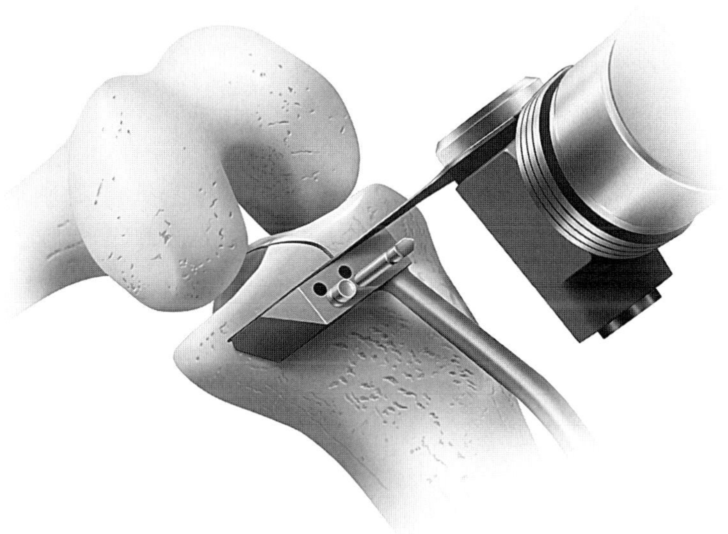

Figure 17.6. The horizontal cut is made with an oscillating saw. The medial collateral ligament must be protected with a retractor during this cut.

is complete when the anterior aspect of the resected bone is seen to move. The specimen is lifted with an osteotome and grasped with a Kocker's forcep. The resected bone is pulled out of the wound, releasing any retained soft tissue attachments. The resected specimen should show the typical pattern of antero-medial arthritis. An estimate of the correct tibial base plate size can then be made by comparing the width of the cut specimen to the base plate trial.

The joint is washed out and remnants of the medial meniscus removed. The base trial is inserted, checking that the size is appropriate. With the trial base plate in situ the 4-mm thick feeler gauge is inserted (3 mm is acceptable in small patients). If this does not pass easily a further cut should be made from the tibia, by reattaching the tibial cutting jig using pins passed through the same holes in the tibia and moving the block down with the pins now passing through the upper holes on the block. This allows a further 3-mm resection to be made. A further check is made that the resection is adequate.

Creating Femoral Drill Holes

With the knee flexed to about 45 degrees the entry hole for the intramedullary rod is made using an awl. The entry point is 1 cm anterior to the anteromedial corner of the intercondylar notch. After passing the rod the knee is flexed to 90 degrees, taking care to ease the passage of the patella against the rod. The rod abuts the patella displacing it laterally. The femoral drill guide, together with the tibial template and a feeler gauge 1 mm narrower than the gap, are placed into the knee

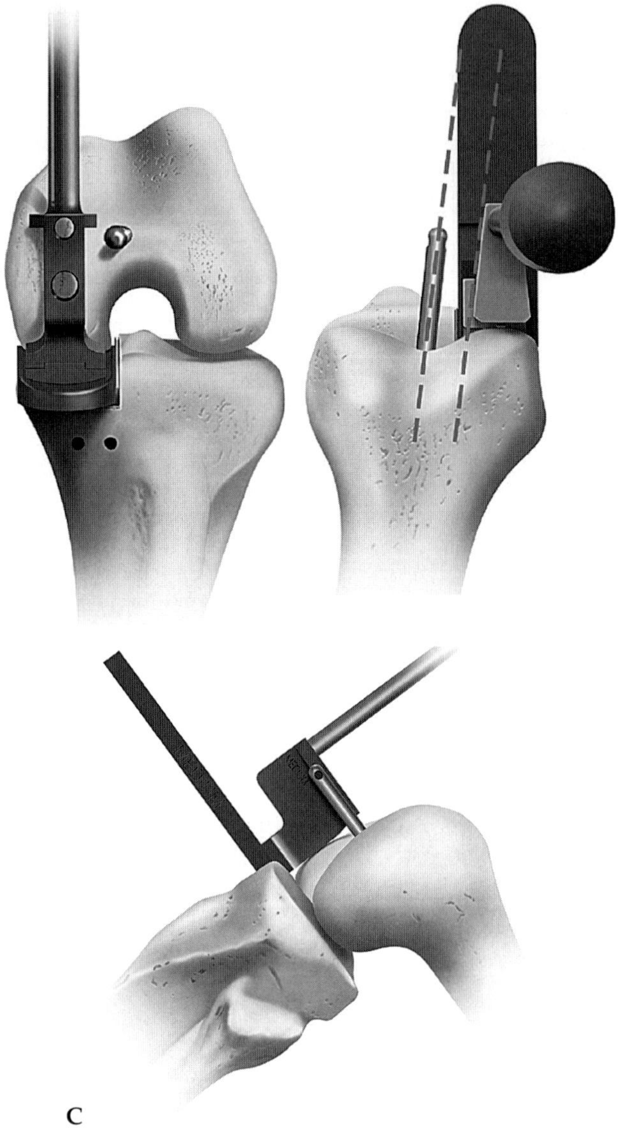

A B C

Figure 17.7. Using the femoral drill guide: (A) anterior view of the guide inserted into the knee, in addition to the tibial template and a feeler gauge, with the handle parallel to the long axis of the tibia, (B) as seen from above, the 7 degrees wing on the tibial guide should be parallel to the intramedullary rod and (C) in the sagittal plane the upper surface of the guide is parallel to the intramedullary rod.

(Figure 17.7). The position of the guide and leg are adjusted until: (1) in the sagittal plane the upper surface of the guide is parallel to the intramedullary rod, (2) in the coronal plane the 7 degrees wing on the tibial guide is parallel to the intramedullary rod, (3) the feeler gauge touches the vertical wall of the tibial template, (4) the center of the 6 mm hole on the jig lies in the central third of the condyle, and (5) the handle of the guide is aligned with the long axis of the tibia. When these conditions are met drill holes are then made through the upper (4 mm) and lower (6 mm) holes on the guide. If it is not possible to get the feeler gauge touching the wall, a narrower feeler gauge should be used. In addition if there is a posteromedial femoral osteophyte displacing the feeler gauge it should be removed with a chisel.

Femoral Condyle Preparation: Posterior Facet Saw Cut and Initial Milling

With the femoral guide removed a femoral cutting block is positioned into the drill holes and the posterior facet of the femoral condyle is resected with an oscillating saw, taking great care not to cut anteriorly (Figure 17.8). The accuracy of the cut is confirmed with a chisel. The femoral mill, guided by a series of spigots, is now used to resect bone from the distal femur. A zero spigot is tapped into the 6-mm guide hole on the femur and the mill is advanced onto it, avoiding soft tissues (Figure 17.9). Milling is performed under power, until the mill is stopped by the collar on the spigot and will not advance further. The mill is removed and any protruding collar or corners of bone are resected with a chisel.

Balancing the Flexion and Extension Gaps

Trial femoral and tibial tray components are inserted. With the knee at 90 degrees, the flexion gap is measured with feeler gauges. The correct

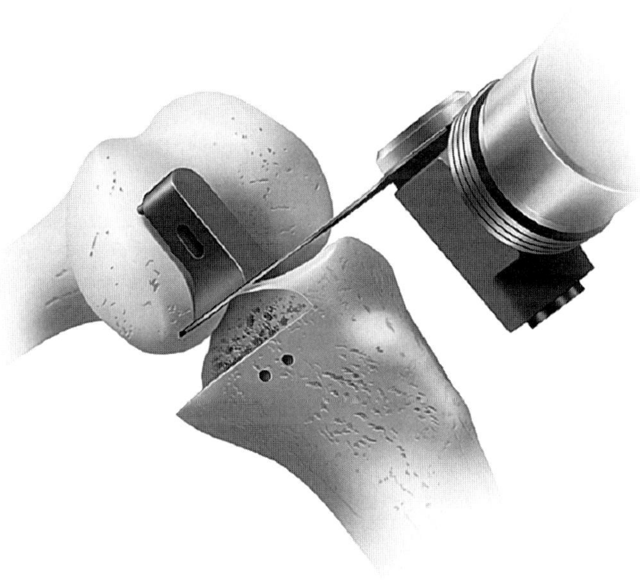

Figure 17.8. The posterior femoral facet cutting block is inserted and the cut made with an oscillating saw.

gauge slides in and out easily, without tilting, holding the medial collateral ligament at its physiological tension. The gauge is removed, the knee extended to 20 degrees of flexion and the extension measured in similar fashion. The initial measurement will usually demonstrate that the flexion gap is bigger than the extension gap. The following formula is then applied to calculate the thickness of bone to be milled from the distal femur:

Flexion gap feeler gauge result – Extension gap feeler gauge result
= Thickness (mm) of bone to be resected
= Spigot number to be used

The chosen spigot is inserted into the knee and the knee milled. The feeler gauges are reinserted into the knee in flexion and extension to ensure correct balance has been achieved (Figure 17.10). If the knee is not balanced, the gap measurement is repeated. The equation above is used to calculate how much more bone should be removed and the appropriate spigot used. When ligament balance has been achieved the knee is washed out with saline.

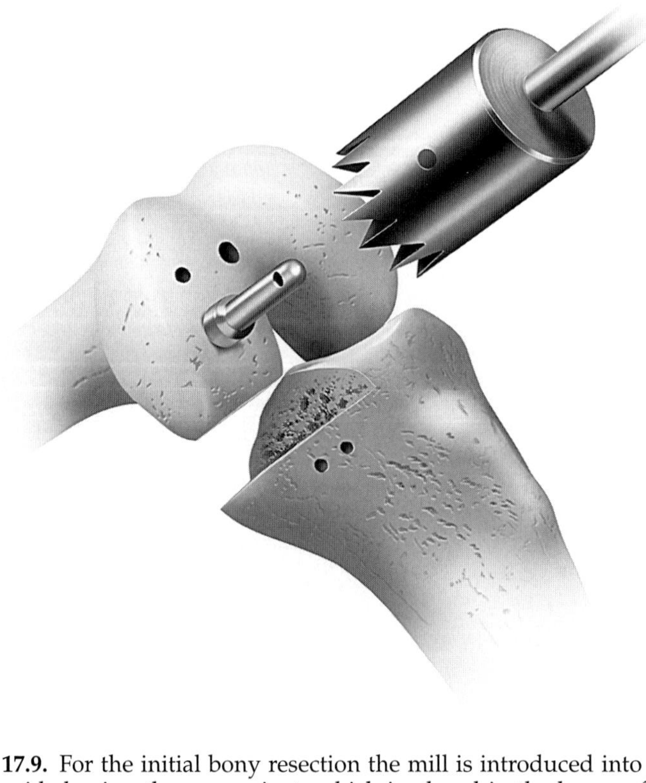

Figure 17.9. For the initial bony resection the mill is introduced into the joint and is guided using the zero spigot, which is placed in the larger of the two femoral drill holes.

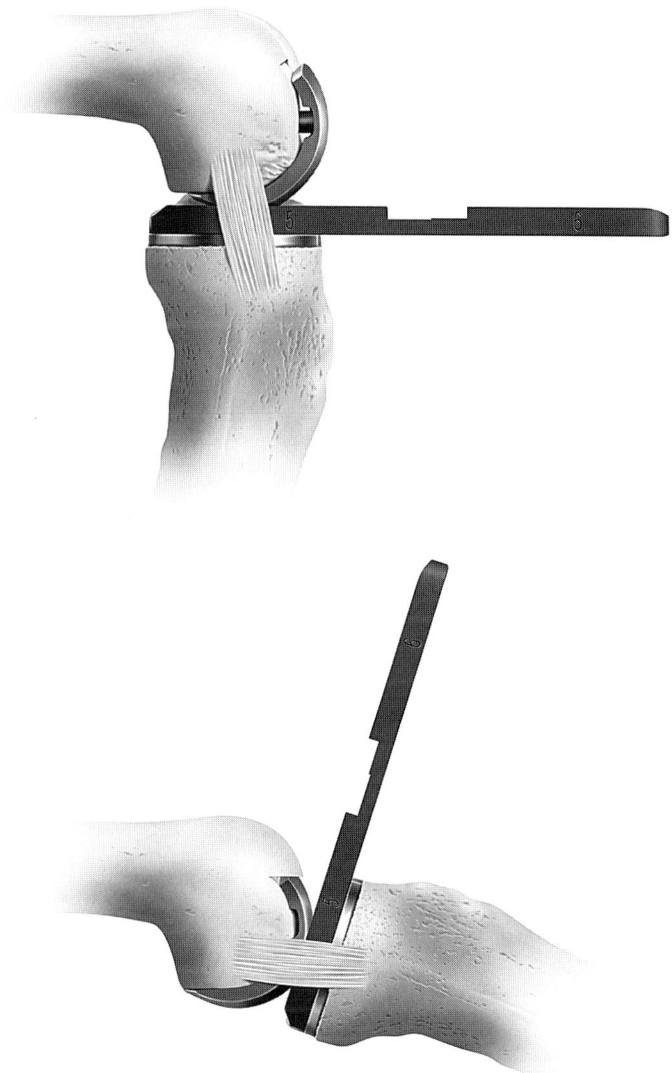

A

B

Figure 17.10. Equality of the flexion and extension gaps is confirmed by inserting the same feeler gauge at both (A) 90 degrees and (B) 20 degrees of flexion.

Final Bony Preparation: Prevention of Impingement and Cutting the Keel Slot

Final preparation of the femur requires insertion of the femoral posterior trimming block and use of the osteophyte chisel to remove posterior osteophytes (Figure 17.11A). A finger is inserted to palpate posteriorly, checking that all osteophytes have been removed. Approximately 5 mm of bone is removed with a chisel from the anterior aspect of the milled femur to prevent anterior bony impingement of the bearing in extension (Figure 11B).

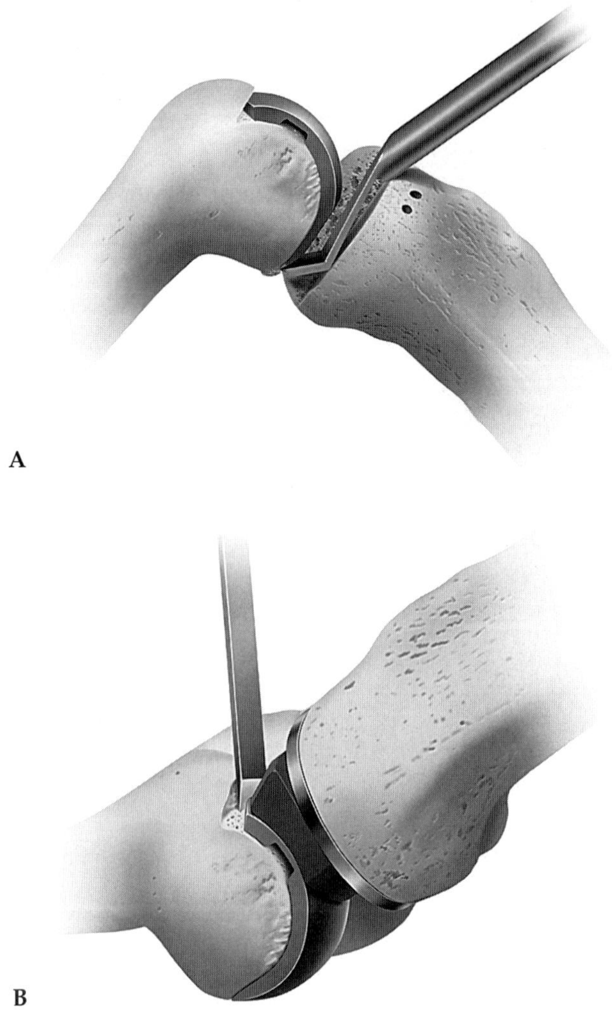

Figure 17.11. (A) To prevent postoperative impingement, posterior osteophytes are removed using a femoral posterior trimming block and the osteophyte chisel. (B) In addition, a chisel is used to remove bone from the anterior aspect of the femur, preventing impingement of the bearing on bone, when the knee is in full extension.

The rim of the cut tibia is inspected and all retained tibial osteophytes removed. The tibial template is reinserted into the knee and a hook used to feel the posterior cortex and ensure that the template reaches the posterior cortex margin. The width of the template is now assessed. It should either be aligned with the medial cortex or overhang by up to 2 mm. If overhang is greater a smaller tibial template is selected. The correctly sized and positioned template is held in position with a nail placed anteriorly. A reciprocating saw is used through the template to cut along each side of the slot at a depth of approximately 10 mm. Care is taken not to cut too deep as this may predispose to tibial fracture. With the template removed a gouge is used remove bone from the slot.

The joint is washed out and the tibial trial base plate inserted to ensure it sits within the keel slot.

Trial Reduction

With both trial femur and tibia in the knee, a trial meniscal bearing of the same thickness as the previously used feeler gauge is inserted (Figure 17.12). The knee is flexed and extended to check the range of movement and to ensure there is no evidence of impingement. The balance of the knee is assessed at 90 degrees and 20 degrees of flexion. A correctly balanced knee allows the prosthetic joint surface to open a few millimeters when a valgus force is applied.

Cementing Components and Final Reduction

The trial components are removed and the joint washed out with saline. Small cement keyholes are drilled into the femoral and tibial joint surfaces. The components are then inserted separately, each with one mix of cement.

A sausage-shaped piece of cement is placed onto the tibial plateau and flattened with a moist chisel to produce a thin layer of cement that extends to the posterior margin of the cut tibial surface. The component is inserted and the keel pressed into the posterior aspect of the slot and then finally anteriorly. In this way excess cement is extruded

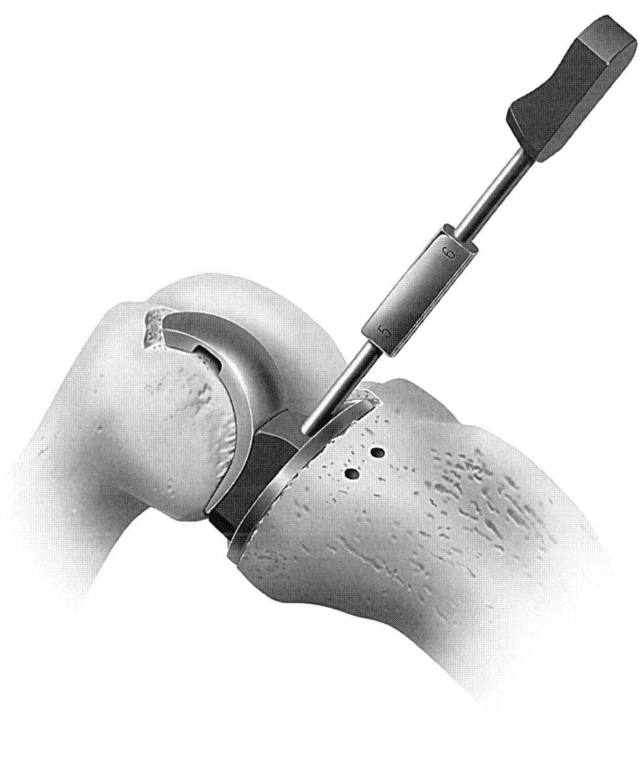

Figure 17.12. A trial reduction is performed with the appropriate trial bearing inserted between the femoral and tibial components, instead of a feeler gauge.

anteriorly and not posteriorly. The right-angled tibial impactor and a small mallet are used to ensure the component is seated properly. Care must be taken to ensure no soft tissue lies under the component. Any excess cement is removed with a curette. The femoral trial component and the correct size of feeler gauge are inserted with the knee held at 45 degrees of flexion, while the cement cures. When the cement is set the feeler gauge is removed together with the femoral trial. The knee is washed out and a detailed inspection of the margins of the implant made to allow removal of any unwanted retained cement.

The second mix of cement is prepared and is loaded onto the concave surface on the femoral component. An additional small amount is pushed into the large femoral drill hole. The femoral component is then pushed onto the prepared femur and is then impacted with a punch at 45 degrees to the long axis of the femur. The feeler gauge is inserted and the knee held flexed to 45 degrees, pressurizing the cement. Excess cement is removed from around the prosthesis.

The knee is washed out with saline. The definitive bearing is inserted into the joint, completing the final reduction of the device (see Figure 17.2). The bearing should move freely as the knee is flexed and extended.

Wound Closure

The wound is closed in layers over one drain. Clips are applied to the skin. Dressings, wool and crepe bandage are applied.

Postoperative Recovery

The patient can be mobilized from the immediate postoperative period, working on establishing a straight-leg raise and knee flexion. Standing, fully weight bearing, is introduced as early as possible and walking encouraged from the first postoperative day. However, we have found that aggressive early mobilization can be counterproductive, causing pain and swelling, which slows recovery. Patients usually have a fixed flexion deformity in the immediate postoperative period, which tends to correct spontaneously during the first year. In addition, some patients have residual pain, stiffness, swelling and numbness lateral to the wound at two months postoperation. Again these symptoms usually settle in the first year.

Summary

We have found this technique to be reliable and with good assistance, generally straightforward. The short incision results in decreased perioperative morbidity, faster recovery and a better outcome for the patient.[11] We have shown that components can be implanted as precisely as with an open technique.[11] Over the past six years we have implanted over 600 mobile bearing unicompartmental arthroplasties in Oxford using this technique and have encountered very few problems.

References

1. Goodfellow J, O'Connor J. The anterior cruciate ligament in knee arthroplasty. A risk-factor with unconstrained meniscal prostheses. Clin Orthop. 1992;276:245–252.
2. Goodfellow J, O'Connor JJ, Murray D. Principles of meniscal bearing arthroplasty for unicompartmental knee replacement. In: Cartier P, Epinette J, Deschamps G, Hernnigou P, eds. Unicompartmental Arthroplasty. Expansion scientific francaise; 1997.
3. Goodfellow JW, Kershaw CJ, Benson MK, O'Connor JJ. The Oxford Knee for unicompartmental osteoarthritis. The first 103 cases. J Bone Joint Surg Br. 1988;70(5):692–701.
4. Murray DW, Goodfellow JW, O'Connor JJ. The Oxford medial unicompartmental arthroplasty: a ten-year survival study. J Bone Joint Surg Br. 1998;80(6):983–999.
5. O'Connor JJ, Goodfellow JW. Theory and practice of meniscal knee replacement: design against wear. Proc Inst Mech Eng [H]. 1996;210(3):217–222.
6. Price AJ, Rees JL, Beard DJ, et al. Sagittal plane kinematics of a mobile bearing unicompartmental knee arthroplasty at ten years. J Arthroplasty. In press, 2004.
7. Price AJ, Webb J, Topf H, et al. Rapid recovery after Oxford unicompartmental arthroplasty through a short incision. J Arthroplasty. 2001;16: 298970–976.
8. Psychoyios V, Crawford RW, O'Connor JJ, Murray DW. Wear of congruent meniscal bearings in unicompartmental knee arthroplasty: a retrieval study of 16 specimens. J Bone Joint Surg Br. 1998;80(6):976–982.
9. Rees JL, Price AJ, Lynskey TG, et al. Medial unicompartmental arthroplasty after failed high tibial osteotomy. J Bone Joint Surg Br. 2001;83(7):1034–1036.
10. Svard UC, Price AJ. Oxford medial unicompartmental knee arthroplasty. A survival analysis of an independent series. J Bone Joint Surg Br. 2001; 83(2):191–194.
11. White SH, Ludkowski PF, Goodfellow JW. Anteromedial osteoarthritis of the knee. J Bone Joint Surg Br. 1991;73(4):582–586.

Section IV

The Knee: Total Knee Arthroplasty

18

Minimal Incision Total Knee Arthroplasty with a Limited Medial Parapatellar Arthrotomy

Giles R. Scuderi

The early description of the medial parapatellar approach to the knee is often credited to von Langenbeck, who described directly detaching the vastus medialis muscle from its insertion onto the quadriceps tendon and continuing the arthrotomy along the medial aspect of the patella. Insall introduced a midline capsular incision that divides the quadriceps tendon in its medial third, and peels the quadriceps expansion from the patella.[1] This approach, or a slight variation thereof, is the most popular approach for total knee arthroplasty.

The traditional medial parapatellar arthrotomy consists of a straight anterior midline skin incision, extending 8 cm proximal to the superior pole and 2 cm distal to the tibial tubercle. The proximal arthrotomy divides the quadriceps tendon along its medial third. The arthrotomy can either curve around the medial border of the patella or can be taken straight over the medial aspect of the patellar bone. Insall preferred a straight medial arthrotomy because it minimizes the disruption of the vastus medialis attachment to the patella, resulting in a straight pull of the extensor mechanism with less tension on the closure. Alternatively, one can use a curved approach, leaving a cuff of tissue medial to the patella for later repair. Once the arthrotomy is made and appropriate releases are performed, the patella is everted and the knee is flexed. Closure is accomplished by anatomic reapproximation with simple sutures placed in an oblique fashion to exploit the vector pull of the vastus medialis muscle.

The popularity of the medial parapatellar arthrotomy is based mainly on its familiarity, simplicity, and on the excellent exposure of all three compartments of the knee. The approach is quite extensile and can be applied to almost any deformity, especially with the ability to perform a quadriceps snip if there is any difficulty with exposure of the joint. In addition, the medial parapatellar arthrotomy approach allows for the greatest distance from the neurovascular structures. The minimal incision technique has evolved from the traditional approach. As experience is gained in performing total knee arthroplasty, the extent of the skin incision and medial parapatellar arthrotomy can be reduced, so that the procedure can be performed safely and accurately through a limited exposure.[2]

Technique

Minimal incision total knee arthroplasty is performed with a limited skin incision and limited medial parapatellar arthrotomy.[2] The 10-cm to 14-cm midline skin incision is strategically placed from the superior aspect of the tibial tubercle and to the superior border of the patella (Figure 18.1). Following subcutaneous dissection, medial and lateral flaps are developed, along with proximal and distal dissection to expose the extensor mechanism. This permits mobilization of the skin and subcutaneous tissue as needed during the procedure. In addition, due to the elasticity of the skin, with the knee in flexion the incision will stretch 2 cm to 4 cm allowing broader exposure.

The intention of minimal incision surgery is to limit the surgical dissection, but not compromise the procedure. The medial parapatellar arthrotomy is used to expose the joint, but the proximal division of the quadriceps tendon should only be of a limited length to permit lateral subluxation of the patella without eversion (Figure 18.2). Initially the quadriceps tendon is incised for a length of 2 cm to 4 cm. If there is difficulty displacing the patella laterally or if the patella tendon is at risk of tearing, the arthrotomy is extended proximally along the quadriceps tendon until adequate exposure is achieved.

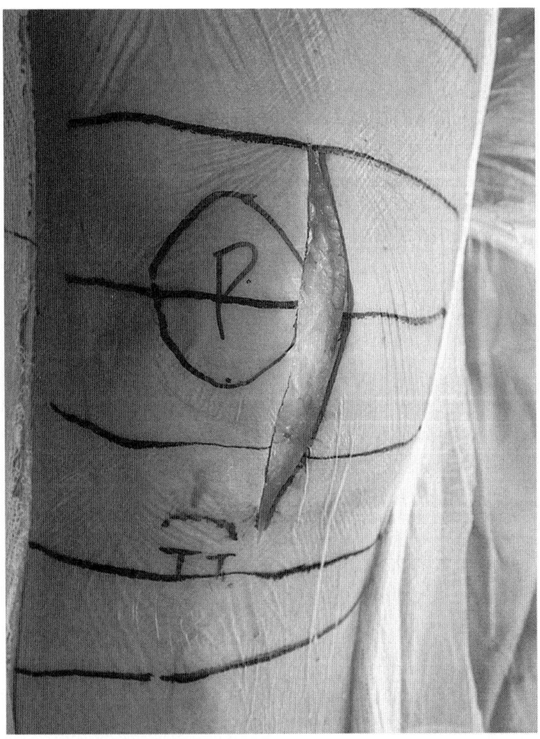

Figure 18.1. The skin incision is carefully placed from the superior pole of the patella to the tibial tubercle. (By permission of Scuderi GR, Tria AJ [eds]: Minimal Incision Total Knee Arthroplasty in MIS of the Hip and Knee: A Clinical Perspective. New York: Springer, 2004.)

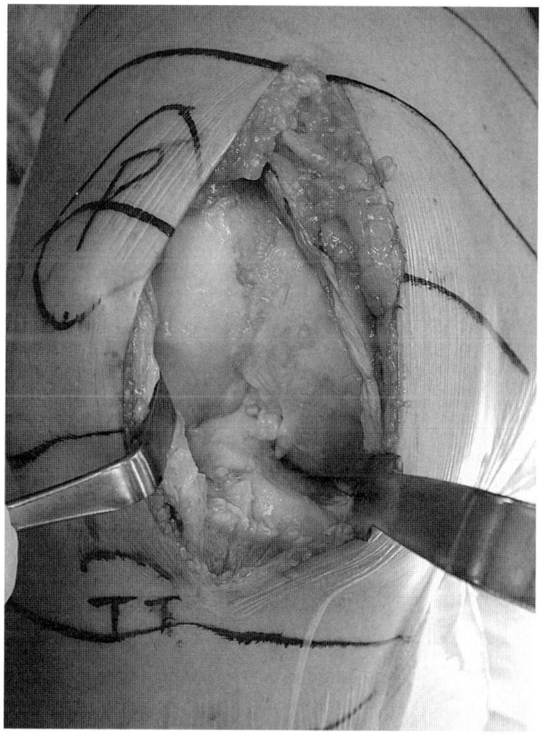

Figure 18.2. The limited medial parapatellar arthrotomy. (By permission of Scuderi GR, Tria AJ [eds]: Minimal Incision Total Knee Arthroplasty in MIS of the Hip and Knee: A Clinical Perspective. New York: Springer, 2004.)

Once the knee is exposed and the patella subluxed laterally, the bone cuts are made. The patella does not have to be everted during the procedure, since lateral subluxation provided adequate exposure. There is no difference from the traditional approach in the bone resection; however, the instrumentation has been modified to fit in a smaller space and also permit accurate bone resection. The author uses the NexGen Multi-Reference 4 in 1 Instrumentation (Zimmer, Warsaw, IN), which has been modified for the minimal incision approach.

Careful placement of retractors protects the supporting soft tissue structures. The incision can be moved as a mobile window from medial to lateral and from superior to inferior as necessary to aid in visualization without applying undue force to the skin and subcutaneous tissues. The order of the bone resection is dependent on the surgeon's preference, but the author recommends cutting the tibia first. Once the proximal tibia bone is removed, there is laxity of the joint in both the flexion and extension gaps permitting easier exposure of the knee and placement of the femoral instrumentation.

With the knee in 90 degrees of flexion and the patella subluxed laterally, the tibia is resected perpendicular to the mechanical axis with an extramedullary cutting guide set at the appropriate depth and slope (Figure 18.3). The retractors are strategically placed to protect the collateral ligaments and the patellar tendon. The retractors also permit

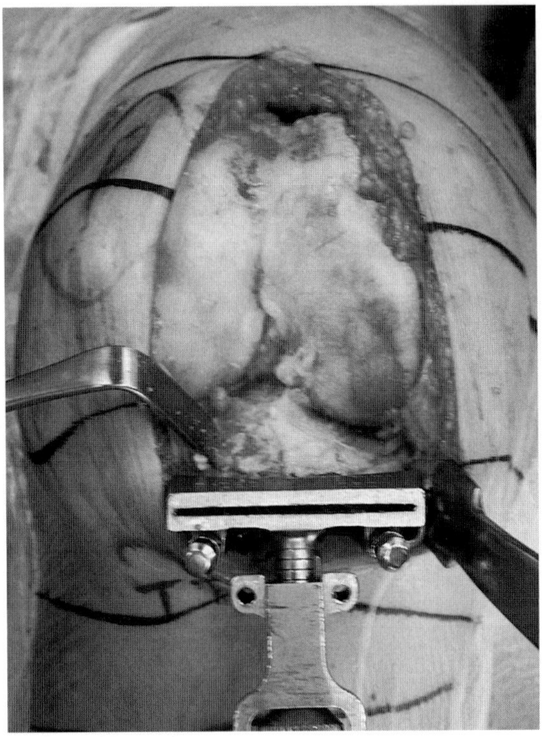

Figure 18.3. Tibial resection. (By permission of Scuderi GR, Tria AJ [eds]: Minimal Incision Total Knee Arthroplasty in MIS of the Hip and Knee: A Clinical Perspective. New York: Springer, 2004.)

mobilization of the arthrotomy to facilitate exposure by applying traction on one side and relaxing the opposite side. This mobile window is moved medially when the medial side is resected and laterally when the lateral tibia is cut since pulling on both the medial and lateral retractors at the same time limits exposure. To remove the resected proximal tibia, it may be necessary to bring the knee to 60 degrees to 70 degrees of flexion. The tibial bone is then brought forward through the arthrotomy with external rotation as the soft tissue attachments are released.

Following removal of the proximal tibial bone, attention is directed to the femur. The knee is once again brought to 90 degrees of flexion and a limited amount of synovial tissue and fat is resected from the anterior cortex. Very little dissection is performed in the suprapatellar pouch in an effort to reduce bleeding and scar tissue formation. I also try to preserve the infrapatellar fat pad for the same reason. The distal femur is resected with the modified intramedullary cutting guide, which is set at the appropriate valgus alignment (Figure 18.4). The next step is to identify either the transepicondylar axis or the anteroposterior axis of the distal femur, which can be done with the knee flexed and careful positioning of the retractors (Figure 18.5). Once the femoral rotation is determined, the femur is sized (Figure 18.6). With the current inventory of femoral component sizes, it is preferable to

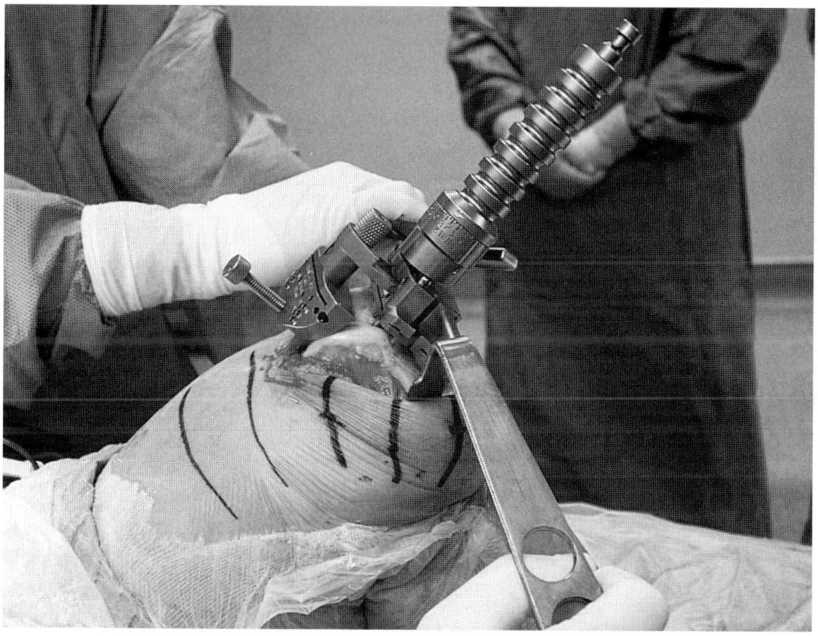

A

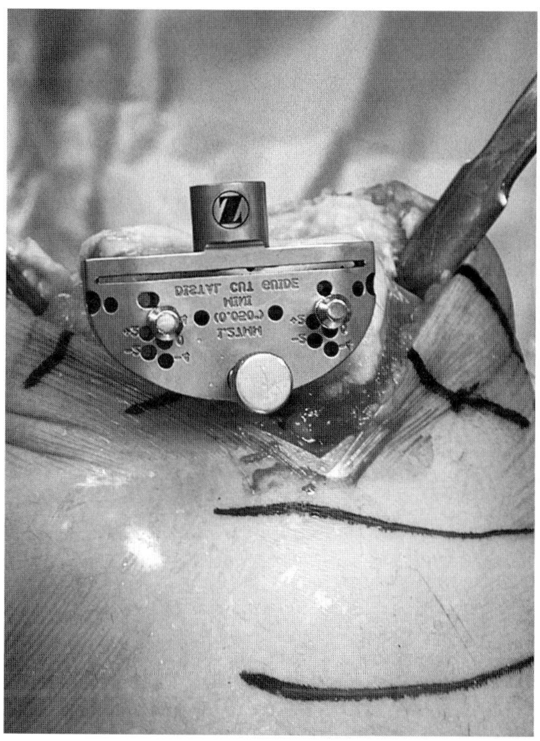

B

Figure 18.4. Distal femoral resection. A. The intramedullary guide in place. B. The distal cutting guide. (By permission of Scuderi GR, Tria AJ [eds]: Minimal Incision Total Knee Arthroplasty in MIS of the Hip and Knee: A Clinical Perspective. New York: Springer, 2004.)

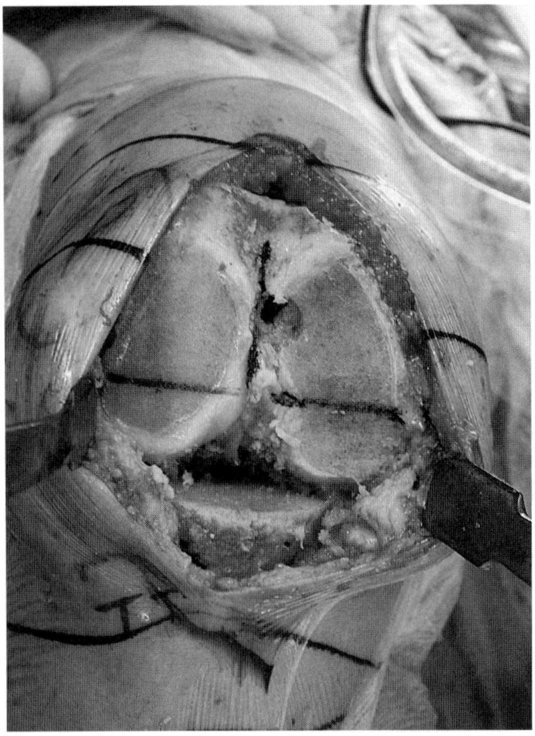

Figure 18.5. The epicondylar axis and the anterior-posterior axis are used for determining the femoral component rotation. (By permission of Scuderi GR, Tria AJ [eds]: Minimal Incision Total Knee Arthroplasty in MIS of the Hip and Knee: A Clinical Perspective. New York: Springer, 2004.)

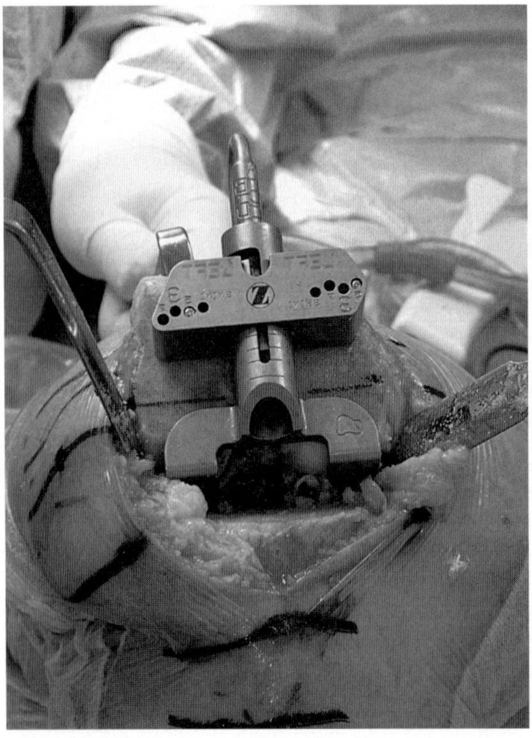

Figure 18.6. The femur is measured and the closest femoral component is chosen. (By permission of Scuderi GR, Tria AJ [eds]: Minimal Incision Total Knee Arthroplasty in MIS of the Hip and Knee: A Clinical Perspective. New York: Springer, 2004.)

select the component that is closest to the measured femur. Following resection of the anterior cortex and posterior femoral condyles, the menisci are removed and if a posterior stabilized prosthesis is being implanted, the posterior cruciate ligament is completely resected. The flexion and extension gaps are now measured and balanced with the spacer block technique (Figure 18.7). After balancing the knee, the final finishing cuts are made on the distal femur and the tibia is sized and prepared to accept the final component. The appropriate tibial template is selected to cover the resected tibial surface and set in the correct rotation. Tibial rotational landmarks include the tibial tubercle and the anterior tibial cortex.

It is my preference to prepare the patella last. With the knee in extension or slight flexion, the patella is everted and resected at the appropriate depth with either a saw or reamer. The patella can easily be prepared with minimal disruption of the extensor mechanism because following the distal femoral and proximal tibial resections there is a great deal more laxity and space in the knee joint cavity (Figure 18.8).

Once the bone has been prepared, the provisional components are implanted. The trial tibial tray is implanted first. The knee is hyperflexed and externally rotated so that the tibia is introduced forward through the arthrotomy. The tibial tray is then inserted. The knee is

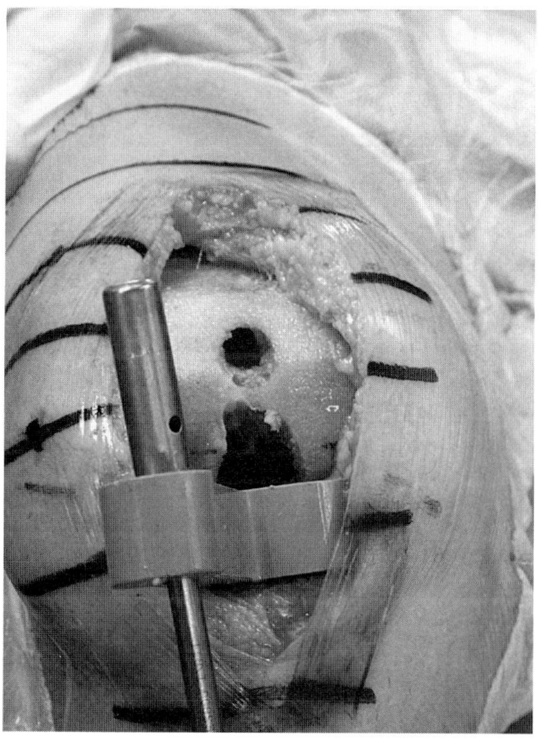

Figure 18.7. The flexion and extension gaps are checked with a spacer block. (By permission of Scuderi GR, Tria AJ [eds]: Minimal Incision Total Knee Arthroplasty in MIS of the Hip and Knee: A Clinical Perspective. New York: Springer, 2004.)

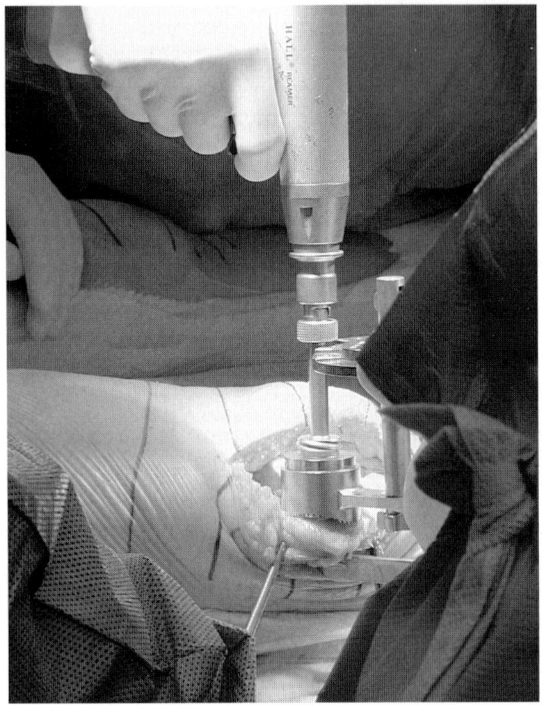

Figure 18.8. The patella is prepared with a reamer.

brought back to 90 degrees of flexion and with distraction of the joint, the flexion space opens and the femoral component is impacted in place. If there is difficulty inserting the tibial polyethylene insert at 90 degrees of flexion, I have found it easier to place the knee at 45 degrees to 60 degrees of flexion and then insert the tibial component. This is the advantage of a front loading tibial component, such as the NexGen LPS prosthesis (Zimmer, Warsaw, IN). The knee is then reduced and assessed for balance and range of motion. If the trial tests are satisfactory, the provisional components are removed and the bone surfaces are cleaned with pulsatile lavage. The final components are cemented in a sequential fashion as described previously, the tibia first, followed by the femur and patella. All excess cement is removed and the knee is reduced (Figure 18.9). The wound is then irrigated with an antibiotic solution. The arthrotomy is closed over a suction drain and the subcutaneous layer and skin are closed in routine fashion.

Soft Tissue Releases

Soft tissue balancing is critical to a successful total knee arthroplasty. The basic principles do not change with minimally invasive surgery. The fixed varus deformity is corrected by release of the deep and superficial medial collateral ligament, the posteromedial capsule and the semimembranosus.[3] Similar to the standard approach, these structures are subperiosteally released from the proximal medial tibia. The one

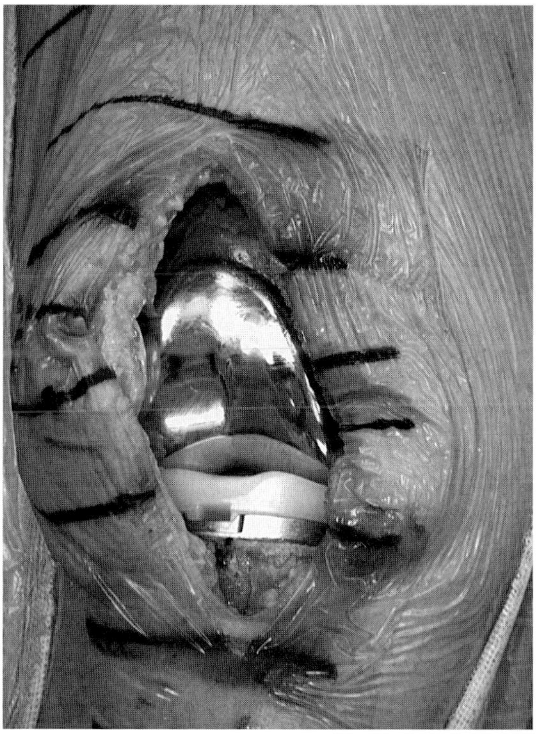

Figure 18.9. The final components are in place. (By permission of Scuderi GR, Tria AJ [eds]: Minimal Incision Total Knee Arthroplasty in MIS of the Hip and Knee: A Clinical Perspective. New York: Springer, 2004.)

difference is that the subcutaneous layer is not dissected from the medial collateral ligament. The medial release is deep to the medial collateral ligament and the entire soft tissue sleeve is subperiosteally elevated from the medial tibia (Figure 18.10).

The fixed valgus deformity is corrected after the primary bone cuts are made. The pie crust release of the lateral capsule and the iliotibial band can be readily completed through the minimal approach[4] (Figure 18.11).

Postoperative Management

Following surgery, the knee is placed in a light compressive dressing and continuous passive motion is initiated in the recovery room. The patient begins a standardized physiotherapy program the day following surgery. The focus is early mobilization and range of motion. Anticoagulation is similar to a standard total knee arthroplasty.

Clinical Observations

Not all arthritic knees are candidates for less invasive surgery. A compromised soft tissue envelope limits the ability to perform a mini-incision technique. This may occur in rheumatoid or inflammatory

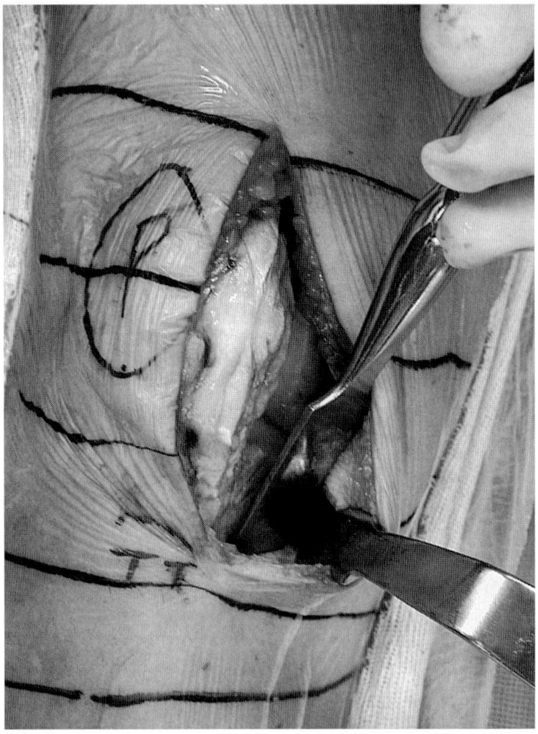

Figure 18.10. The varus release. (By permission of Scuderi GR, Tria AJ [eds]: Minimal Incision Total Knee Arthroplasty in MIS of the Hip and Knee: A Clinical Perspective. New York: Springer, 2004.)

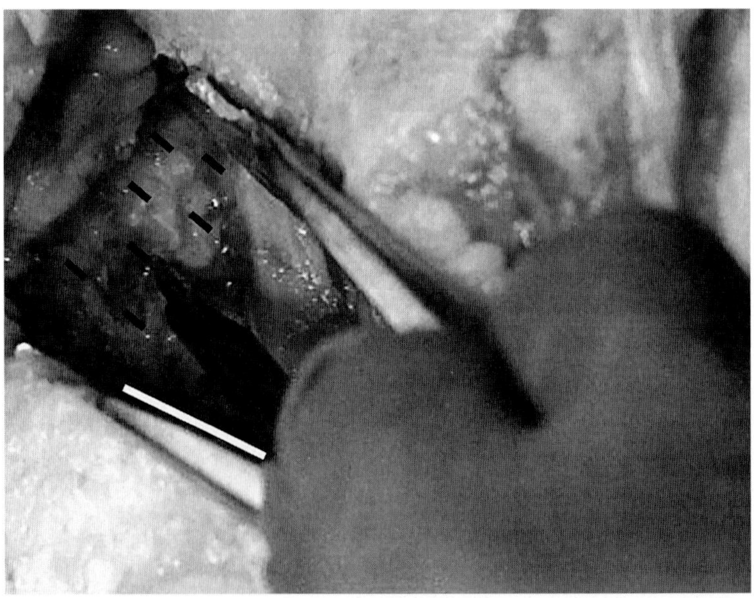

Figure 18.11. The valgus release with the pie crust technique (solid line—release of the posterior lateral capsule at the joint line; dashed line—pie crust release of the iliotibial band). (By permission of Scuderi GR, Tria AJ [eds]: Minimal Incision Total Knee Arthroplasty in MIS of the Hip and Knee: A Clinical Perspective. New York: Springer, 2004.)

arthritis, diabetic patients, patients on chronic steroids, or in the setting of prior skin incisions and prior surgery. The deformity of the knee should be limited to 10 degrees of varus, 15 degrees of valgus, or a flexion contracture less than 10 degrees, with a minimum range of motion of 90 degrees. This is because of the fact that greater deformity and limited motion require greater soft tissue dissection and release to correct the deformity.

As noted previously, my TKA incisions have been reduced by approximately 50%, and usually fall in the 10-cm to 14-cm range. Clinical observations that affect the length of incision and arthrotomy include size of the femur, length of the patella tendon, and body habitus.[2] I have observed that the wider the femur, as measured by the epicondylar width, the longer the incision. This is intuitive because the bigger the femur, the greater the exposure needed for implantation of the larger femoral component. Another observation is that a short patellar tendon requires a longer incision and longer arthrotomy. When the patellar tendon is shortened, it is more difficult to subluxate the patella laterally with a limited arthrotomy without compromising the insertion on the tibial tubercle. Therefore, I measure the Insall–Salvati ratio on the preoperative lateral radiograph and determine the preoperative length of the patellar tendon. Muscular patients, especially men with a prominent vastus medialis, require a longer incision because of the bulk of the quadriceps muscle. Similarly, obese patients may require a more traditional approach.

For more than 2 years, I have been using the minimal-incision approach with a limited medial parapatellar arthrotomy. Using the inclusion criteria mentioned above, the length of the skin incision has been 9.4 cm to 14.0 cm with a 2-cm to 6-cm division of the quadriceps tendon. Although I have had no wound complications, there was one small skin tear, <10 mm, of the proximal wound in one of the initial cases, which healed uneventfully. It is now our recommendation to lengthen the skin as needed to avoid this problem. The radiographic and clinical results are comparable to my previous experience performed with a standard approach.

Adhering to meticulous surgical technique and being aware of the limitations of the exposure can avoid complications. Briefly, the incision or arthrotomy should be extended if there is (1) difficulty with exposure or visualization, (2) difficulty with placement of instruments or implants, and/or (3) undue skin tension. In these situations the medial parapatellar approach has an advantage over the subvastus or midvastus approaches. It can easily be extended into a more extensile approach.

Struggling to gain exposure by pulling or retracting a limited skin incision causes unnecessary soft tissue trauma, including tearing and bruising. It is simpler to extend the skin incision 1 cm to 2 cm proximally or distally as needed to gain exposure. The skin edges must also be watched while the bone is being resected. Careful placement of retractors prevents the saw blade from inadvertently coming in contact with the skin and causing an undue laceration. Excessive retraction or poor visualization can also lead to patellar tendon compromise or even to patellar tendon avulsion. Extending the medial parapatellar arthrotomy is a simple solution that can be performed quickly and without meaningful change in the postoperative result. Intraoperative and postoperative complications can be avoided by emphasizing the use of the mobile window incision and proper visualization of the anatomy throughout the entire procedure.

References

1. Insall JN. A midline approach to the knee. J Bone Joint Surg. 1971;53A:1584.
2. Scuderi GR, Tria AJ. Minimal Incision Total Knee Arthroplasty. In: Scuderi GR, Tria AJ, eds. A MIS of the Hip and Knee: A Clinical Perspective. New York: Springer Verlag; 2004.
3. Yasgur DJ, Scuderi GR, Insall JN. Medial release for fixed varus deformity in Surgical Techniques. In: Scuderi GR, Tria AJ, eds. Total Knee Arthoplasty. New York: Springer Verlag; 2002:189–196.
4. Griffin FM, Scuderi GR, Insall JN. Lateral release for fixed valgus deformity in Surgical Techniques. In: Scuderi GR, Tria AJ, eds. Total Knee Arthoplasty. New York: Springer Verlag; 2002:197–204.

19

Minimally Invasive Total Knee Replacement with the Quadriceps-Sparing Subvastus Approach

Mark W. Pagnano and Giles R. Scuderi

The subvastus approach to the knee offers several distinct advantages when applied to minimally invasive total knee replacement. With minor modifications to the technique as described by Hoffman, the subvastus approach becomes an exposure that is optimized for minimally invasive surgery (MIS).[1–3] The MIS-optimized subvastus approach provides excellent exposure through a small incision, preserves all four attachments of the quadriceps to the patella, does not require patella eversion, minimizes disruption of the suprapatellar pouch, and facilitates rapid and reliable closure of the knee joint at the conclusion of the procedure. With the MIS-optimized subvastus approach, the patella and distal portion of the extensor mechanism are retracted into the lateral gutter of the knee where they remain out of the way to allow visualization of the distal femur during surgery. Additionally, the broad, triangular tendinous attachment of the vastus medialis to the patella is preserved with this approach and provides an ideal region to place retractors without damaging the quadriceps muscle itself. Those advantages have made the MIS-optimized subvastus approach the exposure of choice for both small incision (4 in. to 5 in.) and very small incision (2.5 in. to 3.5 in.) total knee replacement for the two authors.

The utility of the traditional subvastus approach to the knee has been limited because it can be difficult to evert the patella in very muscular or obese patients.[4] Because many patients who present for total knee arthroplasty are substantially overweight, most total knee surgeons have not adopted the subvastus approach despite clear evidence that the subvastus approach leads to less postoperative pain and a stronger extensor mechanism than a traditional medial parapatellar approach.[5–7] As MIS techniques for knee replacement have evolved it has become accepted that surgeons avoid eversion of the patella and limit dissection in the suprapatellar pouch to minimize damage to that richly innervated region of the knee. Fortuitously, when the subvastus approach is modified to avoid everting the patella and to limit dissection in the suprapatellar pouch the exposure is, in fact, enhanced and becomes optimized for MIS total knee surgery. At first this will strike the reader as counterintuitive. However, one quickly recognizes that when the patella is simply retracted laterally and not everted that the extent of dissection can be minimized and the exposure improved. With the MIS-optimized subvastus approach even obese and heavily muscled patients can be handled in a relatively straightforward manner.

Surgery

The knee is prepped and draped in a standard fashion. The tourniquet is inflated after elevating the limb and then hyperflexing the knee to ensure that full excursion of the quadriceps muscle and tendon is allowed. The skin incision is made from the superomedial border of the patella to the top of the tibial tubercle and typically measures 3.5 in. or less in extension (Figure 19.1). The incision is not directly over the midline but instead is made slightly medial. That medial position is preferred as all of the soft tissues will be pulled laterally when the patella is retracted into the lateral gutter of the knee. The subcutaneous tissue is dissected down to but not through the fascial layer that overlies the vastus medialis muscle itself. The inferior border of the vastus

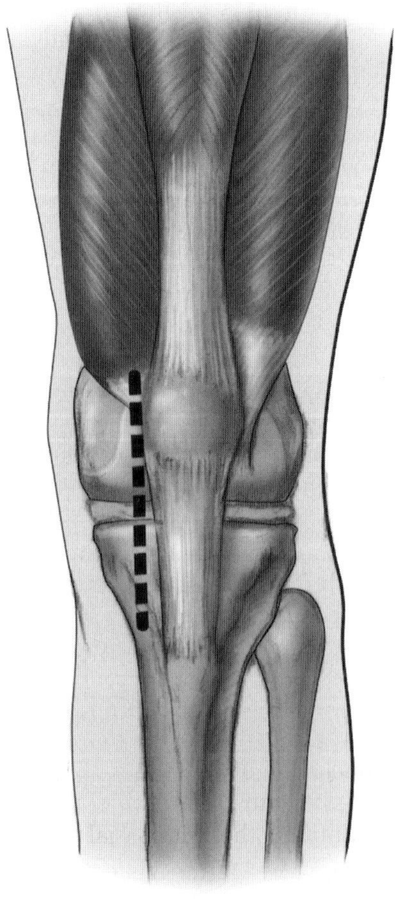

Figure 19.1. A 3.5-in. incision is made from the superomedial border of the patella to the top of the tibial tubercle. The incision should be slightly medial as it will be pulled laterally when the patella is retracted into the lateral gutter later in the case.

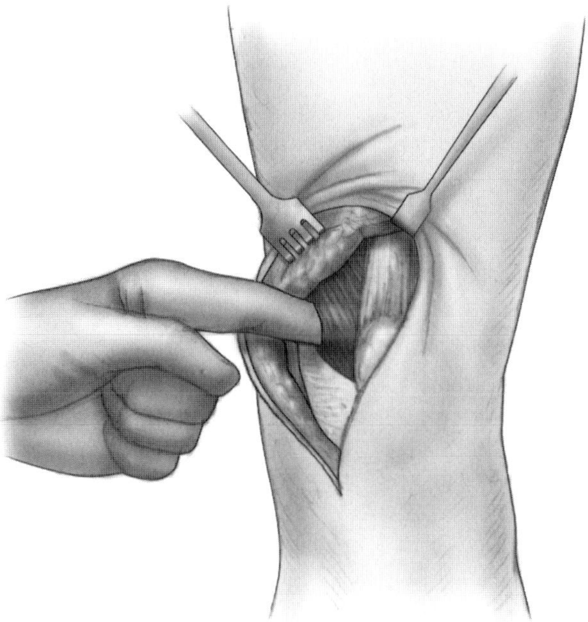

Figure 19.2. The inferior border of the vastus medialis muscle is identified and the surgeon slides his finger under the muscle belly but stays on top of the synovium and out of the knee joint itself. The vastus is then freed using electrocautery being careful to leave a thin edge of myofascial tissue attached to the inferior border of the vastus medialis muscle.

medialis muscle is identified and at a point 5 to 8 cm medial to the patellar border the fascia is incised to allow the surgeon's finger to slide under the muscle belly but on top of the underlying synovial lining of the knee joint (Figure 19.2). The vastus medialis obliquus muscle is pulled superiorly and put under slight tension with the underlying finger. The inferior border of the vastus medialis is then freed from its confluence with the medial retinaculum using electrocautery with care to leave a small cuff of myofascial tissue still attached to the inferior border of the vastus medialis for later repair.

The surgeon must recognize that the tendinous portion of the vastus medialis extends distally to insert at the midpole of the medial border of the patella. Care must be taken to preserve that triangular portion of the tendon to protect the vastus medialis muscle itself from damage later in the case (Figure 19.3). If instead the surgeon incises along the inferior border of the medialis across to the superior pole of the patella, the vastus medialis muscle will be torn, split, or macerated by retractors during the remainder of the operation.

The underlying synovium is then incised to enter the knee joint itself. By incising the synovium at a slightly more proximal position, a 2-layer closure of the knee can be done at the conclusion of the surgery (Figure 19.4). The deep layer of the closure is the synovium itself and the more superficial layer is the medial retinaculum and the myofascial sleeve of tissue that has been left attached to the inferior border of the vastus

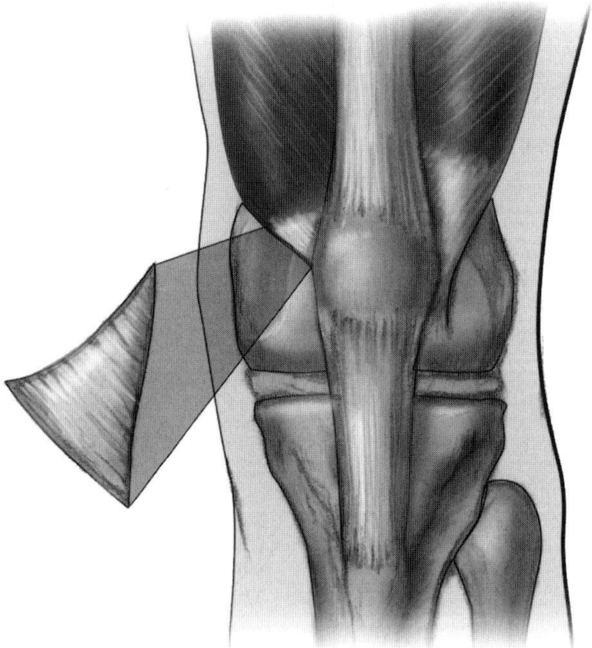

Figure 19.3. It is very important to preserve the triangular portion of quadriceps tendon that extends from the superomedial aspect of the patella distally to the midpole of the patella and then back to the edge of the vastus medialis muscle. This robust portion of tendon is where the retractors need to be placed to pull the patella into the lateral gutter. If this triangular portion of tendon is not preserved, then the retractors rest against muscle tissue itself and macerate or tear the vastus medialis.

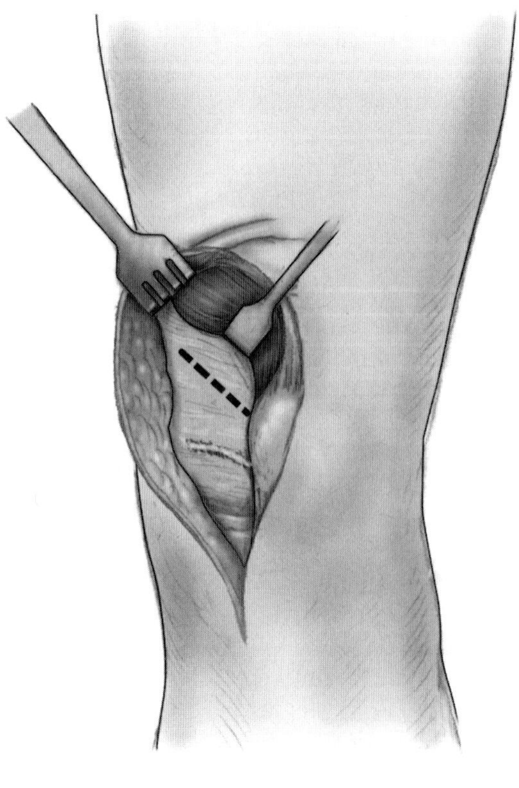

Figure 19.4. With the vastus medialis muscle retracted superiorly the incision through the synovium and into the knee joint is made a slightly more proximal location, thus allowing a 2-layer closure at the end of the procedure.

medialis. The synovial incision is carried to the medial border of the patella and then turned directly inferiorly to course along the medial border of the patella tendon to the proximal portion of the tibia. The medial soft tissue sleeve along the proximal tibia can be elevated in a standard fashion.

A bent Hohmann's retractor is placed in the lateral gutter and levered against the robust triangular portion of tendon that has been preserved just medial and superior to the patella. The patella and extensor mechanism are then retracted into the lateral gutter (Figure 19.5). In most cases this retraction is simple. In some stiff knees or very muscular thighs it may be necessary to mobilize the vastus medialis either from its underlying attachments to the synovium and adductor canal or at its superior surface when there are firm attachments of the overlying fascia to the subcutaneous tissue and skin.

With the patella retracted into the lateral gutter the fat pad can be excised or preserved according to surgeon preference. The knee is then flexed. The patella stays retracted in the lateral gutter behind the bent Hohmann retractor while the quadriceps tendon and vastus medialis lie over the distal anterior portion of the femur (Figure 19.6). Two maneuvers can be used to facilitate visualization of the distal anterior portion of the femur during the remainder of the MIS TKA procedure. First, a thin knee retractor can be placed along the anterior femur to gently lift the extensor mechanism and improve visualization during

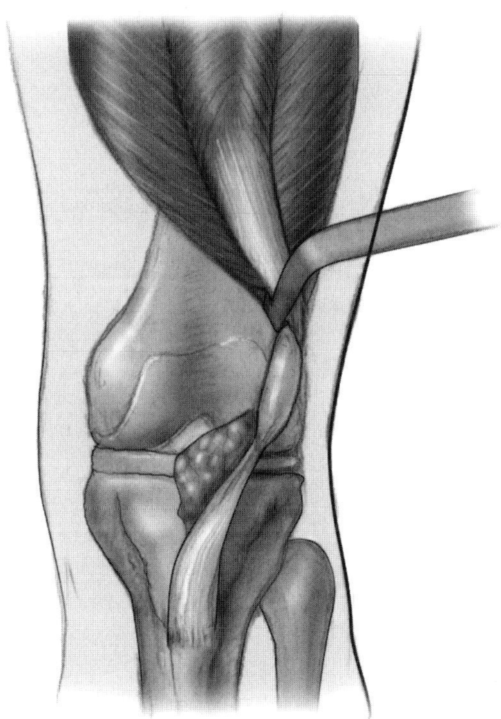

Figure 19.5. The patella and distal portion of the extensor mechanism can be retracted into the lateral gutter of the knee using a bent Hohmann's retractor.

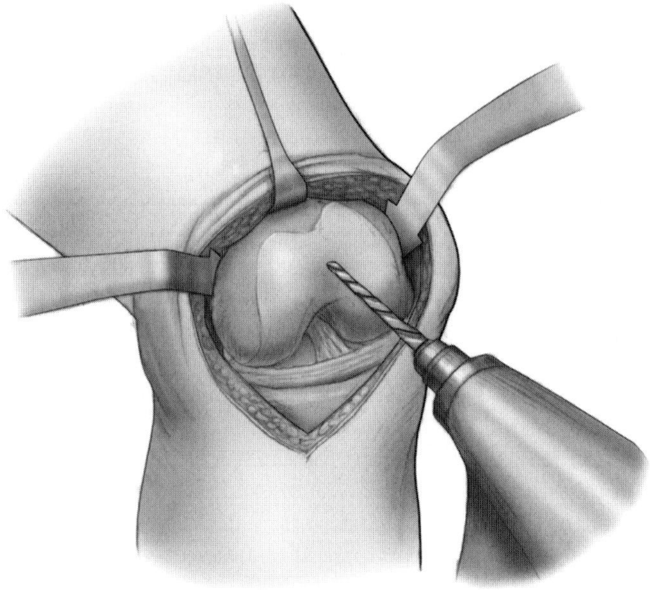

Figure 19.6. With a bent Hohmann's retractor in the lateral gutter the patella remains out of the way as the knee is flexed to 90 degrees. Good visualization of the distal femur is obtained for initial preparation of the femur.

critical steps such as femoral sizing, anterior resection and cementation. Second, the surgeon can bring the knee into varying degrees of extension whenever a better view of the distal femur is needed. Small degrees of knee extension markedly decrease the tension on the extensor mechanism and allow a direct view of the distal anterior femur through even the smallest of MIS TKA incisions.

The distal femur is cut next using the surgeon's MIS instrumentation of choice. The proximal tibia is cut using care to protect the lateral sided structures and the patella tendon (Figure 19.7). A bent Hohmann's or other retractor should be placed directly against the lateral edge of the tibia to protect against an errant saw blade. A so-called pickle-fork retractor can be placed around the tibial attachment of the posterior cruciate ligament and used to help sublux the tibia anteriorly by levering against the distal femur. Even small degrees of anterior subluxation of the tibia substantially improve visualization of the proximal tibia and improve the margin of safety when making this cut. A narrow saw blade is of substantial value during this type of surgery. The narrow saw blade improves maneuverability and tactile feedback to the surgeon working through the small incision and around the patella tendon. After the distal femur and proximal tibia are cut there is substantial room in the extension space and that further diminishes tension on the extensor mechanism whenever the knee is brought into slight extension. Femoral rotation can be assessed accurately at this point with the surgeon's technique of choice. We prefer to check rotation in all cases relative to the trans-epicondylar axis and the view of the distal femur afforded by the MIS-optimized subvastus approach readily allows that. Similarly, the AP axis of the knee and the posterior femoral condyles can be referenced with this approach. The femur is sized and cut after ensuring that the block is appropriately positioned anterior to posterior to avoid femoral notching (Figure 19.8).

The remaining menisci are excised with electrocautery and osteophytes are carefully excised. The tibial and femoral finishing cuts are made, trial components are assembled and ligament balance, alignment and rotation are assessed carefully. The patella is resurfaced at this stage by turning it up 90 degrees but not everting it. The preresection thickness is measured and the patella is cut freehand with a broad thin saw blade from subchondral bone medially to subchondral bone laterally using care to leave a symmetric bone remnant. The patellar component is sized and positioned to recreate the original patellar thickness and high point. Patellar tracking is assessed with the trials in place. Using a no-thumbs test, the patella button should track centrally without tilt or subluxation and the patella button should be in contact with both the medial and lateral femoral condyles at 90 degrees of flexion.

Inserting the real tibial and femoral components can occasionally present a challenge when very small incisions are used. When using a posterior-stabilized knee, we cement the femur first and then hyperflex

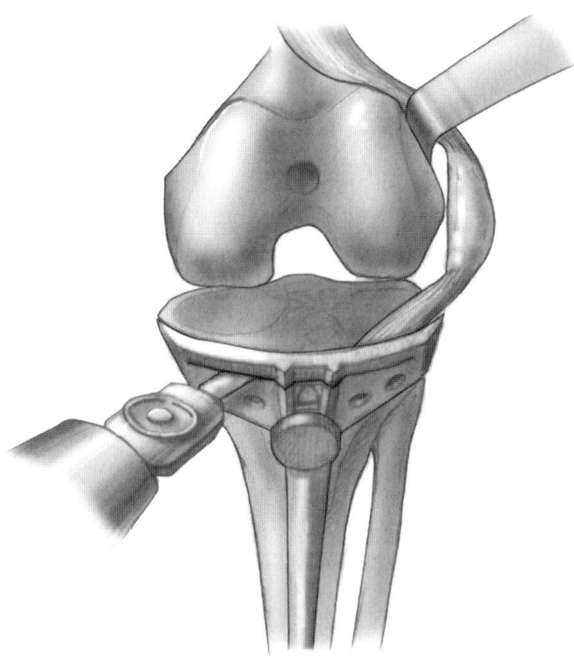

Figure 19.7. After the distal femoral cut the proximal tibia can be resected. An effort should be made to sublux the tibia anteriorly and to position retractors that protects the medial and lateral collateral ligament. A narrow saw blade gives the surgeon better maneuverability and tactile feedback in this situation than does the typical broad blade.

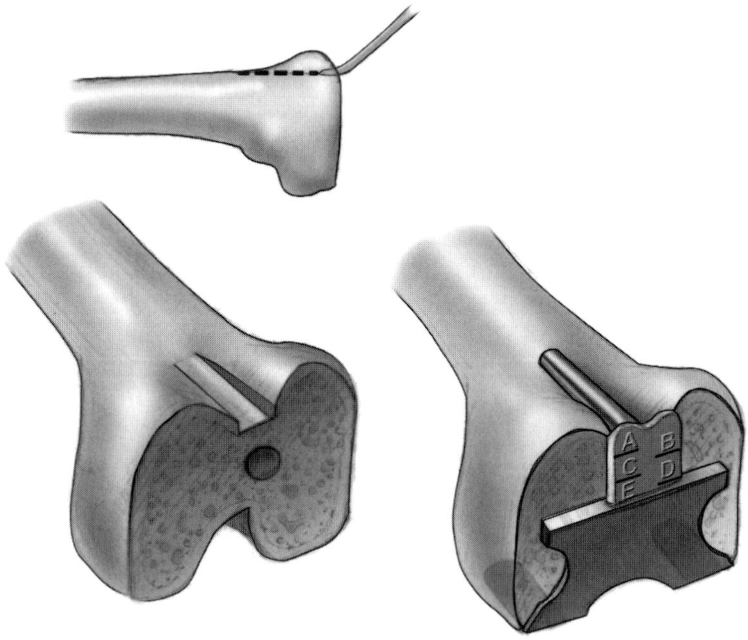

Figure 19.8. Anteroposterior sizing and cutting of the femur can be difficult in any minimally invasive total knee procedure. A useful technique is to use a 13-mm osteotome to cut a channel in the trochlea that is flush with the anterior cortex of the femur. Even when the extensor mechanism is tented over the femur, the surgeon can then palpate the anterior femur or slide an instrument through the slot and ensure that the femur will not be notched anteriorly.

the knee and sublux the tibia forward to allow adequate visualization of the proximal tibia. A bent Hohmann's retractor is placed against the lateral edge of the tibia to hold the patella out of the way. In some cases it is necessary to place a posterior or so-called pickle-fork retractor behind the tibia to lever the proximal tibia anteriorly. When the pickle-fork retractor is used, one must protect the femoral component with a lap-sponge so that it is not scratched. Inserting a posterior-cruciate retaining knee through a small incision is somewhat easier as the tibia with the real tibial insert can be placed first and then the femoral component is impacted with the knee flexed 90 degrees. The knee is brought into extension, excess cement is removed and the patella component is then placed.

Closure

The tourniquet is let down and hemostasis is obtained. Care must be taken to look under the vastus medialis muscle belly for bleeding. There are vessels that course from the adductor canal up through the synovium and into the vastus medialis muscle that if left to bleed will cause a subvastus hematoma. A drain can be left in the subvastus space above the synovium and below the vastus medialis muscle if the surgeon is concerned about hemostasis in that area. The joint is closed in two layers by first reapproximating the synovium on the medial side of the knee. Typically, that synovial layer is closed with 2 or 3 interrupted absorbable sutures. Layer two of the closure begins by anatomically positioning the apex of the L-shaped capsular incision. The oblique limb of the incision is closed by reapproximating the myofascial sleeve left attached to the vastus medialis muscle with the robust medial retinacular tissue using multiple interrupted sutures. The vertical limb is closed by suturing the medial retinaculum to the medial border of the patellar tendon in the standard fashion.

Complications

The MIS-optimized subvastus approach has only one unique potential complication and that is a subvastus hematoma. There are a series of blood vessel that course from the adductor canal and branch through the vastus medialis muscle. Whenever more extensive mobilization of the muscle is done, these vessels can be torn and bleed. In every case the surgeon is advised to let the tourniquet down at the conclusion of the procedure and look carefully in the subvastus space to cauterize any bleeding vessels. A deep drain should be placed in the subvastus space if the surgeon is concerned about further oozing from those vessels postoperatively.

References

1. Gore DR, Sellinger DS, Gassner KJ, Glaeser ST. Subvastus approach for total knee arthroplasty. Orthopedics. 2003;26:33–35.
2. Hoffman AA, Harlow ML. Submedialis Approach. In: Lotke PA, ed. Master Techniques in Orthopedic Surgery: Knee Arthroplasty. New York: Raven Press; 1995.
3. Hoffman AA, Plaster RL, Murdock LE. Subvastus (southern) approach for primary total knee arthroplasty. Clin Orthop. 1991;269:70–77.
4. Cushner FD. The subvastus approach to the knee. J Knee Surg. 2003; 16:52–54.
5. Chang CH, Chen KH, Yang RS, Liu TK. Muscle torques in total knee arthroplasty with subvastus and parapatellar approaches. Clin Orthop. 2002;398:189–195.
6. Faure BT, Benjamin JB, Lindsey B, Volz RG, Schutte D. Comparison of the subvastus and paramedian approaches in bilateral total knee arthroplasty. J Arthroplasty 1993;8:511–516.
7. Roysam GS, Oakley MJ. Subvastus approach for total knee arthroplasty: a prospective, randomized, and observer-blinded trial. J Arthroplasty 2001; 16:454–457.

20

Mini-Midvastus Total Knee Arthroplasty

Steven B. Haas, Andrew P. Lehman, and Mary Ann Manitta

Total knee arthroplasty (TKA) has been a successful modality in the treatment of end-stage arthritis of the knee. Numerous long-term clinical studies have demonstrated the success of total knee arthroplasty in regard to improving both pain and function of the knee.[1–4] The medial parapatellar arthrotomy is the most commonly used approach to expose the knee.[5] This approach was first described by von Langenbeck in 1874[6] and has proven itself with a successful track record in long-term follow-up studies. However, the incision through the quadriceps tendon can contribute to a long and painful recovery. Additionally, there have been reports of complications related to this approach, including subluxation or dislocation of the extensor mechanism.

Alternative exposures include the subvastus[7] and the midvastus approaches.[8] Like the medial parapatellar approach to the knee, both of these exposures involve patella eversion and are generally performed through 20-cm to 30-cm incisions.

Reports of unicompartmental arthroplasty (UKA) through a smaller arthrotomy without patella eversion have shown more rapid functional recovery than the use of larger, more extensile exposures.[9,10] Similar results have been reported for total hip arthroplasty (THA) performed through a less invasive approach.[11,12]

With this in mind the authors developed a minimally invasive total knee arthroplasty (MIS-TKR) technique using a modification of the midvastus approach. With the use of smaller instrumentation and cutting guides, this technique allows the total knee replacement to be performed through a smaller incision. We entitled this modified surgical approach the mini-midvastus approach.

Standard Midvastus Approach

In the standard midvastus approach, by not incising the quadriceps tendon, there is less surgical trauma to the extensor mechanism, and this has translated into early clinical improvements.[13] In this exposure, the distal portion of the arthrotomy is performed the same as the medial parapatellar arthrotomy. However, after splitting the medial parapatellar retinaculum from the tibial tubercle distally to the level of the superomedial corner of the patella proximally, instead of splitting the quadriceps tendon, the vastus medialis obliquus muscle (VMO) is divided in the line of its fibers. The muscle is divided sharply for up to 4 cm and then bluntly if further exposure is required.

Several studies have compared the traditional medial parapatellar arthrotomy with a midvastus approach to the knee during routine total knee arthroplasty.[8,14,15] Dalury and Juranek[14] performed a prospective, double-blinded study of 24 patients with bilateral knee osteoarthritis undergoing bilateral TKAs. In all patients, one TKA was performed with a medial parapatellar approach and the other with a standard midvastus arthrotomy. At six weeks postoperatively, the patients' quadriceps strength was greater, their pain was less, the need for a lateral retinacular release was lower, and there was no evidence of radiographic patellar tilting in the TKAs performed with a midvastus approach. Additionally, 17 of the 24 patients preferred the results in their knee that had a midvastus approach, five patients did not favor either knee, and only two patients preferred the knee that underwent a medial parapatellar arthrotomy.

White et al.[15] looked at 109 patients who underwent bilateral TKAs. Similar to the study by Dalury and Juranek, one TKA was performed with a medial parapatellar approach and the other with a standard midvastus approach. They found four statistically significant postoperative improvements by using a midvastus exposure: fewer lateral retinacular releases, less pain at eight days, less pain at six weeks, and a higher incidence of straight leg raise at eight days. All of these parameters were equal in both knees at six months postoperative. The authors also found no increased difficulty in exposure using a midvastus approach when compared with a medial parapatellar approach, even in patients with severe varus or valgus deformities.

One of the concerns that has been raised regarding the midvastus approach is the potential for denervation of the VMO. The VMO is innervated by the terminal branches of the saphenous nerve, which is a branch of the femoral nerve.[16] A study by Parentis et al.[17] demonstrated that a portion of the VMO was denervated in 9 of 21 patients (43%) undergoing the midvastus approach for a TKA, whereas the postoperative electromyograms on 21 patients undergoing a medial parapatellar arthrotomy were all normal. Despite this finding, the patients who had a midvastus exposure showed a trend toward faster postoperative recovery of quadriceps strength than those patients who received the medial parapatellar approach. This study also demonstrated that fewer lateral releases were performed and there was a lower intraoperative blood loss in patients who underwent a midvastus approach when compared to patients who underwent a medial parapatellar approach.

Cooper et al.[18] demonstrated in a cadaver study that the VMO can be sharply dissected safely to at least 4.5 cm from the patellar margin without denervation of the VMO distally. If further exposure is necessary, the remaining fibers can then be bluntly split to the level of the vastoadductor membrane and adductor magnus tendon without neurovascular injury.

In addition to the superior results obtained in these studies, the midvastus approach is ideally suited for MIS-TKR. Unlike the medial parapatellar approach, a mini-midvastus approach requires no excessive retraction, and the dissection takes place without the need for undermining the skin.

Mini-Midvastus Approach

In 2001, to further decrease the trauma to the extensor mechanism, the senior author (SBH) began using a modified midvastus approach for routine total knee arthroplasty. The modification to the midvastus approach involves lateral dislocation of the patella, rather than eversion. Theoretically, by not everting the patella, it is not necessary to split the VMO as far medially and less stress is placed on the extensor mechanism. This modification was designed to further increase the already accelerated patient recovery rate that occurs when using a midvastus approach for total knee arthroplasty.

Another potential advantage of the mini-midvastus approach is the need for a smaller skin incision. The incision with the traditional medial parapatellar arthrotomy is generally carried proximally to the end of the split in the quadriceps tendon. This is not necessary with the mini-midvastus technique (Figure 20.1). In fact, we have found that with improvements in instrumentation a total knee arthroplasty can be performed through an 8.5-cm to 12-cm skin incision.

A 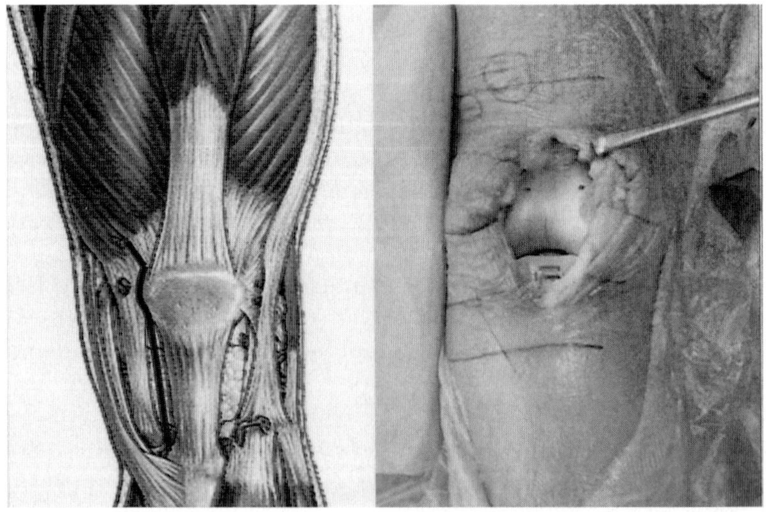 B

Figure 20.1. (A) An illustration of the modified midvastus arthrotomy. (B) The trial implants in place.

Preoperative Assessment

As with any major operation, a thorough preoperative evaluation is imperative prior to performing a total knee arthroplasty through a mini-midvastus approach. Important things to note are the patient's size, musculature, knee range of motion, presence of scars on the operative leg, deformity of the extremity, and the limb's neurovascular status.

Not all patients are good candidates for a mini-midvastus total knee arthroplasty. MIS-TKR is generally not indicated in revision, although the authors have performed one revision of a UKA to a TKA successfully. In a knee that has had previous open surgery performed on it, the surgeon may want to make a longer skin incision, but the deep dissection can still be done using the technique described below.

While the size of the patient poses no absolute contraindication, the surgery is more difficult to accomplish in larger patients. In the authors' experience, exposure is more difficult in men with a large amount of thigh muscle mass. In these patients, some cutting of the quadriceps tendon may be required, although patellar eversion can still be avoided.

Additionally, performing the mini-midvastus technique on patients with excessive deformity of the knee or a limited range of knee motion can also be difficult. The authors generally do not use a MIS-TKR technique in patients with a knee flexion contracture greater than 25 degrees or a limitation of knee flexion of less than 80 degrees.

Instrumentation

An integral part of performing the MIS-TKR is to use downsized instrumentation. In the past, traditional instruments have forced the surgeon to make a longer arthrotomy or to over-retract the skin. To meet the demands of the mini-midvastus approach, not only were guides and cutting blocks made smaller (Figure 20.2), but the edges of the instruments were rounded, and a separate set of instruments was made for both the right and left side. Additionally, the authors use a saw blade that is rigid with a narrow body that fans at the distal tip to facilitate the bone cuts.

The first change that was made was to the tibial cutting guide. With standard instrumentation, the lateral wing of the tibial cutting guide is rarely used during the tibial cut because the patellar tendon is at risk of iatrogenic injury. Hence, the tibial guide was made without a lateral wing. Instead, both a left and right guide were made to wrap around the tibia medially. This modification allows the lateral tibial plateau to be cut from both anterior to posterior as well as medial to lateral.

The second modification was made to the femoral cutting blocks and valgus alignment guides. Again, a separate guide was made for each side. This way the bulk of the guide can be placed medially where there is plenty of exposure. The anterior femoral cutting guide, distal femoral cutting block, and the four-in-one femoral finishing block were made

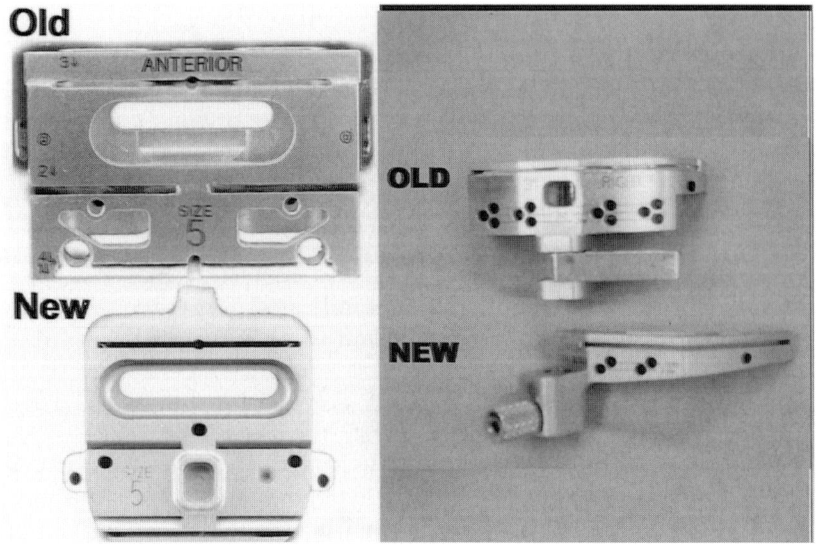

A B

Figure 20.2. (A) A comparison of the modified four-in-one cutting guide to the standard instrumentation. (B) A comparison of the modified tibial cutting guide to the standard instrumentation.

narrower in the medial to lateral dimension and the corners were rounded. This allows easy placement of the guides without impingement on the patella laterally. The cutting blocks were also designed to allow more freely angled cuts when using the saw.

The remainder of the instruments, including the anterior resection stylus, the distal resection stylus, the housing resection block (for posterior stabilized knees), and the femoral sizing guide, also have been downsized to fit the smaller incision. Additionally, the anterior stylus is angled to allow placement under the skin proximally when referencing the anterior femoral cut, and the distal femoral cutting block is wedge-shaped to better fit in the incision and retract the skin without the need for additional retractors.

Surgical Technique

Positioning

After adequate anesthesia is obtained, the patient is positioned supine on the operating table, and a tourniquet is placed on the ipsilateral thigh. The knee should be flexed to only between 70 degrees and 90 degrees of flexion for the majority of the procedure. Unlike a standard total knee arthroplasty, hyperflexion of the knee is performed only intermittently for certain portions of the procedure, such as preparation of the tibia and insertion of the final tibial implant. To aid in holding the leg during the procedure, the authors use a sandbag that is placed under the drapes and across from the contralateral ankle.

Exposure

With the leg fully extended, a longitudinal incision is made over the anterior aspect of the knee along the medial border of the patella. The incision should measure between 8.5 and 12 cm and extend from the superior pole of the patella proximally to the proximal half of the tibial tubercle distally. If the skin appears tight at any point during the operation, the surgeon should not hesitate to lengthen the incision. Excessive tension on the skin edges can cause skin necrosis and lead to devastating long-term complications. However, a longer skin incision, particularly distally, should have little to no effect on your results if the remainder of the principles in this chapter are followed.

A medial arthrotomy is then performed from the proximal border of the patella to about 5 mm medial to the tibial tubercle. The suprapatellar pouch is identified, separated from the underside of the quadriceps tendon, and preserved. The distal extent of the VMO is identified at the superomedial corner of the patella. The fascia of this muscle is incised obliquely along the line of the muscle fibers for approximately 2 cm. The muscle fibers are then bluntly spread by hand.

While keeping the leg fully extended, the patella is retracted laterally. A portion of the fat pad is excised both medially and laterally. The anterior horn of the medial meniscus is divided and excised. Subperiosteal dissection is performed around the proximal medial tibia in standard fashion. The anterior cruciate ligament and the anterior horn of the lateral meniscus are excised. This allows a thin, bent Hohmann's retractor to be placed laterally, facilitating retraction of the patella. A small window is then made along the anterior surface of the distal femur to reference the anterior cortex during femoral preparation.

In patients with tight extensor mechanisms, large patellae, or an abundance of patellar osteophytes, the patella can be cut first to facilitate exposure. This is generally not necessary in female patients. If this is done, however, care must be taken to avoid intraoperative damage to the cut patella surface with retractors in patients with osteoporotic bone. If it is not opted to cut the patella first, the authors prefer to prepare the femur first. However, either the femur or tibia can be prepared first without altering the technique. Patellar preparation is discussed later in the chapter.

Femoral Preparation

Femoral preparation should be accomplished with the knee flexed to only 70 degrees to 90 degrees. Limiting knee flexion allows the soft tissue window to be mobile, and thus, move proximally without difficulty for the surgeon to reference the anterior femoral cortex. Hyperflexion should be avoided because this will not only tighten the extensor mechanism, but also limit the exposure. A thin, bent Hohmann's retractor is placed laterally to hold the patella dislocated.

Rotation for the anterior cut is determined using the traditional rotation landmarks of the anteroposterior axis (Whiteside's line), the epicondylar axis, or the posterior condylar axis. The authors prefer to use Whiteside's line as a primary reference to femoral rotation and the posterior condylar axis as a secondary reference (Figure 20.3). The epicondylar axis can be evaluated, but it may be more difficult requiring retraction of the patella laterally.

After determining femoral rotation, a 9.5-mm intramedullary drill is used to enter the femoral canal from a starting point in the notch just anterior to the posterior cruciate insertion on the femur. An intramedullary referencing guide is placed in the femoral canal after sucking out the marrow contents. The appropriate valgus angle collar, with or without modular posterior paddles, is placed on the rod (Figure 20.4). If paddles are used for posterior condylar referencing, the knee must be hyperflexed to more than 100 degrees during insertion. This will allow the paddles to be positioned under the posterior condyles. Once the paddles are inserted and the rotation guide is secured, the paddles are removed and the knee is returned to between 70 degrees and 90 degrees of flexion for the remainder of femoral preparation. This allows the soft tissue window to move superiorly to allow exposure of the anterior femur. The anterior resection guide is then placed, and an anterior stylus is used to reference the preliminary anterior femoral resection. The stylus is placed in the small window that was created during exposure, and it is placed flush on the highest point of the anterior femoral cortex. The anterior cutting guide is secured in place with pins. The saw blade cuts under the skin, but a right angle retractor may be used for additional protection while the cut is made.

At this time, the distal femoral resection is performed. Additional retractors generally are not necessary for placement of the guide as the guide's wedge shape usually retracts the proximal soft tissues adequately. Once the cutting block is placed on the anterior femur and secured in place, the valgus angle collar and intramedullary guide are removed. The distal femoral cut is made and the bone removed (Figure 20.5).

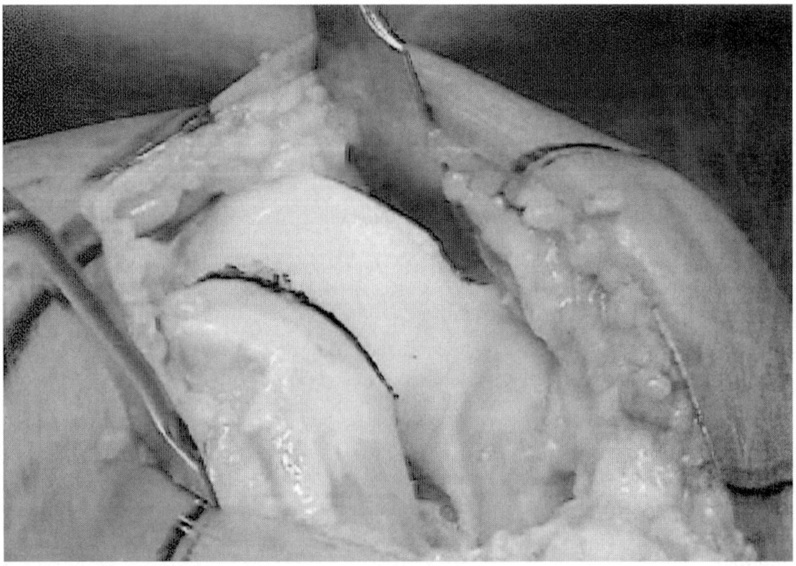

Figure 20.3. Exposure of the distal femur with Whiteside's line drawn.

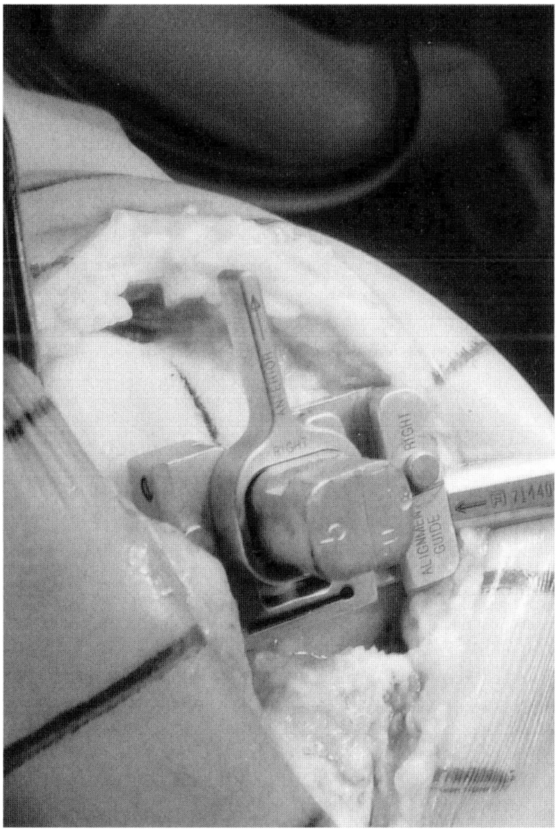

Figure 20.4. The intramedullary referencing guide with valgus angle collar in place.

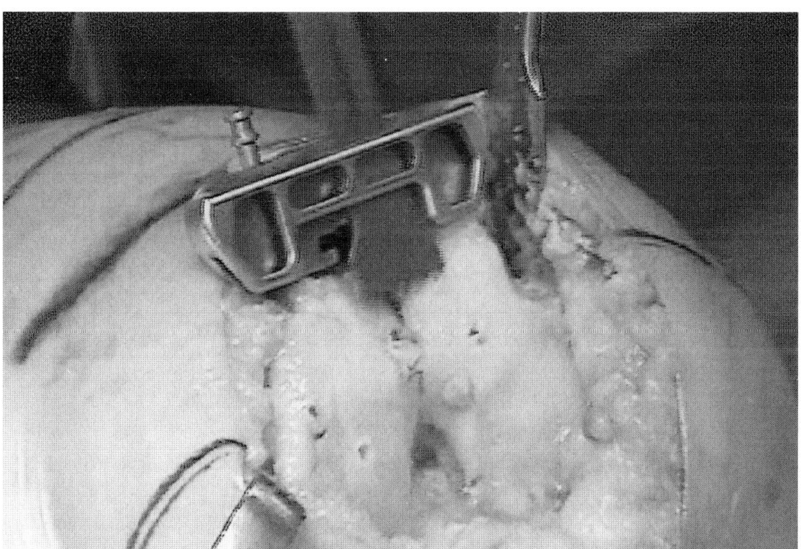

Figure 20.5. The distal cutting guide in place.

The size of the femoral component is determined using a sizing guide. The knee may require more flexion to place it under the posterior femoral condyles. The appropriate sized anteroposterior femoral cutting block is placed on the distal femur and secured in place. The femoral cuts are made in the following order: posterior condyles, posterior chamfer, anterior resection, and anterior chamfer.

Tibial Preparation

The tibia is prepared next. Either intramedullary or extramedullary tibial alignment guides can be used. The authors prefer an extramedullary technique, although both methods are acceptable. Again, the two thin, bent Hohmann's retractors are in place medially and laterally, protecting the medial collateral ligament and the extensor mechanism, respectively. An Aufranc retractor is also placed posteriorly. A rongeur is used to excise any osteophytes from the anteromedial and medial tibia. After the tibial alignment guide is placed parallel to the tibial crest, it is secured to the tibia with pins (Figure 20.6). The authors typically reference the guide over the tibial crest proximally and over the second metatarsal distally. A stylus can be used to measure the amount of tibia to be removed from the least deficient tibial condyle. For varus knees, the stylus is placed on the anterior lateral tibial plateau. In general, the authors set the stylus to measure 11 mm of proximal tibial bone resection from the most normal side. However, this can be adjusted at the surgeon's discretion.

The tibial cut is made perpendicular to the tibial shaft. First, the saw blade should be directed in a posterior direction, then it should be directed laterally. After the tibial cut is made and the bone removed, extension of the knee can provide a better perspective when inspecting the cut tibial surface for cortical ridges. The knee is then placed in

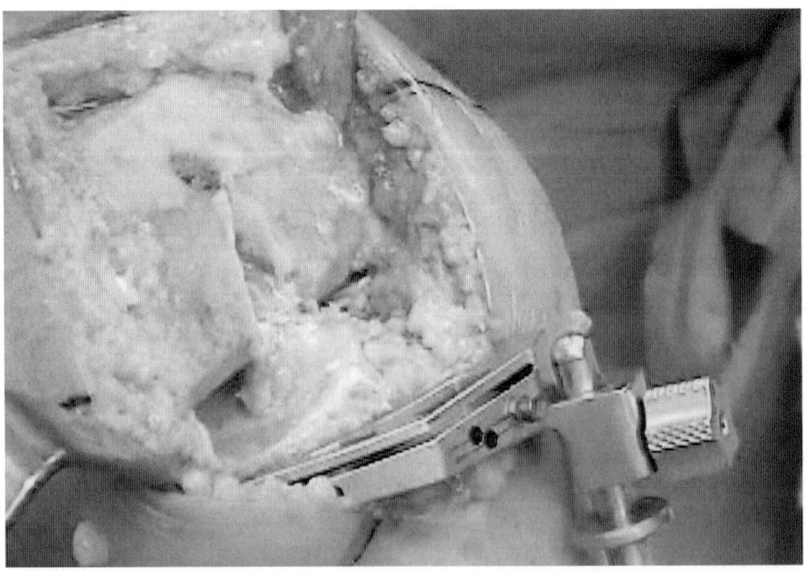

Figure 20.6. The tibial cutting guide in place.

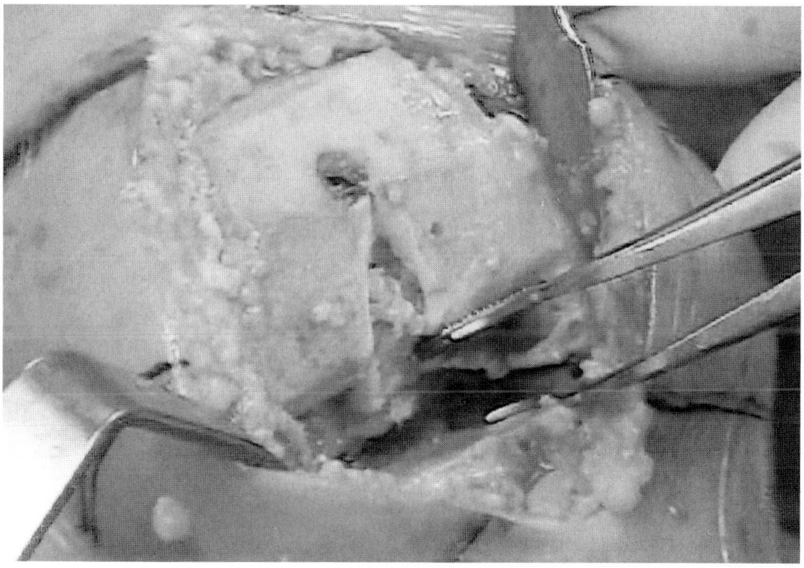

Figure 20.7. The laminar spreaders in place providing access to the posterior knee.

90 degrees of flexion and a laminar spreader is placed in the joint to distract the surfaces (Figure 20.7). This allows easy removal of the posterior horns of both the medial and lateral menisci as well as the posterior cruciate ligament (if a posterior stabilized knee system is being used). Also, any posterior femoral osteophytes can be removed with an osteotome at this time. The tibial preparation is completed by measuring the surface, and drilling and broaching the tibial canal to fit the prosthesis (Figure 20.8).

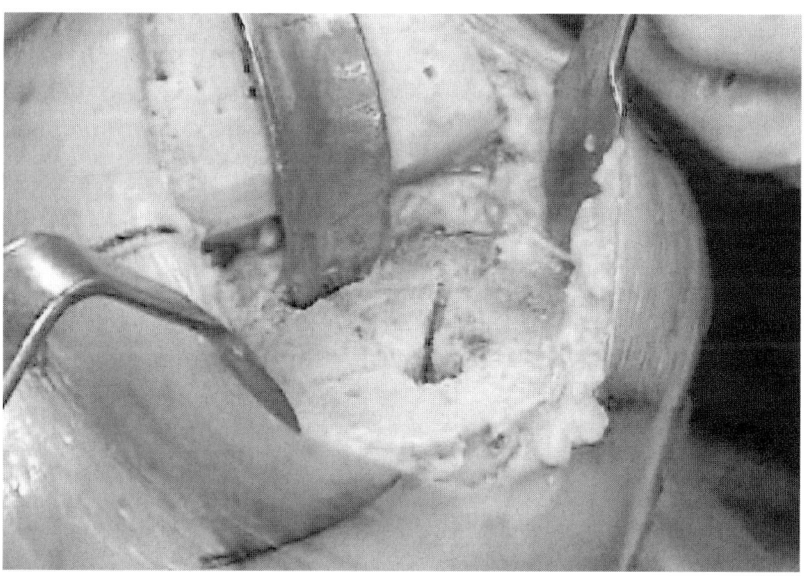

Figure 20.8. Exposure of the prepared tibial surface.

Final Preparation

At this time, spacer blocks are placed to measure the extension and flexion gaps and ligament balance. If there is asymmetry, the appropriate ligamentous releases are performed in standard fashion in order to create a balanced knee. If a posterior stabilized prosthesis is being used, the posterior stabilized resection block is placed on the distal femur and the femoral preparation is completed at this time.

If patellar resurfacing is desired, the patella is prepared following the final preparation of the femur and tibia, unless it is required earlier for adequate exposure. It is easier to wait until after both the femoral and tibial cuts have been made to perform this step, as the leg is shortened and the extensor mechanism is relaxed. With the knee in full extension, the patella can be everted and cut in routine fashion. Occasionally, the patella will not completely evert, but it will routinely rotate more than 90 degrees to allow preparation.

Component Insertion

Once all the bony surfaces have been prepared, the trial components are placed. To clear the femoral condyles with the tibial trial component, the knee must be maximally flexed. In addition to the two thin, bent Hohmann's retractors medially and laterally, an Aufranc retractor can be placed posteriorly to subluxate the tibia anteriorly. The tibial trial is then placed, the knee is returned to 90 degrees of flexion, and the femoral trial component is placed. Once the size of the polyethylene insert is confirmed and the placement of the trial components is deemed satisfactory, the trials are removed and the final implants placed using the same techniques as placement of the trials.

The authors prefer to use cemented implants; however, cementless implants can also be used. The tibial component should be placed first. Doing this allows access to the posterior aspect of the knee and complete removal of excess cement. The posterolateral overhang, which frequently occurs with symmetric tibial implants, can lead to difficulty with implant insertion and cement removal. For this reason, the senior author prefers to use an asymmetric tibial base plate to facilitate clearance of the femoral condyle during placement and subsequent cement removal from the posterior knee (Figure 20.9). Once the tibial implant has been placed, the femoral (Figure 20.10) and patellar components are placed.

Excessive retraction of the proximal tissues for proximal cement removal with the knee flexed should be avoided. Excess cement in the suprapatellar area is more easily removed with the leg in extension. The trial polyethylene insert is placed at this time. The leg is kept in full extension to pressurize the cement while it is hardening. The patellar component is cemented onto the prepared patella and clamped in place until the cement has hardened. All excess cement should be removed at this time. The final polyethylene insert is then placed. If using a posterior stabilized insert, the surgeon should begin insertion of the polyethylene with the knee in 90 degrees of flexion. The knee should then be brought into full extension to engage the locking mechanism.

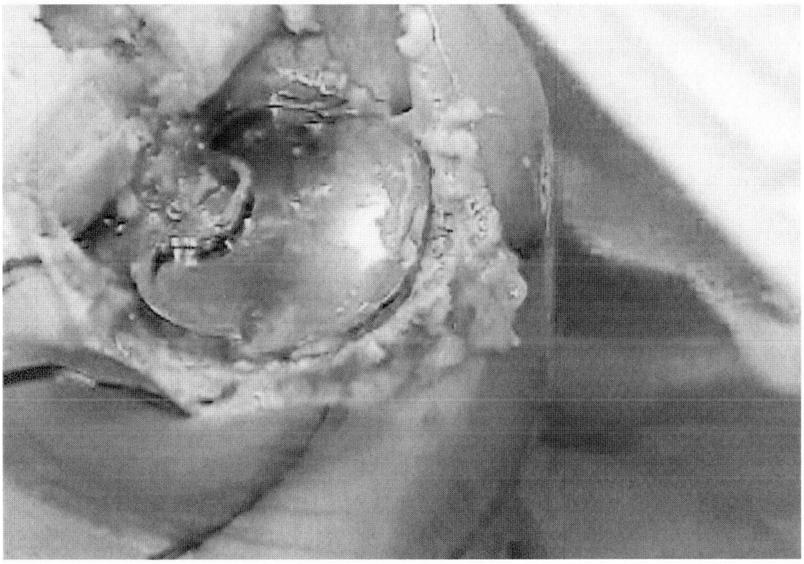

Figure 20.9. The tibial component in place after cement removal.

Closure

The authors recommend that the tourniquet be deflated after the cement has polymerized to achieve hemostasis. Once all bleeding has been controlled, the wound is copiously irrigated and closure begins. Two deep drains are placed. The arthrotomy is closed by initially placing 0-Vicryl sutures in the VMO tendon and fascia. Three to five sutures will usually suffice. The remainder of the arthrotomy, the sub-

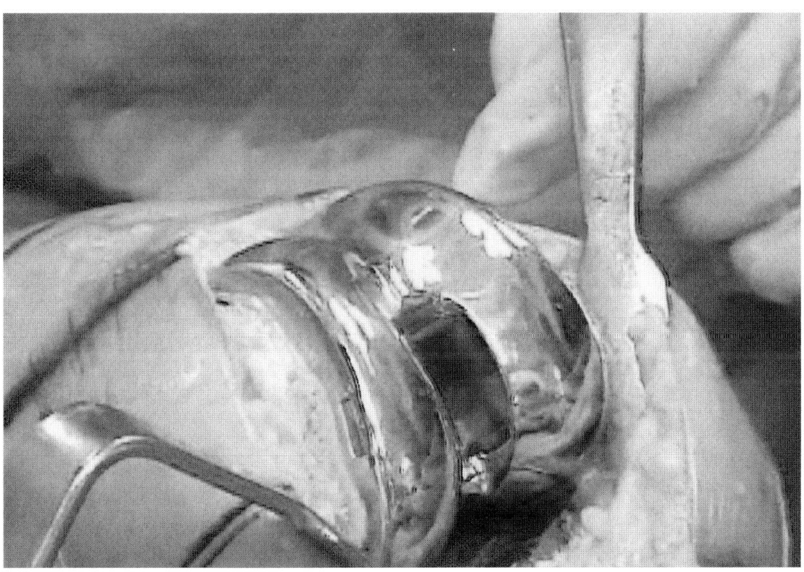

Figure 20.10. The femoral component in place.

cutaneous tissues, and the skin are closed in standard fashion. The authors prefer to use 0-Vicryl suture for both the arthrotomy closure and the closure of the deep subcutaneous tissues. For the superficial closure, 3-0 Vicryl is used.

Results

As of February 2004, the senior author (SBH) has performed over 250 MIS-TKRs using the mini-midvastus technique. The initial 40 TKAs in 37 patients in which this technique was used were evaluated and compared with an age- and sex-matched cohort of 36 patients who received 40 TKAs (control group) through a standard medial parapatellar arthrotomy by the same surgeon the previous year.[19] All patients received the same posterior stabilized condylar knee (Genesis II, Smith and Nephew, Memphis, TN). Both groups also received the same postoperative physical therapy protocol, including the use of a continuous passive motion machine in the recovery room.

There were no statistically significant differences in the patients' demographics between the two groups. The average length of the incision in the MIS-TKR group was 10.3 cm (8.7 cm to 12.0 cm). There were no differences in preoperative tibiofemoral angles or postoperative limb alignment. There were also no statistically significant differences in blood product requirements or postoperative complications between the two groups. Tourniquet time was slightly longer in the MIS-TKR group with a mean of 63 min (32 min to 113 min) compared with the control group with a mean of 49 min (31 min to 89 min). More recent data suggest that in the last 100 MIS-TKRs performed by the senior author, there is no difference in tourniquet time.

The Knee Society preoperative knee and function score averages were 28 and 23, respectively, in the MIS-TKR group and 33 and 24 in the control group. At one year after surgery, the averages were 97 and 92 in the MIS-TKR group and 91 and 90 in the control group.

Preoperative range of motion was similar in both groups. At six weeks after surgery, the average knee flexion was higher in the MIS-TKR group (114 degrees) compared to the control group (96 degrees). This significant difference in knee flexion was still apparent at one year when the mean flexion in the MIS-TKR group improved to 125 degrees and the control group improved to only 116 degrees.

Laskin et al. recently performed a similar study.[20] Thirty-two patients who received a MIS-TKR with a mini-midvastus approach were compared with a cohort of 26 patients (control group) who received a standard medial parapatellar arthrotomy for their TKAs. All patients received the same cruciate-retaining condylar knee (Genesis II, Smith and Nephew, Memphis, TN). Preoperative patient demographics, Knee Society scores, knee flexion, and knee alignment were similar between the two groups.

The patients' postoperative pain level was assessed using a visual analog scale on an hourly basis. The patients who received a MIS-TKR had a statistically significantly lower amount of pain, most remarkable on the day of surgery and postoperative day one. Additionally, the average total dose of morphine sulfate used by each patient was significantly lower in patients who had a MIS-TKR (55 mg) compared with those who underwent a standard medial parapatellar arthrotomy (118 mg).

Several other findings were also statistically significant. Passive knee flexion was consistently higher on a daily basis in the MIS-TKR group. On the third postoperative day, 80% of the patients who had a MIS-TKR were able to achieve knee flexion of greater than 80 degrees, while only 4% of the patients who had a medial parapatellar arthrotomy were able to achieve this amount of knee flexion. Also, the average knee flexion at six weeks postoperative was significantly higher in the MIS-TKR group (124 degrees) compared with the control group (115 degrees). The average postoperative Knee Society score was also significantly higher in the MIS-TKR group at six weeks after surgery.

There was no statistical difference in either the radiographic position of the components or the postoperative leg alignment. No lateral retinacular releases were performed in either group. The mean tourniquet time in the MIS-TKR group was 58 min compared to 51 min in the control group. There were no reported skin complications in either group. Three heavy, muscular male patients in the MIS-TKR group required a modification of the surgical procedure due to the inability to obtain adequate exposure.

To date, more than 350 MIS-TKRs have been performed at the authors' institution. Early results of these patients have mirrored the results found in the above studies.

Conclusion

The MIS-TKR performed with a mini-midvastus approach offers several advantages. First, a midvastus approach to a TKA may lead to a more rapid recovery of motion and a greater ultimate range of motion than a medial parapatellar approach. Smaller, well-designed instruments permit less surgical dissection while avoiding excessive soft tissue retraction, which, in turn, allow the surgeon to avoid patella eversion and reduce the length of the arthrotomy and skin incision. By not everting the patella or disrupting the suprapatellar pouch while using a mini-midvastus approach, early results have demonstrated further improvement in patient recovery, as well as a more favorable cosmetic result, without compromising the radiographic positioning of the implants, the clinical results, or surgical exposure.

References

1. Font-Rodriguez DE, Scuderi GR, Insall JN. Survivorship of cemented total knee arthroplasty. Clin Orthop. 1997;345:79–86.
2. Kelly MA, Clarke HD. Long-term results of posterior cruciate substituting total knee arthroplasty. Clin Orthop. 2002;404:51–57.
3. Pavone V, Boettner F, Fickert S, et al. Total condylar knee arthroplasty: a long-term follow-up. Clin Orthop. 2001;388:18–25.

4. Ranawat CS, Flynn WF, Saddler S, et al. Long-term results of the total condylar knee arthroplasty: a 15-year survivorship study. Clin Orthop. 1993;286:94–102.
5. Hoppenfeld S, deBoer P. The knee. In: Surgical Exposures in Orthopaedics —the Anatomic Approach. 2nd ed. Philadelphia: JB Lippincott Company; 1994:429–482.
6. Von Langenbeck B. Über die Schussverietzungen des Hüftgelenks. Arch Klin Chir. 1874;16:263.
7. Hofmann AA, Plaster RL, Murdock LE. Subvastus (southern) approach for primary total knee arthroplasty. Clin Orthop. 1991;269:70–77.
8. Engh GA, Holt BT, Parks NL. A midvastus muscle-splitting approach for total knee arthroplasty. J Arthroplasty. 1997;12:322–331.
9. Romanowski MR, Repicci JA. Minimally invasive unicondylar arthroplasty: eight-year follow-up. J Knee Surg. 2002;15:17–22.
10. Repicci JA, Eberle RW. Minimally invasive surgical technique for unicondylar knee arthroplasty. J South Orthop Assoc. 1999;8:20–27.
11. Berger R. Two-incision Technique. Presented at: 70th Annual Meeting American Academy of Orthopaedic Surgeons; February 2003; New Orleans, LA.
12. Chimento GF, Pavone V, Sharrock NE, et al. Minimally invasive total hip arthroplasty: a prospective randomized study. Presented at: 70th Annual Meeting American Academy of Orthopaedic Surgeons; February 2003; New Orleans, LA.
13. Engh GA, Parks NL. Surgical technique of the midvastus arthrotomy. Clin Orthop. 1998;351:270–274.
14. Dalury DF, Jiranek WA. A comparison of the midvastus and paramedian approaches for total knee arthroplasty. J Arthroplasty. 1999;14:33–37.
15. White RE, Allman JK, Trauger JA, et al. Clinical comparison of the midvastus and medial parapatellar surgical approaches. Clin Orthop. 1999;367:117–122.
16. Gray H. Anatomy of the human body. Philadelphia: Lea & Febiger; 1959.
17. Parentis MA, Rumi MN, Deol GS, et al. A comparison of the vastus splitting and median parapatellar approaches in total knee arthroplasty. Clin Orthop. 1999;367:107–116.
18. Cooper RE Jr, Trinidad G, Buck WR. Midvastus approach in total knee arthroplasty: a description and a cadaveric study determining the distance of the popliteal artery from the patellar margin of the incision. J Arthroplasty. 1999; 14:505–508.
19. Haas SB. Minimally invasive total knee arthroplasty: a comparative study. Unpublished data.
20. Laskin RS, Beksac B, Phongkunakorn A, et al. Minimally invasive total knee replacement through a mini-midvastus incision: an outcome study. Unpublished data.

21

Minimally Invasive Lateral Approach to Total Knee Arthroplasty

Hari P. Bezwada, Michael A. Mont, Peter M. Bonutti, Sandeep K. Chauhan, Phillip S. Ragland, Craig M. Thomas, and Marc Kester

Standard anterior approaches to total knee arthroplasties have led to both excellent short- and long-term results with overall survivorship rates over 95% at 10 years and longer in multiple series.[1–7] However, when evaluating specific patient-related functional outcomes, it appears that only 20% to 40% of patients are completely satisfied with the results of total knee arthroplasty and that the arthroplasty might limit a variety of functional activities.[8–10] Several authors have described a discrepancy between surgeons' perceptions and the patients' perceptions of outcomes following total knee arthroplasty. In a study by Dickstein et al.,[9] nearly one-third of respondents felt some dissatisfaction with their surgery when evaluated at both 6 and 12 months. Bullens et al.[8] concluded "that surgeons are more satisfied than patients after total knee arthroplasty." In another study of the functional limits of total knee arthroplasty patients with high Knee Society objective knee scores (greater than 90 points) at one year, only 35% of these patients felt that they had no limitations with activity.[11] This finding was even more noticeable in younger patients as only 13% patients under the age of 60 years believed they had no activity limitations.[12] The authors believe that the reasons for these less than favorable results are multifactorial, but may in part have to do with the conventional anterior surgical approach while performing traditional total knee arthroplasties. These procedures are often performed with large anterior incisions (16 cm to 30 cm) and medial parapatellar arthrotomies that are not muscle sparing. The quadriceps extensor mechanism is violated and this may lead to permanent muscle damage, as has been determined by persistent electromyographic changes even a year after the arthroplasty. Dislocation of the tibio-femoral joint may also affect posterior capsular structures and contribute to this long rehabilitative process and permanent knee damage. With these factors in mind, a minimally invasive lateral approach was developed in an attempt to minimize soft-tissue damage when performing total knee arthroplasties.

Special Unique Methods

The surgical technique uses several unique features including:

1. Downsized and unique instrumentation: Cutting blocks have been substantially downsized from traditional cutting blocks. In addition, side-cutting blocks are used to facilitate this approach.
2. Surgical navigation: Cutting blocks have been specially designed for use in conjunction with navigation and to avoid intramedullary instrumentation.
3. Variable leg position: The position of the leg in varying degrees of flexion or extension facilitates exposure for different steps during the knee arthroplasty. For example, flexion exposes the posterior structures and extension of the knee allows visualization of the anterior structures. Retractors are used symbiotically to aid in the exposure of either the medial or lateral side of the knee.
4. Bone platforms: Bone cuts are initially made with cutting blocks and then completed off the initial cut surface as a template and can be used to take out bone in a piecemeal manner when necessary.

Specific Details of the Lateral Approach Procedure

The patient is placed in a supine position on a standard operating room table. A padded tourniquet is applied to the upper thigh followed by standard skin preparation and draping. It is important to drape both the medial and lateral malleoli free, as well as the medial side of the knee, so that appropriate navigational mapping can be performed. A padded valgus leg post may be placed against the distal lateral thigh to allow for opening of the medial part of the joint. The surgical landmarks are outlined including the patella, patellar tendon, lateral tibial plateau, Gerdy's tubercle, fibular head, and distal femur. An approximately 8-cm incision is made from slightly below Gerdy's tubercle to the lateral epicondyle directly lateral to the patella (Figure 21.1). The skin and underlying subcutaneous tissue is sharply incised to the level of the iliotibial band, which is then split from Gerdy's tubercle to the lateral epicondyle. The insertion of the iliotibial band on Gerdy's tubercle is subperiosteally dissected both medially and laterally to expose the proximal tibia. The distal femur is also exposed from the lateral side. Through this lateral arthrotomy, the fat pad is excised along with the anterior horn of the lateral meniscus. This releases the anterolateral knee capsule from the anterior surface of the tibia. Dissection is then continued by placing soft tissue retractors underneath the patellar tendon and across to the medial side of the tibia, releasing any soft tissue that is necessary. The anteromedial surface of the tibia can be visualized and the anterior horn of the medial meniscus, which can also be removed under direct visualization. Attention can then be directed to the proximal soft tissues, with the selective use of retractors and the knee in extension will allow visualization of the suprapatellar pouch. The fat and synovial tissue from the anterior surface of the distal femur can be excised as well as any additional tissue in both the medial and

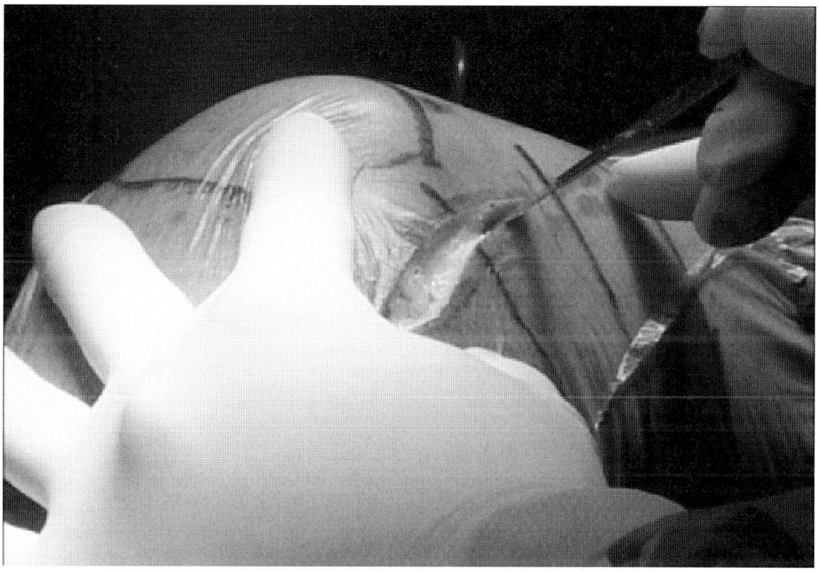

Figure 21.1. The incision is made lateral to the patella just below Gerdy's tubele.

lateral gutters. At this point, there should be sufficient mobilization of the patella to displace it medially.

This is the appropriate time to establish the navigation trackers and registration points. One navigation tracker is set up laterally 10 cm to 12 cm proximal to the distal femur and angled in plane approximately 45 degrees from horizontal. Likewise, another navigation tracker is placed medially approximately 10 cm below the tibial joint line (Figure 21.2). Once the femoral and tibial navigation trackers are anchored, the

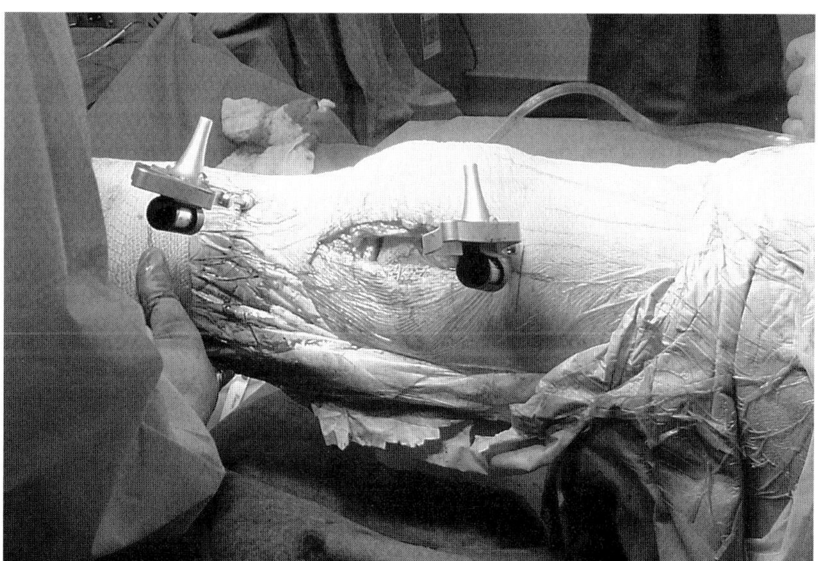

Figure 21.2. Image showing navigation device in place with trackers fixed in the proximal tibia and distal femur.

navigation software is used to map the hip center, femoral landmarks (both epicondyles, center of knee, AP axis [Whiteside's line]), and tibial landmarks (condylar surfaces, tibial spine center, tibia). The ankle is also mapped with respect to the center of the ankle and both the medial and lateral malleoli. The distal femoral resection is made by positioning the resection guide with a navigation tracker in relation to three planes of freedom: varus/valgus, flexion/extension, and distal resection depth. Once the appropriate position has been established, the distal femoral cut is made (Figure 21.3). The proximal tibial resection is made with a similar guide bearing the same three planes of freedom. It is certainly possible to not complete the proximal tibial resection, but to complete only three-quarters of the cut initially to avoid risking injury to the medial collateral ligament. Attention is then directed to the femur where a T-bar device is used to re-map the femoral rotation landmarks. The epicondylar rotation guide should then be used which is based on the 90 degree relationship between Whiteside's AP axis and the surgical transepicondylar axis. The long arm of this alignment guide is placed along Whiteside's AP axis with the tip of the lateral arm aligned with the lateral epicondyle. These points are then marked, which allows for an accurate assessment of rotation during the next step. An idea of the femoral component size is obtained from preoperative radiographic templating and a femoral sizing guide. The anterior femoral cut is then made with a special guide, which is linked to a navigation tracker ensuring the appropriate degree of external rotation. Following the initial anterior femoral cut, a femoral four-in-one cutting guide can be applied to the femur for the finishing cuts. The Scorpio (Stryker, Mahwah, NJ) trochlear recess rasp is then used to prepare the

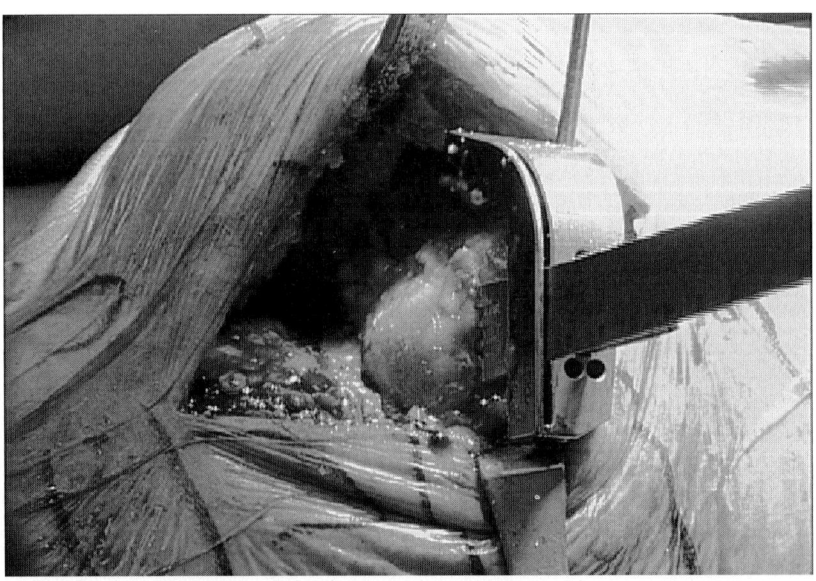

Figure 21.3. The distal femoral resection guide shown after navigation is used to determine the appropriate position.

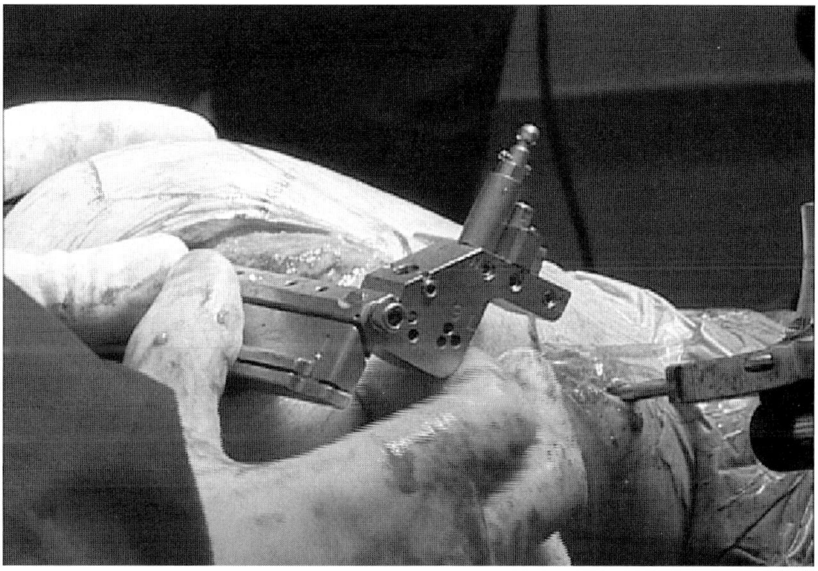

Figure 21.4. The cutting jig for the anterior and posterior chamfer cuts is positioned using navigation.

trochlear recess on the anterior chamfer of the resected femur (Figure 21.4). The surfaces can then be re-checked to ensure appropriate alignment with the navigation devices and both the femur and tibia tested. Appropriate tested rotation can be determined with the navigation unit and with the correctly sized tray, a tibial punch guide can be used for the preparation of a keeled tibial component (Figure 21.5). The femoral

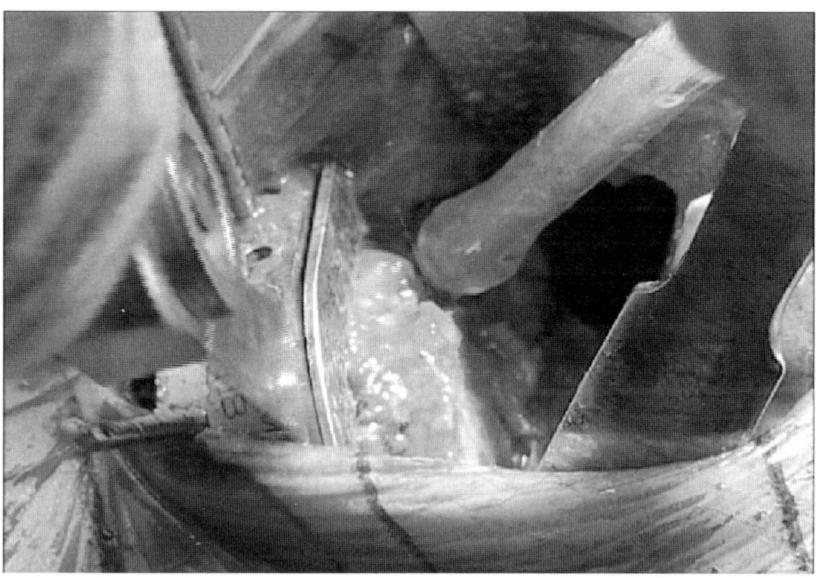

Figure 21.5. Image showing tibial cutting guide in place with adequate exposure allowing implantation of tibial component.

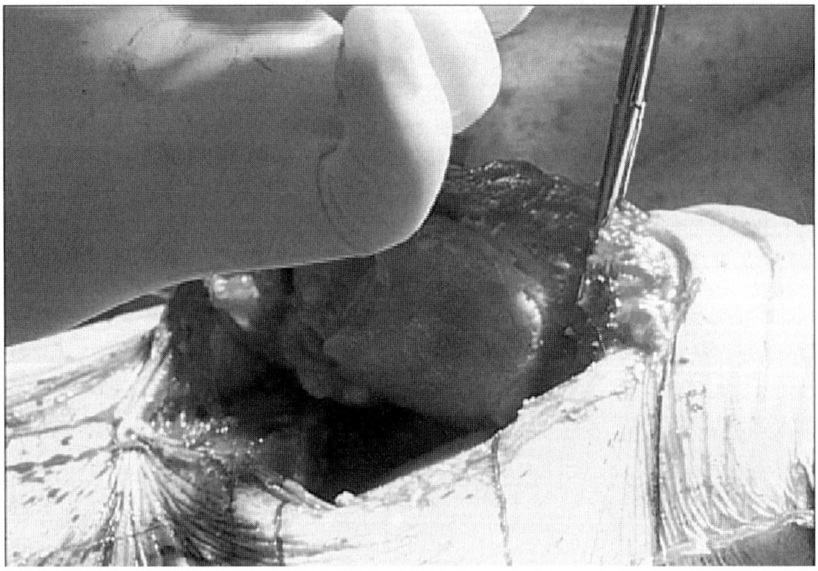

Figure 21.6. The patella is easily prepared without eversion of the quadriceps mechanism.

holes are drilled in preparation for the femoral pegs of the final femoral component. The patella is then osteotomized without eversion, perpendicular to the long axis of the femur and a guide placed for preparing the peg holes (Figure 21.6). The anterior cruciate ligament, remaining meniscal fragments, osteophytes, and excess soft tissues are excised. Trial components are then inserted with an appropriate tibial insert to assess stability in both flexion and extension and patellar tracking.

The trial components are removed and the bone ends are thoroughly irrigated, dried, and cleared of any soft tissue in preparation for cementation. Simplex bone cement (Stryker, Mahwah, NJ) is used for component implantation. Typically in this approach, the tibia is implanted first. A separate step is made to ensure complete removal of any excess cement, especially medially. After this is performed, the femur and patella can then be cemented in place. Initially a trial polyethylene is placed until the cement has cured. A final analysis of knee kinematics from extension to deep flexion using the navigation tools is performed; if the kinematics are appropriate then a final tibial polyethylene insert is impacted into place (Figure 21.7). The joint is then thoroughly irrigated and a single drain is used through the lateral side superior to the skin incision. The lateral arthrotomy and iliotibial band are closed with heavy interrupted absorbable sutures (Figure 21.8) followed by interrupted absorbable sutures in the subcutaneous tissue and closed with staples. A bulky compressive dressing is finally applied.

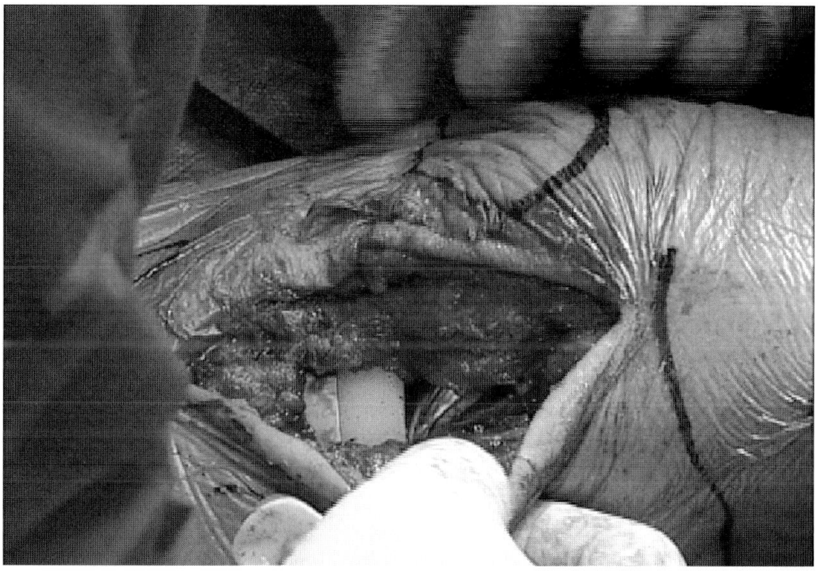

Figure 21.7. Image showing implants in place with incision lateral to the patella.

Results

The results in the initial cohort of 41 patients studied with a prospective IRB sanctioned protocol have shown that almost all patients have minimal anterior knee pain and are able to perform a straight leg raise

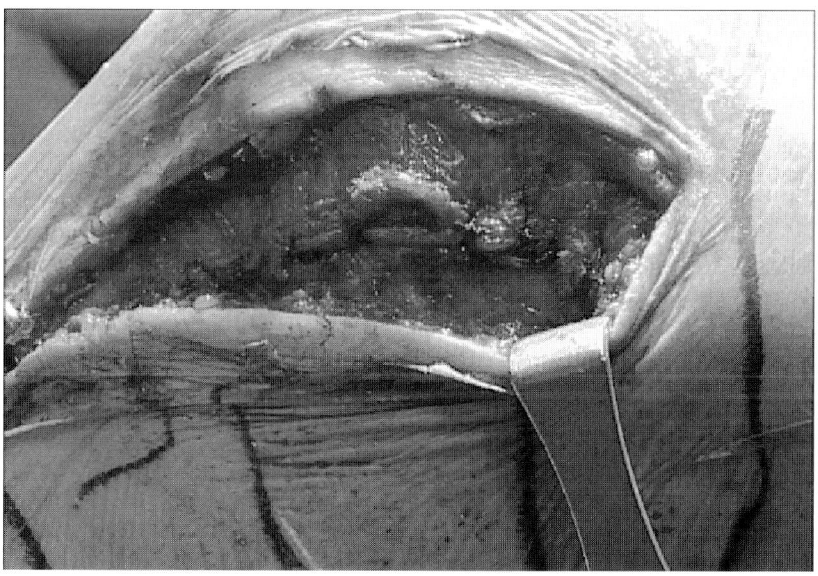

Figure 21.8. Closure of the lateral arthrotomy site.

immediately after surgery. This is quite different from patients with standard knee arthroplasties performed with a conventional anterior approach. The rehabilitation also appears to be rapid with less narcotic analgesic requirement and less use of ambulatory aids (i.e., canes).

Discussion

Many of the techniques for this approach have evolved from a minimally invasive medial approach. This approach involves a small amount of muscle-splitting with incisions typically less than 10 cm long.[12–15] Principles for this approach have included the symbiotic use of retractors with appropriate flexion and extension of the leg, the lack of patellar eversion, and the piecemeal approach to removing osteotomized bone in small incisions. Since reproducible results were obtained in a multicenter study using this approach, the authors felt that it would be worthwhile to further expand on some of these techniques and apply them to the lateral approach to the knee. Patients who have undergone a minimally invasive lateral approach to total knee arthroplasty have so far had superior short-term results when compared with patients with standard total knee arthroplasty techniques. Patients have all been able to straight leg raise almost immediately postoperative or certainly earlier than with standard total knee arthroplasty techniques. Patients have no pain in the anterior part of their knees. At the present time, the authors are evaluating various outcome modalities such as gait analyses and kinematic muscle testing to determine the true effects of this approach and are eager to know if the short-term gains will translate to long-term benefits. In general, patients have been pleased with the size and cosmesis of the small lateral incisions.

This is in contradiction to conventional total knee arthroplasties, which lead to tremendous morbidity with rehabilitative efforts that may take 3 months or more, in the short term. There also is a substantial amount of pain associated with a conventional total knee arthroplasty and patients will often need daily physical therapy for the first several weeks following surgery for optimal results. In addition, some patients need additional operative procedures (i.e., manipulations, to obtain optimal results). Furthermore, the functional outcomes of patients undergoing total knee arthroplasties may not be as favorable as what has been previously reported in the literature.

In summary, this lateral approach has distinct advantages over conventional total knee arthroplasty approaches. It requires a small laterally based incision, which immediately reduces postoperative pain in patients following total knee arthroplasty. The approach does not involve any degree of muscle-splitting, which also has many advantages. In addition, the knee is not dislocated nor is the patella everted. The use of navigation avoids the potential deleterious effects of intramedullary instrumentation. For all of these reasons, the authors believe that this can be an approach that can be used for most patients undergoing total knee arthroplasty. Further refinements to this approach will allow its general application for any knee surgeon.

Technical Summary Highlights of the Lateral Approach

1. Small-incision: The skin incision is generally less than 10 cm. However, it is certainly possible to perform this approach through a larger skin incision.
2. Muscle-sparing: This approach splits the iliotibial band and does not violate the quadriceps extensor mechanism whatsoever. In comparison to less invasive medial approaches, where at best a small portion of the vastus musculature is violated.
3. No patella eversion: The patella is not everted but rather minimally subluxed during both tibial and femoral preparation. Patellar preparation is performed with the patella held perpendicular to the long axis of the femur. It is believed that full patellar eversion may elongate the patellar ligament and may be a contributing factor to extensor mechanism problems following total knee arthroplasty.
4. No tibio-femoral dislocation: The knee joint is not dislocated nor subluxed and the lateral approach allows for the femoral, tibial, and patellar cuts to be made in situ. The tibia does not have to be anteriorly dislocated in front of the femur as in most total knee arthroplasties. This is in part facilitated by the method and the order of the cuts as well as the presence of a short keel on the tibial component.
5. Lateral incision: Although this is a cosmetic feature, it is certainly appreciated by patients. In addition, there are fewer cutaneous nerves on the lateral side of the knee than anteriorly and patients have less pain through their skin afferents. Related to this is that it appears to be very painful in a conventional knee arthroplasty approach to bend the knee through an anterior incision, which is obviously necessary for rehabilitation. This experience has been found in patients undergoing peroneal nerve releases where the pain was far less than an anterior skin incision and were able to range the knee with minimal pain from the lateral side of the knee.
6. Surgical navigation avoids intramedullary instrumentation: Intramedullary rods may lead to embolic phenomena in both the cardiopulmonary system as well as the central nervous system. Surgical navigation may have the advantage of avoiding intramedullary instrumentation without any loss of accuracy or malalignment.

References

1. Buechel FF Sr. Long-term follow-up after mobile-bearing total knee replacement. Clin Orthop. 2002;404:40–50.
2. Font-Rodriguez DE, Scuderi GR, Insall JN. Survivorship of cemented total knee arthroplasty. Clin Orthop. 1997;345:79–86.
3. Hanssen AD, Rand JA. A comparison of primary and revision total knee arthroplasty using the kinematic stabilizer prosthesis. J Bone Joint Surg Am. 1988;70:491–499.
4. Keating EM, Meding JB, Faris PM, Ritter MA. Long-term follow-up of nonmodular total knee replacements. Clin Orthop. 2002;404:34–39.

5. Rand JA, Ilstrup DM. Survivorship analysis of total knee arthroplasty: Cumulative rates of survival of 9200 total knee arthroplasties. J Bone Joint Surg Am 1991;73:397–409.
6. Scott WN, Rubinstein M, Scuderi G. Results after knee replacement with a posterior cruciate-substituting prosthesis. J Bone Joint Surg Am. 1988; 70:1163–1173.
7. Stern SH, Insall JN. Posterior stabilized prosthesis: Results after follow-up of nine to twelve years. J Bone Joint Surg Am. 1992;74:980–986.
8. Bullens PH, van Loon CJ, de Waal Malefijt MC, Laan RF, Veth RP. Patient satisfaction after total knee arthroplasty: a comparison between subjective and objective outcome assessments. J Arthroplasty. 2001;16:740–747.
9. Dickstein R, Heffes Y, Shabtai EI, Markowitz E. Total knee arthroplasty in the elderly: patients'self-appraisal 6 and 12 months postoperatively. Gerontology. 1998;44:204–210.
10. Trousdale RT, McGrory BJ, Berry DJ, Becker MW, Harmsen WS. Patients' concerns prior to undergoing total hip and total knee arthroplasty. Mayo Clin Proc. 1999;74:978–982.
11. Mont MA, Ragland P. Functional results of patients with total knee replacements with excellent Knee Society Scores. Unpublished data.
12. Mont MA, Stuchin SA, Paley D, et al. Different surgical options for monocompartmental osteoarthritis of the knee: high tibial osteotomy versus unicompartmental knee arthroplasty versus total knee arthroplasty: indications, techniques, results, and controversies. Instr Course Lect. 2004;53:265–283.
13. Bonutti PM, Neal DJ, Kester MA. Minimal incision total knee arthroplasty using the suspended leg technique. Orthopedics. 2003;26:899–903.
14. Kolisek F, Bonutti P, Hozack W, Purtill J, Sharkey P, Zelicof S. A prospective, randomized comparison of total knee arthroplasties performed by the MIS technique compared to standard technique. Unpublished data.
15. Stryker-Howmedica-Osteonics Technical Monograph on MIS TKA.

22

Minimally Invasive Total Knee Arthroplasty Using the Quadriceps-Sparing Approach

Alfred J. Tria, Jr.

Standard total knee arthroplasty has been in development since the introduction of the first total knee in 1974.[1,2] The techniques of balancing the ligaments, equalizing the flexion-extension gaps, and adjusting the overall alignment have been perfected so that the long-term results are very satisfactory and are now approaching 20 years for the follow-up studies.[3,4,5,6,7,8] Minimally invasive surgery (MIS) for knee arthroplasty began in the late 1990s. Repicci established the MIS approach for unicondylar knee arthroplasty (UKA) and encouraged interest in both limited surgical approaches and partial knee arthroplasty.[9,10] As the MIS UKA became more accepted, surgeons began to experiment with smaller surgical incisions for total knee arthroplasty (TKA). More than 15 years ago, arthroscopic surgeons attempted to implant a TKA with arthroscopic assistance. Unfortunately, no information was ever published concerning their attempts and the modified approach was abandoned. The MIS techniques for unicondylar surgery are now well developed and MIS TKA can now be approached with greater experience and improved techniques.

The author began to explore the possibility of the MIS TKA in the year 2001 with Dr. Thomas M. Coon and Dr. E. Marlowe Goble. The technique continues to evolve along with the instrument design. The surgical approach is now well established with more than 500 cases completed by the three investigators. This is certainly a work in progress and changes are incorporated almost on a weekly basis with the help of Zimmer Orthopaedics (Warsaw, IN) and the fine support teams. The instruments are constantly being upgraded and it is expected that a new prosthetic knee design will follow. The goal of all of this work is to allow a less invasive technique for TKA that will build on the successes of the present knee replacements and that will permit more rapid recovery with less morbidity.

Preoperative Evaluation

The patients are interviewed and evaluated in a similar fashion to standard TKA. To ensure a higher rate of success with a minimal learning curve, the author has applied restrictive indications for the surgical procedure. Over the past two years this has resulted in a 28% incidence of MIS TKA with five cases that required extension of the arthrotomy to complete the arthroplasty.

The patient should be in good medical health to undergo a procedure that presently is about 50 percent longer than the standard operation. The knee deformity should not exceed 10 degrees of anatomic varus (as measured on a standing anteroposterior x-ray of the knee), 15 degrees of anatomic valgus, and a 10 degree flexion contracture. The quality of the bone is also of some concern and one knee was abandoned and converted to a standard approach because of rheumatoid osteoporosis. Weight limitation is 250 pounds. The body mass index is somewhat misleading and the author is developing a ratio of the length of the thigh (measured from the anterior superior iliac spine of the pelvis to the middle of the patella) divided by the circumference of the knee at the level of the patella. It is the actual girth of the knee that affects the level of surgical difficulty and not the overall size of the patient. The deformity of the knee can be fixed or correctable on physical examination and the range of motion should be greater than 110 degrees. Because the anesthesia time is longer, few patients over the age of 80 are considered.

Surgical Approach

A curvilinear medial skin incision is made from the superior pole of the patella to the tibial joint line (Figure 22.1). This is the same incision that is used for the MIS unicondylar knee arthroplasty. The arthrotomy is in line with the skin incision. It begins at the superomedial border of the patella where the vastus medialis inserts and ends about 2 cm below the tibial joint just medial to the insertion of the patellar tendon. In the valgus knee, the incision may be made on the lateral side of the patella to the tibial joint line; however, the author prefers to avoid this approach because of limited experience with the technique and concerns about increasing the level of difficulty of the surgical exposure. Both the varus and valgus can be readily replaced through the medial arthrotomy. The arthrotomy dose not cut the vastus medialis, the quadriceps tendon, or enter the subvastus space. This concept is important to separate the quadriceps-sparing (QS) MIS surgery from other approaches that are more extensile and are better defined as mini approaches.

There is some variation of the insertion of the vastus medialis into the patella and this can be categorized (Figure 22.2). The type 1 has a very high insertion of the vastus above the medial aspect of the patella. The type 2 inserts just at the superomedial aspect of the patella. The type 3 inserts as low as the middle of the patella. The type 3 insertion

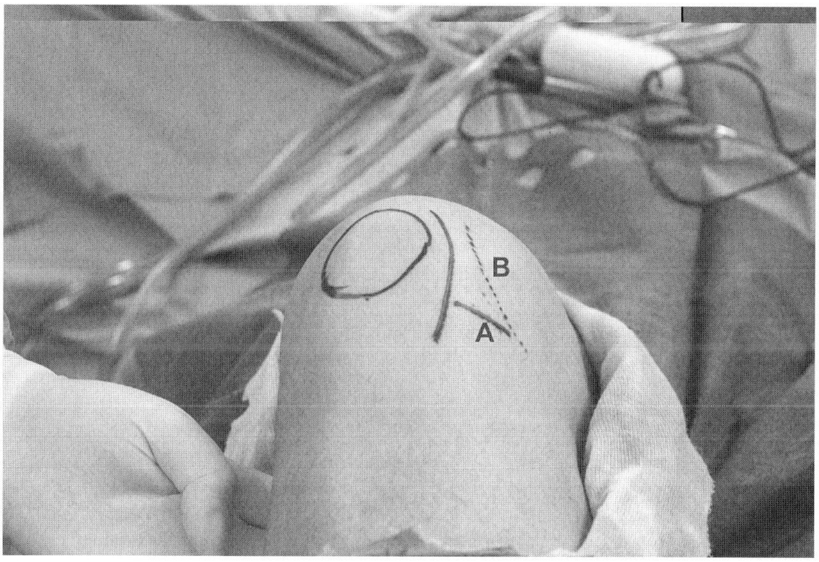

Figure 22.1. Medial incision in a right, varus knee. The dotted line (B) is the outline of the medial femoral condyle and the transverse line (A) is the tibiofemoral joint line. (From Choi YJ, Tanavalee A, Chan APH, et al. Minimally invasive surgery for total knee arthroplasty. In Scuderi GR, Tria AJ, Jr. MIS of the Hip and the Knee. New York: Springer, 2004.)

is usually seen in the muscular male knee. This knee is difficult to replace and the capsular incision does separate the muscle insertion. In this one variation it can be argued that the quadriceps-sparing arthrotomy violates one of the muscles of the quadriceps mechanism.

The knee is placed in full extension, the patellar fat pad is excised, and the posterior surface of the patella is removed with a free hand

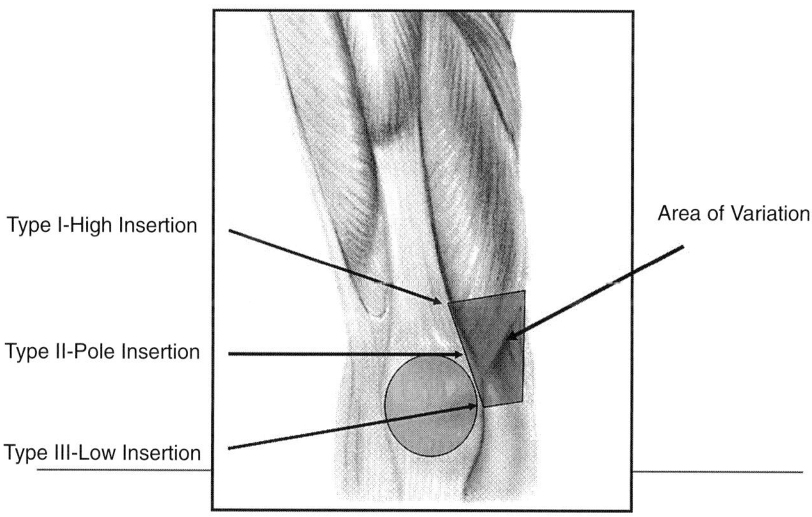

Figure 22.2. The anatomic variations of the vastus medialis muscle insertion.

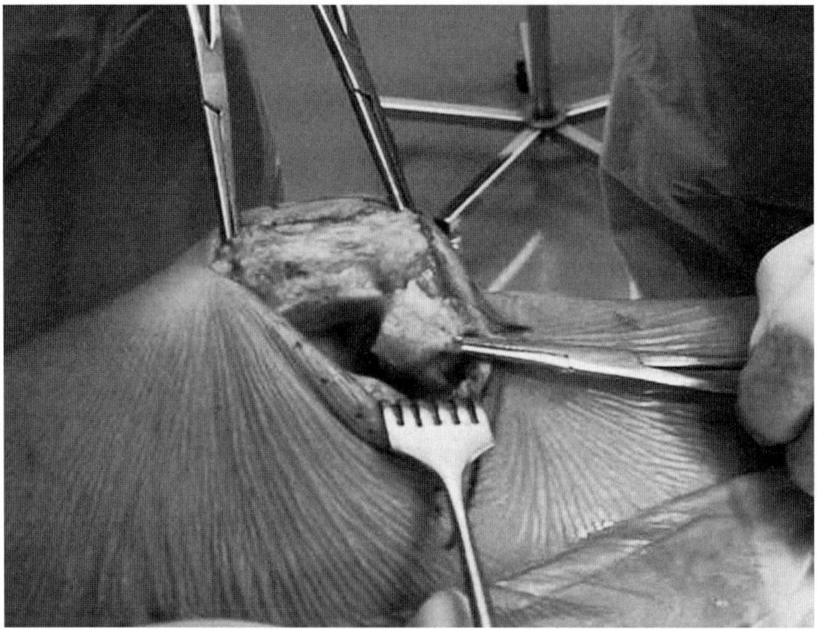

Figure 22.3. The patellar fat pad is completely excised and the patellar surface is removed with an oscillating saw.

saw (Figure 22.3). A guide is now available and can increase the accuracy of this cut but also adds to the time of the surgical procedure. The patella cannot be everted for this step and is cut at a 90-degree angle to the anterior surface of the femur. A metal protector is placed over the patellar surface to protect it from the retractors that are used throughout the remainder of the procedure. The peg holes for the patellar implant are completed at the end of the operation and the thickness is decreased by 1 mm to 2 mm. Early patellar resection increases the overall working room within the knee joint.

The anterior surface of the femur is cleared for about 2 cm above the proximal extent of the femoral sulcus to permit subsequent sizing and positioning of the anterior cut. The anterior and posterior cruciate ligaments are resected from within the intercondylar notch of the femur. The author uses a posterior cruciate substituting total knee design (High Flex Legacy Knee, Zimmer Orthopaedics, Warsaw, IN) but the procedure is also amenable to cruciate retaining total knees. The anteroposterior (AP) axis line of Whiteside's is drawn on the uncut surface of the femur (Figure 22.4); and, then, an intramedullary rod is introduced into the femur through a hole just above the intercondylar notch. A cutting guide is attached to the intramedullary reference (Figure 22.5). The distal cut is made across both femoral condyles and checked with a spacer and a rod versus the anterior superior iliac spine of the pelvis. The lateral condyle resection can be somewhat difficult and care should be taken to assure that the oscillating sawblade does not wander away from the exact cut position.

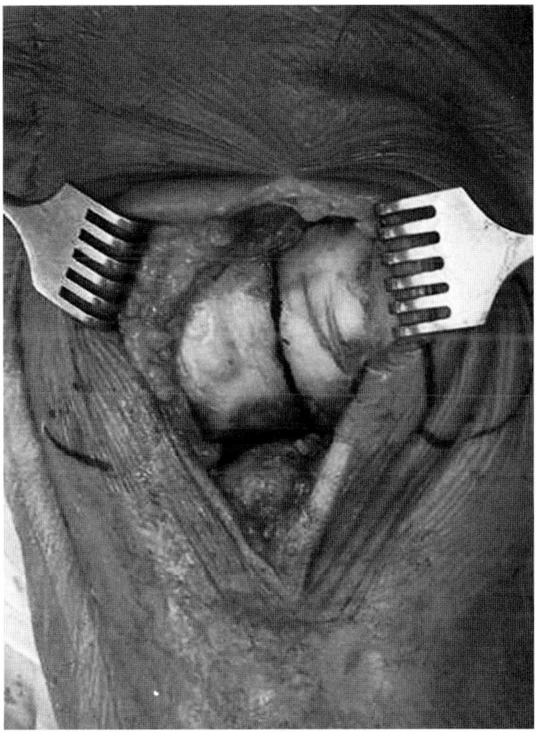

Figure 22.4. Leo Whiteside's anteroposterior axis line is drawn for the rotational femoral reference.

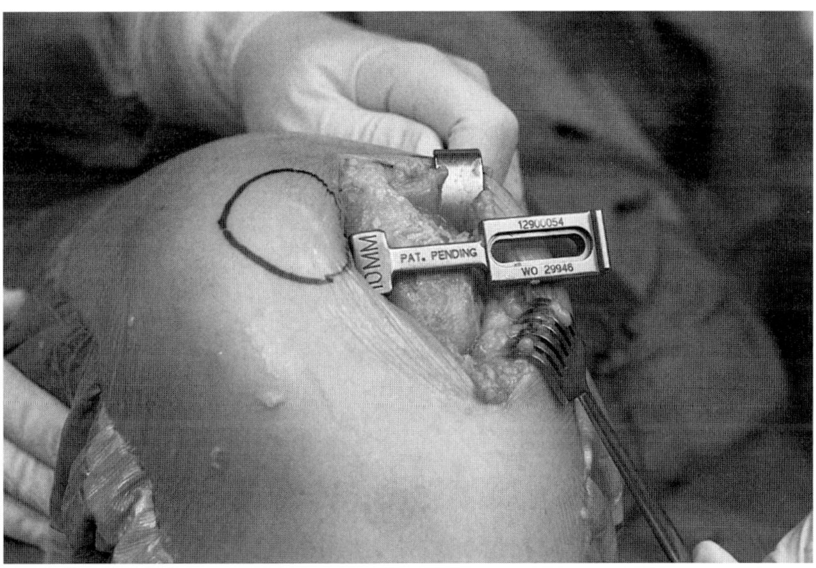

Figure 22.5. The intramedullary guide is used to reference the distal medial femoral condyle. (From Choi YJ, Tanavalee A, Chan APH, et al. Minimally invasive surgery for total knee arthroplasty. In Scuderi GR, Tria AJ, Jr. MIS of the Hip and the Knee. New York: Springer, 2004.)

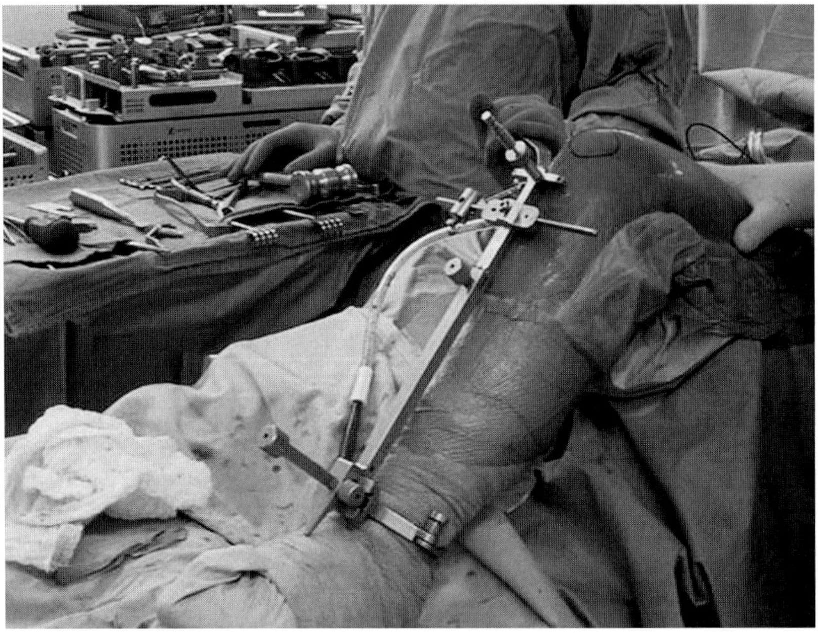

Figure 22.6. The tibial cut is completed with an extramedullary guide that has an outrigger around the medial aspect of the tibial plateau.

The tibial guide is an extramedullary instrument with a cutting head attachment that permits accurate cutting from the medial side (Figure 22.6). The proper adjustments must be made for varus/valgus, flexion/extension, and the anteroposterior slope. This cut must be accomplished with care to avoid injury to the posterior neurovascular structures and the lateral ligaments and peroneal nerve. It is not possible with the QS approach to flex the knee to 90 degrees and force the proximal tibia out of the wound or in front of the femur. Therefore, it is safer to make the cut in about 70 degrees of flexion with the tibia beneath the femur and, then remove the medial one half of the tibial cut in a similar fashion to a UKA surgery (Figure 22.7). The lateral cut can be completed with better visualization and safety after the medial bone is removed. It is simpler to remove the tibial bone in full extension; however, no saw cuts should be made in extension at all.

With both the distal femoral and proximal tibial resections completed, the extension space can be checked with a spacer block and extramedullary rods in the standard fashion to confirm proper valgus alignment with full extension and balanced ligaments (Figure 22.8). If there is a ligament imbalance at this point, the medial or lateral releases can be performed without difficulty because there is a space of almost 20 mm in the knee.

The knee is now flexed to 90 degrees and the femoral *tower* instrument is inserted into the knee with the footpads beneath the medial and lateral femoral condyles for posterior condylar referencing (Figure 22.9). The tower should be parallel to Whiteside's line to confirm proper rotation of the femoral component. The instrument includes

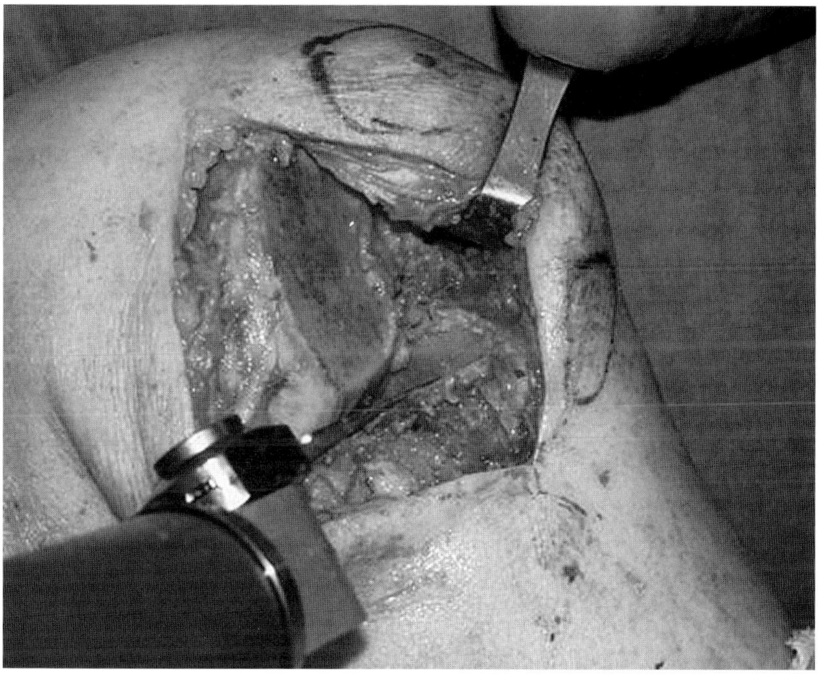

Figure 22.7. The medial one half of the tibia is removed and the saw is gently guided across the remaining lateral tibial bone.

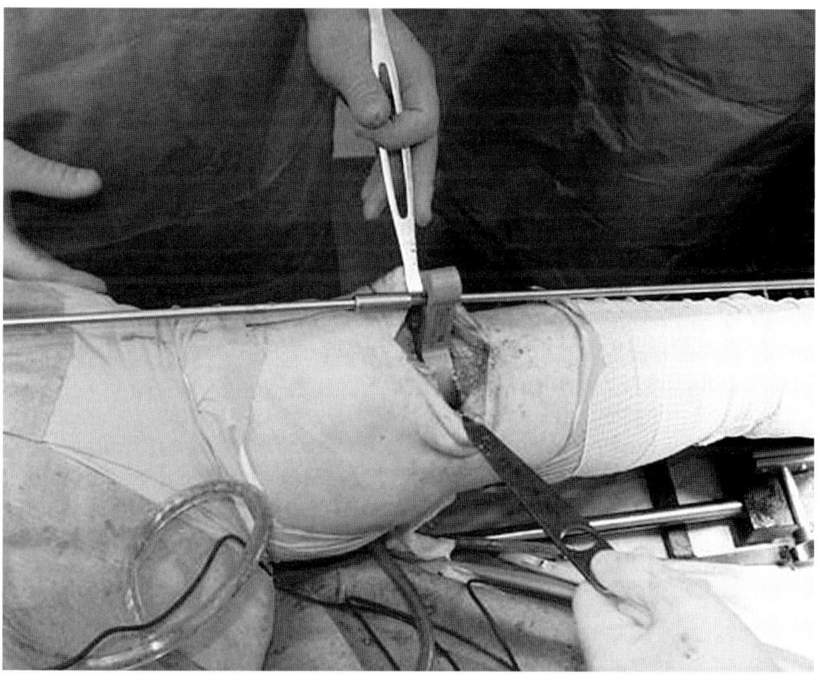

Figure 22.8. The spacer block is inserted in full extension and the extramedullary rods are used to confirm alignment and check the ligament balance.

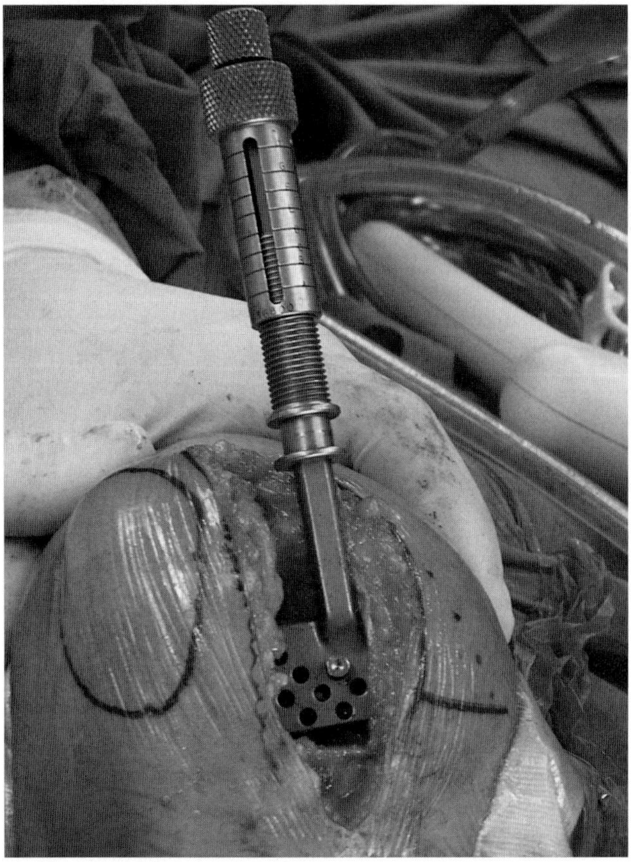

Figure 22.9. The femoral tower references the posterior condylar axis of the femur and should be parallel to Whiteside's line.

three degrees of external rotation versus the posterior condylar line. If there is a deficiency of either the medial or lateral condyle posteriorly, the tower will have to be rotated to realign it parallel to the AP axis. The instrument is pinned onto the normal condyle side and, then, rotated off the deficient side to correct for the deformity. Once the rotation is set, the knee is placed in about 15 degrees of flexion and the measuring handle is attached to reference the anterior cortex of the femur that was cleared at the beginning of the operation (Figure 22.10). The handle establishes the size of the femoral component and also determines the level of the anterior femoral resection. The external rotation cut is completed and the tower is removed (Figure 22.11). The femoral finishing block is placed into the extension gap and positioned medial to lateral with the attached shelf flat against the external rotation cut (Figure 22.12). The knee is flexed to 90 degrees and the femoral finishing cuts are completed (Figure 22.13). The box cut for the posterior stabilized knee can also be completed at this point.

It is now possible to confirm the size of the flexion and extension gaps and determine if any adjustments need to be made. The two

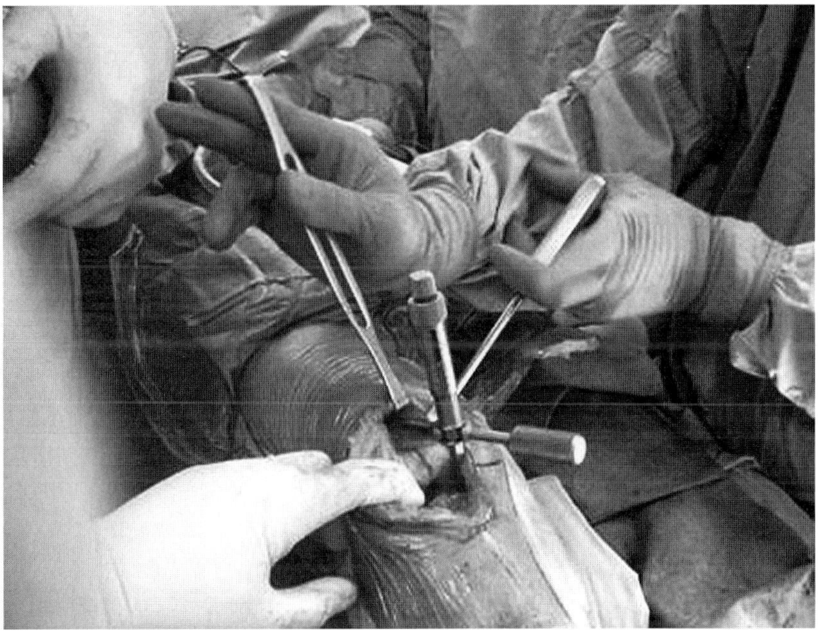

Figure 22.10. The reference handle is locked onto the tower and sets the level of anterior resection.

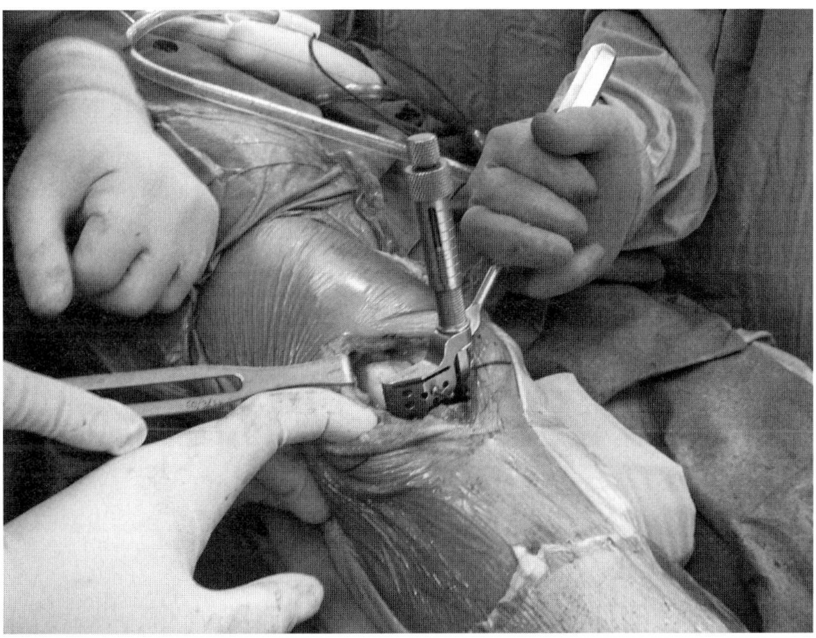

Figure 22.11. The external rotation cut is made with the cutting block locked onto the tower.

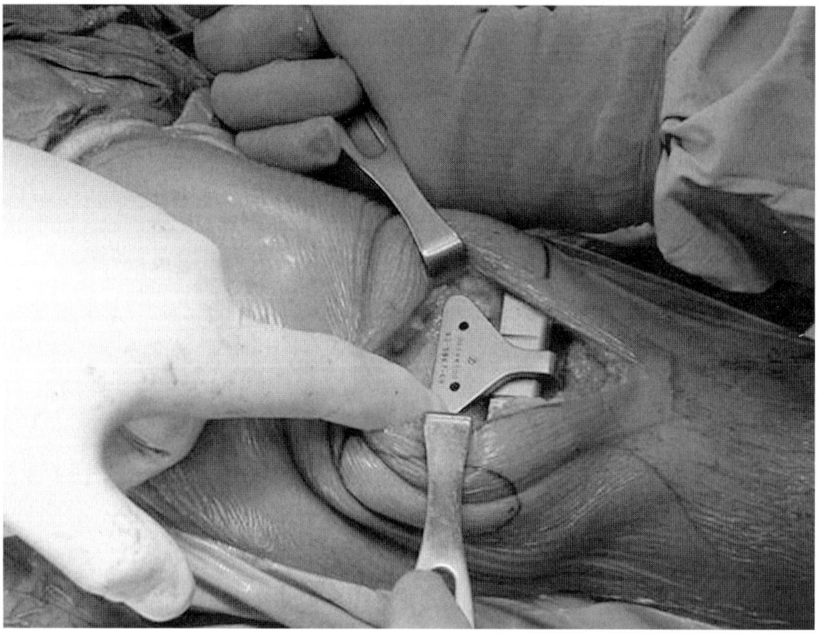

Figure 22.12. The triangular flat plate sits on the external rotation cut for the femur and sets the rotation for the femoral finishing block.

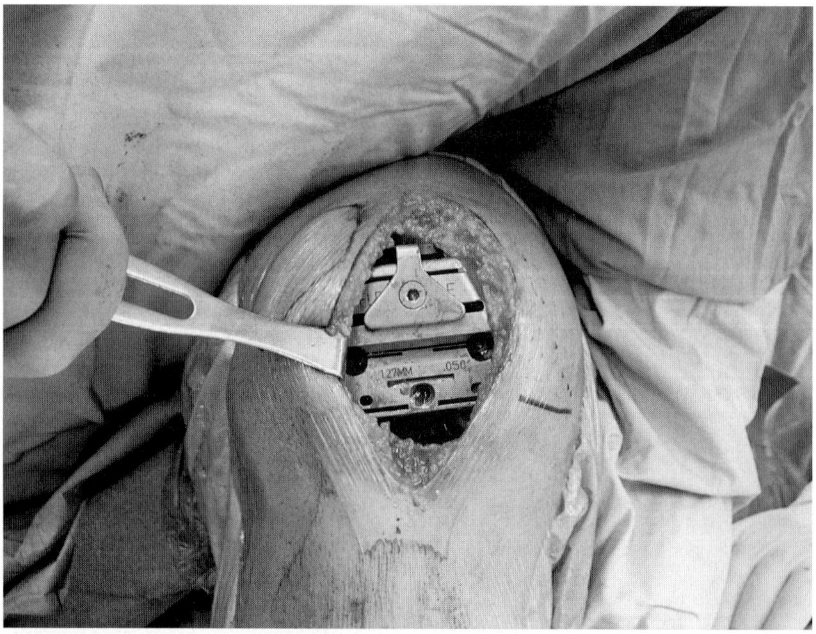

Figure 22.13. The femoral finishing block guides all of the final cuts for the femoral component. In this view the alignment plate is still attached to the block.

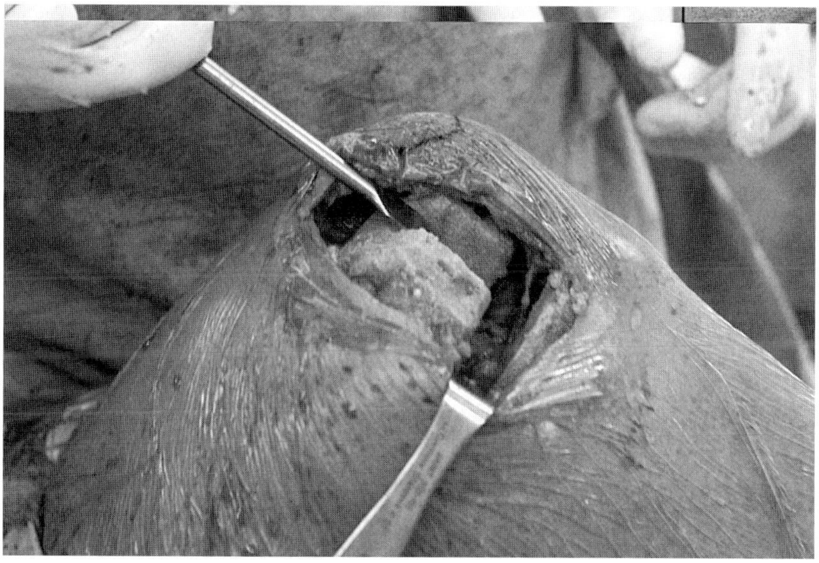

Figure 22.14. This view shows the knee in 90 degrees of flexion with all of the cuts completed. The flexion and extension spaces can now be measured and corrected if necessary.

spaces are checked with a spacer block and extramedullary rods. It is possible at this point to recut the proximal tibia, downsize the femur, or recut the distal femur as indicated. Once again, there is enough bone removed from the joint to allow for proper exposure and adjustments (Figure 22.14).

The tibial cut surface is now sized for placement of the tray. The guide has two posterior hooks that reference the posterior cortex of the proximal tibia (Figure 22.15). The instrument is centered medial to lateral and, then externally rotated referencing the tibial tubercle. After the guide is pinned to the tibia, the position is confirmed versus the tibial tubercle, the femoral box cut, and the malleoli of the ankle. The broaching and stem holes are now completed.

The trial components are inserted: the femoral component, the polyethylene insert with the stemless tibial tray, and the patella, in that order. After the patellar tracking, ligament balance, and range of motion are confirmed, the components are removed and the surfaces are prepared for cementing. All of the components are cemented using standard bone cement. The tibial tray (without the polyethylene insert) is implanted first. The stem of the tray is somewhat difficult to insert at this time and a modular component is in development for later in this calendar year (Figure 22.16). The femoral component is cemented second and is inserted with the patella subluxed to the lateral side, but not everted. The patella is cemented into position last. The polyethylene insert is locked into position after the cementing is completed (Figure 22.17). It is critical to be sure at this point that the flexion extension spaces are equal and acceptable.

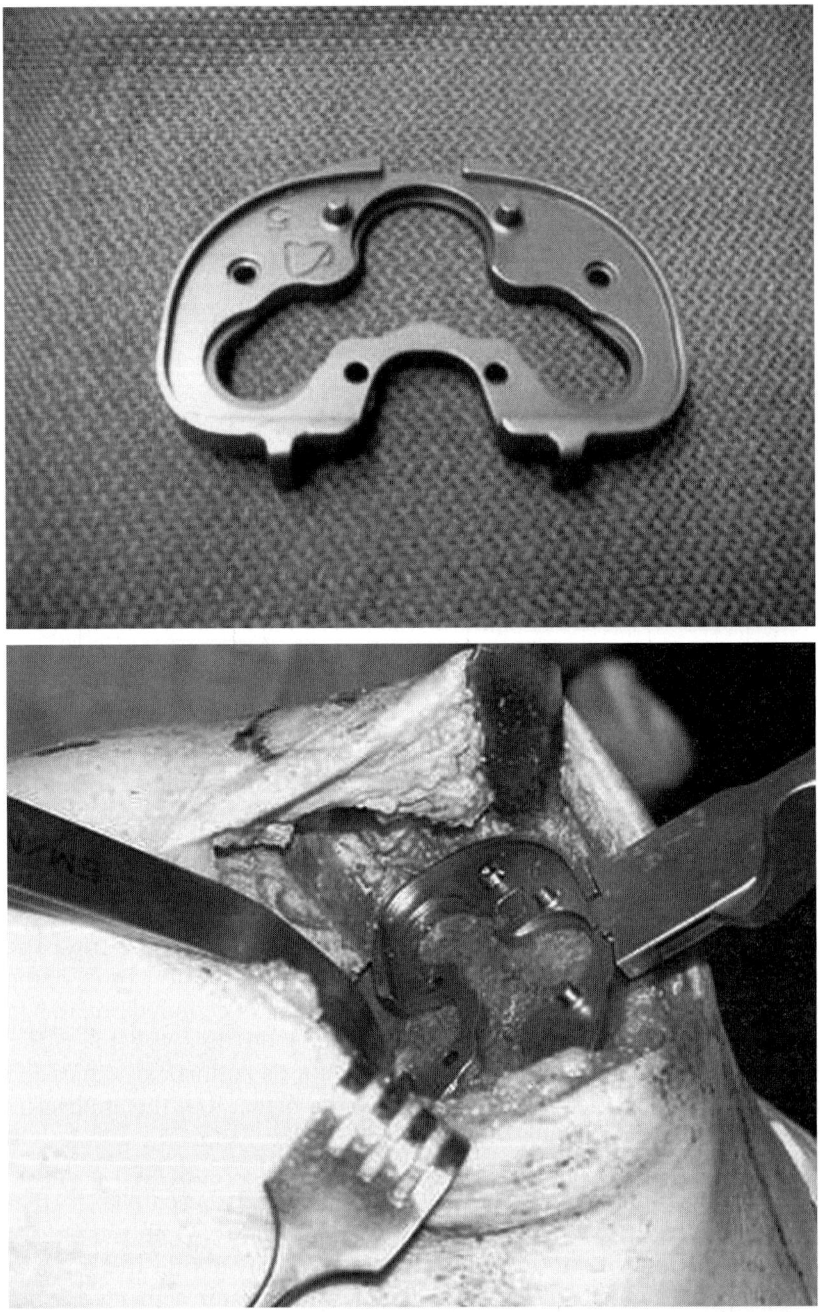

A

B

Figure 22.15. (A) The tibial cutting guide has posterior hooks that contact the posterior cortex of the tibia. (B) This view shows the tibial cutting guide on the top of the tibial cut surface in about 80 degrees of flexion. (B, from Choi YJ, Tanavalee A, Chan APH, et al. Minimally invasive surgery for total knee arthroplasty. In Scuderi GR, Tria AJ, Jr. MIS of the Hip and the Knee. New York: Springer, 2004.)

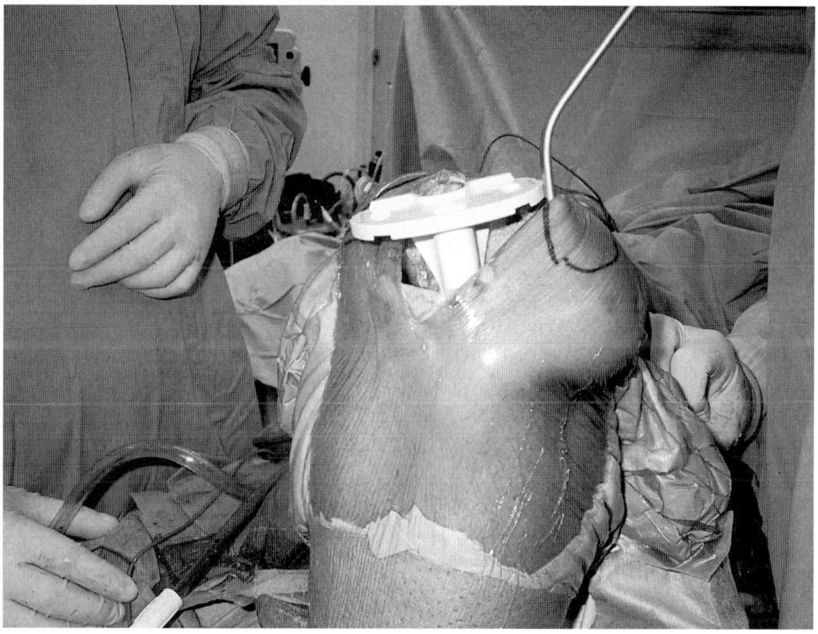

Figure 22.16. The tibial posterior stabilized component is difficult to insert because of the intramedullary stem. A modular component would make this step much easier.

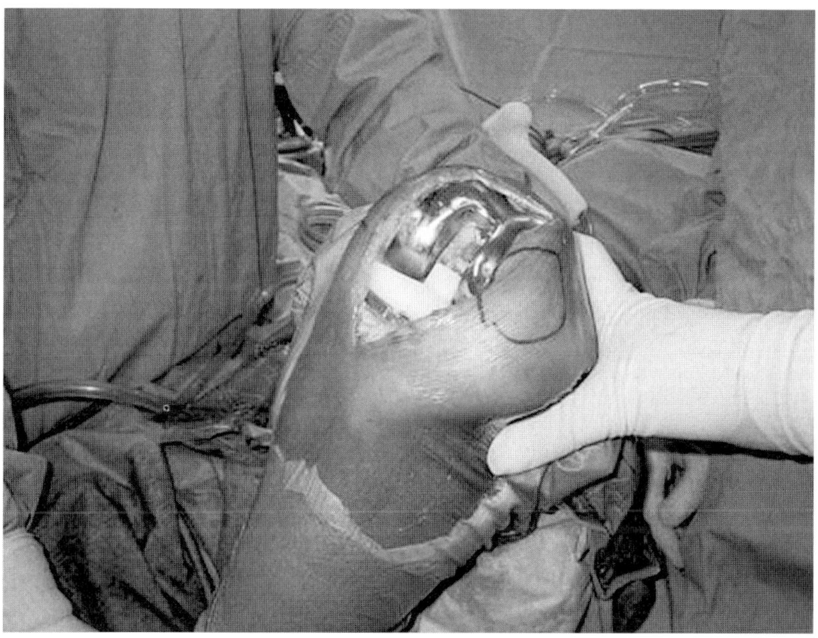

Figure 22.17. The final components in the knee after completion of the cementing.

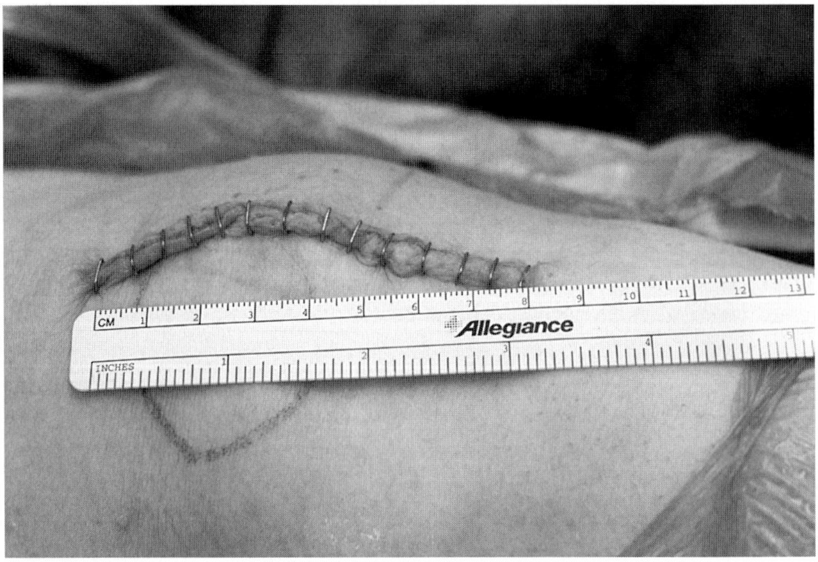

Figure 22.18. The typical skin incision is about 8 cm to 10 cm in length.

Surgical drains can be used if desired. The arthrotomy is closed in the standard fashion along with the skin. It is important to secure the attachment of the vastus medialis to prevent disruption of the medial closure and subluxation of the patella. The skin incision is typically 8 cm to 10 cm long (Figure 22.18).

Postoperative Management

The patient receives one unit of autologous blood during the surgical procedure and the hemoglobin is monitored after the operation. Full weight bearing ambulation and range of motion exercises are started within 2 to 4 hours after the surgery. Fonduparinux (Arixtra, Sanofi-Synthelabo) is started for DVT prophylaxis on the morning after surgery and is continued for 10 days with a Doppler-ultrasound study of both lower extremities before discontinuation.[11,12] The patient is discharged on the second day after surgery to rehabilitation centers.

Results

One hundred sixty-four QS MIS TKAs have now been completed in 169 attempts. One case was discontinued because of obesity. One was discontinued for posterior bleeding. One case could not be included because of inadvertent extension of the quadriceps incision and two cases required quadriceps extension to allow the femoral component insertion. The average age is 67 with a range from 51 to 86 years; 25 of the patients underwent bilateral procedures. The surgical procedure requires about fifty percent more time than the standard open TKA. The average intraoperative blood loss is 375 cc, measured by cell saver technique. This loss is about 20% less than the standard knee arthroplasty. The level of pain is 20% less than the standard approach.

The average length of stay is 2 days compared to for the standard TKA. The complications include one nonfatal pulmonary embolism, one nonfatal myocardial infarction, and two transient cardiac arrhythmias at 2 and 3 days postsurgery. One patient required a manipulation of the knee and is the only patient with poor motion (flexion limited to 70 degrees). The postoperative x-rays show an average distal femoral valgus of 6 degrees, a tibial varus of 2 degrees, and an overall alignment of 4 degrees of valgus. These x-rays were compared with a matched group of patients who underwent unilateral high flex posterior stabilized knee arthroplasty during the same period of time using the standard arthrotomy incision and no statistically significant differences were found. There were no infections, wound complications, reoperations, or component malpositioning in the entire series.

The QS MIS knees have 20 degrees more motion at the first office visit than the matched group. The difference persists for the first six months. At the end of the first year, the MIS QS knees have the same motion as the matched high flex knees with the standard arthrotomy incision. However, it should be emphasized that the QS knees started with 10 degrees less motion; therefore, the QS knees gain motion after the surgery.

Conclusions

MIS TKA is in the early stages of development. There are many opponents who believe that the technique is nothing more than a cosmetic modification of the standard TKA that will lead to more complications and less patient satisfaction. It is important to respect these comments and to thoroughly address them. MIS surgery is a surgery that is not determined by the length of the incision or the cosmetic result. The term *minimally invasive* should refer to the extent of violation of the anatomic structures about the involved joint. In the knee, the MIS approach should not violate the extensor mechanism and should not violate the suprapatellar pouch. MIS should be a capsular approach and, as such, it should produce less discomfort and a faster recovery. Modifications of the MIS technique that extend the arthrotomy into the extensor mechanism, violate the suprapatellar pouch, and evert the patella while using a limited incision are not minimally invasive. There will certainly be a learning curve to this procedure and a smaller incision with standard TKA techniques may be the interim step for the surgeon attempting to master the new approach. At present, the QS MIS TKA does appear to provide excellent results with minimal morbidity. Further studies will certainly be necessary to compare all of the techniques and to place each one in the spectrum of MIS knee arthroplasty.

References

1. Insall J, Ranawat C, Scott WN, Walker P. Total condylar knee replacement. Preliminary report. Clin Orthop. 1976;120:149–154.
2. Insall J, Tria A, Scott W. The total condylar knee prosthesis. The first five years. Clin Orthop. 1979;145:68–77.
3. Ranawat C, Flynn W, Saddler S, Hansraj K, Maynard M. Long-term results of the total condylar knee arthroplasty. A 15-year survivorship study. Clin Orthop. 1993;286:96–102.
4. Stern S, Insall J. Posterior stabilized prosthesis. Results after follow-up of nine to twelve years. JBJS. 1992;74:980–986.
5. Colizza W, Insall J, Scuderi G. The posterior stabilized total knee prosthesis: assessment of polyethylene damage and osteolysis after a ten year minimum follow-up. JBJS. 1995;77:1716–1720.
6. Malkani A, Rand J, Bryan R, Wallrich S. Total knee arthroplasty with the kinematic condylar prosthesis. A ten year follow-up study. JBJS. 1995; 77:423–431.
7. Scott RD, Volatile TB. 12 years experience with posterior cruciate retaining total knee arthroplasty. Clin Orthop. 1986;205:100–107.
8. Ritter MA, Herbst SA, Keating EM, Faris PM, Meding JB. Long-term survivorship analysis of a posterior cruciate retaining total condylar total knee arthroplasty. Clin Orthop. 1994;309:136–145.
9. Repicci JA, Eberle RW. Minimally invasive surgical technique for unicondylar knee arthroplasty. Journal of the Southern Orthopaedic Association. 1999;8(1):20–27.
10. Romanowski MR, Repicci JA. Minimally invasive unicondylar arthroplasty: Eight-year follow-up. Journal of Knee Surgery 2002;15(1):17–22, 2002.
11. Eriksson BL, Bauer KA, Lassen MR, Turpie AG. Fondaparinux compared with enoxaparin for the prevention of venous thromboembolism after hip-fracture surgery. N Engl J Med. 2001;345(18):1298–1304.
12. Bauer KA, Eriksson BL, Lassen MR, Turpie AG. Fondaparinux compared with enoxaparin for the prevention of venous thromboembolism after elective major knee surgery. N Engl J Med. 2001;345(18):1305–1310.

Section V

Computer Navigation

23

Computer-Guided Total Hip Arthroplasty

James B. Stiehl

Computed-assisted orthopedic surgery (CAOS) has been recently defined as the ability to use sophisticated computer algorithms to allow the surgeon to determine three-dimensional placement of total hip implants in situ.[1] A rapid ongoing evolution of technical advances have allowed the ability to move from cumbersome systems requiring a preoperative computed tomography of the patient's hip joint to more elegant systems that use image-free registration or the simple use of fluoroscopy at the time of surgery. In total hip replacement, several reports have cited the accuracy with which implants can be placed using computer-aided robotic devices or surgical navigation.

From a historical perspective, ROBODOC was the first modern attempt to use computers to place implants in bones, in this example, a cementless metal femoral stem in the proximal femoral canal. The goal was to improve the precision of implant placement, and eliminate errors from a variety of sources including inaccurate plain radiographic templating, morphological anatomical variation, and problems related to the insertion of the implants. The ROBODOC system was conceived in 1986 by Bargar and Paul, and developed over the next several years with grants from IBM. That team developed proprietary software for the CT imaging to obtain an accuracy of one pixel for the raw data, which then allowed them to create CT three-dimensional reconstructions for choosing the implant sizes and planning the robotic surgical intervention. Originally, the fiducial markers for the robotic system were placed during a separate operative procedure and the marker was used to specifically orient the robotic tool into the inner canal of the proximal femur. This changed with the ability to register the unique anatomy of the patient intraoperatively. With improvements in software, the system could be referenced by using a digitizing probe for the key areas of the proximal femur and small incisions were used about the midshaft of the femur for distal referencing. Currently, referencing may be done using a highly sophisticated combination of local touch point referencing and image overlay. The ROBODOC system is amenable to very small incisions that are limited in length only by the size of the implants.[2,3]

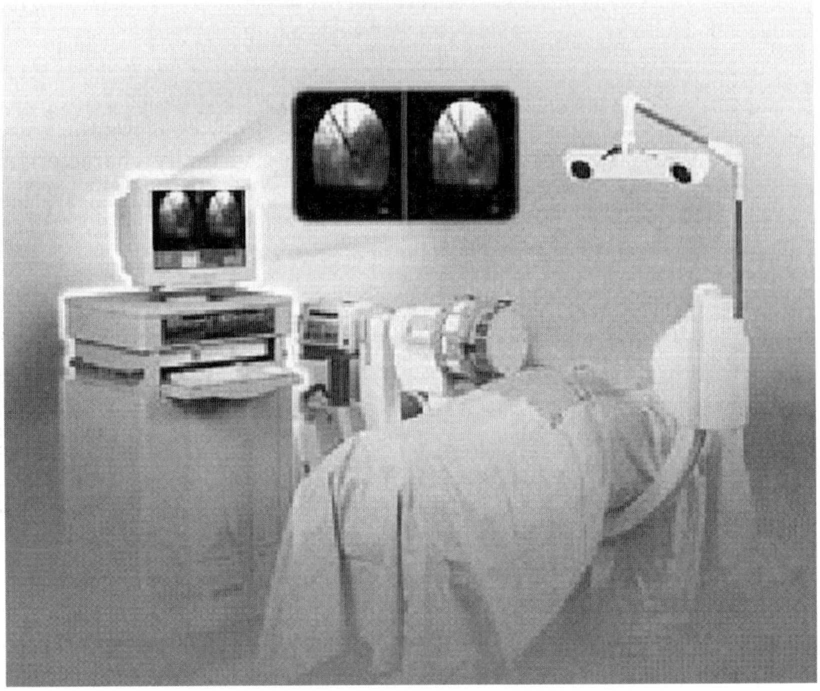

Figure 23.1. Computer navigation system consists of camera, DRBs on the patient, computer platform, and method of image acquisition, in this case, fluoroscopy. (Medtronic Navigation, Inc., Louisville, CO.)

In the early 1990s, other possibilities arose for computer navigation and while *active* or robotic navigation held promise, *passive* navigation developed with the possibility of remotely tracking the instruments and anatomy (Figure 23.1). The idea here was to reference the target object which in this case would be the human acetabulum and then track the instruments passively in space. For navigation about the hip, computed tomography was first used to acquire a digital representation of the structure of the pelvis and femur.[4] Optoelectronic tracking was developed as that system was readily available from other industrial processes. Furthermore, the inputs were not affected by the surgical environment as were other methods such as electromagnetic trackers and ultrasound. A negative feature though is the need for an unobstructed view of the camera and the markers.

In order to determine the exact spatial orientation of the patient or any surgical instrument, at least three non-collinear points on a fixed body (dynamic reference base) must be recognized by a camera system which then inputs data into the computer for virtual referencing. The referencing protocol collects all components including the patient's anatomy and all registered surgical instruments. The dynamic reference bases (DRBs) may be active, consisting of light emitting diodes (LEDs) in which two or three CCD (charged couple devices) of the camera system pick up the light signal, or passive in which reflector balls are placed on the DRB and reflect infrared light originating from a light source on the camera. By differentiating the sphere arrangements on the DRBs, the computer could then detect the specific DRB such as the marker on the pelvis or a reaming instrument.

Registration is the process by which the computer recognizes the various three-dimensional objects that it must virtually characterize. For all DRBs the process is simply finding the appropriately defined DRB with the camera and registering it with the computer. For instruments and implants, the exact dimensions and orientation of the referencing source are encrypted into the software. For the patient, the goal is to reference or *match* the anatomy of the patient into the computer model. Two methods exist for performing this step. Paired-point matching takes prominent anatomical points that have been predetermined on the CT scan and then intraoperatively using a space digitizer (pointer probe) that identifies or matches the same landmark. Surface registration is a secondary referencing method in which a small number of points may be digitized into the system to describe a surface contour such as the dome of the acetabulum. An additional step is verification, which is cross-referencing additional points on the anatomy with the virtual object on the computer. From this information, the surgeon may judge the operational accuracy of the system.

The advantage of the CT scan for referencing is that it provides a three-dimensional data set for creating the virtual model in the computer. However, acquisition of the CT adds additional logistical and financial factors to the process. The CT must be obtained preoperatively and must be digital in format for use on the computer. Additional time will be required by the surgical team to manipulate the data, pick the primary referencing points, templating, etc. Also there are certain examples such as in navigated fracture reduction, in which the bone topology of the CT is intentionally altered during the surgical procedure. Other options exist such as acquiring the images with two-dimensional fluoroscopy or using a direct surgeon defined anatomical approach. Fluoroscopy requires specific calibration to maintain the desired accuracy of the imaging technique. It is known that the earth's magnetic forces significantly distort the image acquired from the fluoroscope camera and this must be accounted for. In practice, a calibrated grid with markers of known size and spatial relationship are combined with the image to create an accurate virtual portrayal on the computer. The images are then acquired with the patient's DRB in position to obtain the virtual model that allows navigation of the fluoroscopic image.[5]

The surgeon defined anatomy approach requires the surgeon to create the virtual model by digitizing the various points of the anatomy with a navigated probe. This is particularly applicable to open total knee replacement where most of the important landmarks are visible and readily identified. A novel kinematic approach has evolved for determining the hip center location in which the center of rotation of the hip joint is determined by simply rotating the lower extremity in a large circular motion. The computer automatically finds the smallest point of movement, which in this case should be the center of the femoral head, if the pelvis is held absolutely rigid. The mechanical axis of the lower extremity is defined by point matching the center of the distal femur, the center of the proximal tibia, and a factored point between the ankle malleoli for the most distal center. Certain proprietary software applications have added surface matching to this direct method to supplement anatomical features.

The applications to minimally invasive surgery will evolve from a unique combination of the previously noted techniques. For example, the two-incision hip approach, which already uses fluoroscopy for identifying the anatomy, will now have a virtual fluoroscopy image on the computer for navigating both the acetabulum and the femur. Direct anatomical landmarks may be point match referenced on such areas as the anterior superior iliac spine, which is readily accessible. For the other landmarks such as the pubic symphysis, indirect referencing may be done by obtaining calibrated fluoroscopic images in two planes. For the total knee arthroplasty, a similar combination of direct and fluoroscopic referencing will be done. While one may easily identify the lower extremity centers for the total knee minimally invasive quad-sparing technique, accessory landmarks such as the distal femoral epicondyles may not be readily obtained. Future applications include newer technologies such as electromagnetic sensors that can be made into miniature DRBs and the use of more sophisticated imaging systems such as ultrasound, three-dimensional C-arms, and the use of intraoperative CT scanners.

Acetabular Component Navigation

Optimal acetabular component orientation in total hip arthroplasty is a complex three-dimensional problem with failure leading to increased wear and instability. Recent publications have demonstrated a connection between the positioning of the prosthesis and the frequency of dislocation.[6,7,8] Lewinnek et al. noted an increase of the hip dislocation rate from 1.5% to 6.1% if a safe range of 15° +/−10° radiographic anteversion or 40° +/−10° acetabular abduction were exceeded.[9] Recent computer simulations have studied range of motion and concluded that the greatest range of motion was noted with acetabular anteversion of 20 to 25°, acetabular abduction of 45°, and femoral stem anteversion of 15°.[10,11]

The positioning of the acetabular component during surgery is dependent on the orientation of the bony acetabulum and position of the patient's pelvis on the operating table. McCollum et al. have stated that patient positioning is not always reproducible in the lateral decubitus position and often leads to pelvic malalignment with resultant improper cup alignment. Pelvic flexion and adduction are virtually unavoidable in this position placing greater demands on the surgical technique for satisfactory outcome.[12] Therefore, improvement in cup implantation occurs if either the pelvis position can be standardized or a method of correctly localizing the anatomical orientation of the acetabulum can be created.

Computed Tomography for Acetabular Navigation

I describe the method of computer-assisted navigation recently used in a group of patients in which computed tomography was the source of image referencing. In patients undergoing computer-assisted navigation of the acetabular components, a preoperative analysis and planning were required (Figures 23.2 and 23.3). The digital computed tomography study was loaded into the Surgigate (Medivision, Oberdorf, Switzerland) software program and the three-dimensional model was then created. The femoral head was extracted from the image and the sagittal plane of view was drawn over the acetabular inlet. This then allowed visualization of the acetabulum in three planes and the three-dimensional model of the pelvis (Figure 23.4). The frontal plane reference was created, which was the landmarking reference subsequently used at the time of surgery. This reference consisted of the plane formed by the points of the anterior superior iliac spines and the pubic symphysis. In most patients, this plane is parallel to the long axis of the patient and is perpendicular to the floor. The Surgigate software automatically creates all images in the sagittal, frontal and axial planes with a 90-degree reference to the frontal plane reference (Figure 23.5). With the three-dimensional model, at least three additional points of reference were identified to be used at the time of surgery. These included the points in the acetabular dome, the acetabular floor, and the cotyloid notch on the lateral wall of the quadrilateral plate. The final step allowed positioning of a virtual acetabular component into the pelvis at the chosen position of 45 degrees acetabular abduction and 20 degrees acetabular anteversion. Additionally, the surgeon has the

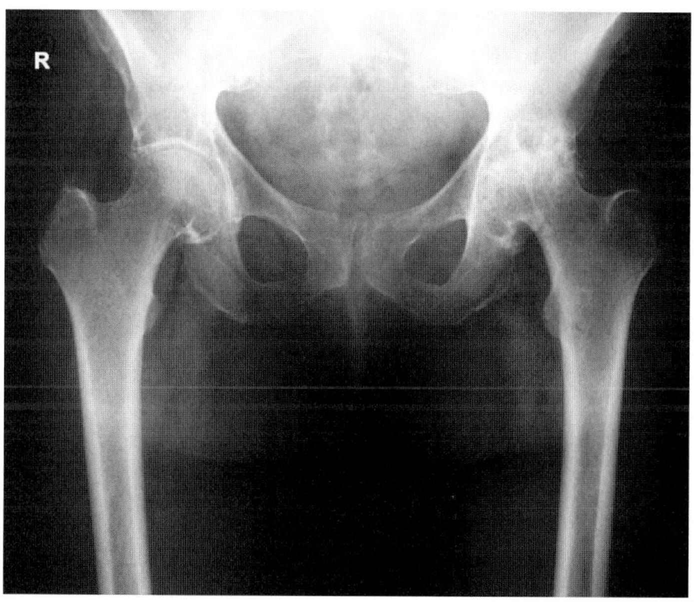

Figure 23.2. Anterior pelvic radiograph of preoperative patient with severe degenerative arthritis of the left hip.

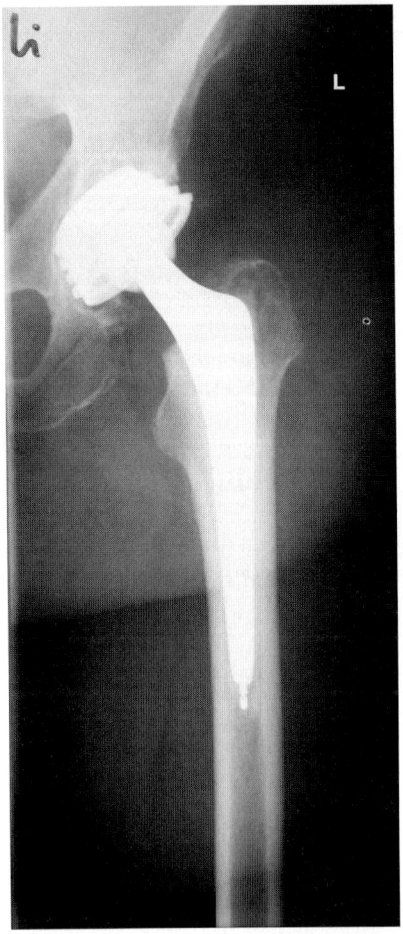

Figure 23.3. Postoperative anterior posterior radiograph of the left hip revealing a screw in cup and press-fit femoral stem.

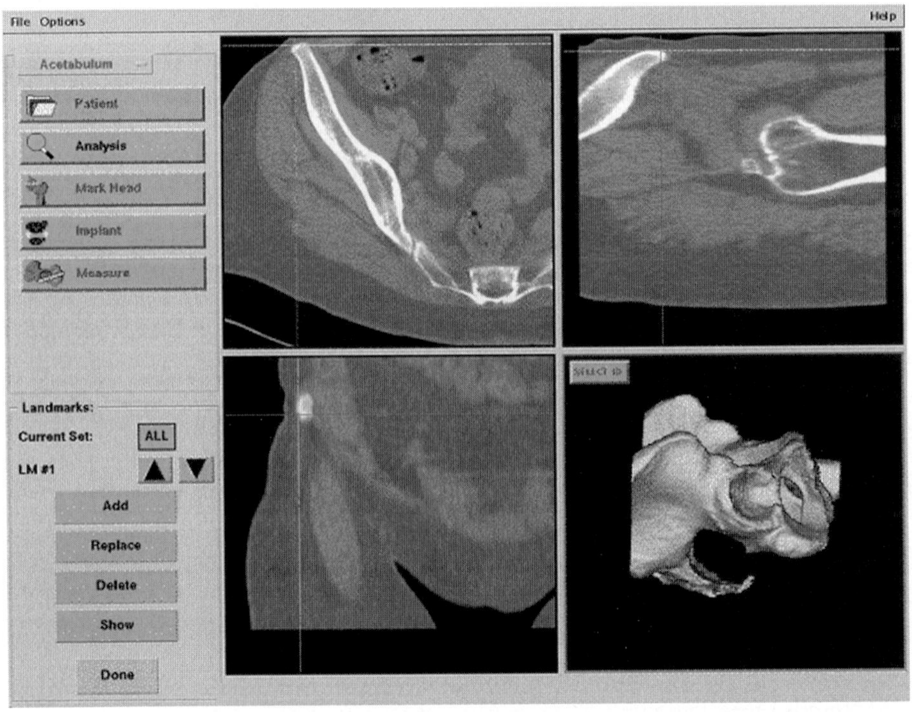

Figure 23.4. Computer screen *analysis* image after acquisition of the computed tomography study, noting position of the ipsilateral anterior superior iliac spine for registration. The point is shown with sagittal, axial and frontal plane views with a composite three-dimensional model of the pelvis.

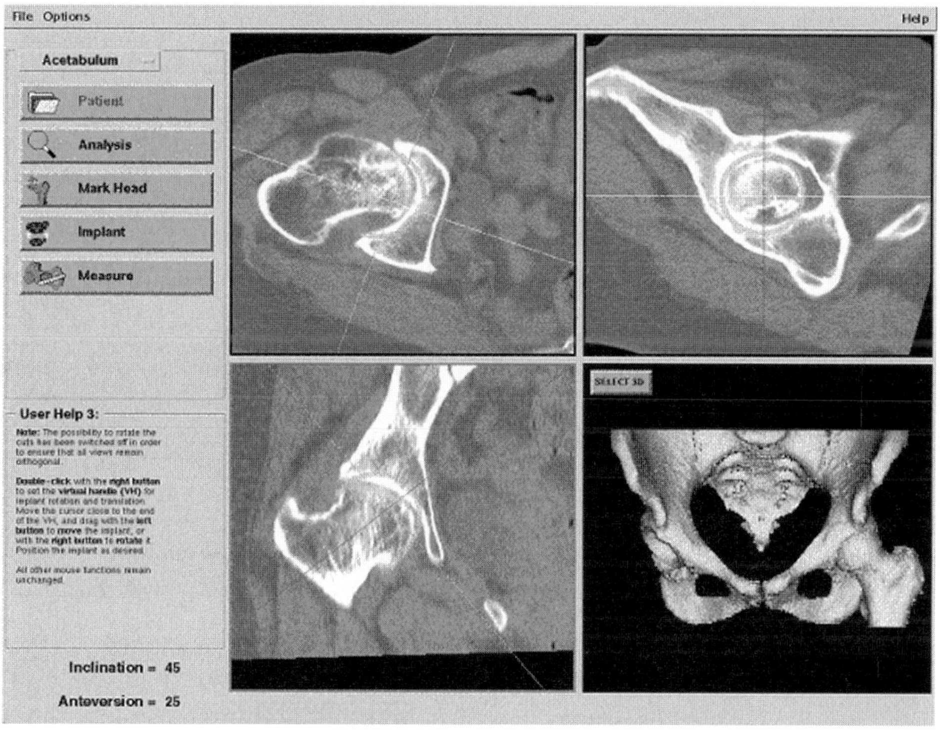

Figure 23.5. In this preoperative planning step, the cup implant in size, design and position is added to the three-dimensional model of the pelvic bone. The position is defined by the anteversion (25 degrees), the inclination (45 degrees) and the depth of the implant.

ability in this planning step to deepen or to make medial the cup position and preferentially position the cup more anteriorly or posteriorly. Final cup position was demonstrated in three planes and also on the three dimensional pelvic model which had the femoral head extracted (see Figure 23.4).

The intraoperative computer-assisted navigation system consisted of an infrared camera (Optotrak 3020, Northern Digital, Waterloo, Canada) on an overhead boom and the Surgigate system including the video with monitor, and Unix Ultra 10 workstation with appropriate Surgigate software. The conventional instruments for the implantation of hip endoprosthes was equipped with infrared transducers or light emitting diodes. With these optoelectronic markers, the position of all instruments was tracked in space by the optical camera and transmitted to the computer system. A special pointer was used to indicate landmarks defined in the preoperative planning phase and now used for referencing those points in the patient's acetabulum. The pointer was also used to initiate certain computer functions by activating or tapping designated areas on a virtual keyboard. In addition a dynamic reference base, an instrument equipped with infrared transducers, was securely fastened to the pelvic skeleton of the patient. This was done by using a Steinmann pin attached approximately 2 cm cranial of the acetabular rim or alternatively, fixed to the anterior superior iliac spine depending on the surgical exposure. Fixation of the DRB must be absolutely rigid as this reference allows the computer system to track the patient's movements on the operating table.

The intraoperative navigation can be divided in two major steps, registration and surgical implantation. First, the instruments and the reference base need to be checked for positional error, which is typically less than 0.5 mm. Following this step, pair point matching was done, which identifies and registers the same landmarks as determined during the preoperative planning phase. Subsequently, surface matching was done, in which a cloud of points consisting of at least 12 separate points were placed on the pelvis of the patient. Preferred areas were the anterior superior iliac spines, acetabular dome, and lateral ilium surrounding the lip of the acetabulum. With this registration process, the Surgigate software attempted to find a best fit between the demonstrated points and the 3D pelvic model generated in the preoperative planning phase. The computer then generated a quality index, which defined the precision of which the patient's pelvis could be matched to that of the virtual pelvis. The manufacturer of the system required a maximum quality index value of 10 after the pair point matching and 2 after the surface point matching. The final step in registration was a verification step during which the software sought the best solution to "align virtual and actual pelvis." The surgeon identified a known point on the pelvis and this point must precisely match the point identified on the virtual pelvic model.

At this point, the surgeon was then capable of navigating both the milling process and the subsequent cup implantation. Both of the instruments used for this process, including the reamer and the cup inserter, were instrumented with a LED, which allowed for precise positioning in the acetabulum. The surgeon used visual cues and numerical positional data displayed on the computer screen to determine the exact reamer and cup position compared with the preoperative planning position. For all patients with acetabular navigation in this study, we recorded the final cup position as indicated on the screen at the conclusion of the procedure (Figure 23.6).

Postoperative Assessment Using CT Computer Analysis

Analysis of all postoperative computed tomography studies was done using the Surgigate Data Analysis software module (Medivision, Oberdorf, Switzerland; now Praxim, Grenoble, France), which allowed for accurate interpretation of implanted acetabular components. Computer hardware used was an Ultra 10 Sun Microsystems workstation (Sun Microsystems, Schwerzenbach, Switzerland). This was a multistep process requiring each CT scan to be loaded into a Surgigate software module. The computer then created a three-dimensional model of the pelvis. From this model the frontal plane was defined by touch pointing the appropriate landmarks, which include the bilateral anterior superior iliac spines and the bilateral pubic tubercles as noted previously. This then defined the reference base of subsequent

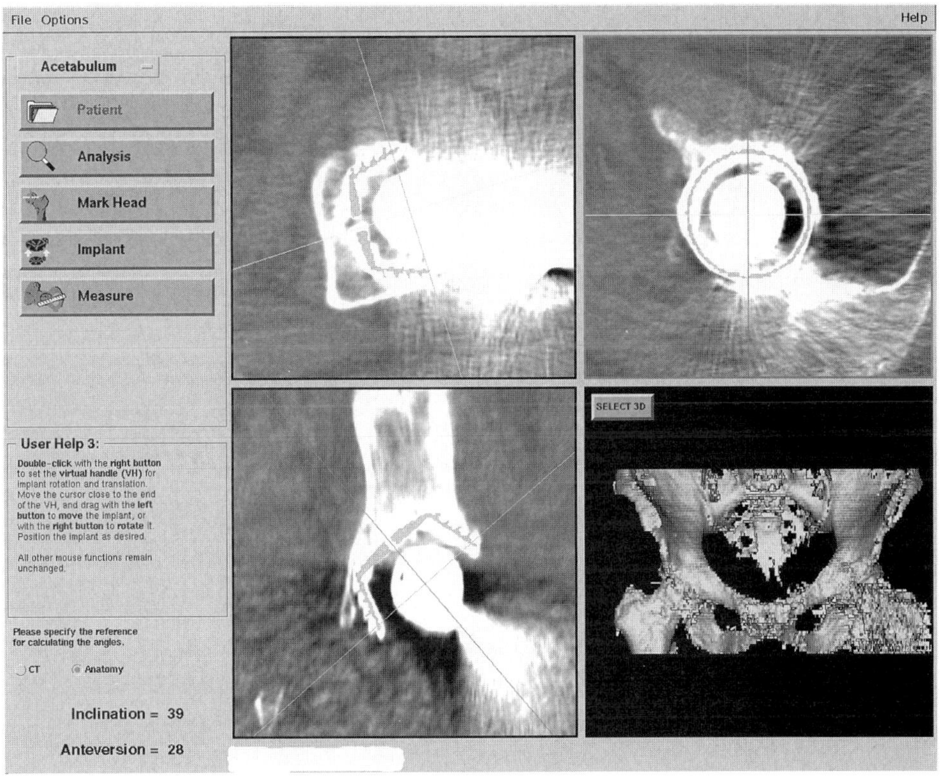

Figure 23.6. Computer screen view demonstrates three postoperative views through the center of the acetabulum from the computed tomographs including the sagittal, axial and frontal views followed by a three-dimensional model of the pelvis. Note the calculated acetabular inclination of 39 degrees and anteversion of 28 degrees.

measurements of acetabular component position. The scans demonstrating the implanted cups were brought into view using the computer touch screen. Using a library of Computer Aided Design models of each specific acetabular component, the appropriately sized and positioned virtual images were then overlaid to the implanted devices (Figure 23.6). After DiGioia et al., operative acetabular abduction and anteversion was described for each implanted device. Specifically, the acetabular abduction was defined as the angle between the projection of the opening plane of the cup in the coronal plane and the sagittal plane; and the anteversion angle was defined as the angle between the projection of the opening plane of the cup in the frontal plane and the sagittal plane.[13,14]

Clinical Experience with CT Navigation

A control group of 69 patients underwent computed tomography for preoperative planning for surgical navigation of the contralateral total hip replacement following a previously placed conventional total hip replacement.[15] Each CT scan was taken through the pelvis with three millimeter slices using a digital format. The cohort of the conventional implanted group was aged 63.4 years (46.5 to 76.8 years). There were 43 women and 26 men. There have been implanted 41 press-fit cups and 28 screw in cups. All patients had reached at least 12 months follow-up at the time radiographic study. Acetabular implant position was assessed in the conventionally placed implants in this group. A second group of 98 patients underwent total hip replacement using the computer assisted navigation system where the acetabular component had been inserted using computer guided indices. In the computer-assisted cup implantation cohort we found an average age of 66.9 years (42.4 to 81.0 years). There have been operated 63 women and 35 men. The implanted prostheses included 64 screw in cups, 26 press-fit cups and 8 cemented cups. The primary diagnosis was osteoarthritis in 86% of cases with the remaining being other including inflammatory arthritis and dysplasia.

From analysis of the posterative computed tomography scans, the average acetabular abduction for computer navigation, was 43.03° (Std Dev. 4.59; 95% CI- 0.97; Range- 30° to 58°); and for acetabular anteversion the average was 22.22° (Std Dev. 7.39; 95% CI- 1.72; Range- 5° to 38°). For the freehand group, the average acetabular abduction was 45.74° (Std Dev. 9.09; 95% CI- 2.63°; Range 26° to 64°). The average acetabular anteversion was 28.51° (Std Dev. 10.25; 95% CI- 3.80°; Range 9° to 53°). The average last saved Surgigate computer navigated acetabular abduction was 43.1° (95% CI- 0.87°; Range 42.22° to 43.98°) and the acetabular anteversion was 22.4° (95% CI- 1.48°; Range 20.94° to 23.92°). Using the F test for comparing the difference in the amount of variation between the two surgical methods, the ratio was 5.56 for abduction ($p < .0001$) and 3.67 for anteversion ($p < .0001$), indicating that the variation could not be attributed to chance for either variable and that computer navigation is significantly more accurate than freehand conventional methods. The F ratio for the last Surgigate computer navigated acetabular abduction position compared to the CT control was 0.30 and that for acetabular anteversion was 1.55, not reaching statistical significance.

Comparing both groups with the anteversion "safe zone" described by Fontes et al., we found that 28% of the freehand cups were placed outside of 11° to 35° anteversion; 4.7% were placed with less than 11 degrees of anteversion and 23.4% have been implanted with an anteversion exceeding 35 degrees. In the computer navigated group, 7% were outside the parameters of 11 degrees to 35 degrees anteversion; there were 4.7% of the cups implanted with less anteversion than 11 degrees and 2.5% exceeded 35 degrees of anteversion.

Fluoroscopic Computer Assisted Navigation

The use of fluoroscopy has been a more recent evolution of CAOS and represents the diversification of other methods used in neurosurgery and ear-nose-throat applications.[16,17] As mentioned previously the technique requires accurate referencing of the fluoroscopic grid, which transfers the images to the computer for point matching and subsequent navigation. I have gained experience with fluoroscopic navigation using the Stealth Universal Hip Application (Medtronic ST, Denver, CO) and describe its use in both the acetabulum and the femur.

Technique of Acetabular Navigation

Fluoroscopic navigation of the pelvis requires that an unobstructed image be acquired in two different planes. This means that the camera must see both the DRB and the grid of the C-arm during the image acquisition. I have used the Jackson operative imaging table for this purpose, which allows the patient to be placed in either the supine or lateral decubitus position. Once the grid has been acquired by the computer, the following images must be acquired for cup navigation: (1) contralateral anterior superior iliac spine in two views; (2) affected acetabulum in two views; (3) pubic tubercle in two views. I have found several modifications helpful for obtaining the contralateral anterior superior iliac spine images, which may be the "downside" with the lateral decubitus minimally invasive lateral approach. First, a simple clamp wrapped in foam tape for insulation may be placed directly adjacent to the ASIS by palpation. The patient is then prepped and draped, and a DRB is applied to the anterolateral wing of the ilium (Figure 23.7).

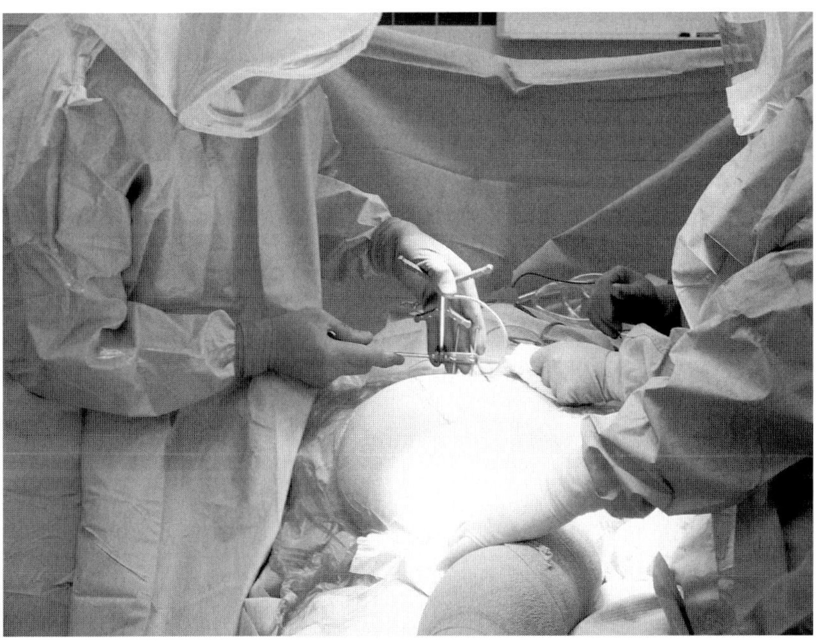

Figure 23.7. Active dynamic reference base (DRB) is placed on a pin pod attached to the superior iliac crest and facing the camera system at the head of the operating table.

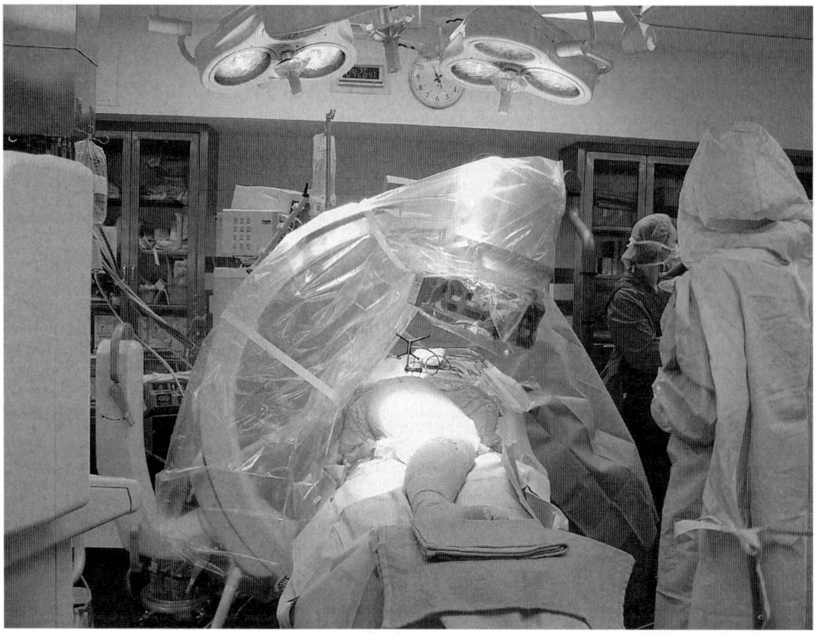

Figure 23.8. Imaging the downside anterior superior iliac spine by tilting the C-arm about 20 degrees oblique to the vertical to bring the ASIS into relief.

The fluoroscope C-arm is then brought over the area, and tilted 15 degrees to 20 degrees oblique to the frontal plane (Figure 23.8). This brings the ASIS into relief compared to the remaining pelvis and with the marker, allows easy identification of the outline of the pelvic ilium, even in obese patients where abdominal contents overlie the image (Figure 23.9). With the C-arm at the same tilt, the affected cup can then be imaged in the oblique view, and the presence of the pins from the DRB in the superior corner confirm the correct side. The image may be moved parallel to the frontal reference plane and the pubic tubercle lateral may be obtained (Figures 23.10 and 23.11). This structure is a bit inferior to the acetabulum and is roughly on a transverse line just above the lesser trochanter and below the infra-cotyloid tubercle. It will be anterior to the acetabulum by roughly 5 cm. The next structure is the anterior-posterior view of the pubic tubercle, which is very easily defined by fluoroscopy. In the lateral decubitus position, the C-arm is parallel to the floor (Figures 23.12 and 23.13). The C-arm is tilted 15 degrees to 20 degrees oblique to the floor and the final images are made, which is the anterior-posterior affected cup view and the anterior-posterior ASIS view (Figure 23.14). Again, the foam-covered clamp enables finding the later structure. The affected side ASIS may be acquired by touch-pointing the anatomical structure in the field.

Referencing the fluoroscopic images that have been acquired is done by touching or mouse pointing the appropriate anatomic structures on the computer screen. This includes the center of the acetabulum or

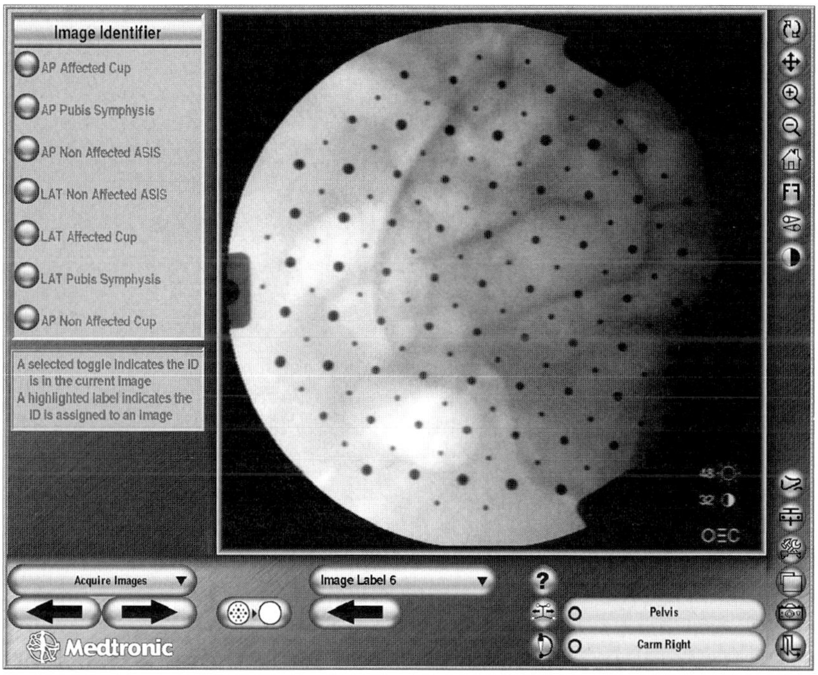

Figure 23.9. Acquired image of the downside anterior superior iliac spine.

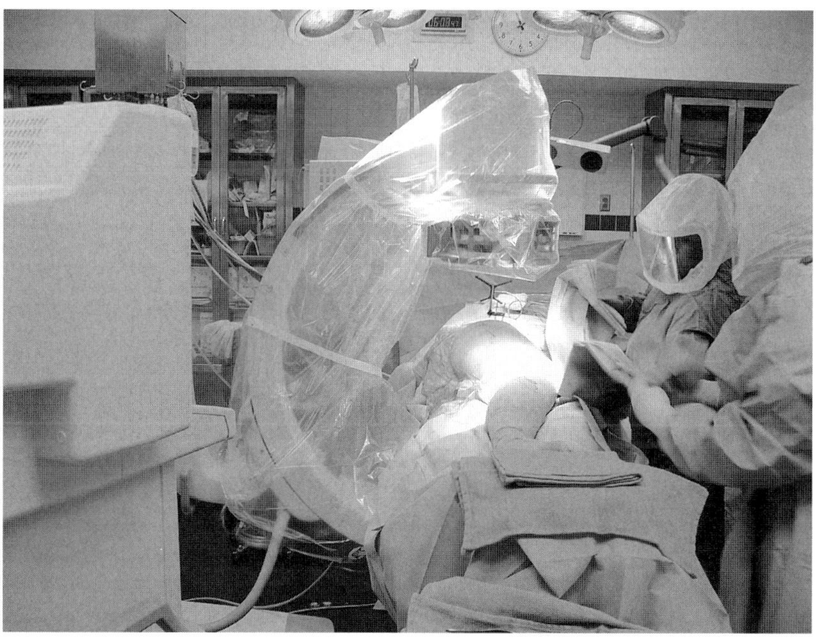

Figure 23.10. Imaging the pubic tubercle from the lateral view of the pelvis with the C-arm vertical to the floor.

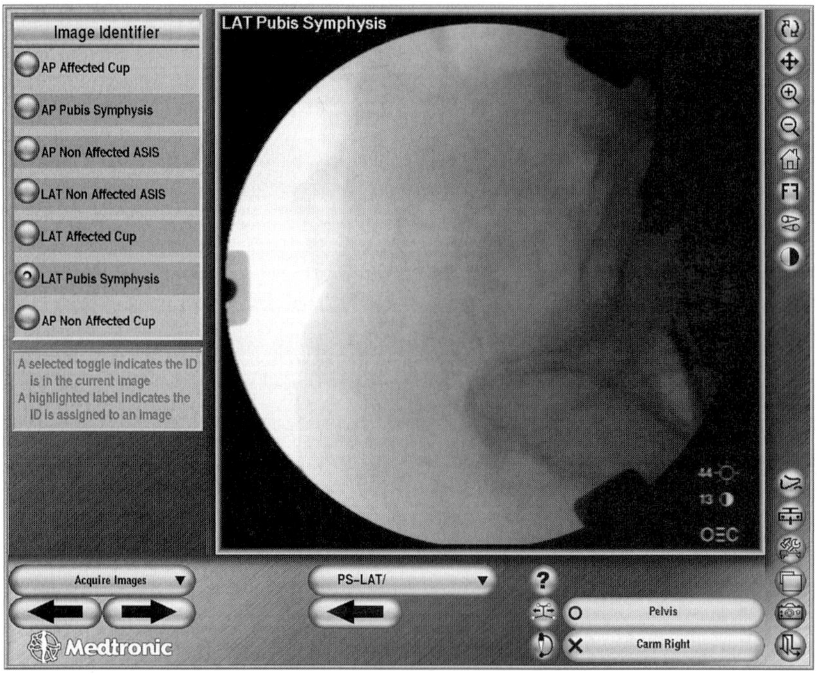

Figure 23.11. Acquired image of the pubic tubercle lateral view.

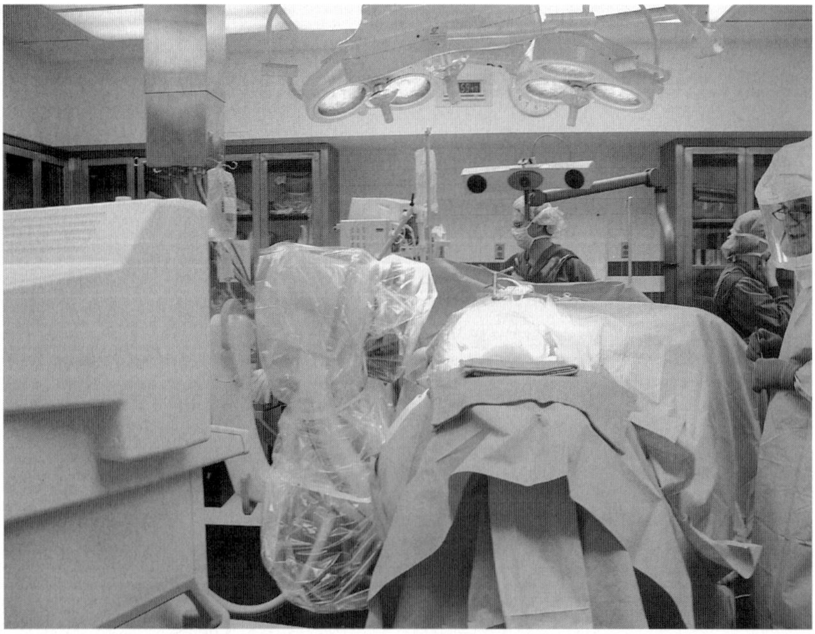

Figure 23.12. Imaging the anterior posterior view of the downside anterior superior iliac spine and the frontal view of the pubic tubercle.

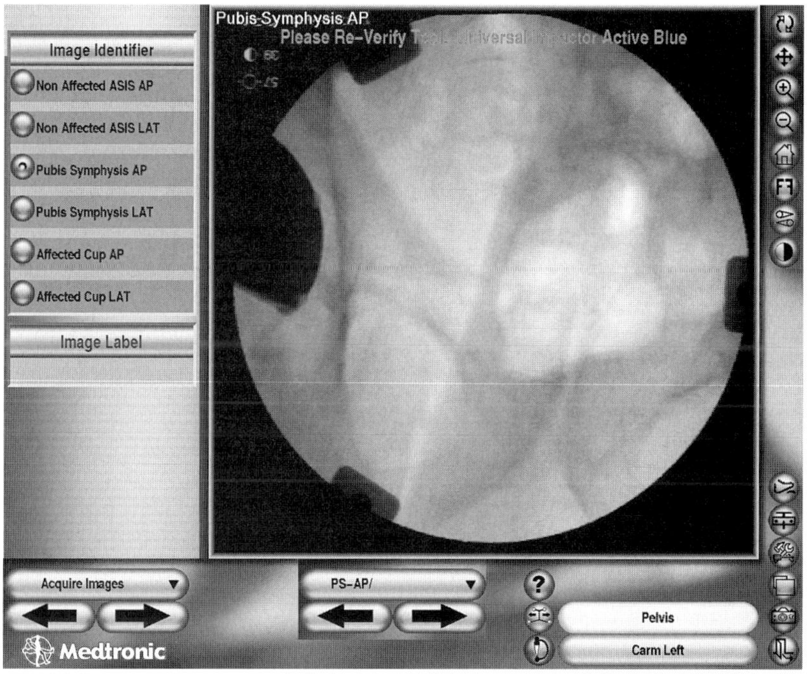

Figure 23.13. Acquired image of the pubic tubercle on the anterior posterior view.

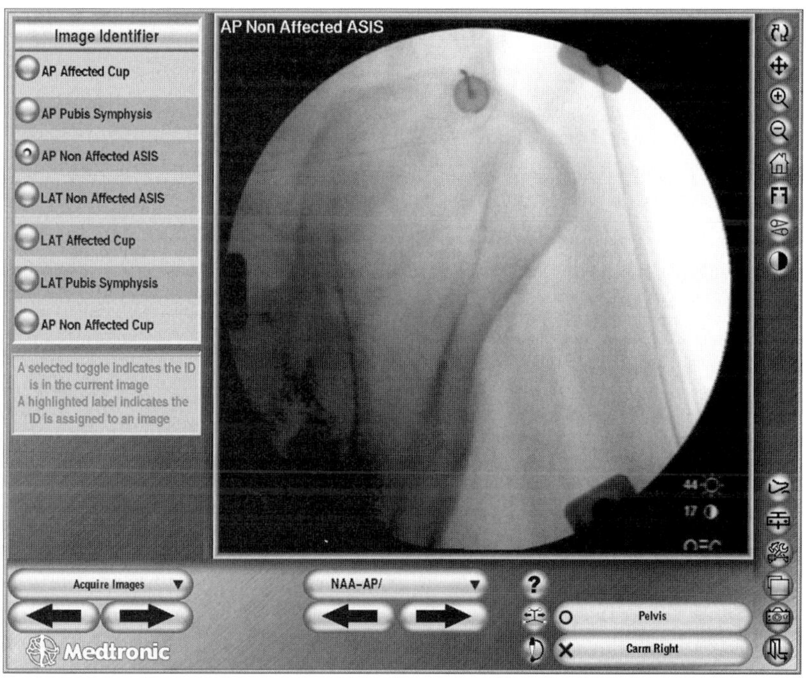

Figure 23.14. Acquired image of the downside anterior superior iliac spine on the anterior posterior view.

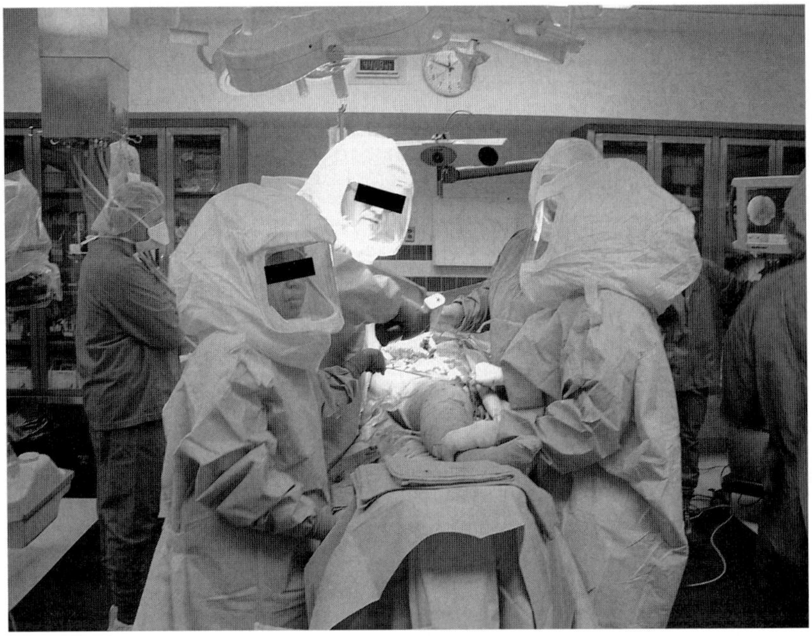

Figure 23.15. Reaming the acetabulum with an active DRB mounted to the reamer. Note camera system at the head of the table and computer screen in upper right-hand corner.

femoral head, pubic tubercle and the contralateral side ASIS. One interesting point is that the easily identified reference points such as the downside lateral ASIS and anterior-posterior pubic tubercle provide a reference line on the other associated view for which the same structure must exist. Thus, the anterior-posterior downside ASIS position, which is difficult to interpret can be more easily identified. For the Stealth system, a final check is to determine if all the reference lines match appropriately with the axes of the extremity.

When referencing is completed the final step before actual navigation is to reference the DRBs attached to the reamers and the cup impactor (Figure 23.15). Navigation then proceeds with the appropriate steps in the operative procedure. As noted previously, the optimal position determined for cup positioning is 45-degree abduction and 20-degree anteversion. The reamer and cup inserter are instrumented with an appropriate DRB. Both reaming and final cup insertion can be virtually observed on the computer, and the operator can carefully match the instruments with the screen calibration targets and numbers (Figures 23.16 and 23.17). I have found the cup insertion usually parallels my "experience" with this effort, but surprisingly little motion of the insertion handle can make a big difference. Postoperative radiographs are difficult to interpret as the frontal pelvic reference frame is not always appropriately positioned.

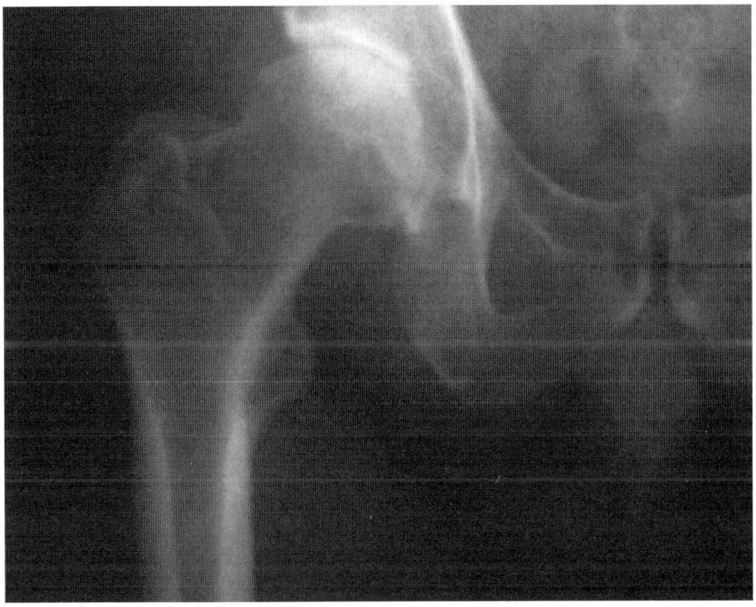

Figure 23.16. Anterior posterior of the affected hip.

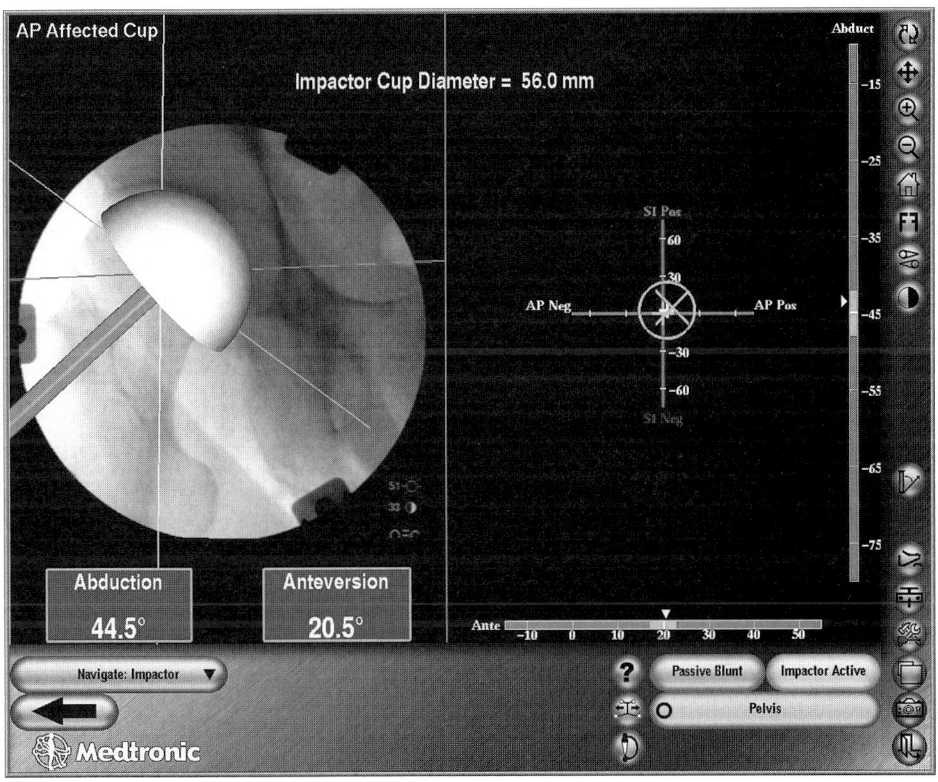

Figure 23.17. Final cup position documented on the computer, with a 56-mm cup inserted at 44-degree abduction and 20-degree anteversion.

Discussion

Acetabular component placement in total hip arthroplasty can be difficult with optimal placement required to prevent chronic instability, exaggerated wear, and implant migration. Recent investigators have sought to define the radiographic analysis of cup position in the clinical setting, prosthetic issues such as range of motion and component impingement, and technical issues at the time of surgery such as body position and how to place the prosthesis in the desired location. Computer-assisted navigation represents a new technology that can be used to deal with all of these problems.[18–24]

The spatial orientation of the natural acetabulum and prosthetic components placed at surgery is a complex three-dimensional problem and most authors have attempted to describe a two-dimensional radiographic answer. Murray has provided the most complete insight into this problem by defining geometrically exactly what these solutions represent (Figure 23.18). For simple comparison, the acetabular abduction is defined as the angle formed to the tranverse plane of the patient when the superior cup is tilted toward the longitudinal axis of the patient, or in the anatomical specimen a line drawn from the superior lip down to the inferior cotyloid notch on the anterior posterior radiograph. The more complex issue is how to determine the acetabular anteversion or flexion, and three possibilities are possible based on how the cup is measured. Operative anteversion occurs when the acetabular component is flexed in the coronal plane of the patient, essentially rotating about a line through the acetabulum, which is perpendicular to the longitudinal axis of the patient. This is the maneuver accom-

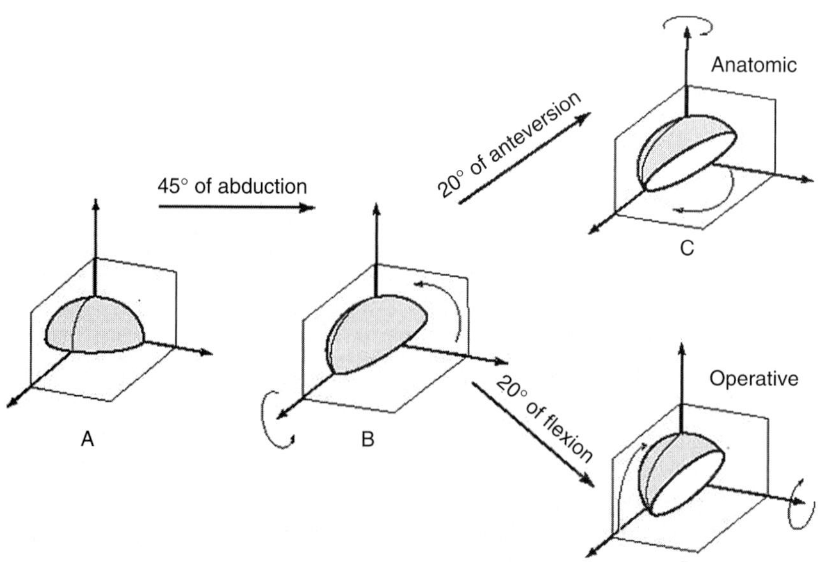

Figure 23.18. Concept of acetabular abduction and anteversion with the various measurement possibilities. (From DiGioia AM, Jamaraz B, Nikou C, et al.,[14] by permission of Operative Techniques in Orthopaedics.)

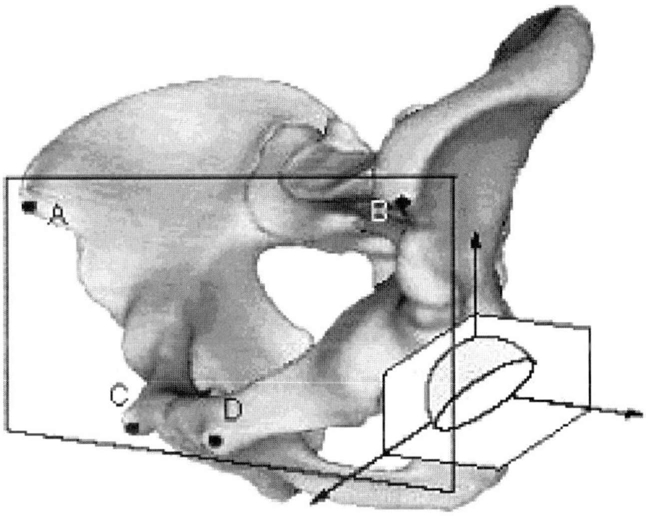

Figure 23.19. Frontal pelvic reference frame marking the anterior superior iliac spine and the pubic promontory. (From DiGioia AM, Jamaraz B, Nikou C, et al.,[14] by permission of Operative Techniques in Orthopaedics.)

plished by most freehand surgical guides and is the planar measurement made by determining the angulation of the cup in the frontal plane compared to the sagittal plane by looking at the coronal section CT scan. Radiographic anteversion occurs when the anterior cup lip is rotated superiorly around the oblique transverse axis of the acetabulum, which lies in the coronal plane of the patient. This measurement was typically used on cemented cups of known dimension that had wire radio-opaque markers. Anatomical anteversion is the position that occurs when the abducted acetabulum position is internally rotated around the longitudinal axis of the patient. This measurement has been used to assess acetabular anatomical position in dysplasia. Murray has concluded that the operative anteversion is the most practical and should be used to describe cup position in total hip arthroplasty.[25] For the computer application, DiGioia et al. have concluded that the operative acetabular abduction and anteversion measurements are the most straightforward reducing the conclusions to strict planar two-dimensional terms.[13,14] We used this method for our abduction and anteversion measurements and have found no other variations in recent publications concerning computer navigation.

Lewinnek et al. were first to describe the concept of the anterior pelvic plane, which is defined as a coronal slice passing through bilateral anterior superior iliac spines and the bilateral anterior pubic tubercles[9] (Figure 23.19). In the normal standing position, this plane is usually parallel to the longitudinal axis of the patient. McCollum et al. have shown that this plane may be altered, especially if patients are placed in the lateral decubitus position, or there is hip flexion reducing the normal lumbar lordosis[12] (Figure 23.20). Lewinnek et al. employed a crude device with three legs and a bubble level applied to the pelvic crests and pubis to make certain that the pelvic plane was

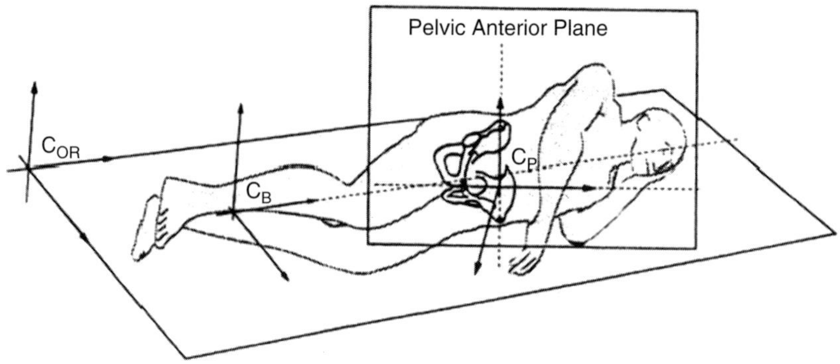

Figure 23.20. Intraoperative tilting of the pelvic reference frame from positioning factors caused at the time of surgery. (From McCollum DE, Gray WJ,[12] by permission of Clin Orthop.)

parallel to the plane of the table prior to taking their anterior posterior radiographs of the pelvis for anteversion measurement[9] (Figure 23.21). An important step in the registration procedure for computer-assisted navigation is to define the anterior pelvic plane using the same references generating a standardized pelvic position.

Numerous investigators have questioned the accuracy of standard radiographic methods for measuring cup position. For radiographic views, the x-ray beam must be carefully directed in a standardized fashion centered over the pelvis and the pelvis must be level with the beam perpendicular to the pelvic frontal plane in each case. However, Ackland et al. stated that an error of as much as 5 degrees could be introduced if the x-ray was centered over the symphysis pubis and not

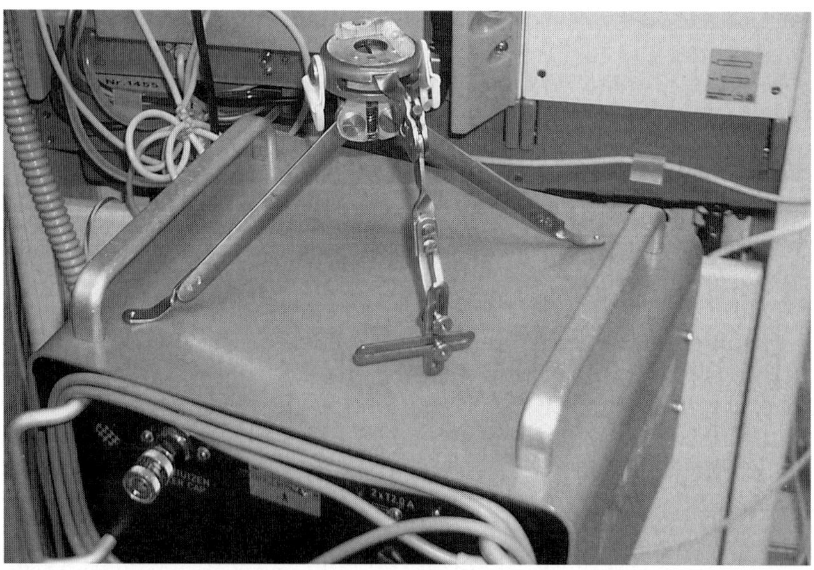

Figure 23.21. Tripod used to establish the pelvic reference frame parallel to the table for a patient undergoing radiography in the supine position.

the hip joint itself.[26] Pelvic rotation certainly is an important consideration, and Thorén et al. demonstrated a 2.5-degree alteration of cup anteversion for 5 degrees of pelvic rotation.[27] Herrlin et al. found that 5 degrees of pelvic flexion or extension could introduce a maxiumum error of 8 degrees in acetabular anteversion.[28] Computed tomography assessments done with computer navigation, on the other hand, have been described as the gold standard for measuring cup abduction and anteversion with an accuracy of about 1 degree to 2 degrees, based on current methodologies.

Optimal acetabular component orientation has been a subject of much debate, but most recent investigations conclude that the approximate position of 45-degree abduction or inclination and 20-degree radiographic anteversion is the ideal target. Obviously, retrospective studies such as those of Lewinnek et al. and Fontes et al. define a "safe" envelope or range about which hip stability after arthroplasty is much greater.[9,29] However, Barrack et al. have used a complex three-dimensional computer analysis to refine the optimization to the above parameters and have shown that certain positions such as cup abduction below 25 degrees or cup anteversion below 0 degrees are clearly unsatisfactory for positions such as sitting or stooping.[10] Acetabular stability and impingement relates not only to component position but also to prosthetic design dimensions and related femoral stem positioning. The average cup position after navigation in our study was acetabular inclination of 43 degrees and cup anteversion of 22 degrees, closely approximating the best position in the majority of cases.

DeGioia et al. used a computer-assisted navigation system similar to the method we used to study the problems of mechanical alignment in the conventional operative setting with the lateral decubitus position and with the use of typical freehand alignment guides.[30] They found that the mean pelvic position was close to the desired anterior pelvic plane prior to dislocation, but after dislocation, the pelvis tilted anteriorly causing a shift of the mean anteversion of the pelvis to 18 degrees. Of 74 cups, 58 were placed outside the desired anteversion of 20° +/− 10° while only one cup was outside of the desired abduction of 45° +/− 10°. In another study, they were able to determine that postoperative radiographs produced variable and inaccurate results compared to their precise intraoperative computer generated measurements.

The use of computer-assisted navigation will be an important asset for surgeons attempting to improve total hip implant insertion. This will be especially true for minimally invasive approaches, which offer a great challenge if the typical landmarks are obscured. The computer offers a virtual image of the pelvis and femur, which is then used for accurate placement of the implants. The current accuracy of most computer navigation systems is within 1 mm or degree. That being said, the true accuracy relates more to the skill of the surgeon in carefully identifying the appropriate landmarks and carefully inserting a stable DRB. A stacking or magnification of errors may occur if simple mistakes are made at several steps. For that reason, both system validation and observer validation is important to maintain system reliability. I presented a recent study where computed tomography was used for reference image acquisition. Interestingly, neither the company developing the system for that study, Medivision, nor the CT technique utilized are currently being sold. I currently favor the use of fluoroscopic referencing using the Medronic ST Stealth station, as the referencing can be done in real time and in a few minutes. Studies are currently in process to validate the clinical in vivo results. In conclusion, recent studies have proven the efficacy of the surgical technique at least to accomplish given surgical goals. Clinical validation and efficacy will require ongoing studies.

References

1. Knolte LP, Langlotz F. Basics of Computer-Assisted Orthopaedic Surgery (CAOS). In: Stiehl JB, Konermann WH, Haaker RG, eds. Navigations and Robotics in Total Joint and Spinal Surgery. New York: Springer-Verlag; 2003.
2. Bargar WL, Bauer A, Bomer M. Primary and revision total hip replacement using ROBODOC. Clin Orthop. 1998;354:82–81.
3. Bargar WL. Robotic surgery and current development with the ROBODOC system. In: Stiehl JB, Konermann WH, Haaker RG. Navigations and Robotics in Total Joint and Spinal Surgery. New York: Springer-Verlag; 2003.
4. Weise M, Schmidt K, Willburger RE. Clinical experience with CT-based Vectorvision system. In: Stiehl JB, Konermann WH, Haaker RG. Navigations and Robotics in Total Joint and Spinal Surgery. New York: Springer-Verlag; 2003.
5. Hagena FW, Kettrukat M, Christ RM, Hackbart M. Fluoroscopy-based navigation in Genesis II total knee arthroplasty with the Medtronic "Viking" system. In: Stiehl JB, Konermann WH, Haaker RG. Navigations and Robotics in Total Joint and Spinal Surgery. New York: Springer-Verlag; 2003.
6. Giurea A, Zehetgruber H, Funovics P, Grampp S, Karamat L, Gottsauner-Wolf F. Risk factors for dislocation in cementless hip arthroplasty—a statistical analysis. Z Orthop. 2001;139:194–199.
7. Kennedy JG, Rogers WB, Soffe KE, Sullivan RJ, Griffen DG, Sheehan LJ. Effect of acetabular component orientation on recurrent dislocation, pelvic osteolysis, polyethylene wear and component migration. J Arthroplasty. 1998;13:530–534.
8. Bader RJ, Steinhauser E, Willmann G, Gradinger R. The effects of implant position, design, and wear on the range of motion after total hip arthroplasty. Hip International. 2001;11:80–90.
9. Lewinnek GE, Lewis JL, Tarr R, Compere CL, Zimmermann JR. Dislocations after total hip replacement arthroplasties. J Bone Joint Surg Am. 1978; 60:217–221.
10. Barrack RL, Lavernia C, Ries M, Thornberry R, Tozakoglou E. Virtual reality computer animation of the effect of component position and design on stability after total hip arthroplasty. Orthopaedic Clinics NA. 2001; 32:569–577.
11. Seki M, Yuasa N, Ohkuni K. Analysis of optimal range of socket orientations in total hip arthroplasty with use of computer-aided design simulation. J Orthop. Res. 1998;16:513–517.
12. McCollum DE, Gray WJ. Dislocation after total hip replacement. Clin Orthop. 1990;159–170.

13. DiGioia AM, Jamaraz B, Blackwell M, et al. Image guided navigation system to measure intraoperatively acetabular implant alignment. Clin Orthop. 1998;354:8–22.
14. Di Gioia AM, Jamaraz B, Nikou C, LaBarca RS, Moody JE, Colgan S. Surgical Navigation for total hip replacement with the use of HipNav. Operative Techniques in Orthopaedics. 2000;10:3–8.
15. Haaker R, Tiedjen K, Ottersbach A, Stiehl JB, Rubenthaler F, Shockheim M. Comparison of Freehand Versus Computer Assisted Acetabular Cup Implantation. J Bone and Joint Surg. B Submitted; 2004.
16. Hofstetter R, Slomczykowski M, Bourquin Y, Nolte LP. Fluoroscopy based surgical navigation. In: Lemke HU, Vannier MW, Inamura K, eds. Computer Assisted Radiology and Surgery. Amsterdam: Elsevier Science B.V.; 1997:956–960.
17. Hofstetter R, Slomczykowski M, Sati M, Nolte LP. Fluoroscopy as an imaging means for computer-assisted surgical navigation. Comput Aided Surg. 1999;4:65–76.
18. Hassan DM, Johnston GHF, Dust WNC, Watson G, Dolovich AT. Accuracy of intraoperative assessment of acetabular prosthesis placement. J Arthroplasty. 1998;13:80–84.
19. Bernsmann K, Langlotz U, Ansari B, Wiese M. Computerassistierte navigierte Pfannenplatzierung in der Hüftendoprosthetik—Anwenderstudie im klinischen Routinealltag. Z Orthop. 2000;138:515–521.
20. Bernsmann K, Langlotz U, Ansari B, Wiese M. Computerassistierte navigierte Platzierung von verschiedenen Pfannentypen in der Hüftendoprosthetik—eine randomisierte kontrollierte Studie. Z Orthop. 2001;139: 512–517.
21. Jarmaz B, DiGioia AM, Blackwell M, Nikou C. Computer assisted measurement of cup placement in total hip replacement. Clin Orthop. 1998; 354:70–81.
22. Jolles BM, Genoud P. Accuracy of computer-assisted placement in total hip arthroplasty. International Congress Series. 2001;1230:314–318.
23. Leenders T, Vandervelde D, Nahiew G, Nuyts R. Reduction in variability of acetabular cup abduction using computed assisted surgery: Prospective and randomized study. Computer Aided Surgery. 2002;7:99–106.
24. Mian SW, Truchly G, Pflum FA. Computed tomography measurement of acetabular cup anteversion and retroversion in total hip arthroplasty. Clin Orthop. 1992;276:206–209.
25. Murray DW. The definition and measurement of acetabular orientation. J Bone and Joint Surg. 1993;75B:228–232.
26. Ackland MK, Bourne WB, Uhthoff HK. Anteversion of the acetabular cup. J Bone and Joint Surg. 1986;68B:409–413.
27. Thoren B, Sahlstedt B. Influence of pelvic position on radiographic measurements of the prosthetic acetabular component. Acta Radiol. 1990;31: 133–136.
28. Herrlin K, Pettersson H, Selvik G. Comparison of two- and three-dimensional methods for assessment of orientation of the total hip prosthesis. Acta Radiol. 1998;29:357–361.
29. Fontes D, Benoit J, Lortat-Jacob A, Didry R. Luxation of total hip endoprosthesis. Statistical validation of a modelization of 52 cases. Rev Chir Orthop. 1991;77:163–170.
30. DiGioia AM, Jaramaz B, Plakseychuk AY, et al. Comparison of a mechanical acetabular alignment guide with computer placement of the socket. J Arthroplasty. 2002;17:359–364.

24

Computer-Guided Total Knee Arthroscopy

Alon Wolf, Branislav Jaramaz, Andrew B. Mor, and Anthony DiGioia III

Total knee arthroscopy is a major concern to an increasing number of people. The World Health Organization estimates that several hundred million people already suffer from bone and joint diseases, with dramatic increases expected due to a doubling in the number of people over 50 years of age by 2020. In Europe, by 2010, for the first time there will be more people over 60 years of age than under the age of 20. A study based on the American National Hospital Discharge Survey (1996–1999) predicts that there will be more than 474,000 total knee arthroplasty (TKA) procedures performed in the United States in 2030. This number is expected to increase in tandem with the life expectancy of the population.

Knee arthroplasty has evolved a great deal since the unsuccessful attempt by Verneuil[1] to modify the articular surfaces of the knee by using soft tissues such as pig bladder, nylon, fascia lata, and so forth.[2] This attempt was followed by an attempted resection of the entire knee by Ferguson in 1860,[3] which resulted in better mobility but less stability of the joint. Ninety years later, in 1940, a more modern approach was reported by Campbell,[4] in which a metallic interposition femoral mold was used. Later in 1958,[5] MacIntosh treated painful varus or valgus deformity of the knee by inserting an acrylic tibial plateau prosthesis into the affected side to correct deformity, restore stability, and relieve pain. However, it took about 85 years to introduce one of the first navigational calculations involving bone in 1974 by Schlondorff et al.,[6] and computer-assisted orthopaedic surgery (CAOS) took almost 115 years to come into being. Indeed orthopedic surgery techniques, in general, and total knee arthroplasty, in particular, have dramatically evolved due to the introduction of computer-assisted surgery techniques and the concept of minimally invasive surgery (MIS).

Classifications for Robotics and Computer-Assisted Surgery Systems

Several classifications for robotics and computer-assisted surgery systems have been tentatively documented in the literature: Cinquin,[7,8] Stulberg,[9] Taylor,[10,11] Troccaz,[12] Bainville,[13] and Nolte.[14] Each of these

Table 24.1. Source of information type versus robotic system

Robotics system Source information systems	Passive	Semiactive	Active
3D (CT, MRI)			
2.5 (Fluoro)			
Image-free			

definitions reflects, to some extent, state-of-the-art technologies that were available at the time. In 2000, Picard et al.[15] suggested combining Nolte's and Cinquin's definitions for computer-assisted knee systems to create a wider definition that is applicable to all CAOS systems. According to Cinquin, there are three categories for robotic systems that reflect the involvement of the robotic component in the operational procedure. The three are passive, semiactive, and active robotic systems. According to Nolte, there are three types of information systems used in the planning phase: preoperative image systems, intraoperative image systems, and image-free systems. The combination of the three robotic systems and the information systems creates a two-dimensional 3×3 table in which each cell is a combination of one type of robotic system with one type of information system; together, the two define a complete system (Table 24.1). For example, the cell that is defined by the intersection of an active robotic system with a preoperative image system defines a system that is based on an active robot that operates according to a preoperative plan, such as the ROBODOC system (Integrated Surgical Systems, Davis, CA).[16] With the evolution in operating rooms (operating rooms of the future) and the availability of CT scanners inside those operating rooms, the preoperative planning can now be performed intraoperatively, hence Picard's definition[15] should be updated to make it more general. Therefore, we suggest categorizing by the source of the information systems (i.e., 3D, 2.5D, and image-free). Table 24.1 shows our modified categorization of the robotic systems versus the source of information.

In the following sections, we define and give examples of each of the categories in Table 24.1. We also review the state of the art medical technologies that are available and categorize each of these systems into the appropriate table cell.

Active Robotic System

Active robotic systems perform surgical tasks, such as drilling or milling, without the direct intervention of the surgeon.[17–27] This group in CAOS includes active robots like ROBODOC, CASPAR, PiGalileo, and MBARS. Perhaps one of the most famous active robots to date is ROBODOC, developed by Paul et al.[28,29] The system was originally used for total hip replacement procedures, but was later modified for use in total knee replacement procedures.

Another robot that is used for cutting the tibia during TKA is the CASPAR by Ortho Maquet GmbH and Co.[30] The robot that is being used is a commercial KUKA 361 industrial serial robot. During the operation, two radiographs of the knee are taken, and then the surgeon determines the location and orientation of the tibial cut on these x-rays. Following this, the tibia is clamped in a bone holder and the resection is performed by the robot.

A somewhat different robotic structure is presented by Brandt et al.[31] In their work, the authors present the CRIGOS-system, which is composed of a 6 degrees-of-freedom parallel robotic structure. The robot is attached to a base clamp along the operating table. The researchers use an intraoperative planning procedure that is based on multiple images taken intraoperatively with a conventional C-arm.

Making use of the advantage of parallel robotic structure, a novel medical robotic concept was introduced by Wolf and Shoham et al.[32,33] In this work, the authors introduced a concept of a miniature bone-attached parallel robot. Taking advantage of a parallel robot's attributes such as low weight, high accuracy, and compactness, they developed a miniature, low mass, bone-attached parallel robot specially designed for spinal operations. The miniature robot was attached to the operative vertebrae by mechanical means, and guided by the surgeon, percutaneously, to selected anatomies in the vertebra. The advantages of this concept over other navigation and robotic systems as was stated are: (1) The operation outcome does not depend on the surgeon's precision, because the system actively guides the surgeon in driving a k-wire to preselected anatomies during the operation. (2) There is no need for an external referencing sensor because the robot is directly attached to the operated vertebrae and moves with the vertebrae as one rigid body. (3) The system is compact and does not consume operating room space.

Though the miniature bone-attached parallel robot for spinal operation operated as a semiactive medical robot (see next section), this miniature bone-attached robot concept was implemented by our team for active use in joint arthroplasty operations. We targeted a reconstructive knee procedure that is well suited for our robotic, less invasive surgical approach. Patellofemoral arthroplasty (PFA) is a technically demanding procedure for the surgeon, and due to the freehand nature of the cutting of the femur, can benefit greatly from the increased accuracy and efficiency of a robotic system. PFA is also an example of a less invasive reconstructive procedure aimed at minimizing the trauma to the patient while relieving pain and improving function, a precursor of where TKA is headed. A mockup of a miniature bone-attached robotic system (MBARS) has been built (Figure 24.1), and construction of the first prototype is completed and first experiments are expected to be conducted soon.

MBARS is based on the classic Stewart-Gough 6 degrees-of-freedom robot. As can be seen in Figure 24.2, the robot is attached to the femur by three pins: one pin is placed into the medial epicondyle, one into the lateral epicondyle, and one into the metadiaphyseal region of the femur. A rigid connection of the robot to the operated bone is obtained through these three pins. The robot is equipped with a milling device, which accurately machines the cavity to fit the femoral component in

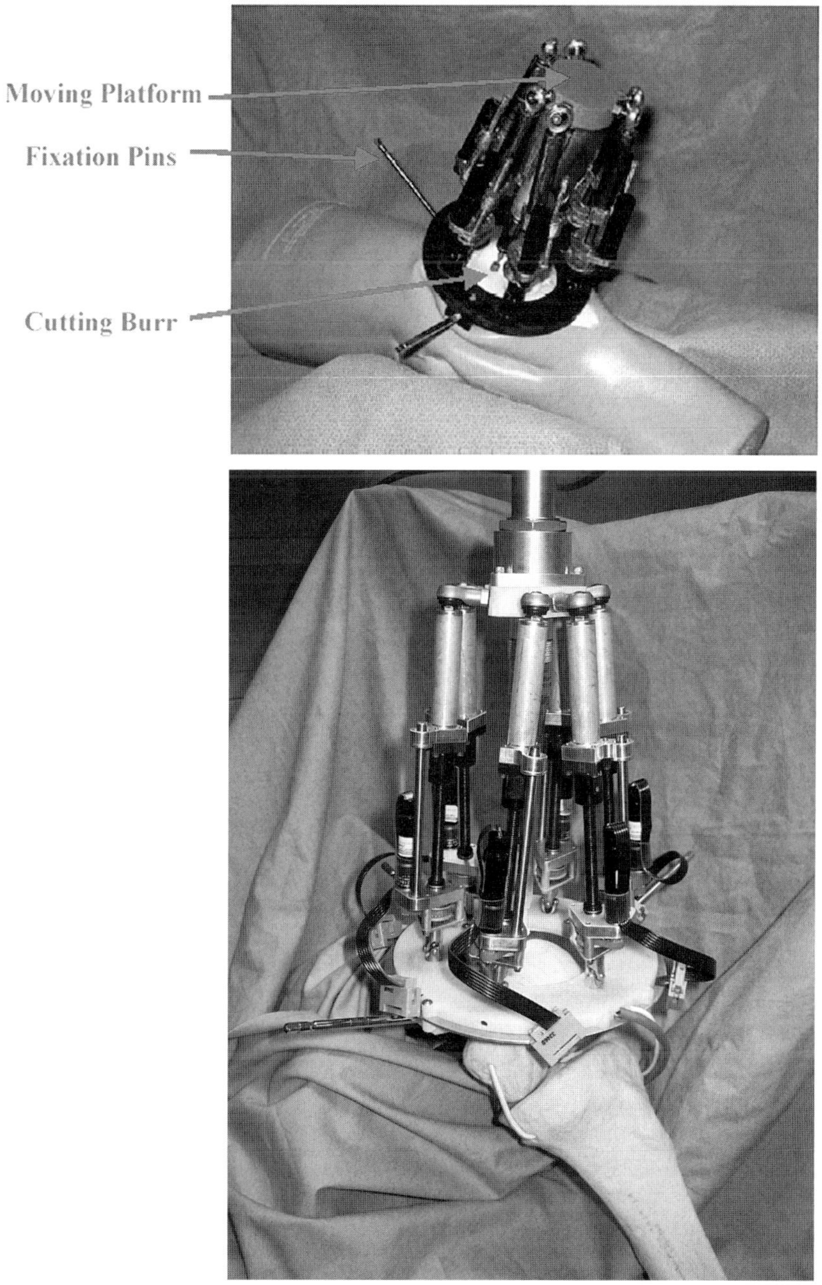

A

B

Figure 24.1. MBARS.

a patellofemoral arthroplasty. It is worth mentioning that MBARS is fully capable of performing other procedures and PFA was chosen to be the first implementation. The planner for MBARS is image-free based, the robot intraoperatively scans the femoral surface to construct the surface model, in its local coordinate system, by using a point probe and a force sensor to detect surface contact (Figure 24.2). The result is

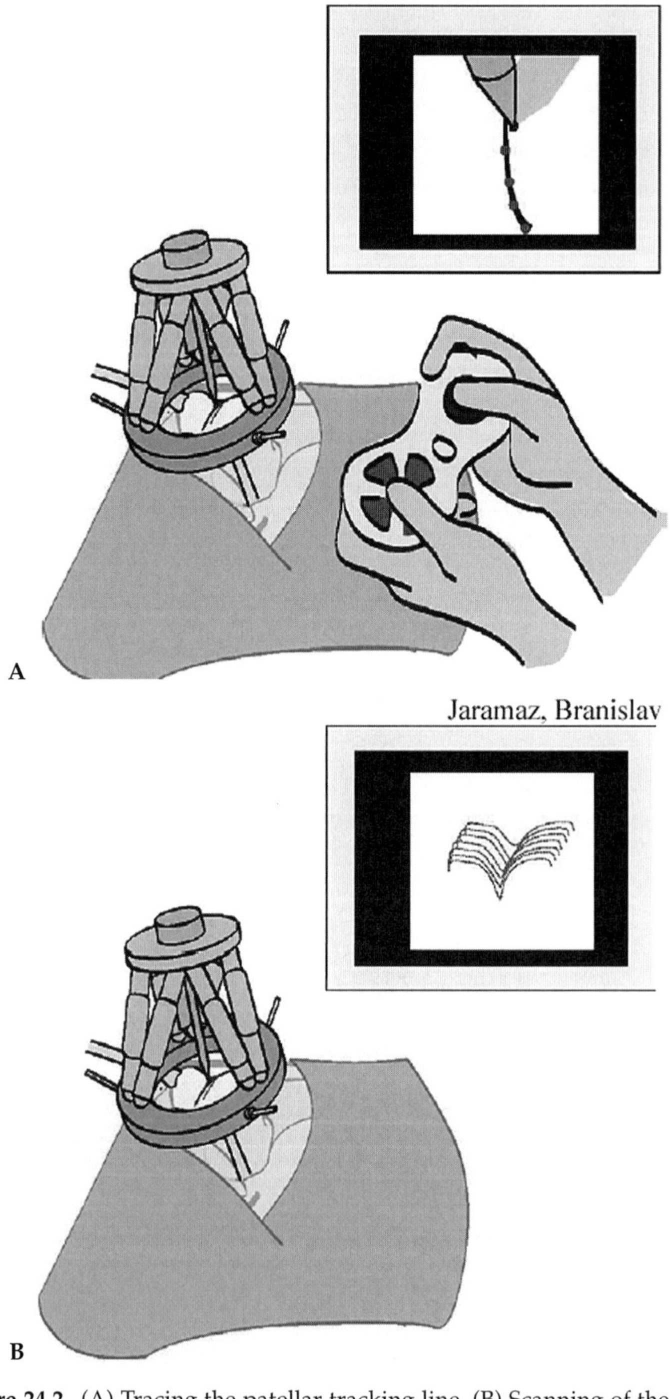

Figure 24.2. (A) Tracing the patellar tracking line. (B) Scanning of the femoral surface to construct the surface model.

a cloud of points given in the robot's fixed coordinate system that are later used for intraoperative planning of implant placement.

Semiactive Robotic System

The defining feature of semiactive robotic systems is that they do not perform any autonomous active acts on the patient's anatomy. Their main purpose is to guide or increase the surgeon's control and accuracy of the operating tool. Such a system may, for example, guide cutting jigs to the correct location during TKA,[34] act to enforce constraints by restricting a task within a pre-determined envelope,[8,34,35] mimic a surgeon's hand motions (telesurgery), or scale and filter hand motion during surgery. The main difference between the semiactive robotic group and the active one is that the control is shared between the robotic tool and the surgeon throughout the operating procedure.

Acrobot (The Acrobot Company, London)[36] is an example of a semiactive robotic system (Figure 24.3). Developed by Davies et al.,[37–41] its core proprietary technology centers on the development of a new type

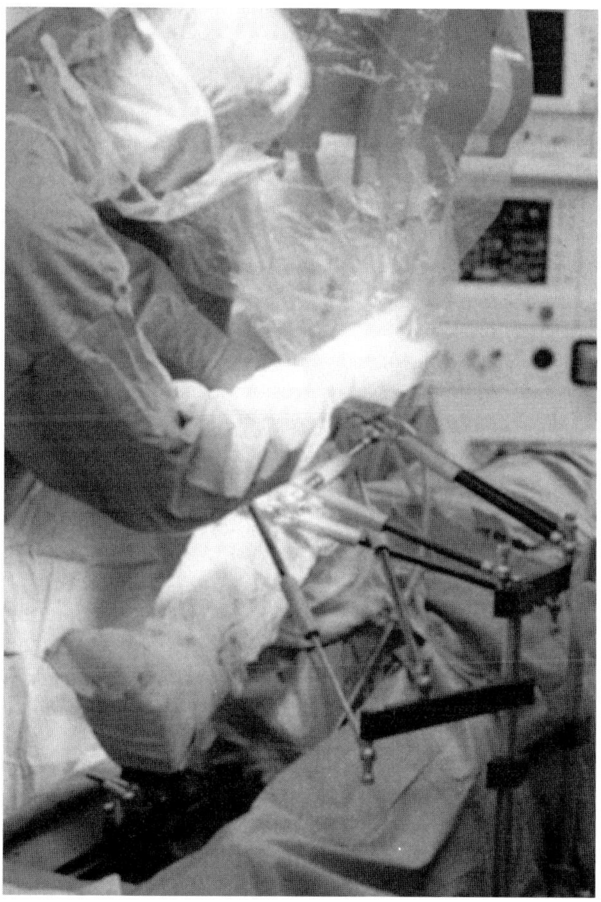

Figure 24.3. Acrobot.

of robotic control: Active Constraint Robotics for orthopedic surgery. This concept facilitates a synergy between the surgeon and the robot, actively assisting the surgeon and helping to prevent surgical error. The surgeon remains in control throughout the procedure, guiding the robot by a handle with a force sensor attached to the robot tip, and thus uses his or her superior human senses and understanding of the overall situation to perform the surgery. The robot provides precise geometric accuracy and increases safety by means of a predefined 3D motion constraint that prevents cutting outside a predefined safe region. This approach, Hands On Robotics, keeps the surgeon in the control loop throughout the surgery. Moreover, the robot is guided by a preoperative imaged-based planning software. This image-based software uses a patient's CT data to facilitate precise planning of the surgery, allowing implant selection and optimal positioning within the joint.

Another semiactive system is presented by Kienzle et al.[34] Their robotic system guides the TKA cutting jigs to the correct location. The surgeon then performs the bone resection conventionally. The robot used is a commercial PUMA 560. For registration, the system uses fiducial registration using preoperatively implanted pins and the center of the femoral head located when the surgeon manually flexes and abducts the thigh. To maintain registration, the ankle and the pelvis are fixed to the operating table, and the distal femur and the proximal tibia are locked to the robot by a 6 degrees-of-freedom arm.

PiGalileo TKR[42] system by PI Systems (Switzerland) assists the surgeon intraoperatively in determining the mechanical axis of the leg, in performing accurate bone resections, and in the correct alignment of the total knee prosthesis. It works strictly CT-free and without extensive preoperative planning. PiGalileo TKR is based on two independent systems that are used stand-alone or jointly, depending on the requirements and the type of surgery. The positioning device consists of a computer-controlled electromechanical device that is used for both the assessment of the anatomical landmarks as well as the positioning of resection guides. The two-axis robotic positioning device, which is fixed to the distal femur, is automatically aligned with the mechanical axis of the femur by the control software. The Photogrammetric Navigation System consists of a camera and active and passive infrared trackers. During surgery, optical trackers are attached to the bones, while other trackers are used to determine anatomical landmarks or to navigate surgical instruments, thereby providing the surgeon with a passive navigation system to assist in the planning and execution of the procedure. The combination of the two components of PiGalileo provides the surgeon with both a semiactive and a passive means of performing TKR procedures.

Another robotic system that was used for guide placement is reported in Matsen et al.[44] In their paper the authors report on a passive robotic system for knee arthroplasty. In their work they use a commercial Unimation PUMA 260 to hold a three-dimensional transparent template that enables the surgeon to indicate the desired position of the prosthetic joint surface. The robot then places the saw guide such that the resulting cut plane agrees with the one indicated by the

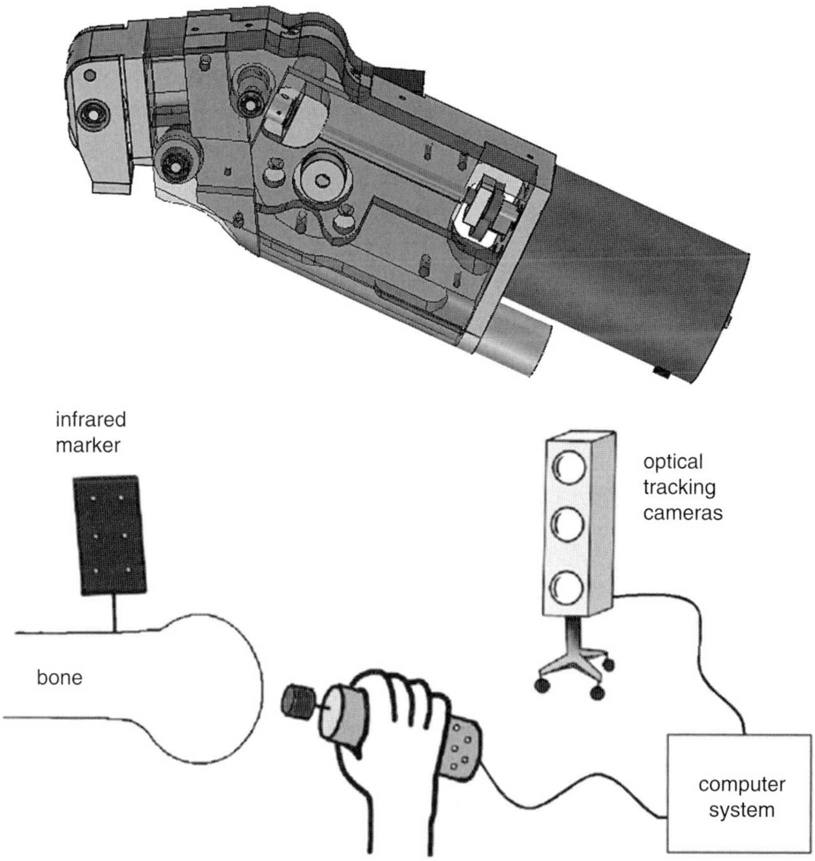

Figure 24.4. Precision freehand sculpting (PFS).

surgeon, who then performs the cuts with the power saw. This system has never been used in the operating room.

The precision freehand sculpting device (PFS)[43] which was developed at Carnegie Mellon University and ICAOS is a handheld semiactive robotic cutting tool. The PFS cutting head is controlled so that it does not cut into areas of the bone that are to be preserved, cutting only sacrificial tissue. This cutting is controlled by retracting the cutting head when it is over areas of good bone, and extending the cutting head past its guard when over areas to be resected. The PFS uses infrared markers on the tool and bone to sense the position of the tool and the bone at all times. The system is imaged based, and depends on a preoperative, CT-based model of the bone (Figure 24.4).

Passive Robotic System

The third category of medical robots is the passive system. This kind of robotic system supports the surgical procedure, but takes no active part during surgery; in other words, the surgeon is in full control of the surgical procedure at all times. There are also a few robotic systems that fall into this category. McEwen et al.[45] use Arthrobot as an assistant in the operating room. The robot is a pneumatically powered, electronically controlled positioning device that intraoperatively holds the limb. The system has no sensing capabilities and is able to move only under explicit human control. The system was used during joint replacements of the knee and hip. Another passive robotic system, although not orthopaedic in nature, is reported by Grace et al.[46] Grace developed a 6 degrees-of-freedom micromanipulator that is used for treatment of retinal venous occlusion. During the procedure, the operator is watching the robot's end-effector through a microscope and guiding it using a multidimensional joystick input device.

However, the most frequent examples of passive robotic systems are surgical navigation systems, as they represent the central element in almost every CAOS system.[47] The basic concept of a surgical navigation system is to ascertain the position (i.e., location and orientation) of the relevant components of the system and the patient's anatomy in a global coordinate system, such that their relative position can be determined. To get a better understanding of the concept of a navigation system think about perhaps one of the most common navigation systems available today: the global positioning system (GPS). This system provides the position of a receiver in earth's global coordinate system. The system does that by determining a set of distances of the receiver with respect to an array of satellites orbiting Earth. The system needs distance readings from three different satellites to determine the position of the receiver. The solution for the receiver position is one of the two points that are defined by the intersection of the three imaginary spheres with the radius equal to the distance to each satellite. One of these two points is usually physically not possible, and is eliminated by the system.

A similar concept to the GPS system is currently in use in operating rooms. In 1974, Schlondorff et al.[48] developed one of the first systems to perform navigational calculations involving bone. The system used a radiographic centimeter scale held between the patient's teeth during a lateral roentgenogram. The measurements enabled the calculation of the distances between several anatomical points. Later, Watanabe et al.[49] from Siemens Corporation, published their work on the first model of the Neuronavigator (Siemens, Munich), a mechanical device based on a multi-joint 3D digitizer. The device is used to track the tip of the sensor arm by indicating its location on preoperative CT or MRI images. But, it was the availability of optical electromagnetic position tracking systems in the 1990s that facilitated large-scale development of surgical navigation. One of the first and most accurate systems available was OptoTrak by Northern Digital Inc. (Waterloo, Ontario). The system is composed of three CCD cameras connected inside a rigid enclosure and a set of active trackers, where each tracker body incorporated a set of LEDs mounted at precise relative positions. By implementing the same concept as the GPS system, each tracker position could be resolved in the OptoTrak coordinate system. The trackers can be affixed to tools, implants, or bones, which enable active tracking of their positions during operative procedures. A follow-on to the OptoTrak system was the Polaris system, also by NDI. This system uses only two cameras, in a smaller enclosure, and can track both active wired tracker bodies, like the OptoTrak, and wireless passive tracker bodies consisting of sets of retroreflective spheres. The Polaris system is able to distinguish between different passive trackers when each tracker body visible has a distinct relative geometry of its set of reflective spheres.

One of the first systems to use this technology was HipNav, developed at Carnegie Mellon University in Pittsburgh, PA, by DiGioia and Jaramaz.[50] The system was the first computer-assisted navigation system for cup placement in total hip replacement (THR) surgery. Beside its significant clinical contribution, it set the standard for preoperative planning and range of motion (ROM) simulation for THR. Moreover, HipNav provides pinless registration capabilities, a new development in CAOS systems. After the patient's pelvis is located relative to the tracking system, the acetabular cup impaction tool, wielded by the surgeon, is guided to the preoperatively planned orientation, and then the surgeon impacts the cup in the conventional manner. This intraoperative guidance greatly increased the accuracy of the final acetabular cup orientation. KneeNav[51,52] for TKR surgery, was subsequently developed by DiGioia and Jaramaz at the Institute for Computer Assisted Orthopedic Surgery (ICAOS) at The Western Pennsylvania Hospital (Pittsburgh, PA). The system relies on the same preoperative planning and intraoperative tracking principles developed for HipNav. Some of the other systems that use this type of technology are VectorVision, Surgigate, Navitrack, StealthStation, Stryker, and Surgetic Systems. Note that the main difference between these systems is the source of information that is used for the planning, i.e., CT, MRI, fluoroscopy, image-free, etc. They all rely on the same basic navigation concept for guidance of the fixation of the cutting guides used by the surgeon. After the anatomical model of the patient's knee is developed, through whichever information source is utilized, the systems optically track the location of the cutting guides relative to that anatomical model. Once the cutting guides are in the correct position, they are fixed to the bones and then the procedure proceeds in a conventional manner. In this manner, the passive navigation systems help the surgeon to place the mechanical guides in the correct position, with the surgeon in total control at all times.

Information System

This section provides a subdivision of the CAOS systems with respect to how the information that is used in planning is acquired. We divide the information systems into three groups, depending on the attributes of the acquisition data: 3D (dimension), 2.5D, and image-free. Next is a short description and examples of systems using each of these information systems.

3D Based Information System

Three-dimensional based image systems rely on models generated preoperatively, or even intraoperatively, usually from large 3D data sets (CT or MRI), and can provide a wealth of detailed information.[53–55] ROBODOC and ORTHODOC were the first active robotic systems to use CT scans for preoperative planning, followed by HipNav, which was the first CT-based navigation system. CT/MRI based systems were the state of the art a few years ago, but the tendency in the past few years has been toward systems that do not depend on preoperative scans, due to their high cost, scheduling issues, and radiation exposure.

ORTHODOC[56] (Integrated Surgical Systems) was the first CT-based preoperative planning workstation to plan the surgical outcome. The CT based system allows the surgeon to preoperatively plan the entire procedure by placing the desired implant in a 3D, virtual, computer-reconstruction of the patient's anatomy. After setting the position of the implant in the computer model, the resulting preoperative plan provides the necessary data for ROBODOC to perform the operation.

Another CT-based system is VectorVision Knee by BrainLab. The system can use CT scans of the leg (femoral head, knee, ankle) acquired preoperatively to generate a 3D surface model of the knee. This model allows precise orientation of the implant components, and allows determination of an optimal alignment of the mechanical limb axis. During the operative procedure, a reference frame is attached to the distal or proximal tibia, following by a surface matching process based on points that are freely digitized by the surgeon both on the femur and on the tibia. Other systems that are CT-based (some are available also in other versions) are: KneeNav (ICAOS), Surgigate (MediVision, Yokneam Elit, Israel) and Navitrack (ORTHOsoft, Montreal).

2.5D Based Information System

A 2.5D based information system relies on intraoperative image data collection to develop anatomical reference models. For example, a set of coordinated fluoroscopic images generated during the surgical procedure can be used to construct a frame of reference and define the surgical plan.[57,58] Hamadeh et al.[59,60] and Weese et al.[61] used images from a calibrated C-arm for coregistration of spinal CT data. Brack et al.[62] used a calibrated C-arm to guide saw cuts for knee arthroplasty. Brandt et al.[31] used intraoperatively acquired C-arm images to guide the CRIGOS-system to position the implants. Yet the first 2.5D based navigation system that implemented fluoroscopy information was the Surgigate system (Medivision, Oberdoirf, Switzerland).

Medtronic Viking is a typical fluoroscopy-based navigation system for total knee arthroplasty.[63] During operation, two fluoroscopic images of the knee are taken, one at a 45 degree AP view of the femoral head and a second lateral view of the knee and ankle joint. Then, the surgeon identifies the center of the femoral head on the monitor, followed by defining the mechanical axis of the femur and the mechanical axis of the tibia by locating landmark points on the femur and tibia with a tracked point probe. After completing the registration steps, the joint surfaces are resected with navigated instruments. The system also intraoperatively displays the alignment of the test implants, dynamic testing of the knee during continuous flexing of the knee, and soft tissues balancing is enabled at 0, 30, and 90 degrees of flexion.

Image-Free Information System

Image-free systems derive all of the patient information required for the task from direct measurements of the bone surface (using, for instance, a tracked probe) or from direct measurement of limb kinematics (e.g., computing rotational centers from relative bone movement).[64,65,66,67,68,69] One of the pioneer systems in the use of the image-free concept is Orthopilot by Aesculap (Tuttlingen, Germany) and Fred Pickard.[70] During the procedure, the mechanical axis of the leg is modeled by three points: the centers of the femoral head, the knee, and the ankle. These points are determined by finding the center of rotation of each joint, by using appropriate movements of the hip, knee and ankle, and then solving the mathematical formulation such that they all lie on a straight line when the leg is in extension. After this process is completed, the mechanical axis of the patient's knee is found, and testing and surgical planning can be done. During the actual procedure, all of the required cutting jigs and tool have a tracker attached, which enables tracking and accurate position and orientation of the blocks on the bones.

The Stryker Navigation System (Stryker-Howmedica-Osteonics, Rutherford, NJ), developed by Kenneth A. Krackow, is an intraoperative, nonimage based navigation system that uses infrared detector arrays to determine the axial, rotational, and translational position of the tibia with respect to the femur. Axial deformity about the knee can be determined without preoperative radiographs. During the procedure, a tracking pin is placed into the patient's ipsilateral iliac crest; this pin is used to identify the center of the femoral head by attaching infrared emitters to the tracking pins, and manipulating the lower extremity in a circular fashion about the hip. Following this, several anatomical landmarks are digitized with a pointing device to determine the center of the knee. Likewise, the geometry of the proximal tibia is digitized as the surgeon identifies the sulcus between the tibial spines, the anteroposterior mid-point, as well as the medial and lateral malleoli, to locate the center of the ankle. Given all the defined points, the tibiofemoral and mechanical axes are determined. This determination then allows accurate depiction of any correction needed to properly align the implant components for that individual patient. Additionally, this navigation system is able to intraoperatively identify the real-time relative position of the tibia with respect to the femur. With this knowledge, the operating surgeon is able to use jigs from any specific instrumentation system to make more accurate cuts.

Bone Morphing, is one of the latest methods used in image-free navigation systems.[71] The method was first demonstrated in the Surgetics Station, by PRAXIM (Walpole, MA). Bone morphing determines the morphology of the knee based on a deformable statistical atlas model of knees. During operation, the physician *paints* the bony and articular surfaces with a point probe by dragging the probe across as much of the accessible surface as possible. These points are then matched with the statistical model stored in the computer, which is deformed, in real time, to fit the patient's knee and points acquired during painting.[72] In this way, even though only a small portion of the patient's knee is accessible during the procedure, the computer can predict the actual shape of inaccessible portions of the knee based on general knowledge of knee anatomy combined with the known shape of portions of that patient's knee. Following registration, navigation is performed based on the computer model, in a similar manner as the other systems described previously.

Vectorvision by BrainLab[70] is also an image free, bone morphing based, knee navigation system that allows correct alignment of the prosthesis, reconstruction of the joint line, optimal balance of the ligaments, and equal extension and flexion gaps. The first step for registration is to define the center of the femoral head by pivoting the head in the acetabulum. Next, several anatomical landmarks are identified using a point probe, including acquisition of multiple points on several bone surface locations. The acquired data is used to create a 3D model of the knee using model morphing techniques. Based on this model, the system automatically calculates the optimum implant size and position which can later be refined by the surgeon.

Cross-Referencing Between Robotic System and Information System

In the previous two sections, we categorized robotic systems and source of information systems into three groups each. These group sets are orthogonal to each other and create a grid in which each node represents a combination of a robotic method with a method in which the necessary information for guiding the robot is acquired. This concept is presented in Table 24.1, in which each cell in the table corresponds to a node on the grid. Next, we take the systems that were presented in previous sections and allocated them into the cell that best represents the robotic system concept and operation mode, as shown in Table 24.2. Note that there is no migration of systems along the horizontal direction (i.e., robotic systems do not tend to change from passive to semiactive or active mode), because it would require a different mechanical concept and design. But, on the vertical grid, there are many changes, and systems that started as 3D based move to 2.5D or even image free. This is mainly because a change in information source does not require significant mechanical changes or a new mechanism design, but is mainly reflected in changes of software. In other words, while the source of the information changes, the final information required to perform the procedure is the same and the actions based on that information do not change. Hence, a few systems could be found in several different cells reflecting their evolution throughout

Table 24.2. Categorization of the robotic systems versus the source of information systems

Robotics system Source information systems	Passive	Semiactive	Active
3D (CT, MRI) ROBODOC	KneeNav VectorVision SurgiGATE Navitrack Surgetics	Acrobot PFS	
2.5 (Fluoro)	SurgiGATE StealthStation VectorVision Surgetics		CASPAR CRIGOS
Image free	OrthoPilot VectorVision Surgetics Stryker	PiGalileo	MBARS

the years. It is worth mentioning that in the last CAOS International meeting held in Chicago in 2004, there was a suggestion to extend this matrix structure to a 3D matrix where the third dimension would correspond to the medical application, such that for every medical procedure there exist a 2D matrix such as Table 24.2, and the general 3D matrix is composed of many 2D layers. We believe that this is a good extension and we would pursue this direction in future works.

This description and categorization of CAOS systems used for total knee replacement is useful in delineating the differences in system design and capabilities, and helped chart the evolution of surgical systems over the past 15 years. It is also useful for the developer and clinician in differentiating between systems, and seeing the positive and negative aspects of the different modalities. CAOS systems have evolved a great deal since their introduction, and as the pace of technologic innovation in the orthopedic community quickens, CAOS systems will change even more in the coming years.

References

1. Verneuil A. De la creation d'une fausse articulation par section ou resection partille de l'os maxillaire inferieur, comme moyen de remedier a l'ankylose vraie ou fausse de la machoire inferieure. Arch Gen Med. 1860;15(ser. 5):174.
2. Insall JN, Windsor RE, Scott WN, Kelly MA, Aglietti P. Surgery of the Knee. 2nd ed. New York: Churchill Livingstone; 1993.
3. Ferguson W. Excision of the knee joint: recovery with a false joint and a useful limb. Med Times. 1961;Gaz 1:601.
4. Campbell WC. Interposition of vitallium plates in arthroplasties of the knee: preliminary report. AM J Surg. 1940;47:639.
5. MacIntosh DL. Hemiarthroplasty of the knee using a space occupying prosthesis for painful varus and valgus deformities. J Bone Joint Surg Am. 1958;40:1431.

6. Schlondorff G. Computer assisted surgery: historical remarks. Computer Aided Surgery. 1998;3:150–152.
7. Cinquin P. Gestes médico-chirurgicaux assistés par ordinateur. Société d'Edition de l'Association d'Enseignement Médical des Hôpitaux de Paris. 1993;63:386–405.
8. Cinquin P, Bainville E. Computer assisted medical intervention: passive and semi-active aids. IEEE. Eng Med. Biol Mag. 1995;14:254–263.
9. Stulberg SD, Picard F, Saragaglia D. Computer assisted total knee arthroplasty. Operative Techniques. Orthopaedics. 2000;10(1):25–39.
10. Taylor RH, Brendt D, Mittelstadt BD, et al. An image directed robotic system for precise orthopaedic surgery. In: Taylor R, Lavallee S, Burdea GC, Mosges R, eds. Computer Integrated Surgery, Technology and Clinical Applications. Cambridge: MIT Press Publishers; 1995:379–391.
11. Taylor RH. Robotics in Orthopedic Surgery. In: Nolte LP, Ganz R. Computer Assisted Orthopaedic Surgery (CAOS). 1998:35–41.
12. Troccaz J. Man-machine interfaces in computer augmented surgery. In: Ranz R, Nolte LP, eds. Computer Assisted Orthopaedic Surgery. Hogrefe & Huber Publishers, Bern; 1999:53–68.
13. Bainville E, Bricault I, Cinquin P, Lavallee S. Concepts and methods of registration for computer integrated surgery. In: Ranz R, Nolte LP, eds. Computer Assisted Orthopedic Surgery (CAOS). Hogrefe & Huber Publishers, Bern; 1999:15–34.
14. Hofstetter R, Slomczykowski M, Sati M, Nolte LP. Fluoroscopy as an Imaging Means for Computer-Assisted Surgical Navigation. Computer Aided Surgery 1999;4:65–76.
15. Picard F, Moody J, Jaramaz B, DiGioia A, Nikou C, LaBarca S. A classification proposal for Computer Assisted Knee systems. Medical Image Computing and computer assisted intervention. MICCAI 2000, 3rd International conference. Pittsburgh, PA: Springer; 2000:1145–1151.
16. Kazanzides P, Mittelstands BD, Musits BL, et al. An Integrated System for Cementless Hip Replacement. IEEE Engineering in Medicine and Biology. 1995; 14:307–312.
17. Bargar W, Bauer A, Borner M. Primary and revision total hip replacement using the Robodoc system. Clin Orthop. 1998;354:82–91.
18. Bauer A. Robot assisted total hip replacement in primary and revision cases. Techniques. Orthopaedics. 2000;10(1):9–13.
19. Fadda M, Bertelli D, Martelli S, Marcacci M, et al. Computer assisted planning for total knee arthroplasty. First Joint Conference of CVRMed and MRCAS. Springer; 1997:619–628.
20. Glozman D, Shoham M, Fischer A. Efficient registration of 3-D objects in Robotic-Assisted Surgery. Proceedings CAOS/USA 1999. Editor UPMC Shadyside Medical Center (A. DiGioia): 248–252.
21. Gotte H, Roth M, Brack CH, et al. A new less-invasive approach to knee surgery using a vision-guided manipulator. IARP workshop on Medical Robotics; 1996; Vienna, Austria:99–106.
22. Kober R, Meister D. Total knee replacement using the Caspar-system. Computer assisted total knee arthroplasty. International Symposium on CAOS; February 2000; Davos:17–19.
23. Martelli S, Beltrame F, Dario P, Fadda M. A system for computer and robot assisted knee implantation. Proc. 14th IEEE Medicine and Biology Conf; 1992; Paris.
24. Peterman J, Kober R, Heinze, et al. Computer assisted planning and robot assisted surgery in the reconstruction of the anterior cruciate ligament. Operative Techniques. Orthopaedics. January 2000;10(1):50–55.

25. Picard F, Leitner F, Raoult O, Saragaglia D. Computer assisted knee replacement. Location of a rotational center of the knee. Total Knee Arthroplasty. International Symposium on CAOS; February 2000; Davos:17–19.
26. Sati M, Staubli H, Bourquin Y, Kunz M, Kasermann S, Nolte LP. Clinical integration of computer-assisted technology for arthroscopic anterior cruciate ligament reconstruction. Operative Techniques Orthopaedics. 2000;10:40–49.
27. Van Ham G, Denis K, Vander Sloten J, et al. Machining and accuracy studies for a tibial knee implant using a force controlled robot. Computer Aided Surgery. 1998;3:123–133.
28. Mittelstadt B, Paul H, Kazanzides P, et al. Development of a surgical robot for cementless total hip replacement, Robotica. 1983:3.
29. Paul H, et al. A surgical robot for total hip replacement surgery, In: Proceedings of the 1992 IEEE International conference on Robotics and Automation; 1992:606–611.
30. Van Ham G, Denis K, Sloten JV, et al. Machining and accuracy studies for a tibial knee implant using a force controlled robot. Computer Aided Surgery. 1998;3:123–133.
31. Brandt G, Radermacher K, Lavallee S, Staudte HW, Rau G. A Compact Robot for Image Guided Orthopedic Surgery: Concept and Preliminary Results. Lecture notes in: Troccaz J, Grimson R, Mosges R, eds. Computer Science 1205, CVRMed-MRCAS'97. 1997:767–776.
32. Wolf A, Shoham M, Shnider M, Roffman M. Morphometric Study of the Human Lumbar Spine for Operation-Workspace Specifications. Spine. 2001;26(22).
33. Wolf A, Shoham M, Michael S, Moshe R. Feasibility Study of a Mini, Bone-Attached, Robotic System for Spinal Operation: Analyses and Experiments. Spine. 2004;29.
34. Kienzle MT, Stulberg D, Peshkin M, et al. A Computer-Assisted Total Knee Replacement Surgical System Using a Calibrated Robot. In: Taylor R, Lavallee S, Burdea GC, Mosges R, eds. Computer integrated surgery. Cambridge: MIT Press; 1996:410–416.
35. Davies BL, Harriss J, Lin WJ, et al. Active compliance in Robotic Surgery—The use of force control as a dynamic constraint. Journal of Engineering in Medicine, Proceedings of the Institution of Mechanical Engineers. 1997; 211:H4.
36. Davies BL, Cobb JP, Gomes SF. Acrobot® System for Robotic MIS Arthroplasty by The Acrobot Company Limited, c/o Imperial College London, London SW7 2AZ.
37. Davies BL, Harris S, Jakopec M, Fan KL, Cobb J. A Special-Purpose Robotic System for Knee Surgery Davies. CAOS 99. 4th Int Conf. On Computer-Assisted Orthopaedic Surgery; March 1999; Davos, Switzerland:49.
38. Davies BL, Harris SJ, Jakopec M, Cobb J. Computer-Assisted Surgery for TKR IMechE—International Conference on Knee Replacement Surgery 1974–2024. Institution of Mechanical Engineers, PEP Ltd; April 1999: 256–259.
39. Davies B, Harris S, Jakopec M, Cobb J. A Novel Hands-on Robot for Knee Replacement Surgery. Proceedings of the CAOS USA '99 Conference on Computer Assisted Orthopaedic Surgery 1999; UPMC, Shadyside Hospital, Pennsylvania, PA: 70–74.
40. Harris SJ, Jakopec M, Cobb J, Davies BL. Intra-operative Application of a Robotic Knee Surgery System. Proceedings of MICCAI '99. Lecture notes in Computer Science 1679. Springer Verlag; September 1999:1116–1124.
41. Davies B, Harris S, Jakopec M, Cobb J. A Novel Hands-on Robot for Knee Replacement. Proceedings of European Robotic Systems Workshop on

Medical Robotics, Scuola Superiore Sant'Anna 56127. September 1999; Pisa, Italy:98–102.
42. Ritschl P, Machacek J, Fuiko R, Zettl R, Kotte B. The Galileo System for Implantation of Total Knee Arthroplasty, Navigation and Robotics in Total Joint and Spine Surgery. New York: Springer, 2004.
43. Brisson G, Kanade T, DiGioia AM III, Jaramaz B. Precision freehand sculpting of bone. Computer Assisted Orthopedic Surgery CAOS International. 2003;36.
44. Matsen FA III, Garbini JL, Sidles JA, Prat B, Baumgarten D, Kaiura R. Robotic assistance in orthopedic surgery. Clin Orthp. Rela Res. 296. 1993: 178–186.
45. McEwen C, Bussani CR, Auchinleck GF, Breault MJ. Development and initial clinical evaluation of pre robotic and robotic retraction systems for surgery. 2nd Annual Int Symposium Custom Orthopaedic Prosthetics; October 1989; Chicago.
46. Grace KW, Colgate JE, Gluksberg MR, Chun JH. A Six Degree of Freedom Micromanipulator for Ophthalmic Surgery. IEEE International Conference on Robotics and Automation. 1993:630–635.
47. Nolte LP, Langlotz F. Basics of computer assisted orthopedic surgery (CAOS). Navigation and robotics in total joint and spine surgery. New York: Springer; 2004.
48. Schlondorff G. Computer assisted surgery: historical remarks. Computer Aided Surgery. 1998;3:150–152.
49. Watanabe E, Watanabe T, Manaka S, Mayanagi Y, Takakura K. Three dimensional digitizer (Neuronavigator): New equipment for computerized tomography-guided stereotactic surgery. Surg. Neurol. 1987;27:543–547.
50. DiGioia A, Jaramaz B, Nilou C, Labarca R, Moody JE, Colgan B. Surgical navigation for total hip replacement with the use of Hipnav. Operative Techniques in Orthopaedics, Medical Robotics and Computer-assisted Orthopaedic Surgery. January 2000;10(1).
51. Picard F, Leitner F, Raoult O, Saragaglia D. Computer assisted knee replacement. Location of a rotational center of the knee. Total Knee Arthroplasty. In: International Symposium on CAOS; 2000; Davos:17–19.
52. Picard F, Moody J, Jaramaz B, DiGioia A, Nikou C, LaBarca S. A classification proposal for Computer Assisted Knee systems. Medical Image Computing and computer assisted intervention. MICCAI 2000, 3rd International conference 2000. Pittsburgh, PA: Springer, 2000:1145–1151.
53. Amiot LP, Labelle H, DeGuise JA, et al. Computer-assisted pedicle screw fixation: a feasibility study. Spine. 1995;10:1208–1212.
54. Jaramaz B, DiGioia A, Blackwell M, Nikou C. Computer assisted measurement of cup placement in total hip replacement. Clin Orthop and Rel Res. 1998;354:70–81.
55. Tucker, A. Analysis of the Orthopedic Industry Equity Research 11.
56. Knabe K, Hurschler C, Stukenborg-Colsman C, Gosse F. An anatomical shaped prosthesis stem—in vitro comparison between robot-assisted and manual implantation, Navigation and robotics in total joint and spine surgery. New York: Springer; 2004.
57. Hofstetter R, Slomczykowski M, Sati M, Nolte LP. Fluoroscopy as an Imaging Means for Computer-Assisted Surgical Navigation. Computer Aided Surgery. 1999;4:65–76.
58. Klos TVS, Banks AZ, Banks SA, et al. Computer and radiographic assisted anterior cruciate ligament reconstruction of the knee. In: Nolte LP, Ganz R. Computer Assisted Orthopaedic Surgery. Hogrefe & Huber Publishers; 1999:184–189.

59. Hamadeh A, Sautot P, Lavallee S, Cinquin P. Towards automatic registration between CT and X-ray images: cooperation between 3D/2D registration and 2D edge detection. In: Proceedings of the 2nd MRCAS symposium; 1995:39–46.
60. Hamadeh A, Lavallee S, Cinquin P. Automated 3-dimensional computed tomographic and fluoroscopic image registration. Comp Aided Surg. 1998; 3:11–19.
61. Weese J, Buzug TM, Lorenz C, Fassnacht C. An approach to 2D/3D registration of a vertebrae in 2D X-ray fluoroscopies with 3D CT images. In Troccaz J, Grimson E, Mosges R, eds. Proceedings of the 1st joint conference on computer vision, virtual reality and robotics in medicine and medical robotics and computer assisted surgery (CVRMed-MRCAS'97); 1997; Grenoble, France. Berlin: Springer-Verlag; 1997:119–128.
62. Brack C, Gotte H, Gosse F, Moctezuma J, Roth M, Schweikard A. Towards accurate X-ray camera calibration in computer assisted robotic surgery. In: Proceedings of the international symposium on computer and communication systems for image guided diagnosis and therapy (CAR'96); 1996; Paris. Amsterdam: Elsevier; 1996:721–728.
63. Hagena FW, Kettrukat M, Christ RM, Hackbart M. Fluroscopy-based navigation in genesis II total knee arthroplasty with the Medtronic Viking system. Navigation and robotics in total joint and spine surgery. New York: Springer; 2004.
64. Dessenne V, Lavallee S, Julliard R, et al. Computer assisted knee anterior cruciate ligament reconstruction: first clinical tests. Journal of Image Guided Surgery. 1995;1:59–64.
65. Krackow K, Serpe L, Phillips MJ, et al. A new technique for determining proper mechanical axis alignment during total knee arthroplasty. Orthopedics. 1999;22(7):698–701.
66. Kuntz M, Sati M, Nolte LP, et al. Computer assisted total knee arthroplasty. In: International Symposium on CAOS; February 2000; Davos:17–19.
67. Leitner F, Picard F, Minfelde R, et al. Computer-assisted knee surgical total replacement. In: First Joint Conference of CVRMed and MRCAS 1997; Grenoble, France. Springer: 629–638.
68. Picard F, Moody J, Jaramaz B, DiGioia A, Nikou C, LaBarca S. A classification proposal for Computer Assisted Knee systems. Medical Image Computing and computer assisted intervention. MICCAI 2000, 3rd International conference, Pittsburgh, PA. Springer Publishers; 2000.
69. Taylor RH, Brendt D, Mittelstadt BD, et al. An image directed robotic system for precise orthopaedic surgery. In: Taylor R, Lavallee S, Burdea GC, Mosges R, eds. Computer Integrated Surgery, Technology and Clinical Applications. Cambridge, MIT Press; 1995:379–391.
70. Saragaglia D, Picard F. Computer-Assisted Implantation of total knee Endoprosthesis with no pre-operative imaging: the kinematic model.
71. Julliard R, Plaweski S, Lavallee S. ACL Surgetics: an efficient computer assisted technique for ACL reconstruction. Navigation and robotics in total joint and spine surgery. New York: Springer; 2004.
72. Fleute M. Shape reconstruction for computer assisted surgery based on non rigid registration of statistical models with intraoperative point data and X-ray images. TIMC IMAG laboratory; 2001.

Index

A

AARROM exercises. *See* active assisted range of motion exercises
Abductor injury, 110
ACL. *See* anterior cruciate ligament
Acrobot, 395
Active assisted range of motion (AAROM) exercises, 28
Active Constraint Robotics, 396
Active range of motion (AROM) exercises, 28
Ahlback classification, 195
Ahlback disease, 195
American National Hospital Discharge Survey, 390
Anesthesia
  for bone-sparing UKA, 196, 202, 204
  for docking procedure on MCL of elbow, 79
  for intramedullary UKA, 217, 227
  for mini-open repair of rotator cuff tear, 23
  for operative treatment of glenohumeral instability, 12
  for two-incision approach to THA, 159
  for UniSpacer knee arthroplasty, 273
Anterior (Heuter) approach, to THA, 121–139
  benefits of, 122–123
  BMI and, 124
  conclusions regarding, 138–139
  image intensifier for, 124
  patient selection for, 124
  PROfx table for, 123–124
  statistics regarding, 138
  surgical technique for
    acetabular prosthesis insertion for, 130, 132
    acetabulum preparation for, 130–131
    acetabulum reaming for, 130–131
    anterior capsulotomy for, 127
    broach insertion for, 135–136
    cancellous bone removal for, 136
    cobra retractors and, 126, 128
    draping for, 125
    fascia lata vulnerability and, 130
    fascial incision placement for, 125–126
    femoral cork screw and, 128
    femoral head extraction for, 130
    femoral hook placement for, 131–133
    femoral mobility and, 133
    femoral neck cut for, 128–129
    femoral neck cut, in situ v. dislocated, 130
    femoral offset and, 136–138
    femoral preparation for, 132, 134
    femoral prosthesis insertion for, 138–139
    hip dislocation for, 127–128
    hip stability and, 138
    Hohmann retraction of vastus and, 128
    lateral hip capsule palpation for, 126
    leg length, 136–138
    patient placement and, 124–125
    pneumatic compression boots and, 125
    postoperative precautions after, 138
    PROfx table and, 124–125, 134
    prosthesis choice for, 134–135
    proximal femoral exposure for, 132, 134
    skin incision placement for, 125–126
    trial reduction for, 136
    trochanteric retraction for, 132–133
    wound closure for, 138
    x-ray length and offset assessments for, 136–137
Anterior cruciate ligament (ACL) of knee, 193
  ACL deficiency and UniSpacer knee arthroplasty, 272

Anterior cruciate ligament (ACL) of knee (*cont.*)
  evaluation for Oxford TKA, 289
  excision for lateral TKA, 344
  excision for mini-midvastus TKA, 329
  laxity and intramedullary approach to UKA, 214
  resection for quadriceps-sparing TKA, 352
Anterolateral mini-incision approach, to THA
  conclusions regarding, 120
  preoperative planning for, 103
  surgical technique for, 103–120
    abductor injury and, 110
    acetabular component placement for, 113–114
    acetabulum preparation for, 111–113
    acetabulum reaming for, 112–113
    Charnley retractor and, 104
    fascia detachment for, 106
    fascia lata incision for, 104, 106
    femoral component placement for, 116–117
    femoral head placement for, 116, 118
    femoral neck cut for, 110
    femur preparation for, 113
    femur retraction for, 110–111
    femur retractor placement for, 115
    gluteus medius detachment for, 106, 108
    gluteus medius muscle division for, 106–107
    gluteus minimus detachment for, 106, 108
    gluteus minimus tendon incision for, 106, 108
    greater trochanter and, 104, 106–107
    hip capsule excision for, 109
    hip capsule exposure for, 108–109
    hip dislocation for, 109–110
    lateral trochanter medial portion removal for, 115
    leg length measurements for, 109
    Low-Profile reamer and, 112–113
    patient placement for, 104
    provisional prosthesis for, 115–116
    skin incision placement for, 104–105
    wound closure for, 116, 118–120
Anterolateral resurfacing approach, to THA, 181–187
  acetabular component placement for, 185
  acetabular exposure for, 184–185
  acetabular preparation for, 184
  acetabular reaming for, 185
  anterior capsule dissection for, 183
  anterior capsulectomy for, 183
  bone hook use for, 183
  chamfer cuts for, 187
  chamfer reaming for, 187
  circumferential guide use for, 186
  Cobb elevator use for, 182, 183
  concentric reaming and, 185
  cylindrical reaming and, 186
  deep exposure for, 182–183
  donut tower guide use for, 186
  electrocautery use for, 182, 183
  fascia lata incision for, 182
  femoral component placement for, 187–188
  femoral component sizing for, 184
  femoral head reaming for, 186–187
  femoral neck dissection for, 183
  femoral neck measurement for, 183–184
  femoral neck notches and, 184, 185
  femoral resurfacing for, 185–187
  gluteus medius muscle detachment for, 183
  guide pin placement for, 186
  hemostatic device use for, 182
  hip dislocation for, 183
  Hohmann retractor use for, 183, 184
  mobile window and, 182
  osteophyte excision for, 185
  postoperative care for, 187–188
  radiographs for, intraoperative, 185
  radiographs for, preoperative, 182
  self-retaining retractor use for, 182
  skin incision placement for, 181–182
  Smillie meniscal knife use for, 183
  smooth Bennett retractor use for, 185
  smooth Richardson retractor use for, 186
  spiked Mueller retractor use for, 184–185
  Tissue Link use for, 182
  trial head component placement for, 187
  wound closure for, 187
AO/ASIS classification system, 32
Apprehension test, 8–9
AROM exercises. *See* active range of motion exercises
Arthritis. *See* glenohumeral arthritis; osteoarthritis
Arthrobot, 398
Arthroscopic stress test, 74, 76
Arthroscopy
  for bone-sparing UKA, 197, 207
  for docking procedure on elbow MCL, 79–80
  of the elbow, 74, 76
  magnetic resonance, 10
  of the shoulder, 21–24

for UniSpacer knee arthroplasty, 273–275, 280–281
Arthrotomy. *See also* Medial parapatellar arthrotomy, limited, to TKA; Medial parapatellar arthrotomy, traditional, to TKA
for bone-sparing UKA, 197
cutting guides for, 305–307
for extramedullary UKA, 258
for intramedullary UKA, 217–218
for knee arthroplasty with UniSpacer, 277
for lateral TKA, 340
for mini-midvastus TKA, 329
for quadriceps-sparing TKA, 350
for standard midvastus TKA, 325
Aufranc retractor, 332, 334
Avascular necrosis, 32–34, 41–42, 57–58

B

Bankart lesion, 4, 14, 17
Bankart repair, 11, 12
Barrel stitch, 14, 15
Bennett retractor, 185
Biceps. *See* distal biceps tendon repair
BMI. *See* body mass index
Body mass index (BMI), 124
Bone and joint diseases, 390
Bone-sparing approach, to UKA, 193–210
common errors with, 205
posterior femoral condyle resection for, 197–198, 205
tibial component size and, 205
tibial surface resection and, 205
complications with, 205–206
learning curve and, 205
training for, 206
conclusions regarding, 209–210
conservative management and, 209
proper surgical technique and, 210
nonoperative treatment and, 195
patient selection for
Ahlback classification for, 195
Ahlback disease and, 195
contraindications for, 195
patient choice and, 196
patient selection for, 195–196
physical examination for, 195
Repicci II unicondylar knee system use for, 206
surgical technique for
0-prolene suture use for, 205
0-Vicryl suture use for, 205
anesthesia for, 196
articular defect and, 197–198
bupivacaine use for, 202
capsular closure after, 205
depth gauge for, 200
diagnostic arthroscopy for, 197
distracter joint use for, 199
distracter pin use for, 199
draping for, 197
epinephrine use for, 202
exposure for, 197–198
femoral component insertion for, 202, 204–205
femoral drill guide use for, 202
femoral preparation for, 200–202
femoral resection for, 200–202
femoral-tibial alignment for, 202–203
final preparation for, 202, 205
high-speed burr use for, 199
local anesthesia for, 202, 204
medial parapatellar capsular arthrotomy for, 197
methylene blue marks for, 202–203
methylmethacrylate cement use for, 202
operating table choice for, 197
patellar eversion and, 197
patient placement for, 197
radiographic assessment before, 195
round burr use for, 200
sagittal saw use for, 202
sclerotic bone preservation and, 200
side-cutting burr use for, 202
skin incision placement for, 197–198
subcutaneous dissection for, 197
tibial bone resection for, 199
tibial inlay component for, 200
tourniquet use for, 197, 205
trial reduction for, 202, 204
wound closure after, 205
Bupivacaine, 202

C

CAOS. *See* computer assisted orthopedic surgery
Capsule
arthrotomy for bone-sparing UKA, 197
closure for bone-sparing UKA, 205
closure for posterolateral THA, 155
excision for anterolateral MI THA, 108–109
extension for intramedullary UKA, 217
incision and retraction for two-incision THA, 163–165, 167
palpation for anterior THA, 126
release for shoulder arthroplasty, 63
Capsulectomy
for anterolateral resurfacing THA, 183
medial, 289

Capsulorrhaphy, 11–17
  inferior capsular shift procedure and, 11–12
  laterally-based T capsulorrhaphy and, 12
  results of, 17
Capsulotomy
  anterior for anterior (Heuter) THA, 127
  medial for Oxford insertion UKA, 289
  radial for posterolateral THA, 144–145
CASPAR, 391
Chamfer cuts
  for anterolateral resurfacing approach to THA, 187
  for extramedullary tensor approach to UKA, 248
  for lateral approach to TKA, 342–343
Charnley awl, for two-incision approach to THA, 171
Charnley retractor
  for anterolateral total hip arthroplasty, 104
  for posterolateral total hip arthroplasty, 144
Chondromalacia, 273–274
Circumferential guide, 186
Cobb elevator
  for resurfacing approach to THA, 182–183
  for two-incision approach to THA, 163
Cobra retractor, 126, 128
Computer-assisted orthopedic surgery (CAOS), 367–388
  2.5D information systems (for TKA) and
    C-arm use and, 400
    CRIGOS and, 400
    fluoroscopy and, 400
    intraoperative image data collection and, 400
    Medtronic Viking and, 400–401
    SurgiGATE and, 400
  3D information systems and
    CT/MRI navigation and, 400
    KneeNav and, 400
    Navitrack and, 400
    ORTHODOC (Integrated Surgical Systems) and, 400
    preoperative scans and, 400
    ROBODOC and, 400
    SurgiGATE and, 400
    VectorVision Knee and, 400
  active (robotic) navigation v. passive navigation and, 368
  active robotic system (for TKA), 391–395
    CASPAR and, 391
    CRIGOS-system and, 392
    MBARS and, 391–392
    parallel robotic structures and, 392
    patellofemoral arthroplasty using MBARS and, 392–394
    PiGalileo and, 391
    ROBODOC and, 391
    Stewart-Gough 6 degrees-of-freedom robot and, 392
    surface modeling with MBARS and, 393–394
    tibial cutting and, 391
  classifications of (TKA related) robotic systems for, 390–399
    information systems and, 391
    robotic system/information system matrix and, 402–403
  electromagnetic tracking and, 368
  image-free information systems (for TKA) and
    bone morphing and, 401–402
    bone surface measurements for, 401
    deformable statistical atlas model of knees and, 402
    infrared detector arrays and, 401
    limb kinematics measurements for, 401
    Orthopilot and, 401
    point probe use for, 402
    Stryker Navigation System and, 401
    Surgetics Station and, 401
    tracking pin use for, 401
    Vectorvision and, 402
  opteoelectronic tracking and, 368
    DRBs for, 368–369
  passive robotic systems (for TKA), 397–399
    Arthrobot and, 398
    Carnegie Mellon University and, 399
    global positioning system and, 398
    HipNav and, 399
    multi-joint 3D digitizer and, 398
    Navitrack and, 399
    Neuronavigator and, 398
    optical electromagnetic position tracking systems and, 398
    OptoTrak and, 398–399
    pin-less registration and, 399
    six degrees-of-freedom micromanipulator and, 398
    StealthStation and, 399
    surgical navigation system and, 398
    SurgiGATE and, 399
    VectorVision and, 399
  registration for, 369
    CT scans for, 369
    fluoroscopy for, 369
    paired-point matching for, 369
    surface registration for, 369
    verification and, 369
  ROBODOC and, 367
    CT imaging for, 367
    digitizing probe for, 367
    image overlay for, 367
    touch point referencing for, 367
  semiactive robotic system (for TKA), 395–397
    Acrobot and, 395
    Active Constraint Robotics and, 396
    bone resection and, 396

Carnegie Mellon University and, 397
guide placement and, 396
Hands On Robotics and, 396
ICAOS and, 397
Photogrammetric Navigation System and, 396
PiGalileo and, 396
precision freehand sculpting device and, 397
PUMA 560 and, 396
telesurgery and, 395
Unimation PUMA 260 and, 396
surgeon defined anatomy approach to, 369–370
THA and, 384–388
accuracy of, 387
acetabular abduction and, 384
acetabular anteversion and, 384
acetabular component orientation and, 387
anatomical anteversion and, 385
anterior pelvic plane and, 385–386
conclusions regarding, 387–388
mechanical alignment and, 387
operative anteversion and, 384–385
pelvic reference tripod use for, 385–386
pelvic rotation and, 387
radiographic accuracy and, 386
radiographic anteversion and, 385
two dimensional radiography and, 384
THA using CT navigation, 370–376
3D pelvic modeling for, 371–373
acetabular abduction comparison and, 376
acetabular anteversion comparison and, 376
acetabular component orientation and, 370
bony acetabulum orientation and, 370
clinical experience with, 375–376
CT scans for, 374
DRB use for, 373–374
infrared camera use for, 373
LED equipped instruments for, 373–374
patient position and, 370
postoperative computed tomography for, 374–375
preoperative analysis for, 371–373
registration for, 374
surgical implantation and, 374–375
SurgiGATE software use for, 371–372, 374–375
Unix Ultra 10 workstation use for, 373
THA using fluoroscopic navigation, 376–383
acetabular navigation for, 377
acetabular reaming for, 382–383
acetabulum views for, 377
anterior superior iliac spine views for, 377–381
cup insertion for, 382–383
DRB application for, 377
fluoroscopic C-arm use for, 378–379
image referencing for, 378, 382
Jackson operative imaging table use for, 377
patient preparation for, 377–378
pubic tubercle views for, 377–381
Stealth Universal Hip Application use for, 377
Troccaz and, 390
ultrasound and, 368
Computerized tomography (CT)
and 3D information systems, 400
CT navigation for CAOS THA, 370–376
and ROBODOC, 367
Conserve Plus device, 180
CRIGOS, 392, 400
Crowe classification, 144
CT. *See* computerized tomography
Cutting guides
for extramedullary approach to UKA, 258
for extramedullary tensor approach to UKA, 236–237
for medial parapatellar arthrotomy, limited, to TKA, 305–307
for mini-midvastus approach to TKA, 327–328, 332
for quadriceps-sparing approach to TKA, 359–360

D

Dead-arm syndrome, 5
Distal biceps tendon repair, 90
bone sutures for, 90
complications with, 98
history of, 90
mini-incision technique for, 90, 93–97
biceps tendon reduction for, 94–96
biceps tendon retraction for, 94
cancellous trough and, 94
cortical bone roughening and, 94
dissection and, 94
modified Krackow stitch and, 94–95
postoperative radiograph and, 96–97
repair evaluation for, 96–97
skin incision placement for, 93
subcutaneous flaps and, 93–94
suture anchors for, 94, 95
tuberosity preparation and, 94–95
wound closure for, 96
patient history and, 91

Distal biceps tendon repair (*cont.*)
physical examination for, 91, 92
flexion strength and, 92
MRIs and, 92
proximal retraction of biceps and, 91
radiography and, 92, 96
range of motion and, 91–92
supination and, 92
rehabilitation after, 98
summary for, 99
Distal biceps tendon rupture
endurance fatigue from, 91
etiology of, 90–91
eccentric muscle contraction and, 91
mechanical processes and, 91
pathogenesis and, 91
tendon hypovascularity and, 91
operative v. nonoperative treatment of, 92–93
pain from, 91
persistent weakness from, 91
Docking procedure on elbow MCL, 73–87
MRI and, 76–78
3-dimensional volumetric gradient-echo, 76
coronal, 77
fast spin-echo, 76
saline-enhanced, 76
patient history and, 73–74
acute event and, 74
acute on chronic event and, 74
ulnar neuritis and, 74, 78
physical examination of, 74–76
arthroscopic stress test in, 74, 76
O'Brien's milking test in, 74–75
O'Driscoll's moving valgus stress test, 74–75
range of motion in, 74
Tinsel's test in, 74
valgus extension overload test in, 74
valgus stress test in, 74–75
postoperative management of
physical therapy for, 86
throwing program for, 86
surgical technique for
anesthesia for, 79
anterior bundle of MCL and, 78
anterior compartment arthroscopy and, 79–80
arthroscopic evaluation for, 79–80
flexor carpi ulnaris and, 78
flexor mass and, 78
fragmented spurs and, 80
graft harvesting for, 81
graft passage for, 84–85
graft tensioning for, 84–85
humeral tunnel creation for, 83
instrumentation for, 81
Krackow stitch and, 81, 84
MCL exposure for, 81
MCL incision for, 81–82
medial opening and, 80
muscle splitting incision, 78
native ligament repair for, 83–84
palmaris longus and, 81
patient position for, 79–80
posterior compartment arthroscopy and, 80
results of, 87
skin incision for, 81–82
splint placement after, 84
submuscular ligament exposure for, 81–82
suture fixation for, 84, 86
tendon graft reconstruction and, 79
tourniquet use for, 81, 84
ulnar nerve and, 79
ulnar tunnel creation for, 83
valgus stress test and, 79
wound closure for, 84
Donut tower guide, 186
Doppler-ultrasound, 362
DRBs. *See* dynamic reference bases
Drill guides
for bone sparing approach to UKA, 202
for Oxford insertion approach to UKA, 291–292
for percutaneous pinning of proximal humerus fractures, 42
Dynamic reference bases (DRBs), 368–369
in THA (CT navigation), 373–374
in THA (fluoroscopic navigation), 377

E

Elbow. *See* Medial collateral ligament of elbow
Electrocautery
for anterolateral resurfacing approach to THA, 182–183
for extramedullary tensor approach to UKA, 239
for MIS-optimized subvastus approach to TKA, 317, 321
for two-incision approach to THA, 163, 169
Epinephrine
for bone-sparing approach to UKA, 202
for knee arthroplasty with UniSpacer, 273
for two-incision approach to THA, 175
Extension gap disease, 193–194
Extramedullary approach, to UKA, 257–268
principles of, 257
summary regarding, 268
surgical technique for
alignment tower use for, 262
distal femoral resection for, 263–264
femoral finishing guide selection for, 263–264
femoral preparation for, 261–263
femoral resection guide use for, 263
medial parapatellar arthrotomy for, 258

MG femoral component placement and cementing for, 267
MG tibial template selection for, 265–266
MG uni prosthesis use for, 257
osteophyte removal for, 258
retractor use for, 258, 267
skin incision placement for, 258
spacer block technique and, 258
spacer block use for, 258, 260, 261
subperiosteal dissection for, 258
tibial component placement and cementing for, 267
tibial cutting guide use for, 258
tibial resection for, 258–260
trial reduction for, 265–266
water pick lavage use for, 267
Extramedullary tensor approach, to UKA, 230–255
conclusions regarding, 252
extremity alignment and, 234
eye ball revisions and, 231
insert thickness and, 234
instrument systems for, 230
mechanical axis of lower extremity and, 234
MG uni prosthesis and, 230, 232
MIS goals for, 231
postoperative radiography of, 255
soft tissue balance and, 234
soft tissue release for, 235
space filling tensioner use for, 233
surface cut orientation for, 233
surgical technique for, 235–255
alignment correction for, 239, 241–242
anterior femoral marking for, 247–248
anterior tibial boss removal for, 239, 241
chamfer cut for, 248
cutting block use for, 236–237
cutting guide use for, 236–237
distal femoral resection for, 242–243
electrocautery use for, 239
extension/flexion gap gauge use for, 245, 247
femoral component placement and cementing for, 252–254
femoral finishing guide sizing and positioning for, 248–249
femur sizing for, 245, 247
flexion gap balancing for, 236
Hohmann retractor use for, 239
keying off of distal femur for, 236–237
Kocher clamp use for, 244
medial unicompartmental degenerative joint disease and, 235–236
oscillating saw use for, 242, 245
osteophyte excision for, 239
patient selection for, 238
post hole drilling for, 248
posterior condyle fragment removal for, 248, 250
pulsatile lavage use for, 252
reciprocating saw use for, 244–245
retractor use for, 242
skin incision placement for, 238–240
surgical steps for, 238–239
tensor device use for, 241–243
tibial cuts for, 244–246
tibial cutting block use for, 244
tibial implant placement and cementing for, 252–254
tibial plate placement for, 250–251
tibial sizing for, 250
trial femoral component placement for, 252
variable spacing block use for, 236–237
wound closure for, 252, 255
tensor device use for, 231
unicompartmental pathology and, 234

F
Fascia lata incision
for anterior (Heuter) approach to THA, 125–126
for anterolateral mini-incision approach to TKA, 104, 106
for anterolateral resurfacing approach to THA, 182
for mini-midvastus approach to TKA, 329
for MIS-optimized subvastus approach to TKA, 317
for posterolateral approach to THA, 144
for two-incision approach to THA, 161
Femoral elevator, 150, 152–154
Finishing guides
for extramedullary approach to UKA, 263–264
for extramedullary tensor approach to UKA, 248–249
Fluoroscopic navigation, for THA, 376–383. *See also* computer-assisted orthopedic surgery
Fluoroscopy
CAOS 2.5D information systems and, 400
for CAOS registration, 369
for knee arthroscopy with UniSpacer, 282–283
for proximal humerus fractures, 39–40
for two-incision approach to THA, 161, 163, 168–173
Fonduparinux, 362
Fukuda retractor
for glenoid exposure in shoulder arthroplasty, 63

Fukuda retractor (*cont.*)
  for treatment of glenohumeral instability, 14–15

G
Glenohumeral arthritis, shoulder arthroplasty for, 59–63
Glenohumeral instability, 3, 4
  check-reins and, 4
  MRI and, 10
  multiple etiologies for, 5
  nonoperative treatment of, 11
  operative treatment of, 11–17
    anesthesia for, 12
    arm position for, 17
    axillary incision for, 12–13
    Bankart repair and, 11
    barrel stitch for, 14–15
    components of instability and, 14
    Fukuda retractor use for, 14–15
    inferior capsular shift and, 11–12
    T capsulorrhaphy and, 12
  pain from, 5–6
  patient history of, 4–5
  physical examination of, 5–10
    anterior apprehension test and, 8–9
    deformity and, 5
    Jobe's relocation test and, 9
    laxity and, 5–7
    load-and-shift tests and, 7–8
    posterior stress test, 10
    range of motion and, 7
    strength and, 5
    sulcus test and, 7
  postoperative care for, 17
  radiographic features of, 10
  results of treatment for, 17
  trauma and, 4
  voluntary control of, 5
Glenohumeral joint, 3, 10
  inspection of, 22
Glenohumeral ligaments, 3
  avulsion of, 16
Glenoid, 3, 11, 14
Glenoid deficiency, 16
global positioning system, 398

H
Hemiarthroplasty, 33, 51–52
High Flex Legacy Knee (Zimmer), 352
Hills-Sachs lesion, 10, 16–17
Hip. *See* Total hip arthroplasty
HipNav, 399
Hohmann retractor
  for extramedullary tensor UKA, 239
  for Heuter approach to THA, 128
  for mini-midvastus TKA, 329, 332, 334
  for MIS-optimized subvastus TKA, 319–320, 322
  for resurfacing approach to THA, 183–184
  for two-incision approach to THA, 163, 167, 174
Heuter approach, to THA. *See* anterior (Heuter) approach, to THA
Humeral head, 3

I
Intramedullary approach, to UKA, 214–228
  ACL laxity and, 214
  anteroposterior x-ray, 215
  conclusions regarding, 228
  deformity limits and, 215
  lateral x-ray, 215–216
  pain in tibiofemoral compartment and, 214
  patellar x-ray, 215
  patient history and, 214
  patient selection for, 214
  physical examination for, 214
  preoperative planning for, 214–217
  radiography for, 214–217
  results of, 227–228
  standing x-ray and, 214–215
  surgical technique for, 217–227
    anesthesia for, 217, 227
    arthrotomy for, 217–218
    capsular extension and, 217
    deep MCL release for, 217
    distal femoral cut for, 220–221
    extramedullary instrument use for, 222
    femoral component position for, 223–224
    final component placement for, 227–228
    flexion contractures and, 222–223
    flexion-extension balance and, 223, 226
    flexion-extension gap and, 225
    intramedullary guide use for, 220–221
    intramedullary hole placement for, 219–220
    intramedullary retractor use for, 223–224
    knee valgus and, 226
    knee varus and, 226
    leg holding device and, 217–218
    osteophyte removal for, 218
    patella retraction for, 223–224
    skin incision placement for, 217, 219
    soft tissue sparing and, 218
    tibial cut for, 222–223
    tibial tray position for, 223
    tourniquet use for, 217, 227
    trial component placement for, 225
    UKA spacing and, 226
    valgus knee deformity and, 222
    wound closure for, 227
  tibial slope and, 215–216
  tibial translocation and, 215–216

J
Jackson operative imaging table, 377
Jobe procedure, 78
Jobe's relocation test, 9

K
Knee. *See* Knee arthroplasty, with UniSpacer; Total knee arthroplasty; Unicondylar knee arthroplasty

Knee arthroplasty, with UniSpacer, 270–284
contraindications for, 271–273
ACL deficiency and, 272
chondromalacia and, 273–274
femoral sulcus degeneration and, 274
lateral compartment degeneration and, 273
medial subluxation of femur and, 271–272
medial tibial bone loss and, 274
patellofemoral compartment degeneration and, 273
posterior femoral osteophytes and, 273
osteoarthritis treatment and, 270
patient selection for, 270, 273–274
physical examination for, 271–273
MRI scans for, 273
x-ray evaluation for, 271
surgical technique for
anesthesia for, 273
anteromedial meniscectomy for, 278
antibiotic prophylaxis use for, 273
arthroscopic probe use for, 280–281
arthroscopy and, 273–275
cartilage removal for, 279–280
chondroplasty for, 278–279
epinephrine use for, 273
femoral condyle contour and, 280
femoral sculpting for, 278
final UniSpacer implantation, 284
fluoroscopy for, 282–283
measurement of tibial plateau AP dimension, 280–281
mobile window and, 275–276
osteophyte resection after arthrotomy, 277
osteophyte resection, arthroscopic, 275
osteotome use for, 277
patient position for, 273
posterior meniscectomy, arthroscopic, 275
rasp use for, 278
retractor use for, 277
rongeur use for, 277
skin incision placement for, 275–276
step-by-step summary of, 273
thickness gauge use for, 280
tibial sculpting for, 278
trial implant for, 280–281
tweenplasty for, 279–280
UniSpacer insertion and, 281–282
UniSpacer kinematics and, 278–279
UniSpacer sizing for, 280
wound closure for, 284
tibial plateau deformity and, 271–272
UniSpacer design and, 270–271
KneeNav (ICAOS), 400
Kocher clamp, 244
Kocker's forceps, 291
Krackow stitch
for distal biceps tendon repair, 94–95
for docking procedure on elbow MCL, 81, 84

L

Labrum, 3, 14
Langer's line, 24, 25
Lateral approach, to TKA, 339–340
anterior knee pain and, 345–346
bone platforms for, 340
instrumentation for, 340
lateral incision with, 347
muscle-sparing with, 347
patellar eversion and, 347
rehabilitation and, 346
results of, 345–346
skin incision size and, 347
surgical navigation for, 340, 347
surgical technique for, 340–345
ACL excision for, 344
chamfer cuts for, 342–343
distal femoral resection for, 342
draping for, 340
femoral component placement for, 344
femoral landmark mapping for, 342
femoral preparation for, 344
Gerdy's tubercle and, 340
hip center mapping for, 342
knee kinematics and, 344
landmarks for, 340
lateral arthrotomy for, 340
navigational tracker placement for, 341–342
osteophyte excision for, 344
patellar component placement for, 344
patellar osteotomy for, 344
patient position for, 340
physical therapy and, 346
polyethylene insert placement for, 344–345
proximal tibial resection for, 342
resection guide use for, 342
retractor use for, 340
Scorpio trochlear recess rasp use for, 342
Simplex bone cement use for, 344
skin incision placement for, 340–341
subcutaneous dissection for, 340
suprapatellar pouch visualization for, 340
tibial component placement for, 344
tibial landmark mapping for, 342
tibial preparation for, 343
tibial punch guide use for, 343
tibial rotation measurement for, 343
tourniquet use for, 340

Lateral approach, to TKA (*cont.*)
trial component placement for, 344
valgus leg post use for, 340
Whiteside's AP axis mapping for, 342
wound closure after, 344–345
tibio-femoral dislocation and, 347
variable leg position for, 340
Load-and-shift tests, 7–8
Low-Profile reamer, 112–113

M

Magnetic resonance (MR) arthroscopy, 10
Magnetic resonance imaging (MRI)
CT/MRI navigation for CAOS, 400
for distal biceps tendon repair, 92
of elbow MCL, 76–78
for glenohumeral instability, 10
for UniSpacer knee arthroplasty, 273
Marcaine, 175
MBARS. *See* miniature bone-attached robotic system
MCL. *See* medial collateral ligament, of elbow
Medial collateral ligament (MCL), of elbow, 71–87
biomechanics and anatomy of, 71–73
anterior bundle and, 71, 73
flexor carpi ulnaris and, 73, 78
ulnar nerve and, 73
docking procedure on, 78–87
anesthesia for, 79
anterior bundle of MCL and, 78
anterior compartment arthroscopy and, 79–80
arthroscopic evaluation for, 79–80
flexor carpi ulnaris and, 78
flexor mass and, 78
fragmented spurs and, 80
graft harvesting for, 81
graft passage for, 84–85
graft tensioning for, 84–85
humeral tunnel creation for, 83
instrumentation for, 81
Krackow stitch and, 81, 84
MCL exposure for, 81
MCL incision for, 81–82
medial opening and, 80
muscle splitting incision, 78
native ligament repair for, 83–84
palmaris longus and, 81
patient position for, 79–80
posterior compartment arthroscopy and, 80
results of, 87
skin incision for, 81–82
splint placement after, 84
submuscular ligament exposure for, 81–82
suture fixation for, 84, 86
tendon graft reconstruction and, 79
tourniquet use for, 81, 84
ulnar nerve and, 79
ulnar tunnel creation for, 83
valgus stress test and, 79
wound closure for, 84
elbow arthroscopy and, 76
Jobe procedure on
complications with, 78
flexor pronator mass and, 78
MRI and, 76–78
3-dimensional volumetric gradient-echo, 76
coronal, 77
fast spin-echo, 76
saline-enhanced, 76
patient history and, 73–74
acute event and, 74
acute on chronic event and, 74
ulnar neuritis and, 74, 78
physical examination of, 74–76
arthroscopic stress test in, 74, 76
O'Brien's milking test in, 74–75
O'Driscoll's moving valgus stress test, 74–75
range of motion in, 74
Tinsel's test in, 74
valgus extension overload test in, 74
valgus stress test in, 74–75
postoperative management of
physical therapy for, 86
throwing program for, 86
radiographs and, 76–77
throwing athletes and, 71, 73
valgus load and, 71–72
Medial collateral ligament (MCL), of knee, deep MCL release for intramedullary approach to UKA, 217
Medial collateral ligaments (MCL), of knee, 193
Medial parapatellar arthrotomy, limited, to TKA, 303–314
anterior cortex resection for, 309
anteroposterior axis of distal femur and, 306, 308
bone resection for, 305
complications with, 313–314
contraindications for, 311, 313
distal femoral resection for, 306–307
extramedullary cutting guide use for, 305
femoral component insertion for, 310–311
femoral component sizing for, 306, 308
femoral rotation and, 306, 308
flexion-extension gap balancing for, 309
instrumentation for, 305
intramedullary cutting guide use for, 306–307
joint exposure for, 304–305
mobile window and, 305–306
NexGen LPS prosthesis use for, 310
NexGen Multi-Reference 4-in-1 use for, 305

patella eversion and resection for, 309–310
posterior femoral condyle resection for, 309
postoperative management after, 311
retractor use for, 305
skin incision extension and, 313
skin incision placement for, 304
skin incision size and, 313
soft tissue balancing and, 310–312
spacer block technique and, 309
subcutaneous dissection for, 304
tibial component insertion for, 310
tibial resection for, 305–306
tibial template selection for, 309
tibial tray insertion for, 309–310
transepicondylar axis and, 306, 308
trial component insertion for, 309–310
wound closure after, 310
Medial parapatellar arthrotomy, traditional, to TKA, 303
Medtronic Viking, 400–401
Meniscectomy
for knee arthroplasty with UniSpacer, 274, 278
for mini-midvastus approach to TKA, 329
for MIS-optimized subvastus approach to TKA, 321
Metal-on-metal resurfacing approach, to THA, 180–189
bone conservation and, 188
contraindications for, 181
dislocation rate and, 188
gait analyses for, 189
incision downsizing for, 189
indications for, 180
proximal femor stress transfer and, 188
proximal femoral deformity and, 180–181
range of motion and, 188
results of, 188–189
Methylene blue marks, 202–203
Methylmethacrylate cement, 202
MG. *See* Miller Galante Unicondylar prosthesis (Zimmer)
MI instrument set (Zimmer), for two-incision approach to THA, 163
Miller Galante (MG) Unicondylar prosthesis, 257
for extramedullary tensor approach to UKA, 230, 232
femoral component placement for extramedullary UKA, 267
tibial template selection for extramedullary UKA, 265–266
Miniature bone-attached robotic system, 391–394
Mini-midvastus approach, to TKA, 324, 326–328
4-in-1 cutting guide and, 327–328
conclusions regarding, 337
contraindication of, 327
femoral cutting blocks and, 327
instrumentation for, 327–328
knee flexion contracture and, 327
patellar dislocation and, 326
patient selection for, 327
patient size and, 327
postoperative pain level and, 336
postoperative range of motion and, 336–337
preoperative evaluation for, 327
results of, 336–337
skin incision size and, 326
stylus shape and, 328
surgical technique for, 328–336
ACL excision for, 329
anterior resection guide use for, 330–331
Aufranc retractor use for, 332, 334
cement use for, 334
distal femoral resection for, 330–331
extension-flexion gap measurement and balancing for, 334
extramedullary alignment guide use for, 332
fascia incision for, 329
femoral component placement for, 334–335
femoral component sizing for, 332
femoral cuts for, 332
femoral rotation and, 329–330
Hohmann retractor use for, 329, 332, 334
intramedullary drill use for, 330–331
laminar spreader use for, 333
medial arthrotomy for, 329
medial meniscus division and excision for, 329
osteophyte excision for, 332–333
patellar component placement for, 334
patellar pouch preservation for, 329
patellar resurfacing for, 334
patellar retraction for, 329
patient position for, 328
polyethylene insert placement for, 334
skin incision placement for, 329
skin necrosis and, 329
spacer block use for, 334
stylus use for, 330, 332
subperiosteal dissection for, 329
tibial canal drilling and broaching for, 333
tibial component placement for, 334–335
tibial cuts for, 332
tibial cutting guide use for, 332
tibial resection for, 332–333

Mini-midvastus approach, to TKA (*cont.*)
- trial femoral component placement for, 334
- trial tibial component placement for, 334
- Vicryl suture use for, 335–336
- Whiteside's line and, 329–330
- wound closure after, 335–336

tibial cutting guide and, 327
tourniquet time and, 337
valgus alignment guides and, 327

MIS-optimized subvastus approach, to TKA, 315–323
overweight patients and, 315
patellar eversion and, 315–316
surgical technique for, 316–323
- complications with, 323
- distal femoral visualization for, 319–320
- electrocautery use for, 317, 321
- extensor mechanism retraction for, 319
- fascia incision for, 317
- femoral component insertion for, 321–322
- femoral cut for, 320–322
- femoral rotation assessment for, 320–321
- femoral sizing for, 321–322
- Hohmann retractor use for, 319, 320, 322
- meniscectomy for, 321
- no-thumbs test and, 321
- osteophyte excision for, 321
- patellar component placement for, 321–322
- patellar resurfacing for, 321
- patellar retraction for, 319
- patient position for, 316
- pickle-fork retractor use for, 320
- quadriceps tendon preservation for, 317–318
- saw blade selection for, 320–321
- subcutaneous dissection for, 316
- subvastus hematoma and, 323
- synovium incision for, 317–319
- tibial component insertion for, 321–322
- tibial cut for, 320–321
- tourniquet use for, 316, 322
- vastus medialis muscle freeing for, 317
- wound closure after, 322–323

MR. *See* magnetic resonance arthroscopy
MRI. *See* magnetic resonance imaging
Mueller retractor, 184–185

N

Navitrack (ORTHOsoft), 399–400
Neuronavigator (Siemens), 398
NexGen LPS prosthesis (Zimmer), 310
NexGen Multi-Reference 4-in-1 (Zimmer), 305
No-thumbs test, 321

O

O'Brien's milking test, 74–75
O'Driscoll's moving valgus stress test, 74–75
OptoTrak (Northern Digital), 398–399
ORTHODOC, 400
Orthopilot (Aesculap), 401
Oscillating saw
- for extramedullary tensor approach to UKA, 242, 245
- for Oxford insertion approach to UKA, 290–291, 293
- for quadriceps-sparing approach to TKA, 351–352

Osteoarthritis, 193–194. *See also* glenohumeral arthritis
- anteromedial, 193–194
- nonoperative treatments of, 270
- tricompartmental, 194
- unicompartmental, 193–194, 209

Osteophyte removal
- for anterolateral resurfacing THA, 185
- for extramedullary UKA, 239, 258
- for intramedullary UKA, 218
- for knee arthroplasty with UniSpacer, 275, 277
- for lateral TKA, 344
- for mini-midvastus TKA, 332–333
- for Oxford insertion UKA, 289, 295–296
- for two-incision THA, 171

Osteotome
- for knee arthroplasty with UniSpacer, 277
- for Oxford insertion UKA, 291
- for two-incision THA, 163

Osteotomy
- patellar for lateral TKA, 344
- trochanteric for THA, 121–122

Oxford insertion approach, to UKA, 285–298
- contraindications for, 285
- operative technique for, 287–298
  - ACL evaluation for, 289
  - bearing insertion for, 298
  - cement keyhole drilling for, 297
  - chisel use for, 289, 293, 295–296
  - distal femur resection for, 293–294
  - extramedullary jig use for, 290
  - feeler gauge use for, 291, 294–295, 297
  - femoral component placement for, 298
  - femoral condyle resection for, 293
  - femoral drill guide use for, 291–292
  - femoral drill hole creation for, 291–293

femoral mill use for, 293–294
flexion-extension gap balancing, 293–295
keel slot cutting for, 296–297
knee milling for, 294
Kocker's forceps use for, 291
medial capsulotomy for, 289
oscillating saw use for, 290–291, 293
osteophyte removal for, 289, 295–296
osteotome use for, 291
patient position for, 287–288
postoperative recovery and, 298
preoperative radiograph templating for, 287
reciprocating saw use for, 290, 296
resected bone removal for, 291
retractor use for, 290–291
skin incision placement for, 287, 289
spigot selection for knee milling, 294
spigot use for, 293–294
tibial component placement for, 297–298
tibial cut for, 290–291
tibial saw guide and, 291
trial base plate insertion for, 291
trial reduction for, 297
wound closure for, 298
patient selection for, 285
Phase 3 Oxford UKA and, 286–287
summary regarding, 298
survival rates for, 285

P

Passive range of motion (PROM) exercises, 28
PCL. *See* Posterior cruciate ligament of knee
Percutaneous pinning, 32–35. *See also* proximal humerus fractures
Photogrammetric Navigation System, 396
Pickle-fork retractor, 320
PiGalileo (PI Systems), 391, 396
Pneumatic compression boots, 125
Posterior cruciate ligament (PCL) of knee, 352
Posterior stress test, 10
Posterolateral approach, to THA, 141–158
modified instruments for, 141
posterolateral surgical technique for, 141–157
acetabular component selection for, 150
acetabular exposure for, 147–148
acetabular labrum resection for, 147
acetabular liner insertion for, 150–151
acetabular reaming for, 147, 149–150
acetabular shell insertion for, 150–151
adipose tissue and, 144
broach abrasion avoidance, 153–154
broach removal for, 154
Crowe I-II type hips and, 144
doglegged acetabular inserter for, 150–151
enhanced posterior capsular closure for, 155
fascia lata incision for, 144
femoral broaching for, 153
femoral elevator for, 150, 152–154
femoral head placement for, 155–156
femoral head removal for, 147
femoral head trials for, 155
femoral neck cut for, 145–146
femoral reaming for, 152
femoral stem insertion for, 154–155
gluteus maximus fascia incision for, 144
hip dislocation for, 145–146
hip hyperextension and, 154–155
incision extension and, 142
incision landmarks for, 142–143
incision placement for, 142–144
lateral subluxation and, 144
leg length and, 142
mobile window and, 144, 147
modified Charnley retractors and, 144
osteophytes and, 147, 150–151
patient position for, 142
patient selection for, 141
piriformis fossa reaming for, 152–153
posterior capsular flap development for, 144–145
postoperative protocol for, 157
preoperative templating for, 142
provisional reduction for, 154
proximal femur extraction for, 147–148
radial capsulotomy for, 144–145
reciprocating saw use for, 145
skin protector for, 150, 152
varus neck angle and, 141
wound closure for, 155, 157
prostheses for, 141
summary notes regarding, 157–158
Precision freehand sculpting device, 397
PROfx table, 123–125, 134
PROM exercises. *See* passive range of motion exercises
Propofol, 159
Prostheses
Judet acrylic, 121
MG Unicondylar, 230, 232, 257, 265–267
NexGen LPS, 310

Prostheses (*cont.*)
  Repicci II unicondylar knee system, 206
  trabecular metal, 57–58
Proximal humerus fractures, 32–43, 51
  anatomic considerations of, 34
  avascular necrosis and, 32–34, 41–42
  closed reduction of, 33
  fixation of, 32, 41
  four-part, 32, 51–58
    alignment rods for, 55–56
    hemiarthroplasty and, 51–52
    humeral head removal for, 52
    prosthesis design and, 51
    prosthesis height for, 55–56
    prosthesis placement for, 52–54
    prosthesis version for, 55–56
    provisional prosthesis for, 53–55
    skin incision placement for, 52–53
    trabecular metal prosthesis and, 57–58
  hemiarthroplasty of, 33
  humeral head and, anatomic position of, 37–38
  open reduction of, 32, 36
  percutaneous pinning of, 32–33
    anatomic reduction for, 35
    bone stock quality and, 35
    complications with, 42
    conclusions regarding, 43
    contraindications for, 35
    drill guides and, 42
    nerve injury and, 42
    patient compliance and, 35
    pin migration and, 42
    results of, 41–42
    soft tissue management for, 35
    stable fixation for, 35
    superficial infections and, 43
  physical examination for, 35–36
  postoperative management of, 41
    pin removal for, 41
  preoperative consent and, 36
  radiograph of, 34
  radiographic evaluation for, 36
  surgical procedure for, 36–40
    fluoroscopic guidance for, 39–40
    instrumentation for, 39
    patient position and, 36–37
    percutaneous reduction for, 37
    pin placement for, 39–40
    reduction portal for, 37–38
    results of, 41
  valgus impacted four-part, 32
    blood supply and, 34
Punch guide, 343

Q

Quadriceps-sparing approach, to TKA, 349–362
  blood loss and, 363
  bone quality and, 350
  complications with, 363
  conclusions regarding, 363
  knee deformity and, 350
  patient selection for, 350
  patient weight and, 350
  range of motion and, 363
  results of, 362–363
  surgical technique for, 350–362
    ACL resection for, 352
    arthrotomy for, 350
    distal femoral cuts for, 352
    Doppler-ultrasound use for, 362
    external rotation cuts for, 356, 358
    extramedullary guide use for, 354
    femoral component placement for, 359, 361
    femoral component sizing for, 356
    femoral tower use for, 354, 356–357
    flexion-extension gap measurement for, 356, 359
    Fonduparinux use for, 362
    High Flex Legacy Knee use for, 352
    intramedullary guide use for, 352–353
    ligament balance and, 354–355
    oscillating saw use for, 351–352
    patellar component placement for, 359, 361
    patellar fat pad excision for, 351–352
    patellar resection for, 352
    PCL resection for, 352
    polyethylene insert placement for, 359, 361
    postoperative management for, 362
    retractor use for, 352
    skin incision placement for, 350–351
    tibial broaching for, 359
    tibial cuts for, 354–355
    tibial cutting guide use for, 359–360
    trial component insertion for, 359
    valgus alignment and, 354–355
    vastus medialis muscle insertion for, 350–351
    Whiteside's AP line and, 352–353
    wound closure after, 362
  Zimmer Orthopaedics and, 349
Quadriceps-sparing subvastus approach, to TKA. *See* MIS-optimized subvastus approach, to TKA

R

Radiography
  for anterolateral resurfacing approach to THA, 182, 185
  for bone-sparing approach to UKA, 195
  and CAOS THA, 384–386
  for distal biceps tendon repair, 92, 96–97

for extramedullary tensor approach to UKA, 255
for glenohumeral instability, 10
for intramedullary approach to UKA, 214–217
for Oxford insertion approach to UKA, 287
for two-incision approach to THA, 178
Radiolucent operating table, 159
Range of motion
AAROM exercises, 28
AROM exercises, 28
distal biceps tendon repair and, 91–92
docking procedure on elbow MCL and, 74
glenohumeral instability and, 7
metal-on-metal resurfacing approach to THA and, 188
mini-midvastus approach to TKA and, 336–337
PROM exercises, 28
quadriceps-sparing approach to TKA and, 363
shoulder arthroplasty and, 59
Reciprocating saw
for extramedullary tensor approach to UKA, 244–245
for Oxford insertion approach to UKA, 290, 296
for posterolateral approach to THA, 145
Relocation test, 9
Repicci II unicondylar knee system, 206
Resection guides
for extramedullary approach to UKA, 263
for lateral approach to TKA, 342
for mini-midvastus approach to TKA, 330–331
Resurfacing arthroplasty, 180
Retractor
Bennett retractor for anterolateral THA, 185
Charnley retractor
for anterolateral total hip arthroplasty, 104
for posterolateral total hip arthroplasty, 144
cobra retractor for anterior THA, 126, 128
for extramedullary tensor UKA, 239, 242
for extramedullary UKA, 258, 267
Fukuda retractor
for glenoid exposure in shoulder arthroplasty, 63
for treatment of glenohumeral instability, 14–15
Hohmann retractor
for extramedullary tensor UKA, 239
for Heuter approach to THA, 128
for mini-midvastus TKA, 329, 332, 334
for MIS-optimized subvastus TKA, 319–320, 322
for resurfacing approach to THA, 183–184
for two-incision approach to THA, 163, 167, 174
for intramedullary UKA, 223–224
Mueller retractor for anterolateral resurfacing THA, 184–185
for Oxford insertion UKA, 290–291
pickle-fork retractor for MIS-optimized TKA, 320
for quadriceps-sparing TKA, 352
Richardson retractor for anterolater resurfacing THA, 186
Richardson retractor, 186
ROBODOC, 367, 391, 400
Rotator cuff, 3
Rotator cuff tear
mini-open repair of, 21–30
anesthesia for, 23
arthroscope and, 23, 24
deltoid origin and, 22
deltoid split and, 24, 25
glenohumeral joint inspection and, 22
Langer's line and, 24, 25
portal placement for, 23, 25
postoperative protocol for, 28–29
results of, 29
surgical technique for, 23–28
open repair of, 21
shoulder arthroscopy and, 21
tendon healing after, 26, 27
Rotator interval, 3, 14

S

Sagittal saw, 202
Scapular stabilizers, 3, 4, 11
Scorpio trochlear recess rasp, 342
Shoulder arthroplasty, 45
avascular necrosis and, 57
surgical procedure for, 58
concealed axillary approach to, 46–49, 60
axillary incision for, 46
clavipectoral fascia incision for, 47–48
conjoint tendon retraction for, 47, 49
coracoacromial ligament resection for, 47, 49
deltoid retraction for, 47–48
pectoralis major retraction for, 47–48
subcutaneous dissection for, 46–47
conclusions regarding, 69
four-part proximal humerus fractures and, 51–58
alignment rods for, 55–56
hemiarthroplasty and, 51–52
humeral head removal for, 52
prosthesis design and, 51
prosthesis height for, 55–56
prosthesis placement for, 52–54
prosthesis version for, 55–56
provisional prosthesis for, 53–55

Shoulder arthroplasty (*cont.*)
skin incision placement for, 52–53
trabecular metal prosthesis and, 57–58
glenohumeral arthritis and, 59–63
concealed axillary incision for, 60
humeral component placement for, 60
humerus preparation for, 60–61
pain relief and, 59
patient selection and, 59
range of motion and, 59
skin incision placement and, 59
subscapularis detachment for, 59–60
subscapularis repair for, 60, 62
wound closure for, 60, 63
glenoid exposure in, 63–68
capsular release for, 63
cement and, 64
Fukuda retractor use and, 63
glenoid components and, 64
glenoid preparation and, 64–68
patient selection and, 63
mini-incision approach to, 47–51
skin incision placement for, 50
subcutaneous dissection for, 50–51
patient age and, 45
postoperative care after, 64
Shoulder biomechanics
dynamic stabilizers in, 4
static stabilizers in, 3, 4, 14
Shoulder instability, operative treatments of, 3, 11–17
Side-cutting reamer, 171
Simplex bone cement, 344
Skin necrosis, 329
Smillie meniscal knife, 183
Smith-Peterson incision, for two-incision approach to THA, 159
Stealth Universal Hip Application, 377
StealthStation, 399
Stewart-Gough 6 degrees-of-freedom robot, 392
straight reamer, 172
Stryker Navigation System, 401
Subscapularis, 11, 12
Sulcus test, 7
Surgetics Station (PRAXIM), 401
SurgiGate (MediVision), 371–372, 374–375, 399–400
Sutures
0-prolene sutures for bone-sparing UKA, 205
bone sutures for distal biceps tendon repair, 90
suture anchors for distal biceps tendon repair, 94–95
suture fixation for docking procedure on elbow MCL, 84, 86
Vicryl sutures for bone-sparing UKA, 205
Vicryl sutures for mini-midvastus TKA, 335–336

T

THA. *See* total hip arthroplasty
Tinsel's test, 74
Tissue Link, 182
TKA. *See* total knee arthroplasty
Total hip arthroplasty (THA), 103
acetabular posterior defects and, 124
anterior (Heuter) approach to, 121–139
benefits of, 122–123
BMI and, 124
conclusions regarding, 138–139
image intensifier for, 124
patient selection for, 124
PROfx table for, 123–124
statistics regarding, 138
anterior (Heuter) surgical technique for
acetabular prosthesis insertion for, 130, 132
acetabulum preparation for, 130–131
acetabulum reaming for, 130–131
anterior capsulotomy for, 127
broach insertion for, 135–136
cancellous bone removal for, 136
cobra retractors and, 126, 128
draping for, 125
fascia lata vulnerability and, 130
fascial incision placement for, 125–126
femoral cork screw and, 128
femoral head extraction for, 130
femoral hook placement for, 131–133
femoral mobility and, 133
femoral neck cut for, 128–129
femoral neck cut, in situ v. dislocated, 130
femoral offset and, 136–138
femoral preparation for, 132, 134
femoral prosthesis insertion for, 138–139
hip dislocation for, 127–128
hip stability and, 138
Hohmann retraction of vastus and, 128
lateral hip capsule palpation for, 126
leg length, 136–138
patient placement and, 124–125
pneumatic compression boots and, 125
postoperative precautions after, 138
PROfx table and, 124–125, 134
prosthesis choice for, 134–135
proximal femoral exposure for, 132, 134
skin incision placement for, 125–126

trial reduction for, 136
trochanteric retraction for, 132–133
wound closure for, 138
x-ray length and offset assessments for, 136–137
anterolateral mini-incision technique for, 103–120
abductor injury and, 110
acetabular component placement for, 113–114
acetabulum preparation for, 111–113
acetabulum reaming for, 112–113
Charnley retractor and, 104
conclusions regarding, 120
fascia detachment for, 106
fascia lata incision for, 104, 106
femoral component placement for, 116–117
femoral head placement for, 116, 118
femoral neck cut for, 110
femur preparation for, 113
femur retraction for, 110–111
femur retractor placement for, 115
gluteus medius detachment for, 106, 108
gluteus medius muscle division for, 106–107
gluteus minimus detachment for, 106, 108
gluteus minimus tendon incision for, 106, 108
greater trochanter and, 104, 106–107
hip capsule excision for, 109
hip capsule exposure for, 108–109
hip dislocation for, 109–110
lateral trochanter medial portion removal for, 115
leg length measurements for, 109
Low-Profile reamer and, 112–113
patient placement for, 104
preoperative planning for, 103
provisional prosthesis for, 115–116
skin incision placement for, 104–105
wound closure for, 116, 118–120
anterolateral resurfacing approach to, 181–187
acetabular component placement for, 185
acetabular exposure for, 184–185
acetabular preparation for, 184
acetabular reaming for, 185
anterior capsule dissection for, 183
anterior capsulectomy for, 183
bone hook use for, 183
chamfer cuts for, 187
chamfer reaming for, 187
circumferential guide use for, 186
Cobb elevator use for, 182, 183
concentric reaming and, 185
cylindrical reaming and, 186
deep exposure for, 182–183
donut tower guide use for, 186
electrocautery use for, 182, 183
fascia lata incision for, 182
femoral component placement for, 187–188
femoral component sizing for, 184
femoral head reaming for, 186–187
femoral neck dissection for, 183
femoral neck measurement for, 183–184
femoral neck notches and, 184, 185
femoral resurfacing for, 185–187
gluteus medius muscle detachment for, 183
guide pin placement for, 186
hemostatic device use for, 182
hip dislocation for, 183
Hohmann retractor use for, 183, 184
mobile window and, 182
osteophyte excision for, 185
postoperative care for, 187–188
radiographs for, intraoperative, 185
radiographs for, preoperative, 182
self-retaining retractor use for, 182
skin incision placement for, 181–182
Smillie meniscal knife use for, 183
smooth Bennett retractor use for, 185
smooth Richardson retractor use for, 186
spiked Mueller retractor use for, 184–185
Tissue Link use for, 182
trial head component placement for, 187
wound closure for, 187
CAOS (CT navigation) approach to, 370–376
3D pelvic modeling for, 371–373
acetabular abduction comparison and, 376
acetabular anteversion comparison and, 376
acetabular component orientation and, 370
bony acetabulum orientation and, 370
clinical experience with, 375–376
CT scans for, 374
DRB use for, 373–374
infrared camera use for, 373
LED equipped instruments for, 373–374
patient position and, 370

Total hip arthroplasty (THA) (*cont.*)
postoperative computed tomography for, 374–375
preoperative analysis for, 371–373
registration for, 374
surgical implantation and, 374–375
SurgiGATE software use for, 371–372, 374–375
Unix Ultra 10 workstation use for, 373
CAOS (fluoroscopic navigation) approach to, 376–383
acetabular navigation for, 377
acetabular reaming for, 382–383
acetabulum views for, 377
anterior superior iliac spine views for, 377–381
cup insertion for, 382–383
DRB application for, 377
fluoroscopic C-arm use for, 378–379
image referencing for, 378, 382
Jackson operative imaging table use for, 377
patient preparation for, 377–378
pubic tubercle views for, 377–381
Stealth Universal Hip Application use for, 377
Harding approach to, 122
hip deltoid biomechanics and, 122
history of, 121–122
Judet acrylic prosthesis, 121
Judet table, 121, 123
metal-on-metal resurfacing approach to, 180–189
bone conservation and, 188
contraindications for, 181
dislocation rate and, 188
gait analyses for, 189
incision downsizing for, 189
indications for, 180
proximal femor stress transfer and, 188
proximal femoral deformity and, 180–181
range of motion and, 188
results of, 188–189
posterolateral approach to, 141–158
modified instruments for, 141
prostheses for, 141
summary notes regarding, 157–158
posterolateral surgical technique for, 141–157
acetabular component selection for, 150
acetabular exposure for, 147–148
acetabular labrum resection for, 147
acetabular liner insertion for, 150–151
acetabular reaming for, 147, 149–150
acetabular shell insertion for, 150–151
adipose tissue and, 144
broach abrasion avoidance, 153–154
broach removal for, 154
Crowe I-II type hips and, 144
doglegged acetabular inserter for, 150–151
enhanced posterior capsular closure for, 155
fascia lata incision for, 144
femoral broaching for, 153
femoral elevator for, 150, 152–154
femoral head placement for, 155–156
femoral head removal for, 147
femoral head trials for, 155
femoral neck cut for, 145–146
femoral reaming for, 152
femoral stem insertion for, 154–155
gluteus maximus fascia incision for, 144
hip dislocation for, 145–146
hip hyperextension and, 154–155
incision extension and, 142
incision landmarks for, 142–143
incision placement for, 142–144
lateral subluxation and, 144
leg length and, 142
mobile window and, 144, 147
modified Charnley retractors and, 144
osteophytes and, 147, 150–151
patient position for, 142
patient selection for, 141
piriformis fossa reaming for, 152–153
posterior capsular flap development for, 144–145
postoperative protocol for, 157
preoperative templating for, 142
provisional reduction for, 154
proximal femur extraction for, 147–148
radial capsulotomy for, 144–145
reciprocating saw use for, 145
skin protector for, 150, 152
varus neck angle and, 141
wound closure for, 155, 157
trochanteric osteotomy and, 121–122
two-incision approach to, 159–179
complication rate of, 179
IM femoral nail and, 159
radiographs of, 178
Smith-Peterson incision and, 159
summary regarding, 178–179
two-incision surgical technique for, 159–177
acetabular component insertion for, 170
acetabular preparation for, 167

acetabular reaming for, 168–169
acetabular screw placement for, 171
acetabular shell placement for, 170–171
acetabular visualization for, 167–168
anesthesia for, 159
anterior dissection for, 161–163
anterior incision placement for, 161
capsule incision for, 163–165
capsule retraction for, 167
Charnley awl use for, 171
Cobb elevator osteotome use for, 163
dogleg acetabular inserter use for, 170
draping for, 160
electrocautery use for, 163, 169
epinephrine use for, 175
fascia lata incision for, 161
femoral broaching for, 172–173
femoral head component placement for, 175
femoral head removal for, 163, 166, 175
femoral neck and, 161
femoral neck cut for, 163, 166
femoral neck resection for, 163, 167
femoral reaming for, 172–173
femoral stem component placement for, 174–176
fluoroscope use for, 161, 163, 168–173
hip stability assessment for, 174
Hohmann retractor use for, 163, 167, 174
labrum excision for, 168
lateral femoral vessel coagulation for, 163
Marcaine use for, 175
MI instrument set (Zimmer) use for, 163
osteophyte removal for, 171
patient position for, 159
posterior incision lateralization for, 171–172
posterior incision placement for, 171
preparation for, 160
Propofol use with, 159
radiolucent table use for, 159
rasp use for, 172–173
redundant synovium excision for, 168
sartorius retraction for, 161–162
side-cutting reamer use for, 171
straight reamer use for, 172
superior acetabulum excision for, 168
tensor fascia lata retraction for, 161–162
threaded Steinmann pin use for, 163
trial reduction for, 172, 174, 175
Vicryl stitch use for, 175
wound closure for, 175, 177
total knee arthroplasty (TKA), 194–195
American National Hospital Discharge Survey predictions for, 390
history of, 390
lateral approach for, 339–340
anterior knee pain and, 345–346
bone platforms for, 340
instrumentation for, 340
lateral incision with, 347
muscle-sparing with, 347
patellar eversion and, 347
rehabilitation and, 346
results of, 345–346
skin incision size and, 347
surgical navigation for, 340, 347
tibio-femoral dislocation and, 347
variable leg position for, 340
lateral approach surgical technique for, 340–345
ACL excision for, 344
chamfer cuts for, 342–343
distal femoral resection for, 342
draping for, 340
femoral component placement for, 344
femoral landmark mapping for, 342
femoral preparation for, 344
Gerdy's tubercle and, 340
hip center mapping for, 342
knee kinematics and, 344
landmarks for, 340
lateral arthrotomy for, 340
navigational tracker placement for, 341–342
osteophyte excision for, 344
patellar component placement for, 344
patellar osteotomy for, 344
patient position for, 340
physical therapy and, 346
polyethylene insert placement for, 344–345
proximal tibial resection for, 342
resection guide use for, 342
retractor use for, 340
Scorpio trochlear recess rasp use for, 342
Simplex bone cement use for, 344
skin incision placement for, 340–341
subcutaneous dissection for, 340
suprapatellar pouch visualization for, 340
tibial component placement for, 344
tibial landmark mapping for, 342
tibial preparation for, 343
tibial punch guide use for, 343
tibial rotation measurement for, 343
tourniquet use for, 340

total knee arthroplasty (TKA) (*cont.*)
trial component placement for, 344
valgus leg post use for, 340
Whiteside's AP axis mapping for, 342
wound closure after, 344–345
medial parapatellar arthrotomy, limited, 303–314
anterior cortex resection for, 309
anteroposterior axis of distal femur and, 306, 308
bone resection for, 305
complications with, 313–314
contraindications for, 311, 313
distal femoral resection for, 306–307
extramedullary cutting guide use for, 305
femoral component insertion for, 310–311
femoral component sizing for, 306, 308
femoral rotation and, 306, 308
flexion-extension gap balancing for, 309
instrumentation for, 305
intramedullary cutting guide use for, 306–307
joint exposure for, 304–305
mobile window and, 305–306
NexGen LPS prosthesis use for, 310
NexGen Multi-Reference 4-in-1 use for, 305
patella eversion and resection for, 309–310
posterior femoral condyle resection for, 309
postoperative management after, 311
retractor use for, 305
skin incision extension and, 313
skin incision placement for, 304
skin incision size and, 313
soft tissue balancing and, 310–312
spacer block technique and, 309
subcutaneous dissection for, 304
tibial component insertion for, 310
tibial resection for, 305–306
tibial template selection for, 309
tibial tray insertion for, 309–310
transepicondylar axis and, 306, 308
trial component insertion for, 309–310
wound closure after, 310
medial parapatellar arthrotomy, traditional, 303
mini-midvastus approach to, 324, 326–328
4-in-1 cutting guide and, 327–328
conclusions regarding, 337
contraindication of, 327
femoral cutting blocks and, 327
instrumentation for, 327–328
knee flexion contracture and, 327
patellar dislocation and, 326
patient selection for, 327
patient size and, 327
postoperative pain level and, 336
postoperative range of motion and, 336–337
preoperative evaluation for, 327
results of, 336–337
skin incision size and, 326
stylus shape and, 328
tibial cutting guide and, 327
tourniquet time and, 337
valgus alignment guides and, 327
mini-midvastus surgical technique for, 328–336
ACL excision for, 329
anterior resection guide use for, 330–331
Aufranc retractor use for, 332, 334
cement use for, 334
distal femoral resection for, 330–331
extension-flexion gap measurement and balancing for, 334
extramedullary alignment guide use for, 332
fascia incision for, 329
femoral component placement for, 334–335
femoral component sizing for, 332
femoral cuts for, 332
femoral rotation and, 329–330
Hohmann retractor use for, 329, 332, 334
intramedullary drill use for, 330–331
laminar spreader use for, 333
medial arthrotomy for, 329
medial meniscus division and excision for, 329
osteophyte excision for, 332–333
patellar component placement for, 334
patellar pouch preservation for, 329
patellar resurfacing for, 334
patellar retraction for, 329
patient position for, 328
polyethylene insert placement for, 334
skin incision placement for, 329
skin necrosis and, 329
spacer block use for, 334
stylus use for, 330, 332
subperiosteal dissection for, 329
tibial canal drilling and broaching for, 333
tibial component placement for, 334–335

tibial cuts for, 332
tibial cutting guide use for, 332
tibial resection for, 332–333
trial femoral component placement for, 334
trial tibial component placement for, 334
Vicryl suture use for, 335–336
Whiteside's line and, 329–330
wound closure after, 335–336
MIS-optimized subvastus approach to, 315–316
overweight patients and, 315
patellar eversion and, 315–316
MIS-optimized subvastus surgery for, 316–323
complications with, 323
distal femoral visualization for, 319–320
electrocautery use for, 317, 321
extensor mechanism retraction for, 319
fascia incision for, 317
femoral component insertion for, 321–322
femoral cut for, 320–322
femoral rotation assessment for, 320–321
femoral sizing for, 321–322
Hohmann retractor use for, 319, 320, 322
meniscectomy for, 321
no-thumbs test and, 321
osteophyte excision for, 321
patellar component placement for, 321–322
patellar resurfacing for, 321
patellar retraction for, 319
patient position for, 316
pickle-fork retractor use for, 320
quadriceps tendon preservation for, 317–318
saw blade selection for, 320–321
subcutaneous dissection for, 316
subvastus hematoma and, 323
synovium incision for, 317–319
tibial component insertion for, 321–322
tibial cut for, 320–321
tourniquet use for, 316, 322
vastus medialis muscle freeing for, 317
wound closure after, 322–323
quadriceps-sparing approach to, 349–350
blood loss and, 363
bone quality and, 350
complications with, 363
conclusions regarding, 363
knee deformity and, 350
patient selection for, 350
patient weight and, 350
range of motion and, 363
results of, 362–363
Zimmer Orthopaedics and, 349
quadriceps-sparing surgical technique for, 350–362
ACL resection for, 352
arthrotomy for, 350
distal femoral cuts for, 352
Doppler-ultrasound use for, 362
external rotation cuts for, 356, 358
extramedullary guide use for, 354
femoral component placement for, 359, 361
femoral component sizing for, 356
femoral tower use for, 354, 356–357
flexion-extension gap measurement for, 356, 359
Fonduparinux use for, 362
High Flex Legacy Knee use for, 352
intramedullary guide use for, 352–353
ligament balance and, 354–355
oscillating saw use for, 351–352
patellar component placement for, 359, 361
patellar fat pad excision for, 351–352
patellar resection for, 352
PCL resection for, 352
polyethylene insert placement for, 359, 361
postoperative management for, 362
retractor use for, 352
skin incision placement for, 350–351
tibial broaching for, 359
tibial cuts for, 354–355
tibial cutting guide use for, 359–360
trial component insertion for, 359
valgus alignment and, 354–355
vastus medialis muscle insertion for, 350–351
Whiteside's AP line and, 352–353
wound closure after, 362
skin incision placement for, 316
standard anterior approaches to
permanent knee damage from, 339
permanent muscle damage from, 339
surgeons' perceptions v. patients' perceptions of, 339
standard midvastus approach, 324–325
standard midvastus approach to
medial parapatellar arthrotomy and, 325
studies of, 325
VMO denervation and, 325
traditional subvastus approach to, 315
von Langenbeck and, 303, 324
trochanteric retraction
for anterior (Heuter) approach to THA, 132–133

trochanteric retraction (*cont.*)
for anterolateral mini-incision approach to THA, 104, 106–107, 115
two-incision approach, to THA, 159–179
complication rate of, 179
IM femoral nail and, 159
radiographs of, 178
Smith-Peterson incision and, 159
summary regarding, 178–179
surgical technique for, 159–177
acetabular component insertion for, 170
acetabular preparation for, 167
acetabular reaming for, 168–169
acetabular screw placement for, 171
acetabular shell placement for, 170–171
acetabular visualization for, 167–168
anesthesia for, 159
anterior dissection for, 161–163
anterior incision placement for, 161
capsule incision for, 163–165
capsule retraction for, 167
Charnley awl use for, 171
Cobb elevator osteotome use for, 163
dogleg acetabular inserter use for, 170
draping for, 160
electrocautery use for, 163, 169
epinephrine use for, 175
fascia lata incision for, 161
femoral broaching for, 172–173
femoral head component placement for, 175
femoral head removal for, 163, 166, 175
femoral neck and, 161
femoral neck cut for, 163, 166
femoral neck resection for, 163, 167
femoral reaming for, 172–173
femoral stem component placement for, 174–176
fluoroscope use for, 161, 163, 168–173
hip stability assessment for, 174
Hohmann retractor use for, 163, 167, 174
labrum excision for, 168
lateral femoral vessel coagulation for, 163
Marcaine use for, 175
MI instrument set (Zimmer) use for, 163
osteophyte removal for, 171
patient position for, 159
posterior incision lateralization for, 171–172
posterior incision placement for, 171
preparation for, 160
Propofol use with, 159
radiolucent table use for, 159
rasp use for, 172–173
redundant synovium excision for, 168
sartorius retraction for, 161–162
side-cutting reamer use for, 171
straight reamer use for, 172
superior acetabulum excision for, 168
tensor fascia lata retraction for, 161–162
threaded Steinmann pin use for, 163
trial reduction for, 172, 174, 175
Vicryl stitch use for, 175
wound closure for, 175, 177

U
UKA. *See* unicondylar knee arthroplasty
ulnar neuritis, 73–74, 78
unicondylar knee arthroplasty (UKA), 194
anteromedial osteoarthritis and, 193–194
bone-sparing technique for, 193
0-prolene suture use for, 205
0-Vicryl suture use for, 205
Ahlback classification for, 195
Ahlback disease and, 195
anesthesia for, 196
articular defect and, 197–198
bupivacaine use for, 202
capsular closure after, 205
common errors with, 205
complications with, 205–206
conclusions regarding, 209–210
contraindications for, 195
conversion to TKA, 196
depth gauge for, 200
diagnostic arthroscopy for, 197
distracter joint use for, 199
distracter pin use for, 199
draping for, 197
epinephrine use for, 202
exposure for, 197–198
extension gap disease, 193–194
femoral component insertion for, 202, 204–205
femoral drill guide use for, 202
femoral preparation for, 200–202
femoral resection for, 200–202
femoral-tibial alignment for, 202–203
final preparation for, 202, 205
high-speed burr use for, 199
local anesthesia for, 202, 204
medial parapatellar capsular arthrotomy for, 197

methylene blue marks for, 202–203
methylmethacrylate cement use for, 202
nonoperative treatment and, 195
operating table choice for, 197
patellar eversion and, 197
patient choice and, 196
patient placement for, 197
patient selection for, 195–196
physical examination before, 195
physical examination for, 195
posterior femoral condyle resection for, 197–198, 205
prosthesis survivorship of, 196
radiographic assessment before, 195
radiographic assessment for, 195
Repicci II unicondylar knee system use for, 206
round burr use for, 200
sagittal saw use for, 202
sclerotic bone preservation and, 200
side-cutting burr use for, 202
skin incision placement for, 197–198
subcutaneous dissection for, 197
tibial bone resection for, 199
tibial component size and, 205
tibial inlay component for, 200
tibial surface resection and, 205
tourniquet use for, 197, 205
trial reduction for, 202, 204
wound closure after, 205

extramedullary surgical technique for, 257–268
alignment tower use for, 262
distal femoral resection for, 263–264
femoral finishing guide selection for, 263–264
femoral preparation for, 261–263
femoral resection guide use for, 263
medial parapatellar arthrotomy for, 258
MG femoral component placement and cementing for, 267
MG tibial template selection for, 265–266
MG uni prosthesis use for, 257
osteophyte removal for, 258
principles of, 257
retractor use for, 258, 267
skin incision placement for, 258
spacer block technique and, 258
spacer block use for, 258, 260, 261
subperiosteal dissection for, 258
summary regarding, 268
tibial component placement and cementing for, 267
tibial cutting guide use for, 258
tibial resection for, 258–260
trial reduction for, 265–266
water pick lavage use for, 267

extramedullary tensor approach to, 230–255
conclusions regarding, 252
extremity alignment and, 234
eye ball revisions and, 231
insert thickness and, 234
instrument systems for, 230
mechanical axis of lower extremity and, 234
MG uni prosthesis and, 230, 232
MIS goals for, 231
postoperative radiography of, 255
soft tissue balance and, 234
soft tissue release for, 235
space filling tensioner use for, 233
surface cut orientation for, 233
tensor device use for, 231
unicompartmental pathology and, 234

extramedullary tensor surgical technique for, 235–255
alignment correction for, 239, 241–242
anterior femoral marking for, 247–248
anterior tibial boss removal for, 239, 241
chamfer cut for, 248
cutting block use for, 236–237
cutting guide use for, 236–237
distal femoral resection for, 242–243
electrocautery use for, 239
extension/flexion gap gauge use for, 245, 247
femoral component placement and cementing for, 252–254
femoral finishing guide sizing and positioning for, 248–249
femur sizing for, 245, 247
flexion gap balancing for, 236
Hohmann retractor use for, 239
keying off of distal femur for, 236–237
Kocher clamp use for, 244
medial unicompartmental degenerative joint disease and, 235–236
oscillating saw use for, 242, 245
osteophyte excision for, 239
patient selection for, 238
post hole drilling for, 248

unicondylar knee arthroplasty (UKA) (*cont.*)
posterior condyle fragment removal for, 248, 250
pulsatile lavage use for, 252
reciprocating saw use for, 244–245
retractor use for, 242
skin incision placement for, 238–240
surgical steps for, 238–239
tensor device use for, 241–243
tibial cuts for, 244–246
tibial cutting block use for, 244
tibial implant placement and cementing for, 252–254
tibial plate placement for, 250–251
tibial sizing for, 250
trial femoral component placement for, 252
variable spacing block use for, 236–237
wound closure for, 252, 255
intramedullary approach to, 214–228
ACL laxity and, 214
anteroposterior x-ray, 215
conclusions regarding, 228
deformity limits and, 215
lateral x-ray, 215–216
pain in tibiofemoral compartment and, 214
patellar x-ray, 215
patient history and, 214
patient selection for, 214
physical examination for, 214
preoperative planning for, 214–217
radiography for, 214–217
results of, 227–228
standing x-ray and, 214–215
tibial slope and, 215–216
tibial translocation and, 215–216
intramedullary surgical technique for, 217–227
anesthesia for, 217, 227
arthrotomy for, 217–218
capsular extension and, 217
deep MCL release for, 217
distal femoral cut for, 220–221
extramedullary instrument use for, 222
femoral component position for, 223–224
final component placement for, 227–228
flexion contractures and, 222–223
flexion-extension balance and, 223, 226
flexion-extension gap and, 225
intramedullary guide use for, 220–221
intramedullary hole placement for, 219–220
intramedullary retractor use for, 223–224
knee valgus and, 226
knee varus and, 226
leg holding device and, 217–218
osteophyte removal for, 218
patella retraction for, 223–224
skin incision placement for, 217, 219
soft tissue sparing and, 218
tibial cut for, 222–223
tibial tray position for, 223
tourniquet use for, 217, 227
trial component placement for, 225
UKA spacing and, 226
valgus knee deformity and, 222
wound closure for, 227
minimally invasive program of, 206–209
arthroscopy use for, 207
goals for, 207
pain management for, 209
soft tissue preservation for, 207
UKA to TKA conversion and, 208
osteoarthritis and, 193
Oxford insertion approach to, 285–298
contraindications for, 285
patient selection for, 285
Phase 3 Oxford UKA and, 286–287
summary regarding, 298
survival rates for, 285
Oxford operative technique for, 287–298
ACL evaluation for, 289
bearing insertion for, 298
cement keyhole drilling for, 297
chisel use for, 289, 293, 295–296
distal femur resection for, 293–294
extramedullary jig use for, 290
feeler gauge use for, 291, 294–295, 297
femoral component placement for, 298
femoral condyle resection for, 293
femoral drill guide use for, 291–292
femoral drill hole creation for, 291–293
femoral mill use for, 293–294
flexion-extension gap balancing, 293–295
keel slot cutting for, 296–297
knee milling for, 294
Kocker's forceps use for, 291
medial capsulotomy for, 289
oscillating saw use for, 290–291, 293
osteophyte removal for, 289, 295–296
osteotome use for, 291
patient position for, 287–288
postoperative recovery and, 298
preoperative radiograph templating for, 287

reciprocating saw use for, 290, 296
resected bone removal for, 291
retractor use for, 290–291
skin incision placement for, 287, 289
spigot selection for knee milling, 294
spigot use for, 293–294
tibial component placement for, 297–298
tibial cut for, 290–291
tibial saw guide and, 291
trial base plate insertion for, 291
trial reduction for, 297
wound closure for, 298

UniSpacer. *See* knee arthroplasty, with UniSpacer

V

valgus extension overload test, 74
valgus stress test, 74–75, 79
VectorVision (BrainLab), 399–400, 402

W

Whiteside's AP line
  lateral approach to TKA and, 342
  mini-midvastus approach to TKA and, 329–330
  quadriceps-sparing approach to TKA and, 352–353
World Health Organization, 390

X

X-ray, standing, 214–215

Z

Zimmer Orthopaedics, 349
  High Flex Legacy Knee and, 352
  MI instrument set and, 163
  NexGen LPS prosthesis and, 310
  NexGen Multi-Reference 4-in-1 and, 305